PEDIATRIC OPHTHALMOLOGY

A TEXT ATLAS

PEDIATRIC OPHTHALMOLOGY
A TEXT ATLAS

Robert A. Catalano, MD
Executive Vice President and Chief Operating Officer
Olean General Hospital
Olean, NY

Formerly Acting Chairman, Department of Ophthalmology
Associate Professor of Ophthalmology and Pediatrics
Albany Medical College
Ophthalmologist-in-Chief
Albany Medical Center Hospital
Albany, New York

Leonard B. Nelson, MD
Co-director of Pediatric Ophthalmology Services
Wills Eye Hospital

Associate Professor of Ophthalmology and Pediatrics
Jefferson Medical College of Thomas Jefferson University
Philadelphia, PA

Illustrated by Laurie Maimone

APPLETON & LANGE
Norwalk, Connecticut

Copyright © 1994 by Appleton & Lange
Paramount Publishing Business and Professional Group

94 95 96 97 98 / 10 9 8 7 6 5 4 3 2 1

Prentice Hall International (UK) Limited, *London*
Prentice Hall of Australia Pty. Limited, *Sydney*
Prentice Hall Canada, Inc., *Toronto*
Prentice Hall Hispanoamericana, S. A., *Mexico*
Prentice Hall of India Private Limited, *New Delhi*
Prentice Hall of Japan, Inc., *Tokyo*
Simon & Schuster Asia Pte. Ltd., *Singapore*
Editora Prentice Hall do Brasil Ltda., *Rio de Janeiro*
Prentice Hall, *Englewood Cliffs, New Jersey*

Library of Congress Cataloging-in-Publication Data

Catalano, Robert A.
    Pediatric ophthalmology : a text atlas / Robert A. Catalano,
Leonard B. Nelson ; illustrated by Laurie Maimone.
        p. cm.
    Includes bibliographical references and index.
    ISBN 0–8385–7817–9
    1. Pediatric ophthalmology. 2. Pediatric ophthalmology—Atlases.
I. Nelson, Leonard B. II. Title.
    [DNLM: 1. Eye Diseases—in infancy & childhood. WW 610 C357p
1994]
RE48.2.C5C38 1994
618.92′0977—dc20
DNLM/DLC   93–39628
for Library of Congress   CIP

Production Editor: Elizabeth C. Ryan
Designer: Penny Kindzierski
Cover Designer: Elizabeth A. Schmitz

PRINTED IN THE UNITED STATES OF AMERICA

ISBN 0-8385-7817-9

This book is dedicated to our parents, who provided us the opportunity to pursue our academic endeavors.
It is also dedicated to our families for their unending understanding, patience, and support of these endeavors:
Madeline, Christopher, Ruth, Thomas, Matthew, Helene, Jennifer, Kimberly, and Bradley.

CONTENTS

FOREWORD

Pediatric ophthalmology was virtually unheard of thirty years ago. Dr. Frank Costenbader of Washington, DC, whom I first met following World War II, was the first ophthalmologist in the United States who began to devote his practice solely to strabismus and disorders of the child's eye. Judging from my experience at that time, I wondered how he could keep busy in what seemed to be such a limited field.

During the next two decades increasing interest in strabismus was producing much improved clinical results and by 1974, the Association of Pediatric Ophthalmology was formed with approximately 45 charter members, and this subspecialty had come of age.

Now twenty years later the American Association of Pediatric Ophthalmology and Strabismus is comprised of over 400 members in North America, more than 40 international members, and over 50 orthoptists who devote their entire practice to strabismus and ocular disorders of childhood with a strong emphasis on genetic and systemic manifestation of disease.

However, in addition to these specialized ophthal-mologists trained in the nuances of pediatric ocular disorders, there is an essential need for a well-informed referral system. Pediatricians, neonatologists, family physicians, house officers, and non-physician practitioners who initially see most children are in a position to make an appropriate referral. This carefully illustrated text atlas represents a valuable desk reference, especially for them.

The accelerating advances in genetics, immunology, neonatology, metabolic defects, and pharmacology require continuing study and updating so that the best professional care can be provided to those who depend on us.

A text atlas of this quality fulfills its promise in presenting the essentials in pediatric eye care in clear, concise terms and I congratulate the authors on the selectivity of the subject matter, which crosses many disciplines.

Robison D. Harley, MD, PhD, FACS

PREFACE

This book was conceived to fill a need not completely met by existing encyclopedic treatises, scattered review articles, or monographs on visual disorders in children. Our intent was to write a clinically oriented, cohesive text that reviewed the signs, symptoms, and treatment of common ocular diseases and disorders in infants and children. We also intended that the book be useful to pediatricians and family physicians, yet be primarily directed to vision care providers. To this end, information essential to primary care practitioners is provided at the beginning of nearly every chapter, followed by more comprehensive information for those who provide ophthalmic care to children. A final goal was to create a ready resource for publications pertaining to the disorders discussed. Each chapter is thus concluded with an extensive reference list/bibliography.

It was also our desire to write a book that would be easy to read. We therefore avoided long discourses on theoretic considerations that have little clinical relevance. Further, flow diagrams and examination sheets are provided throughout the book to outline the work-up of children with specific signs or symptoms. Finally, the book has been generously illustrated to demonstrate the multitude of ocular conditions encountered in pediatric ophthalmology.

The book is primarily organized by ocular structure. Separate chapters on ocular anatomy and the pediatric eye exam provide an overview for the chapters that follow. Chapter 3, on normal visual development, learning disabilities, and functional disorders, reviews information that cannot be subdivided into specific subjects such as corneal diseases, glaucoma, cataracts, refractive errors, strabismus, retinal disorders, optic nerve abnormalities, eyelid and orbital disorders, and nystagmus. The latter topics constitute the subjects of individual chapters that comprise most of the remainder of the book. Because infections and ocular trauma overlap the anatomic subdivision of the eye, they are treated as separate entities. An appendix completes the book by listing the names, addresses, and telephone numbers of organizations that provide individuals and their families assistance with certain conditions.

It is our hope that this book will provide the necessary information to allow those who provide vision care to children to successfully diagnose and treat their patients. It is also hoped that this work will serve as a helpful teaching and review manual for ophthalmology residents.

Robert A. Catalano, MD
Leonard B. Nelson, MD

ACKNOWLEDGMENTS

It is with great pleasure and gratitude that we acknowledge the efforts of several individuals who made this book possible. Laurie Maimone has illustrated several books for us, and her expertise and talent has again enriched our efforts. Similarly, we are again indebted to Joe Fisher, our photographer, who, as with our previous works, provided invaluable assistance with the photographs and composites used. We also thank Judy Whalen for reviewing much of the text and offering many helpful suggestions. We are also obliged to Annette Rickey, who typed and retyped most of the manuscript. Her cheerful disposition and tireless work was substantially responsible for the timely completion of this book. Finally, we would like to thank Elizabeth Ryan of Appleton & Lange, who worked so diligently to keep this production on schedule.

ANATOMY OF THE EYE

EXTERNAL EYE AND EYELIDS

The **cornea** is a clear, dome-shaped structure that extends across the anterior one fifth of the globe (Fig. 1–1). Its radius of curvature is small (7.8 mm centrally), and its shape is slightly elliptical. Horizontally the cornea is 12 mm in diameter; vertically its diameter is only 11 mm. At its center the cornea is a mere 0.5 mm thick; peripherally its thickness increases to 1.0 mm. Within the cornea are numerous sensory nerve endings, but no blood vessels. Avascularity and the regular arrangement of uniformly sized collagen fibrils renders the cornea transparent.

The optically opaque **sclera** forms the "white" of the eye. Collagen fibrils in the sclera are irregular in diameter and randomly arranged and interwoven. Ground substance is less abundant and of a different composition than in the cornea. This gives the sclera rigidity at the expense of transparency.

The junction of the cornea with the sclera is called the **limbus.** The limbus is also the transition zone between the corneal and conjunctival epithelium. The **conjunctiva** is a mucous membrane that covers the sclera (bulbar conjunctiva) and inner eyelids (palpebral conjunctiva). It has a rich vascular and lymphatic supply and contains goblet cells, which contribute mucin to the tear film. Nasally, a conjunctival fold, the **plica**

semilunaris, represents the vestigal remnant of the nictitating membrane of lower animals. Adjacent to this is a fleshy-appearing mass called the **caruncle.** This structure is derived from a pinched-off part of the lower eyelid, and contains hair and accessory lacrimal, sebaceous, and sweat glands.

The **eyelids** are specialized folds of tissue that protect the eye. Each eyelid contains four layers. The outermost layer is skin, composed of keratinized epidermis and scant subcutaneous tissue. It is loose and elastic, and notable for being the thinnest skin of the body. The second layer is circularly oriented, striated muscle called the **orbicularis oculi** muscle. The third layer, the **tarsus,** is a dense fibrous tissue that gives the eyelid rigidity. Located within the tarsus are the meibomian glands, responsible for producing the oily layer of the tear film. The innermost layer is the tightly adherent palpebral conjunctiva. The mucocutaneous junction of the eyelid coincides with the meibomian gland orifices. This is not the same as the **gray line** visible on the edge of the eyelid. The latter lies anterior to the mucocutaneous junction and represents the junction of the tarsal plate with the orbicularis oculi muscle.

Two muscles, the levator palpebrae and Müller's muscle, raise the upper eyelid. The aponeurosis of the **levator palpebrae muscle** inserts on the anterior sur-

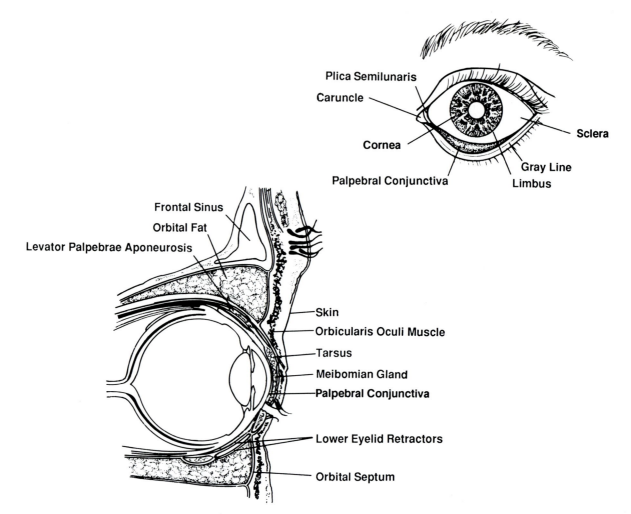

Figure 1–1. The external eye and eyelids.

face of the tarsal plate and the skin. It is supplied by the third cranial nerve. **Müller's muscle** originates on the undersurface of the levator muscle and inserts on the superior edge of the tarsus. It is supplied by the sympathetic system. The **lower eyelid retractors** are less well defined, but extend to the lower tarsal plate from the fused inferior rectus and inferior oblique muscle sheaths.

The **orbital septum** lies posterior to the orbicularis oculi muscle. It encircles the orbit and attaches to the orbital rim, the levator aponeurosis, and the lower eyelid retractors. It serves as a barrier to blood, edema, and infection between the eyelid and the orbit.

EXTRAOCULAR MUSCLES

The eye can be rotated horizontally, vertically or about an anteroposterior axis by the action of six exquisitely balanced extraocular muscles (Fig. 1–2). These extraocular muscles are named for their location and the direction they traverse to insert on the globe.

Six extraocular muscles originate at the apex of the orbit on the bone surrounding the optic canal and the superior orbital fissure. This circular arrangement of origins is called the **annulus of Zinn.** Four of these muscles follow a straight course to the eye and are called **rectus muscles.** The rectus muscles insert on the globe at varying distances from the limbus. The medial rectus muscle inserts closest to the limbus followed sequentially by the inferior, lateral, and superior rectus muscles. The **spiral of Tillaux** describes an imaginary line that connects these non-equidistant insertions.

Two oblique muscles also insert on the eye. Similar to the rectus muscles, the **superior oblique muscle** originates at the annulus of Zinn. It proceeds forward and becomes tendinous just before passing through a fibrocartilaginous loop attached to the frontal bone called the **trochlea.** From the trochlea it inserts underneath the superior rectus muscle in the superotemporal quadrant of the globe. The **inferior oblique muscle** arises from the orbital surface of the maxillary bone, passes below the inferior rectus muscle, and inserts in the inferotemporal quadrant of the eye. Each rectus

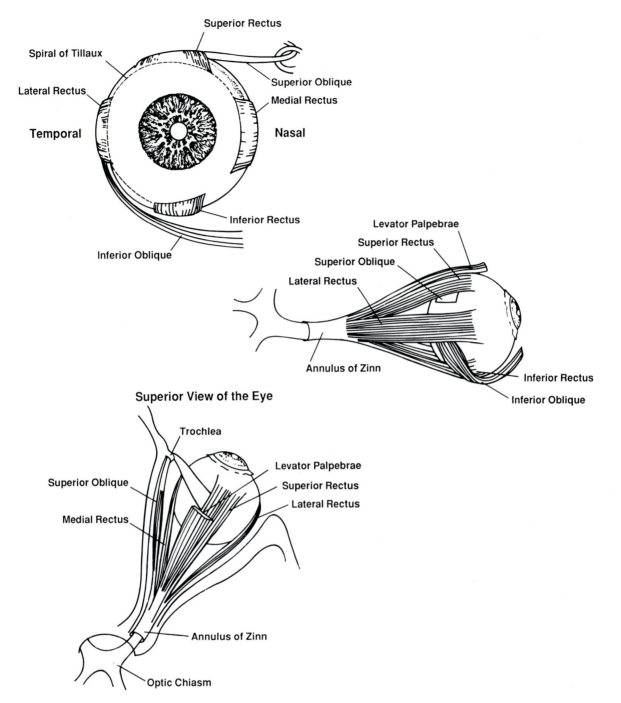

Figure 1–2. The extraocular muscles. **A.** Anterior view of the eye. **B.** Lateral view of the eye. **C.** Superior view of the eye. (Figure 1–2 **A** and **B** modified from Nelson LB, Catalano RA: Atlas of Ocular Motility. Philadelphia, Saunders, 1989, p 3, with permission).

muscle is approximately 37 mm in length and has a tendon of 3 to 7 mm. The superior and inferior oblique muscles are also approximately 40 mm in length. The tendon of the superior oblique muscle, however, is 20 mm in length, and that of the inferior oblique is at most 1 to 2 mm long.

The third (**oculomotor**) cranial nerve innervates the majority of extraocular and intraocular muscles. Its upper division innervates the superior rectus and superior oblique muscles, and its lower division inner-

vates the medial rectus, inferior rectus, and inferior oblique muscles. The third cranial nerve also supplies parasympathetic innervation to the ciliary body (responsible for accommodating the lens for near vision) and iris (pupillary constriction). The fourth (**trochlear**) cranial nerve supplies only the superior oblique muscle. The sixth (**abducens**) cranial nerve supplies only the lateral rectus muscle. Table 1–1 summarizes the innervation of the extraocular muscles and the directions they pull the eye from the straight-ahead position.

TABLE 1–1. ACTIONS AND INNERVATION OF THE EXTRAOCULAR MUSCLES

Muscle	Primary	Secondary	Tertiary	Innervation
Medial rectus	Adduction	—	—	CN III
Lateral rectus	Abduction	—	—	CN VI
Superior rectus	Elevation	Intorsion	Adduction	CN III
Inferior rectus	Depression	Extorsion	Adduction	CN III
Superior oblique	Intorsion	Depression	Abduction	CN IV
Inferior oblique	Extorsion	Elevation	Abduction	CN III

CN = cranial nerve.
Modified from Nelson LB, Catalano RA: Atlas of Ocular Motility. Philadelphia, Saunders, 1989, p 21, with permission.

The levator palpebrae muscle also arises at the annulus of Zinn. It passes above the superior rectus to form an aponeurosis that inserts in the upper eyelid.

LACRIMAL SYSTEM

The lacrimal apparatus can be divided into secretory and collecting systems (Fig. 1–3). The secretory system consists of the lacrimal and accessory lacrimal glands. The collecting portion includes the puncta, canaliculi, lacrimal sac, and nasolacrimal duct.

The **lacrimal gland** is located in the anterior lateral orbit, within the lacrimal gland fossa of the frontal bone. The aponeurosis of the levator palpebrae muscle divides it into a large orbital portion and a smaller palpebral portion. The secretory ducts of both empty into the superior conjunctival fornix. Parasympathetic secretory innervation occurs via the seventh (**facial**) cranial nerve. Sensory fibers from the fifth (**trigeminal**) nerve also supply the gland. The glands of **Krause** and **Wolfring** are accessory lacrimal glands located principally in the superior cul-de-sac. They are responsible for forming the middle (aqueous) layer of the tear film.

Tears pass down over the bulbar and palpebral conjunctiva and the cornea and drain through the puncta of the eyelids. The **puncta** are slightly elevated out-pouchings, with 0.5 mm apertures located on the eyelid margins about 6 mm from the medial angle of the eyelids (**medial canthus**). The eyelid is normally slightly inverted so that the puncta lie against the globe. Each punctum leads into a **canaliculus,** which consists of a vertical portion 2 to 3 mm in length, followed by a horizontal portion 8 to 10 mm in length. The diameter of the canaliculus is about 1 mm. The superior and inferior canaliculi usually fuse to form a common canaliculus just before emptying into the lacrimal sac. The **lacrimal sac** lies within the lacrimal sac fossa, at the level of the middle meatus of the nose. The dome, or fundus, of the sac extends 3 to 5 mm above the medial canthus. The body of the sac is an additional 10 mm long. The lacrimal collection system continues downward as the **nasolacrimal duct.** This opens into the nose through the inferior meatus under the inferior turbinate of the lateral wall. Its course extends about 12 mm and runs slightly laterally and posteriorly (see Fig. 8–16). The distance from the nasolacrimal duct opening to the external nares is approximately 20 to 25 mm.

Tears pass into the puncta by capillary attraction. Blinking or closure of the eyelids creates negative pressure within the lacrimal sac, drawing in fluid from the canaliculus. Positive pressure is placed on the tear sac when the eyelids open, forcing tears into the nose. This process is called the **lacrimal pump.**

Two valves are commonly described in the lacrimal collecting system. The **valve of Rosenmüller** is located at the junction of the common canaliculus with the lacrimal sac. It prevents reflux of tears from the sac back into the canaliculus. The **valve of Hasner** is a mucosal fold that partially covers the ostium of the nasolacrimal duct as it opens into the inferior meatus. It prevents reflux of material from the nose into the nasolacrimal duct, and is the most common site of obstruction in congenital nasolacrimal duct disorders.

INTERNAL STRUCTURE OF THE EYE

The eye can be divided into three compartments: the anterior chamber, the posterior chamber, and the vitreous cavity (Fig. 1–4). The **anterior chamber** is the area between the cornea and the anterior surface of the iris. In the normal adult, this chamber is about 3 mm deep

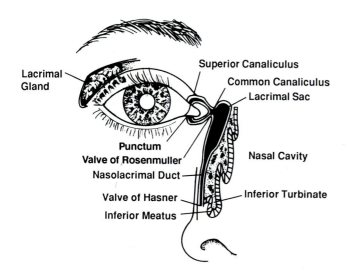

Figure 1–3. The lacrimal system.

Lacrimal Gland
Superior Canaliculus
Common Canaliculus
Lacrimal Sac
Punctum
Valve of Rosenmuller
Nasolacrimal Duct
Valve of Hasner
Inferior Meatus
Nasal Cavity
Inferior Turbinate

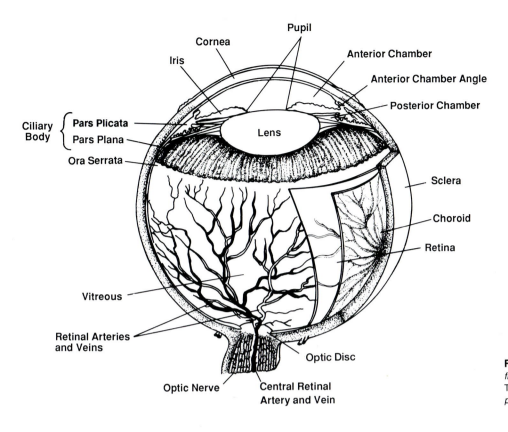

Figure 1–4. The interior eye. *(Modified from an original drawing by Paul Peck in* The Anatomy of the Eye, *reproduced with permission of Lederle Laboratories.)*

centrally and contains approximately 0.20 mL of aqueous humor. The middle compartment, or **posterior chamber,** lies between the posterior surface of the iris and the anterior surface of lens and zonule. It has a volume of only 0.06 mL. Aqueous humor is secreted by the ciliary epithelium in the posterior chamber and passes into the anterior chamber at the pupillary margin (see Fig. 1–5). The **vitreous** cavity contains 4.5 mL of vitreous, which is comprised of over 95% water, and constitutes the posterior four fifths of the eye.

The globe can also be divided into three layers. The cornea and sclera comprise the outermost coat of the eye. A vascular layer with specialized structures, called the **uvea,** lies in the middle and the inner layer consists of the **retina.**

The cornea and sclera contain dense collagenous tissue that gives the eye rigidity and protection. Their junction, the limbus, contains the trabecular meshwork and canal of Schlemm, which function as the aqueous humor drainage system (see Fig. 1–5). The cornea has no external covering. The sclera, however, is covered by the conjunctiva anteriorly and by a smooth-surfaced elastic tissue called **Tenon's capsule** posteriorly. The sclera is thinnest (0.3 mm) just posterior to the rectus muscle insertions and near the equator of the eye. Posteriorly its thickness increases to 1.0 mm. At the sieve-like **lamina cribosa,** the axons of the ganglion cells traverse the sclera to form the **optic nerve.** Numerous other openings for blood vessels and nerves also pierce the sclera.

The middle coat of the globe, or **uvea,** contains vascular tissue and specialized structures necessary for accommodation (the process by which the lens becomes thicker and more curved, increasing the focusing power of the eye for near visual tasks). The uvea can be subdivided into three zones: the iris, ciliary body, and choroid. The **iris** controls the amount of light entering the eye. It contains both dilator muscle innervated by the sympathetic system and sphincter muscle innervated by parasympathetic fibers of the third cranial nerve. The color of the iris is dependent upon the amount of melanin present in the iris stroma. The **ciliary body** is a ring of tissue that extends from a spur of sclera at the limbus to the termination of the retina called the **ora serrata** (see Fig. 1–5). This 6-mm zone is further divided into the pars plicata anteriorly, which contains the ciliary muscle and ciliary processes, and the pars plana posteriorly, which is flat and relatively nonspecialized. The **choroid** is the most posterior part of the uvea. Unlike the epithelium of the ciliary body and iris, which are derived from neuroectoderm, the choroid is of mesodermal origin. It is principally a vascular structure supplying the adjacent retinal pigment epithelium (RPE) and external half of the sensory retina. The choroid is composed of three layers of blood vessels. The innermost layer, the **choriocapillaris,** contains fenestrated, large-diameter capillaries, arranged in a distinct lobular pattern. It is separated from the RPE by a five-layered structure containing basal lamina and elastic tissue called **Bruch's membrane.** Breaks

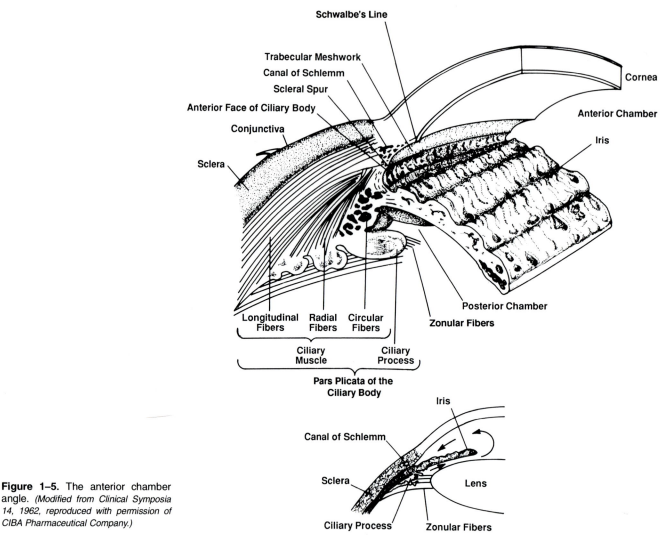

Figure 1–5. The anterior chamber angle. *(Modified from Clinical Symposia 14, 1962, reproduced with permission of CIBA Pharmaceutical Company.)*

in Bruch's membrane lead to the development of neovascular tissue under the retina.

The innermost coat of the eye develops from the invagination of the optic vesicle in embryogenesis. It forms the pigment epithelium of the iris and ciliary body anteriorly, and the sensory retina and RPE posteriorly (described below).

ANTERIOR CHAMBER ANGLE AND CILIARY BODY

Over 90 percent of the **aqueous humor** is resorbed at the **anterior chamber angle.** This specialized structure is composed of tissue derived from the cornea, sclera, iris, and ciliary body (Fig. 1–5). To egress the eye, aqueous first enters the **trabecular meshwork.** This structure is a triangular wedge of tissue that extends from a base at an invagination of sclera called the **scleral spur** to an apex at the termination of Descemet's membrane of the cornea (**Schwalbe's line**). The meshwork is a series of circumferentially oriented, thin, fibrocellular sheets with multiple fenestrations. Beyond the mesh-

work, the aqueous collects in a large venous channel, the **canal of Schlemm.** The cells of this single-layered structure contain micropinocytotic vesicles that likely play a role in aqueous outflow. The aqueous subsequently enters collector channels that drain into the intrascleral venous plexus and aqueous veins.

Posterior to the scleral spur and at the apex of the anterior chamber angle recess lies the **ciliary body.** This structure is divided into the pars plicata anteriorly, and the pars plana posteriorly. The **pars plicata** is a 2-mm zone that contains smooth muscle and 60 to 70 folds of epithelium called **ciliary processes.** Although traditionally divided into inner circular, middle radial, and outer longitudinal layers, the muscle fibers of the ciliary body are interconnected. The entire structure undergoes a three-dimensional inward and anterior movement upon contraction. The circular muscle fibers, at the inner edge of the ciliary body, may help stabilize the attachment of the iris root to the ciliary body and are especially important in relaxing the lens zonule, permitting the lens to assume a more convex shape during accommodation. The longitudinal fibers attach to the scleral spur posteriorly and may counteract a tendency for Schlemm's canal to collapse as the ciliary body moves anteriorly during accommodation.

Each ciliary process in the pars plicata is covered by a single layer of nonpigmented epithelium, which continues posteriorly as the nonpigmented epithelium of the pars plana and eventually as the sensory retina. Aqueous humor is secreted at the apex (scleral side) of these nonpigmented cells and must pass between the cells to get to the posterior chamber. **Zonular fibers** arising posteriorly from the pars plana adhere to the basement membrane of these cells (lens side), closely binding the zonular system to the ciliary body. It is as yet not completely resolved whether some zonules originate or terminate on the pars plicata. Beneath the nonpigmented epithelium lies a layer of pigmented epithelium, which continues posteriorly as a similar layer in the pars plana and eventually as the retinal pigment epithelium.

The **pars plana** of the ciliary body, which is 4 mm in width, extends from the pars plicata to the terminal end of the retina, called the **ora serrata** (see Fig. 1–4). This flat area provides the safest posterior surgical approach to the inside of the eye.

The **zonule** (annular ligament of Zinn) is a complex circumferential arrangement of fibers that interconnects the ciliary epithelium of the pars plana and pars plicata with the lens. The zonular apparatus holds the lens in place and mediates accommodation.

THE RETINA

The retina is the innermost coat of the posterior eye (Fig. 1–6). It is formed entirely of neuroectodermal tissue. The outer pigmented epithelial layer is derived from the outer layer of the invaginated embryonic optic vesicle. The inner, highly specialized, multicellular layer, called the sensory retina, is derived from the inner layer of the optic vesicle.

The outer **retinal pigment epithelium (RPE)** is a monolayer of hexagonal cells. It merges anteriorly with the pigmented epithelium of the pars plana. Its basal lamina forms the inner layer of Bruch's membrane, and its apical border has multiple villous processes that surround the outer segments of the rods and cones. The RPE serves many functions including absorption of light, vitamin A and rhodopsin metabolism, metabolic functions for the rods and cones, and maintenance of the outer blood–retinal barrier. Separation of the RPE from the neurosensory retina is called a **retinal detachment.**

The sensory retina contains three layers of nuclei,

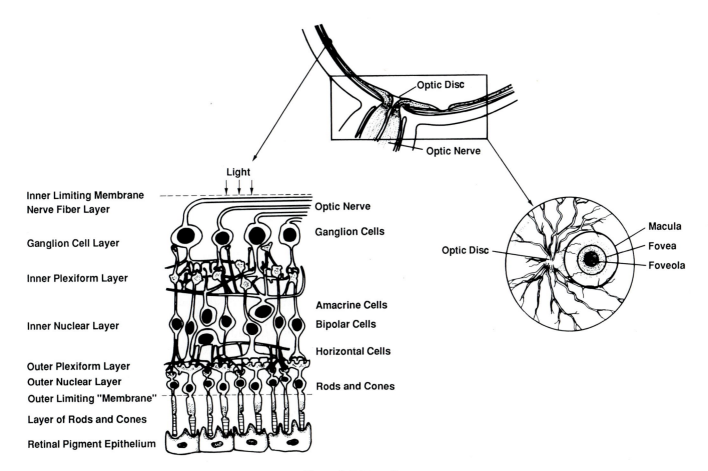

Figure 1–6. The retina.

three layers of fibers, two "limiting membranes," and a layer containing the outer segments of the rods and cones. The innermost layer is the nerve fiber layer. This layer contains the axons of the ganglion cells, which collect to form the optic nerve. Light must pass through this and all the other layers of the sensory retina to reach the layer of rods and cones. Ganglion cells receive impulses from the bipolar cells, which in turn receive impulses from the rods and cones. Interspersed within the inner plexiform zone (comprised of ganglion cell dendrites and bipolar cell axons) are amacrine cells. These modulate the visual impulse. Horizontal cells act similarly, but lie within the outer plexiform zone (comprised of bipolar cell dendrites and photoreceptor axons). Supporting astroglial, or Müller cells, are also present in the retina.

Similar to the uvea, the retina can be divided into regions. The area responsible for the most distinct vision is called the **macula**. The anatomic and clinical definitions of the macula differ. Anatomically, the macula is a 4.5-mm region in which the ganglion cell layer is multicellular and xanthophyll pigment is found. In the center of this area is a 1.5-mm sloping depression called the **fovea**. The 0.4-mm center or floor of this indentation is called the **foveola** (Fig. 1–6, bottom right). Histologically, no rods are found within the fovea, and the foveola is further characterized by the peripheral displacement of all cell layers such that in this area light falls directly on the cone outer segments. The fovea is nurtured solely by the choriocapillaris, and its vascular supply remains intact after a central retinal artery occlusion. This gives it a cherry red appearance (spot) when surrounded by hypoxic whitish retina. The "clinical" macula is defined generally as the area of retina that lies between the temporal vascular arcades.

In the peripheral retina rods predominate. Peripheral cones differ histologically from foveal cones, and peripheral ganglion cell bodies are larger and arranged in a single layer. The **ora serrata** is the anterior termination of the retina. It is located approximately 6 mm posterior to the limbus, and continues forward as the nonpigmented ciliary epithelium.

The inner half of the retina is supplied by branches of the central retinal artery. The outer half is nurtured by the choriocapillaris. Capillaries are distributed in a superficial network in the nerve fiber layer and an inner network in the region of the bipolar cells.

REFERENCES

Anterior Chamber Angle and Ciliary Body

Hayreh SS: The choriocapillaris. Graefes Arch Ophthalmol 192:165, 1974.

Mann I: The Development of the Human Eye. New York, Grune & Stratton, 1964.

Streeten BW: The zonular insertion: A scanning electron microscopic study. Invest Ophthalmol Vis Sci 16:364, 1977.

Tripathi RC, Tripathi BJ: Functional anatomy of the anterior chamber angle. In Duane TD, Jaeger EA (eds): Biomedical Foundations of Ophthalmology. Philadelphia, Lippincott, 1990, vol 1.

Warwick R (ed): Eugene Wolff's Anatomy of the Eye and Orbit, ed 7. Philadelphia, Saunders, 1977.

External Eye and Eyelids

Hornblass A (ed): Oculoplastic, Orbital and Reconstructive Surgery. Volume 1, Eyelids. Baltimore, Williams & Wilkins, 1988.

Kohn R: Textbook of Ophthalmic Plastic and Reconstructive Surgery. Philadelphia, Lea & Febiger, 1988.

Warwich R (ed): Eugene Wolff's Anatomy of the Eye and Orbit, ed 7. Philadelphia, Saunders, 1977.

Yanoff M, Fine BS: Ocular Pathology: A Text and Atlas, ed 3. Philadelphia, Lippincott, 1989.

Extraocular Muscles

Nelson LB, Catalano RA: Atlas of Ocular Motility. Philadelphia, Saunders, 1989.

Parks MM: Eye movements and positions. In Duane TD, Jaeger EA (eds): Clinical Ophthalmology. Philadelphia, Lippincott, 1990.

Von Noorden GK: Binocular Vision and Ocular Motility. Theory and Management of Strabismus, ed 4. St. Louis, Mosby, 1990.

Internal Structure of the Eye

Jakobiec FA, Ozanics V: General topographic anatomy of the eye. In Duane TD, Jaeger EA (eds): Biomedical Foundations of Ophthalmology. Philadelphia, Lippincott, 1990.

Lucas DR (ed): Greer's Ocular Pathology, 4th ed. Boston, Blackwell Scientific, 1989.

O'Connor GR: The uvea: Annual review. Arch Ophthalmol 93:675, 1975.

Snell R, Lemp MA: Clinical Anatomy of the Eye. Boston, Blackwell Scientific, 1989.

Lacrimal System

Hornblass A (ed): Oculoplastic, Orbital, and Reconstructive Surgery. Volume 2, Orbit and Lacrimal System. Baltimore, Williams & Wilkins, 1990.

Jones LT, Wobig JL: Surgery of the Eyelids and Lacrimal System. Birmingham, Aesculapius Publishing Co, 1976.

Viers ER: Lacrimal Disorders. St. Louis, Mosby, 1976.

The Retina

Hogan MJ, Alvarado JA, Weddell JE: Histology of the Human Eye. Philadelphia, Saunders, 1971.

Ryan SJ, Ogden TF, Schachat AP, et al (eds): Retina. St. Louis, Mosby, 1989.

Straatsma BR, Hall MO, Allen RA, Crescitelli F (eds): The Retina: Morphology, Function, and Clinical Characteristics. Berkeley, University of California Press, 1969.

THE PEDIATRIC EYE EXAM

ESSENTIAL INFORMATION FOR PRIMARY CARE PRACTITIONERS

Preschool Vision Screening

In a policy statement in 1992, the American Academy of Ophthalmology recommended preschool vision screening as a means of reducing preventable visual loss. Their recommended screening schedule is reviewed in Table 2–1. Fulton (1992) appropriately as-serted that this testing should "fall under the purview of primary providers, and should be accomplished in conjunction with well-child visits."

Children and infants with an abnormal finding on a screening exam should be referred for formal evaluation. This evaluation includes an ocular and medical history, assessment of vision, and examination of the eye. This section reviews the fundamentals of the exam.

TABLE 2–1. VISION SCREENING SCHEDULE FOR INFANTS AND CHILDREN

Age	Screening Test	Findings Requiring Referral
Newborn to 3 months	Red reflex test (see Chapter 11) Corneal light reflex test External examination	Opacity of the cornea, cataract, retinal detachment or disorder Ocular misalignment (strabismus) Structural defect
6–12 months	Red reflex test Corneal light reflex test Occlusion of each eye separately Fixation and following	As above As above Amblyopia if child resists occlusion unequally Amblyopia if unable to do
3 years	Red reflex test Corneal light reflex test Visual acuity test Stereoacuity	As above As above Refractive error, amblyopia Refractive error, amblyopia
5 years	Same as 3 years	As above

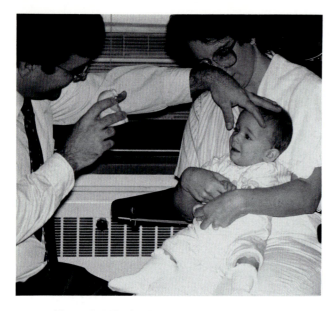

Figure 2–1. Testing fixation and following behavior.

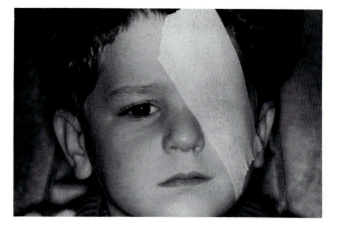

Figure 2–3. Occluding one eye with paper tape to assess vision in each eye separately.

Visual Acuity Testing

Many tests of visual acuity exist. Which is used depends on the child's age and level of cooperation, as well as the clinician's preference and experience with each test. The most commonly used visual acuity test in infants is an assessment of their ability to fixate and follow a target. If appropriate targets are used, this reflex can be demonstrated in most infants by about 6 weeks of age. The test is performed by seating the child comfortably in the parent's lap. The object of visual interest, possibly a bright-colored toy, is slowly moved to the right and to the left. The examiner observes whether the infant's eyes turn toward the object and follow its movements. The examiner can use a thumb to occlude one of the infant's eyes, in order to test each eye separately (Fig. 2–1). Although a sound-producing object might compromise the purity of the visual stimulus, in practice toys that squeak or rattle heighten an infant's awareness and interest in the test.

Although the aforementioned test objects are more commonly used, the human face is, in fact, a more ideal target. The examiner can exploit this by moving his or her face slowly in front of the infant's face. If the appropriate following movements are not elicited, the test should be repeated with the parent moving his or her face as the test stimulus.

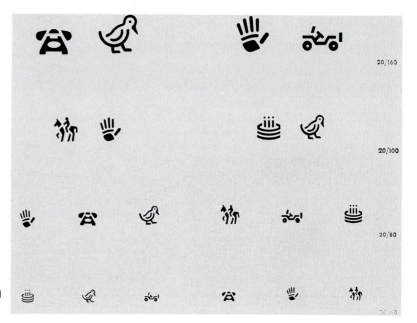

Figure 2–2. Allen picture eye chart used for preschool children.

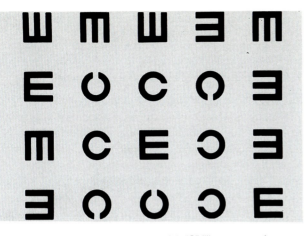

Figure 2–4. Tumbling "E" and Landolt "C" illiterate eye chart.

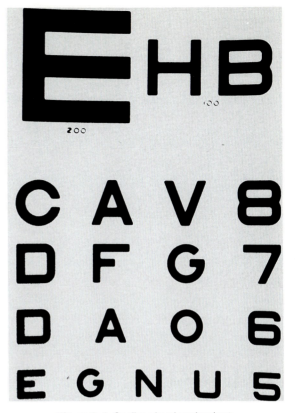

Figure 2–6. Snellen visual acuity chart.

An objective measurement of visual acuity usually becomes possible when children reach 2½ to 3 years of age. Children this age are tested using a schematic picture or other illiterate eye chart (Fig. 2–2). Each eye should be tested separately. This can be accomplished by placing a piece of paper tape over one eye (Fig. 2–3). Tape is less bothersome to a child than a parent's hand. Test symbols should be presented individually, because children in this age group are easily confused.

The tumbling "E" and Landolt "C" tests are the most widely used visual acuity tests for preschool children (Fig. 2–4). The object is for the child to point in the direction of the letter held by the examiner (Fig. 2–5). Right-left presentations are more confusing than up-down presentations. With pretest practice, this test can be performed by most children 3 to 4 years of age.

At about age 5 or 6 years, an adult-type Snellen acuity chart can be used (Fig. 2–6). Before employing this chart, however, the examiner must be sure that the child knows letters. It is better to determine the child's ability to identify letters by presenting them close initially, rather than asking parents if their child has this ability.

An acuity of 20/40 is generally accepted as normal for 3-year-old children. At age 4, 20/30 is typical. By age 5 or 6, most children attain 20/20 vision.

External Examination

The external examination of the eye determines if there are any ocular infections, orbital tumors, or structural defects of the eye or orbit. Techniques used include visual inspection, palpation, and auscultation.

The eyelids are inspected for inflammation, apposition to the globe, and drooping (Fig. 2–7). The lacrimal system is evaluated in infants with obstruction, inflammation, or infection of the tear drainage system. The different tests used are described later in this chapter.

Pupillary Examination

The pupillary exam evaluates the size, shape, reaction, and symmetry of the pupils. Both pupils usually are

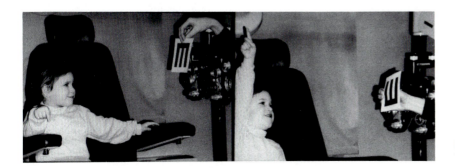

Figure 2–5. Child demonstrating the illiterate "E" test.

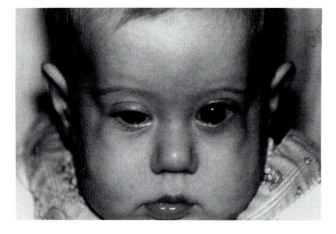

Figure 2–7. Ptosis (droopy upper eyelid), right eye.

the same size, but in 20 to 25 percent of normal individuals, the size differs slightly (anisocoria) (Fig. 2–8).

The direct pupillary response to light is measured by shining a light into one eye while the child fixates on a distant object. Pupillary constriction is not synonymous with visual awareness, but indicates functioning afferent and efferent pupillary pathways. This response can be elicited in premature infants as young as 31 gestational weeks. In the neonate, the resting pupillary size is relatively small, and the pupil constricts and dilates more slowly than an older infant's pupil. To test this response in the newborn nursery, the room should be semidarkened, to moderately dilate the pupil. Other pupillary tests look for atypical dilation of a pupil to light stimulation. This phenomenon suggests an affer-

ent pupillary defect, due to an optic nerve or retinal abnormality (described in the section on Afferent Pupillary Defect.)

Assessment of Ocular Alignment and Motility

Different tests are used to assess ocular alignment. These include corneal light reflex tests and cover tests.

Corneal light reflex tests use the image of incident light on the cornea to assess the status of ocular alignment. They are useful in patients who cannot cooperate for cover testing or who have poor fixation. They are performed by having the infant fixate a light held 33 cm away. A 1-mm decentration of the corneal light reflex corresponds to 7 degrees of deviation (Figs. 2–9 and 2–10). A light reflex at the margin of a midsized pupil would be about 2 mm from the expected position, corresponding to 15 degrees of deviation. A light reflex in the middle of the iris would equal 4 mm of decentration, or about 30 degrees of deviation. A light reflex at the limbus would equal 6 mm of decentration, or about 45 degrees of deviation.

Cover tests provide the most accurate and reproducible measurements of ocular alignment. Prerequisites to cover testing include foveal fixation in each eye, image perception from each eye, absence of restriction of eye movements, and patient cooperation. All cover tests involve covering the apparently fixing eye. The response to cover testing in both the occluded and the nonoccluded eye is observed. If the previously fixating eye moves behind the occluder, a latent strabismus or phoria is present (Fig. 2–11). If the nonoccluded eye rotates to pick up fixation, a manifest strabismus or tropia in the deviating eye is present (Fig. 2–12).

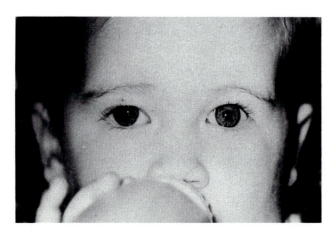

Figure 2–8. Anisocoria (asymmetry of pupil size).

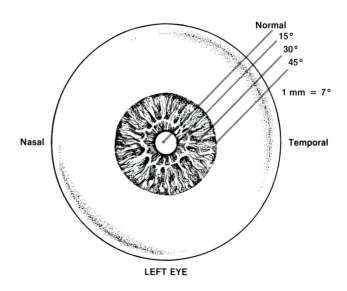

Figure 2–9. The light reflex test of Hirschberg. The degree of ocular misalignment corresponding to the reflection of light on the cornea. *(From Nelson LB, Catalano RA: Atlas of ocular motility. Philadelphia, Saunders, 1989, p 99, with permission.)*

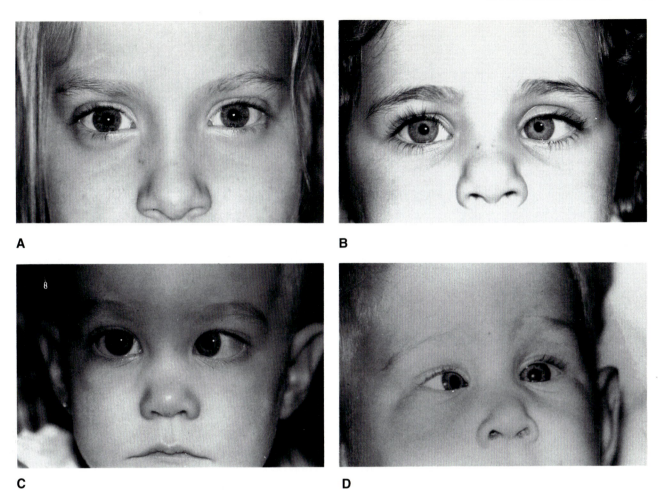

Figure 2–10. Examples of the corneal light reflex test. **A.** Normal. **B.** 15-degree turning in and down of the left eye. **C.** 30-degree turning in of the left eye. **D.** 45-degree turning in of the right eye.

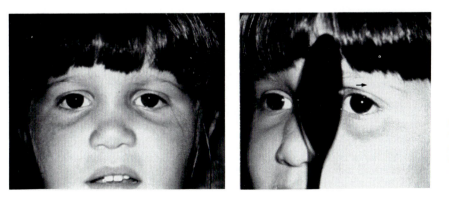

Figure 2–11. Cover test demonstrating a latent strabismus (phoria). When the cover is placed in front of the left eye, it turns outward (left exophoria). *(From Nelson LB, Catalano RA: Atlas of ocular motility. Philadelphia, Saunders, 1989, p 85, with permission.)*

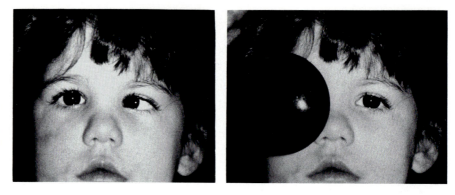

Figure 2–12. Cover test demonstrating a manifest strabismus (tropia). When the cover is placed in front of the right eye, the left eye turns outward (left esotropia). *(From Nelson LB, Catalano RA: Atlas of ocular motility. Philadelphia, Saunders, 1989, p 103, with permission.)*

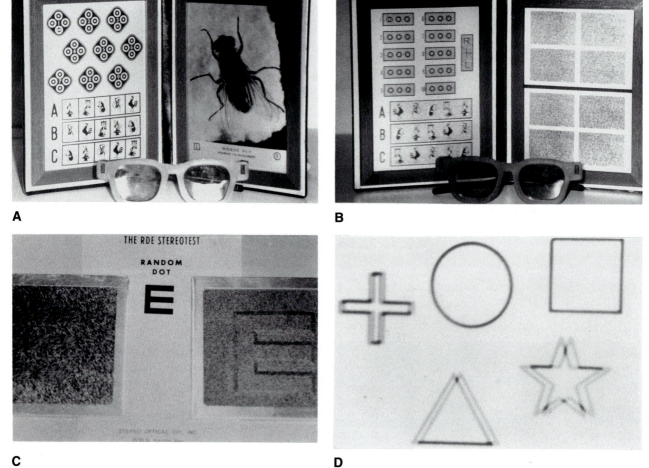

A

B

C

D

Figure 2–13. Stereoscopic tests. **A.** Titmus test. **B.** TNO random dot test. **C.** Random dot E test. **D.** Distance stereoscopic test. In the latter test the least disparate object is in the upper right corner. Disparity increases counterclockwise, with the star appearing to be closest to the subject.

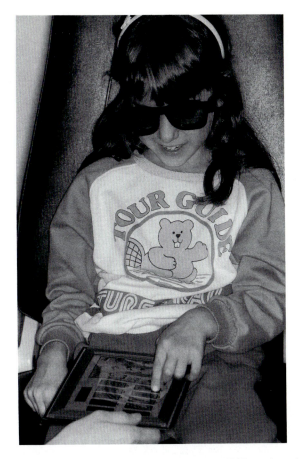

Figure 2–14. Child being tested with the near TNO random dot stereoscopic test.

Ocular rotations are tested by having the child fixate on a near target that is moved into the cardinal positions of gaze (see Fig. 2–45). In younger children, it is usually necessary to restrain the head from moving, especially in extreme fields of gaze. Testing ocular rotations allows the examiner to evaluate under- and over-

action of extraocular muscles, as well as possible restrictions in gaze.

Assessment of Stereopsis

Depth perception (stereopsis) is tested using various tests at near and distant fixation. Near fixation tests, such as the Titmus and TNO random dot tests, use Polaroid glasses and cards upon which slightly disparate objects have been printed (Fig. 2–13). In both tests, the disparate object is grouped with objects without disparity. When viewed through the Polaroid glasses, it appears to project out of the plane of the card, toward the observer. Groups of figures are arranged such that the amount of disparity in the odd object decreases as one descends through the chart (Fig. 2–14). In this way, the degree of stereopsis can be quantitated. The smallest near stereoscopic target subtends approximately 20 seconds of arc. A distant stereoscopic test uses images projected 20 feet.

Examination of the Cornea

In infants, the cornea should be evaluated for diameter and clarity. The cornea measures approximately 10 mm in diameter in the newborn and increases to approximately 12 mm during the first 2 years of life. A large, cloudy cornea suggests infantile glaucoma; a small cornea suggests a small, malformed eye (see Chapter 9).

The cornea should also be carefully examined after an eye injury, particularly if there is any suggestion of a corneal abrasion or foreign body. Either causes acute ocular pain, tearing, and light sensitivity. Young children will usually squeeze their eyelids tightly closed in this situation. If conventional methods of spreading the eyelids, using fingers or cotton-tipped applicators, are unsuccessful, lid retractors may be necessary. Retractors can be made by bending paperclips; infant-sized lid retractors can also be purchased (Fig. 2–15).

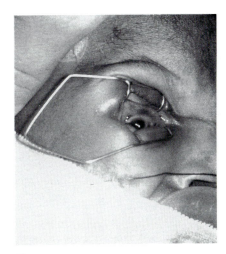

A   **B**

Figure 2–15. Infant eyelid retractors.
A. Solid blade. **B.** Open blade. (Continued)

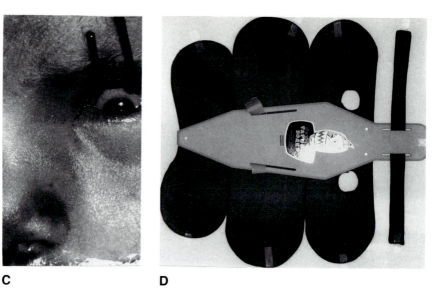

Figure 2–15. (*Continued*) **C.** Bent paper clip.
D. Papoose board (used to restrain infants)

C

D

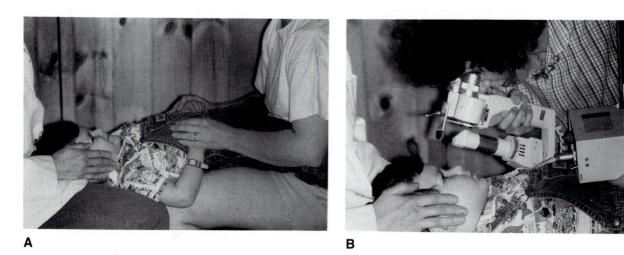

A

B

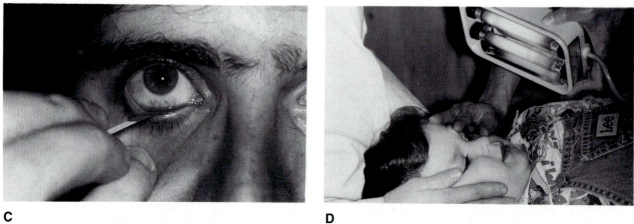

C

D

Figure 2–16. A. Positioning used to restrain a toddler. **B.** Portable slit lamp being used to examine the external eye and eyelids.
C. Instillation of fluorescein dye. **D.** Wood's lamp illumination of the eye to check for a corneal abrasion.

Anesthesia using a topical anesthetic (proparacaine 0.5%, or tetracaine 0.5%) may be helpful, if a corneal abrasion is suspected.

The use of retractors requires total immobilization of the child. A papoose board is useful in restraining infants (Fig. 2–15). A useful position to restrain toddlers is demonstrated in Figure 2–16A. The parent sits facing the physician's assistant. Both should be at the same level, and their knees should be close or touching. The child lies supine in the parent's and assistant's lap with the legs wrapped around the parent's waist and head in the assistant's lap. The parent holds the child's hands folded across the child's waist. The physician's assistant, using both hands, immobilizes the child's head.

Once the cornea has been exposed, the examiner should use a good source of focal illumination and magnification, either loupes or a portable slit lamp. If a superficial corneal injury (corneal abrasion) is suspected, fluorescein dye, which assists in identifying corneal surface irregularities, should be instilled. This is accomplished by applying a fluorescein-impregnated sterile paper strip to the conjunctival surface of an everted lower eyelid. The child is then encouraged to blink, which allows the dye to cover the corneal surface uniformly. The cornea is examined using a blue light source from a hand-held Wood's lamp or a slit lamp (Fig. 2–16). The fluorescein dye accentuates corneal surface irregularities by pooling in the abraded area (Fig. 2–17).

Examination of the Anterior Segment

An adequate examination of the anterior segment of the eye usually requires the use of a slit lamp. This instrument provides superb illumination and magnification (see the section on Anterior Segment Examination, later in this chapter). With it, any inflammatory cells or proteinaceous transudate in the anterior chamber can be identified. The anterior chamber is normally optically empty. The presence of cells or protein indicates an intraocular inflammatory process (uveitis), hemorrhage, or infection.

Ophthalmoscopy

Four instruments are available for viewing the interior eye. These are the direct and indirect ophthalmoscope, and contact and noncontact retinal lenses. Direct ophthalmoscopy provides an upright, magnified (approximately 15X) image. Indirect ophthalmoscopy provides an inverted, reversed, three-dimensional image. Contact and noncontact retinal lenses provide highly magnified, well-illuminated, three-dimensional views of the fundus.

Direct ophthalmoscopy is accomplished in a stepwise fashion. The child should be sitting, and fixating on a distant object. The examiner should approach the child from the side, and use the left eye to examine the left eye of the patient (or the examiner's right eye to examine the patient's right eye). While peering through the observer aperture of the ophthalmoscope, the light beam of the scope should be directed toward the patient's pupil. The examiner's index finger should be on the focusing wheel of lenses as the examiner comes closer to the patient (Fig. 2–18). With proper focusing of the red reflex, the retina becomes visible. When a large retinal vessel is located, it is followed either nasally or temporally to the optic disc, which is usually examined first. The macula is examined by asking the patient to look toward the light of the ophthalmoscope.

The direct ophthalmoscope provides a detailed examination of the optic nerve and macula, but it cannot be used to examine the peripheral retina. The indirect ophthalmoscope is used when evaluation of the retinal periphery is essential (as in examining for retinopathy of prematurity or retinal detachment).

Indirect ophthalmoscopy requires specialized equipment and training, and is usually performed only by ophthalmologists. Its use requires alignment of the observer's eyes, a light source, a lens, and the patient's

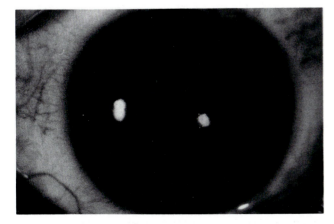
Figure 2–17. Corneal abrasion stained with fluorescein dye.

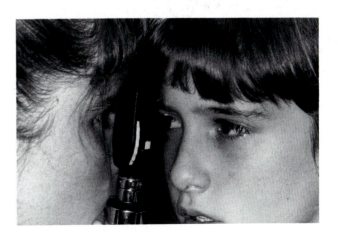
Figure 2–18. Method of direct ophthalmoscopy.

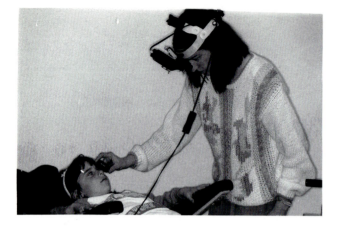

Figure 2–19. Method of indirect ophthalmoscopy.

eye (Fig. 2–19). Although it is difficult to master, its advantages are many. Stronger illumination allows visualization through opacities that the direct ophthalmoscope cannot penetrate. Although the magnification of the indirect ophthalmoscope is less (approximately 2 to 4X), its field of view is considerably larger than the direct ophthalmoscope. With the use of scleral depression, the entire retina can usually be examined. The greatest advantage of indirect ophthalmoscopy, however, is that lesions can be visualized in depth.

Contact and noncontact retinal lenses are used at the slit lamp (Fig. 2–20). Many are available including the Goldmann lens, the Hruby lens (an attachment to many slit lamps), and several hand-held lenses such as the Volk 90 diopter lens.

Indications for Ophthalmologic Referral

The pediatrician or family physician is in a unique clinical setting to recognize ocular disorders in infants and children. Early recognition of many disorders is important. If early identification of infantile glaucoma is made, effective therapy is available that can preserve

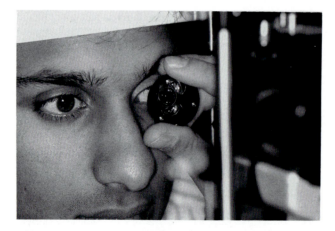

Figure 2–20. Retinal examination using the Goldmann three-mirror lens.

sight in a great majority of cases. Early detection of a retinoblastoma can save a child's life.

Although many ocular disorders are easily managed by primary care physicians, certain conditions should be evaluated by an ophthalmologist. Table 2–2 lists conditions where ophthalmologic referral is suggested. Keeping with the outline of this chapter, the list is divided into historical signs and symptoms, and findings on examination of the eye. Certain entities (such as loss of vision or visual field) merit referral if noted on the history or found on examination.

COMPREHENSIVE INFORMATION ON THE PEDIATRIC EYE EXAMINATION

The proper sequence to conduct the eye examination is listed in Table 2–3. Each of the 11 steps should be conducted in a specific sequence. Measuring the intraocular pressure in a patient with a red eye, prior to the anterior segment examination, risks infectious contamination of the instrument used to measure the pressure. After the pupils have been dilated with a cycloplegic agent (a drug that widens the pupils and prevents the lens from focusing), pupillary responses and near vision cannot be tested. Similarly, corneal sensitivity cannot be assessed after the instillation of topical anesthetics.

If at any time during the examination suspicion of a ruptured globe develops, no further diagnostic examinations should be performed. A protective eyeshield

TABLE 2–2. CONDITIONS THAT MERIT OPHTHALMOLOGIC REFFERAL

- *FINDINGS ON THE HISTORY THAT MERIT REFERRAL*

Loss of vision, whether transient or sustained
Distortion of vision (metamorphopsia)
Constriction or loss of the visual field
Diplopia in any field of gaze
The perception of flashes of light or new floaters
Abnormal sensitivity to light

- *FINDINGS ON THE OCULAR EXAMINATION THAT MERIT REFERRAL*

Any ocular disorder that results in a sustained reduction of vision,
    or loss of the visual field
Perforating injury to the eye or orbit
Laceration involving the eyelid margin
Imbedded corneal foreign body
Blood in the anterior chamber of the eye
Inflammation within the eye
Irregular, asymmetric, or poorly reacting pupil
Relative afferent pupillary defect
Restricted ocular movements with diplopia
Elevated intraocular pressure
Blood in the vitreous
Evidence of diabetic or hypertensive retinopathy
Absence of findings but persistent eye pain or visual complaints

TABLE 2–3. THE 11-PART EYE EXAM

1. Ophthalmic history
    a. Chief complaint
    b. History of present illness
    c. Past ocular history
    d. Family history of ophthalmic disorders
2. Systemic history
    a. Prenatal history
    b. Birth history
    c. Developmental history
    d. Current medications
    e. Allergies
3. Assessment of vision (each eye tested separately)
    a. Corrected/uncorrected visual acuity
    b. Measurement of noncyclopleged refractive error
    c. Contrast sensitivity vision[a]
    d. Color vision[a]
4. External examination
    a. Orbit
    b. Eyelids
    c. Lacrimal system
5. Pupillary examination
    a. Pupillary responses
    b. Relative afferent pupillary defect
    c. Paradoxical pupillary reaction
6. Assessment of ocular alignment and motility
    a. Versions, vergences, and ductions
    b. Ocular rotations into the cardinal positions of gaze
    c. Ocular alignment (light reflex and cover tests)
    d. Dissimilar image and target tests[a]
    e. Stereopsis (depth perception) testing[a]
    f. Oculocephalic and caloric testing[a]
    g. Forced duction and active force generation testing[a]
7. Visual field examination
    a. Confrontational testing
    b. Goldmann/automated field testing
8. Anterior segment examination
    a. Eyelids
    b. Conjunctiva and sclera
    c. Cornea and tear film
    d. Anterior chamber
    e. Iris
    f. Ocular lens
    g. Gonioscopy[a]
9. Measurement of intraocular pressure[b]
    a. Indentation tonometry
    b. Applanation tonometry
    c. Digital tonometry
10. Measurement of refractive errors
    a. Objective refraction (retinoscopy)
    b. Subjective refraction
11. Fundus examination
    a. Direct ophthalmoscopy
    b. Indirect ophthalmoscopy
    c. Contact lens exam[a]

[a]Optional technique for selected disorders.
[b]Deferred in the presence of active infection.
Modified from Catalano RA: Ocular emergencies. Philadelphia, Saunders, 1992, p 4, with permission.

that fits entirely over the bony orbit, completely encasing the eye (without a pressure patch), should be taped to the face (see Fig. 15–12). Further examination and treatment should be carried out only under general anesthesia.

The Ophthalmic History

The **chief complaint** is the patient's reason for seeking medical care. If it is very specific (e.g., "I splashed bleach in my eye"), the examination and treatment can be readily directed. If the complaint is a symptom (e.g., "I woke up with double vision"), a differential diagnosis must be developed.

The **history of present illness** should provide sufficient information for the examiner to reconstruct a sequence of events. The physician should ascertain what, where, when, and how an event occurred. Precipitating influences and associated signs or symptoms should also be elicited. Additionally, any instituted treatment, including self-treatment, should be carefully documented.

The **past ocular history** should elicit any preexisting cause for decreased vision in an eye with an acute problem. Examples include amblyopia, previous trauma, surgery, or infection. The ocular history should also note whether the patient is using, or has

ever used, any eye medications, topically or systemically, and the name of the disorder being treated. For most ocular drugs, the color of the bottle top correlates with the type of medication (Table 2–4). Any previous episodes similar to the current disorder should be thoroughly reviewed, with emphasis on the effectiveness of different treatments. An ocular surgical history should also be recorded.

The **family history** should specifically elicit

TABLE 2–4. BOTTLE TOP COLORS OF EYE MEDICATIONS

Color	Pharmacological Property	Action(s)
Green	Cholinergic	Treats glaucoma Constricts pupil
Red	Anticholinergic	Dilates pupil
	Sympathomimetic	Treats glaucoma (some)
White	Corticosteroid (milky solution)	Reduces inflammation
	Antibiotic (clear solution)	Treats infection
	Artificial tears (clear solution)	Treats dry eye conditions
Yellow	Beta blocker	Treats glaucoma
Blue	Beta blocker	Treats glaucoma

Modified from Catalano RA: Ocular emergencies. Philadelphia, Saunders, 1992, p 6, with permission.

whether other individuals ever had a condition similar to the patient. Detailing the cataract history of every grandparent is not as productive as concentrating on persons with poor vision of undetermined cause, and heritable ophthalmic disorders. If the family history is unavailable, it should be noted as such; it is misleading to record an absence of history as a negative history.

The Systemic History

The **general medical/surgical history** should intelligently review the relevant organ systems of the body. In children, attention should be directed to abnormalities of the cardiac, respiratory, central nervous, and immune systems, as well as any history of benign or malignant tumors. Knowledge of preexisting conditions may modify treatment of the ophthalmic disorder.

A review of **current medications** may prevent the use of incompatible pharmaceuticals, and reveal medications that may have an adverse effect on the eyes. A review of medicinal **allergies** is always appropriate prior to administering any pharmaceutical. Many patients do not distinguish allergic from toxic effects. Signs of true allergy always should be elicited. These include itching, hives, rashes, respiratory distress, and cardiovascular collapse. In children with pruritic "red eyes," a history of environmental allergies should be sought.

ASSESSMENT OF VISION

Acuity is the most widely recognized and understood measure of visual function. It is recorded as an unreduced fraction based on a normal viewing distance of 20 feet. The numerator of the fraction is the viewing distance; the denominator represents the distance at which a person without an ocular abnormality can resolve the same-sized letter. For example, an individual with 20/200 vision can resolve at 20 feet the same sized letter that an individual without ocular abnormality can recognize 200 feet away. In most parts of the world, acuities are given in metric equivalents. Table 2–5 lists these and also gives an estimate of the percentage loss of central vision corresponding to a given level of acuity.

Assessment of Vision in the Preverbal Infant

In recent years, there has been an upsurge of interest in the assessment of visual function in the preverbal child. Several objective techniques (optokinetic nystagmus, visual evoked potentials, and preferential looking) are now available to assess vision in very young children.

Optokinetic nystagmus is a rhythmic two-phase eye movement elicited by the stimulus of a moving

TABLE 2–5. DISTANCE VISUAL ACUITY CONVERSIONS AND PERCENTAGE OF LOSS OF CENTRAL VISION

Snellen Optotypes		
British (ft)	*Metric (m)*	*% Loss*
20/15	6/5	0
20/20	6/6	0
20/25	6/7.5	5
20/30	6/10	10
20/40	6/12	15
20/50	6/15	25
20/60	6/20	35
20/70	6/22	40
20/80	6/24	45
20/100	6/30	50
20/150	6/50	70
20/200	6/60	80
20/300	6/90	85
20/400	6/120	90
20/800	6/240	95

Modified from Catalano RA: Ocular emergencies. Philadelphia, Saunders, 1992, p 8, with permission.

stripe. Alternating light and dark stripes may be presented on a drum rotating in front of an infant's eyes (Fig. 2–21), or by a continuous sheet or tape that is moved past the eyes. The nystagmus generated by an optokinetic stimulus consists of two phases: (1) a slow phase of fixation, during which the eye follows the stimulus across the visual field (smooth pursuit); and (2) a fast corrective phase in the opposite direction (saccade). The resolving power, or visual acuity, of the eye is estimated by presenting a series of striped patterns of smaller width, until nystagmus is no longer elicited.

The visual evoked potential is a measure of change in electrical activity in the visual cortex in response to a patterned stimulus presented to the eye (Fig. 2–22). The patterned stimulus is either phase-alternated checkerboards or square-wave gratings. The macula is overrepresented at the cortical level and therefore domi-

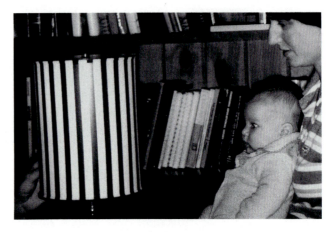

Figure 2–21. Optokinetic nystagmus testing.

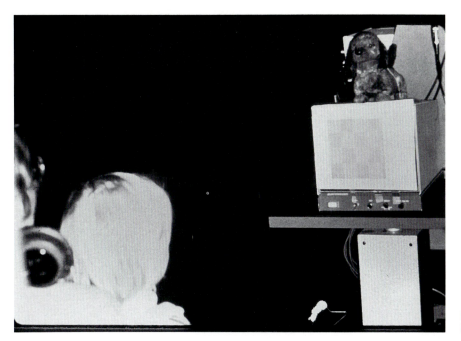

Figure 2–22. Visual evoked potential testing. *(Courtesy of John W. Simon.)*

nates the visually evoked potential response, making this test useful for evaluating visual acuity in infants.

Preferential looking is based on the observation that infants prefer to fixate a patterned stimulus rather than a homogeneous field. The technique involves having the infant gaze at two circular windows. Behind one of the windows is a homogeneous field; behind the other is a grating-like field of black-and-white stripes (Fig. 2–23). Either field may be presented at either window. An observer is masked from knowing to which window the striped pattern will be presented. He is positioned behind a peephole and records the direction of the infant's eyes and head during successive presentations of the pattern. The infant's visual acuity is estimated by determining the smallest stripe width that stimulates preferential fixation. Teller acuity card testing is a modification of preferential looking. This method necessitates only one tester, and uses hand-held cards upon which patterns of varying-width stripes are printed (Fig. 2–24).

Visual Acuity Charts for Literate Individuals

Although the Snellen eye chart is the most widely used visual acuity test (see Fig. 2–6), it has been criticized because the letters on the chart vary in resolvable difficulty (letters with oblique lines and curves are more difficult to resolve). Additionally, the progression of letter size is irregular, and the spacing and number of letters on each line is inconsistent. Newer charts have been developed which use an equal number of letters designed by Sloan, of approximately equal difficulty, with a geometric progression of letter height from line

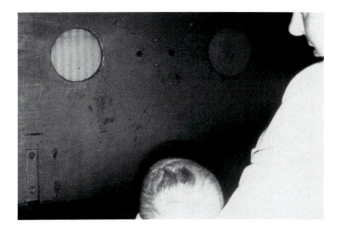

Figure 2–23. Preferential looking testing. *(Courtesy of John W. Simon.)*

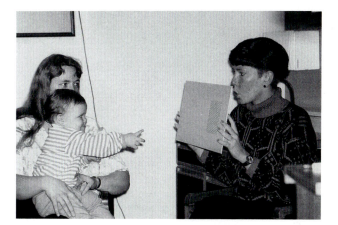

Figure 2–24. Teller acuity card testing.

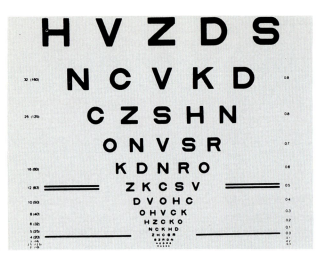

Figure 2–25. Log MAR visual acuity chart.

to line (Fig. 2–25). These charts are called **log MAR,** because they are based on a logarithmic scale of the minimal angle of resolution.

Charts have also been developed that assess a different parameter of vision, **contrast sensitivity** (Fig. 2–26). Reduced contrast sensitivity occurs in patients with optic neuritis, glaucoma, diabetic retinopathy, and compressive lesions of the optic nerve and chiasm. Differences in contrast sensitivity have also been noted in amblyopia.

Several different measures of vision are used for individuals with markedly reduced vision. These include the ability to count fingers presented by the examiner (at a stated distance) or to recognize hand movements or light. The visual quadrants where these are perceived should also be recorded. The abbreviations used to describe these levels of acuity are CF (count fingers), HM (hand motion), LP (light perception), and NLP (no light perception). Because the term "blind" has legal and social connotations, the acuity should never be re-

corded as "blind." The federal government defines **legal blindness** as a best corrected visual acuity in the better eye of 20/200 or less, or a field of vision of 20 degrees or less.

Procedure for Measuring Acuity

The procedure for measuring acuity involves testing each eye individually. Vision can be tested with and without correction, at distance and at near. For most situations, the best corrected vision at distance is of primary importance. A near visual acuity is less reproducible, but should be used when circumstances prevent the determination of distance acuity (Fig. 2–27). If a child's corrective lenses are not available, a pinhole (abbreviated PH) can be used to try to ascertain the best possible acuity. Improvement of vision when looking through a pinhole is strongly suggestive that the reduction in acuity is secondary to a refractive error (need for glasses). Acuity is recorded in terms of the lowest line an individual can read. A plus or minus notation denotes that the patient recognized a certain number of letters on the next line, or missed a certain number of letters on the given line, respectively. The notations and abbreviations used to record visual acuity are listed in Table 2–6.

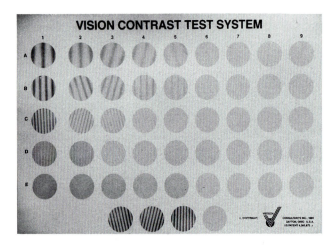

Figure 2–26. Contrast sensitivity chart.

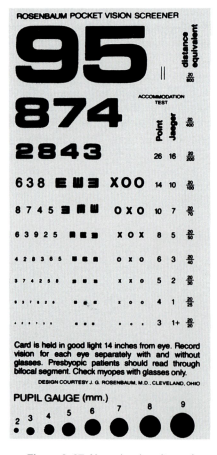

Figure 2–27. Near visual acuity card.

TABLE 2–6. NOTATIONS AND ABBREVIATIONS USED TO RECORD VISUAL ACUITY

V$_A$	=	visual acuity	RE =	right eye
c̄c	=	with correction	LE =	left eye
s̄c	=	without correction	OD =	oculus dexter: right eye
PH	=	acuity looking through a pinhole	OS =	oculus sinister: left eye
NI	=	no improvement	OU =	oculi uterque: both eyes
W	=	wears (spectacle correction)	D =	distance acuity
PC	=	present correction (spectacle)	N =	near acuity
J	=	Jaeger notation (near vision)	E =	E game
+	=	convex lens used to treat hyperopia	Pics =	Allen pictures
–	=	concave lens used to treat myopia	SPH =	spherical lens

- ***ACUITY NOTATIONS IN INFANTS***

F+F	=	fixate and follow
CSM	=	central, steady, maintained fixation
C(S)M	=	central, unsteady, maintained fixation (nystagmus)
CS(M)	=	central, steady, but not maintained fixation (amblyopia)
GCM	=	good, central, maintained fixation
G(C)M	=	eccentric but maintained fixation
GC(M)	=	good, central, but not maintained fixation (amblyopia)

- ***ACUITY NOTATIONS IN OLDER CHILDREN AND ADULTS***

20/50–1	=	missed one letter on 20/50 line	HM at 3′	=	hand motion at 3 feet
20/50+2	=	resolved 20/50 line and two letters on 20/40 line	LP	=	light perception
20/30 Pics	=	20/30 on Allen chart	NLP	=	no light perception
20/25 E	=	20/25 on E game	LP c̄ proj	=	light perception with projection
CF at 1′	=	count fingers at 1 foot			

- ***QUADRANTS***

ST	=	superotemporal
IT	=	inferotemporal
SN	=	superonasal
IN	=	inferonasal

- ***EXAMPLE***

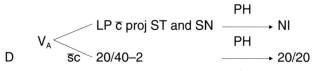

This indicates that without correction the distance vision in the right eye is light perception with projection in the superotemporal and superonasal quadrants. In the left eye the patient could read all but two letters on the distant 20/40 line. No improvement in vision of the right eye was obtained looking through a pinhole, but the vision in the left eye improved to 20/20.

From Catalano RA: Ocular emergencies. Philadelphia, Saunders, 1992, p 12, with permission.

Color Vision

Color vision is tested when the history, signs, or symptoms suggest an optic nerve or retinal abnormality. It should also be tested routinely for boys at the time of their preschool examination. Special pseudoisochromatic plates are available, including illiterate charts for children (Fig. 2–28), to test the ability to discriminate different hues. Different hues are juxtaposed on each plate in such a way that the normal eye recognizes a pattern or number. The absence of this recognition signifies a hereditary deficit or optic nerve or retinal abnormality. More detailed color vision tests are available for specialized testing.

THE EXTERNAL EXAMINATION

The orbit should be examined for proptosis (protrusion of an eye), enophthalmos (recession of an eye within the orbit), pulsations, or periorbital changes. An exophthalmometer (Fig. 2–29) is used to measure protrusion of the eyes. Measurements are made of the distance between the lateral orbital rim and the anterior surface of the eye. A difference between the eyes of 2 mm or more is considered abnormal. To ensure accurate serial measurements, the same base setting of the exophthalmometer should always be used for a given patient.

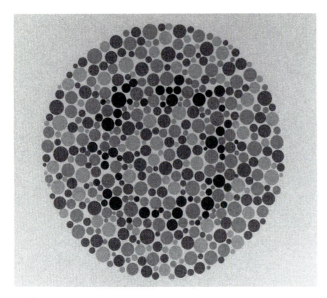

Figure 2–28. Color vision test plate.

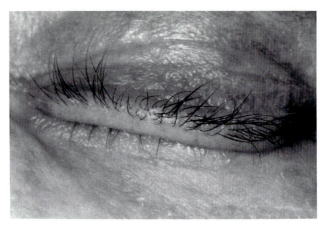

Figure 2–31. Distichiasis (an extra row of lashes in the upper eyelid). *(Courtesy of Dale R. Meyer.)*

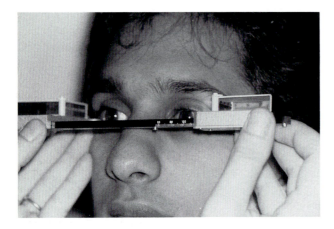

Figure 2–29. Hertel exophthalmometer.

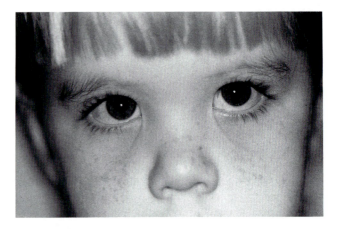

Figure 2–32. Prominent epicanthal folds covering the inner margin of each eyelid.

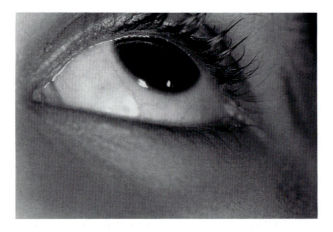

Figure 2–30. Entropion (inward turning of the lower eyelid).

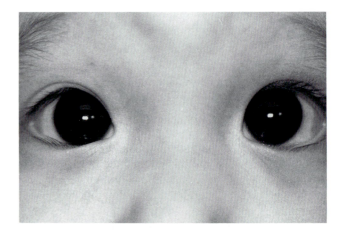

Figure 2–33. Bilateral epiblepharon. Note how the extra skin fold causes the eyelashes to be directed upward and inward.

Palpation of the orbit can detect masses, orbital rim fractures, and subcutaneous emphysema. Orbital rim fractures are suspected when "step-offs" or asymmetries of the bony orbits are found; orbital floor or medial wall fractures are suspected when subcutaneous emphysema (crepitus) is present. Palpation should be performed with the eyes open and gaze directed straight ahead. The anterior orbit is palpated with the examiner's fingers placed between the patient's eye and orbital rim. Pulsation of the globe is most apparent when observing the patient from a lateral position.

The **eyelids** are inspected for symmetry of position, function, apposition to the globe, and inflammation. Unilateral ptosis (drooping of the upper eyelid; see Fig. 2–7) is measured by the difference in size between the two palpebral fissures. Alternatively, it is recorded as the number of millimeters of corneal coverage by the eyelid. Levator function is measured by applying firm pressure to the brow (to prevent elevation of the eyelid by frontalis contraction) and measuring the difference in interpalpebral width between downward and upward gaze. A difference of 4 mm or less is considered poor function; an 8 mm or more increase is good function. The normal span is approximately 15 mm.

Additional eyelid malpositions include eyelid eversion (**ectropion**) and inturning (**entropion**; Fig. 2–30). **Trichiasis** is a condition in which the eyelashes are misdirected and rub against the cornea. It can cause symptoms of ocular irritation, foreign body sensation, tearing, and red eye. **Distichiasis** is a extra row of eyelashes, usually originating near the openings of the meibomian glands (Fig. 2–31). It is usually asymptomatic. **Epicanthus** is a skin fold that runs from the upper to the lower eyelid, covering the medial canthal angle. It is frequently present in infants and young children (Fig. 2–32). Because less sclera (white) is seen on the inside than the outside of the eye, epicanthal folds give a child the appearance of having crossed eyes (pseudoesotropia). **Epiblepharon** is a redundant fold of skin near the lid margin of the lower eyelid (Fig. 2–33). Like epicanthus, it can be prominent in infancy and regress during the first years of life. Occasionally, epiblepharon causes the medial eyelashes of the lower eyelid to turn in against the cornea, requiring surgical correction.

The **lacrimal system** is evaluated in children with obstruction, inflammation, or infection of the tear drainage system (Fig. 2–34). The different tests that can be performed are reviewed in Chapter 8.

PUPILLARY EXAMINATION

The **pupillary light reflex** describes constriction of the pupils to light. The **pupillary near reflex** describes constriction due to fixation of the eye on a near object. The latter reflex is associated with convergence and accommodation of the eyes. Pupillary responses should be evaluated in both bright and dim illumination, with the patient's gaze directed toward a distant object. Common abbreviations and notations to describe pupillary responses are listed in Table 2–7.

A **relative afferent pupillary defect (RAPD)** is characterized by bilateral pupillary dilation with continuous light stimulation to an affected eye. The "swinging flashlight test," used to detect RAPD, is performed in a dim room by alternately illuminating the eyes (Fig. 2–35). A penlight is directed obliquely in one

TABLE 2–7. NOTATIONS AND ABBREVIATIONS USED TO RECORD PUPILLARY RESPONSES

RRL	= round, reactive to light
RAPD	= relative afferent pupillary defect graded from 0 (no RAPD) to 4+ (brisk RAPD)
$4 \rightarrow 2$	= 4-mm wide pupils in dim illumination, constricting to 2 mm in bright illumination
0 to 4+	= briskness of light and near responses graded from 0 (no response) to 4+ (brisk)

▪ EXAMPLES

Pupils: $4 \rightarrow 2$ RRL $\bar{s}$ RAPD
  $5 \rightarrow 3$ RRL $\bar{c}$ RAPD

This indicates that the right pupil is 4 mm wide in dim illumination and constricts to 2 mm in bright illumination. It is also without an afferent pupillary defect. The left pupil is 5 mm wide in dim illumination, constricts to 3 mm, and has a relative afferent pupillary defect.

Pupils:

	Size	Light response	Near response	RAPD
	$4 \rightarrow 2$	4+	4+	0
	$5 \rightarrow 3$	3+	3+	2+
or:	4/5 → 2/3	4+/3+	4+/3+	0/2+

This further indicates that the right pupil responds more briskly by both the light and near reflex than the left pupil. This also grades the relative afferent pupillary defect in the left eye as 2+.

From Catalano RA: Ocular emergencies. Philadelphia, Saunders, 1992, p 17, with permission.

Figure 2–34. Congenital right nasolacrimal duct obstruction.

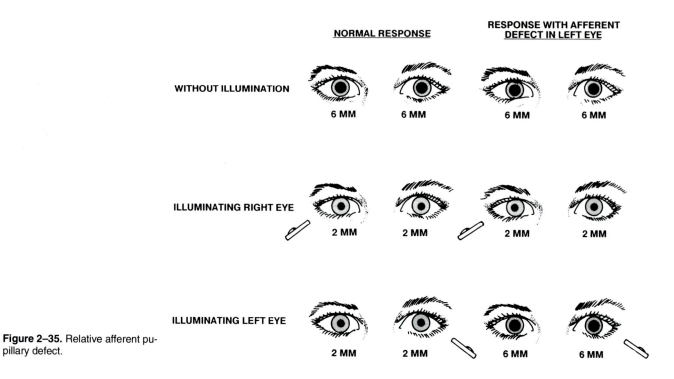

Figure 2–35. Relative afferent pupillary defect.

eye and then the other from below. Constriction of the iris in the illuminated eye is a "direct response." Constriction of the opposite iris is a "consensual response." In the absence of RAPD, pupillary constriction does not vary in either eye when they are alternately illuminated. With RAPD, however, both pupils constrict when light is directed into the unaffected eye, and dilate when directed into the affected eye.

The presence of RAPD is useful in localizing a defect in the visual pathway to anterior to the optic chiasm. It is also useful in determining whether a reduction in visual acuity is due to an optic nerve or a macular disorder. Subtle RAPD can occur with maculopathies, but no macular abnormality can account for a profound RAPD. Similarly, the presence of a cataract or a nontotal hyphema never explains a brisk RAPD. RAPD can be seen in an amblyopic eye even when the visual acuity is not markedly diminished; but similar to a maculopathy, RAPD in amblyopia is generally very subtle.

A **paradoxical pupillary reaction** is defined as pupillary dilation on exposure to light and constriction when the light is removed, or dilation with near vision and constriction with distance vision. It is best appreciated by shining a penlight obliquely on the pupils and then turning off the room lights. Constriction of the pupils, rather than dilation, is confirmatory. A paradoxical pupillary reaction is most frequently noted in patients with congenital stationary night blindness or congenital achromotopsia. The former is characterized by night blindness, decreased vision, and normal or only mildly abnormal color vision. Achromotopsia is characterized by a complete absence of color vision, vi-

sual acuity worse than 20/200, nystagmus (usually pendular), and photophobia. A normal fundus appearance, electroretinogram abnormalities, and lack of progression are characteristics of both. A paradoxical pupillary reaction can also occur with Leber's congenital amaurosis, dominant optic atrophy, and old bilateral optic neuritis. Rare associations include syphilis, tumors of the quadrigeminal region, and barbituate intoxication.

TABLE 2–8. CLASSIFICATION PARAMETERS OF STRABISMUS

Fusional status	Phoria: latent
	Tropia: manifest
	Intermittent: occasionally manifest
Direction of deviation	Horizontal: esodeviation, exodeviation
	Vertical: hyperdeviation, hypodeviation
	Torsional: incyclo- and excyclodeviation
Age of onset	Congenital: prior to 6 months of age
	Acquired: after 6 months of age
Fixation preference	Monocular: definite preference for one eye
	Alternating: no ocular preference
Variation with gaze position	Comitant: does not vary
	Incomitant: varies with direction of gaze
Distant and near fixation relationship	Normal AC/A: same deviation distant and near
	High AC/A: excessive convergence with accommodation
	Low AC/A: deficient convergence with accommodation

Modified from Nelson LB, Catalano RA: Atlas of ocular motility. Philadelphia, Saunders, 1989, p 87, with permission.

TESTS OF OCULAR ALIGNMENT

The direction of the visual axes is referred to as the ocular alignment. When there is no misalignment (the visual axes are parallel), the term orthophoria is used. A deviation is called **strabismus.**

Strabismus is always described with respect to the nonfixating eye. When the visual direction of the deviated eye is inward, the prefix "eso" is used; "exo" describes a divergent position. "Hyper" means that the deviated eye is turned upward, and "hypo" downward. In addition to the direction of misalignment, strabismus is also reported as either latent (phoria) or manifest (tropia). It is classified by the age of onset and the variation of deviation with fixation preference, gaze position, or fixation distance (Table 2–8).

Different tests are used to measure ocular misalignment. (Table 2–9 gives the different notations and abbreviations used to record ocular alignment.) The **Hirschberg corneal light reflex test** measures the devi-

ation based on the decentration of a light reflected on the cornea. A 1-mm decentration corresponds to approximately a 7-degree deviation of the visual axes (see above). Numerous potential pitfalls make this test, at best, crude. A more accurate measurement can be ob-

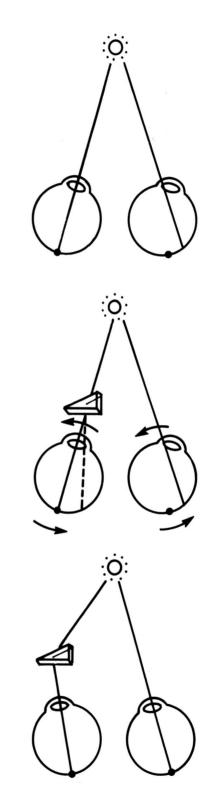

Figure 2–36. The Krimsky test. See text for description. *(From Nelson LB, Catalano RA: Atlas of Ocular Motility. Philadelphia, Saunders, 1989, p 101, with permission.)*

TABLE 2–9. NOTATIONS AND ABBREVIATIONS USED TO RECORD OCULAR ALIGNMENT AND MOTILITY

- **EXTRAOCULAR MUSCLES**

EOM = extraocular movements

RSR	= right superior rectus	LSR	= left superior rectus
RLR	= right lateral rectus	LLR	= left lateral rectus
RIR	= right inferior rectus	LIR	= left inferior rectus
RMR	= right medial rectus	LMR	= left medial rectus
RSO	= right superior oblique	LSO	= left superior oblique
RIO	= right inferior oblique	LIO	= left inferior oblique

- **OCULAR ALIGNMENT**

E	= esophoria	ET	= esotropia
X	= exophoria	XT	= exotropia
DVD	= dissociated vertical deviation	HT	= hypertropia

E(T), X(T) = intermittent esotropia, exotropia
E′, X′, ET′, XT′, E(T)′, X(T)′ = at near fixation
EX = EX′ = 0 : no ocular misalignment
Ortho = orthophoria (no ocular misalignment)

- **OCULAR MEASUREMENTS**

PD   = Δ = prism diopters
°   = degrees
K   = Krimsky test (given in prism diopters)
H   = Hirschberg test (given in degrees)
ROTS = ocular rotations, usually graded from 4– (maximum underaction) to 4+ (maximum overaction)
        OA = overaction of a muscle
        UA = underaction of a muscle

A	= accommodation	AC/A	= accommodative convergence to accommodation ratio
AC	= accommodative convergence		
NPA	= near point of accommodation	NPC	= near point of convergence

From Catalano RA: Ocular emergencies. Philadelphia, Saunders, 1992, p 21, with permission.

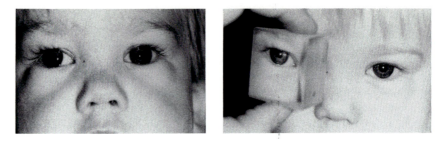

Figure 2–37. Krimsky test being used in a child with exotropia.

tained if prisms are used to align the corneal reflexes (the **Krimsky test**). The optical basis of this test, in a patient with an outwardly deviated eye, is depicted in Figure 2–36. If a base-in prism is placed in front of the fixating eye, the image of the light in this eye will be shifted nasally. The eye will turn out to regain fixation. By Hering's law, the deviating eye makes a simultaneous and equal movement inward. Larger and larger prisms are introduced in front of the fixating eye until the corneal light reflex is centered on the devi-

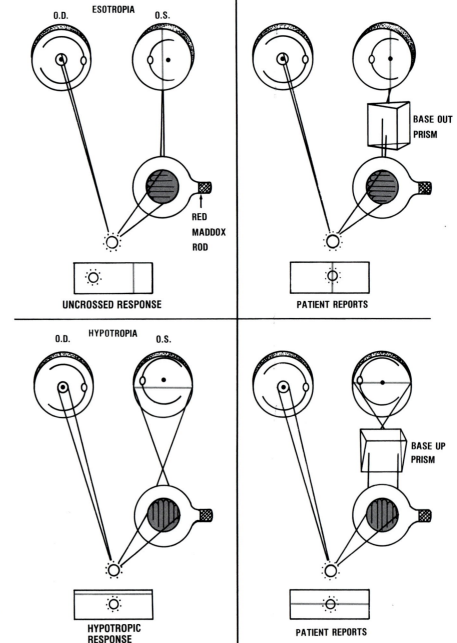

Figure 2–38. The single Maddox rod test. See text for description. *(From Nelson LB, Catalano RA: Atlas of Ocular Motility. Philadelphia, Saunders, 1989, p 111, with permission.)*

ating eye. To perform the test, the examiner should be seated directly in front of the deviating eye, to avoid a parallax error in the estimation. The deviation is recorded in prism diopters corresponding to the prism power needed to center the corneal light reflex in the deviating eye (Fig. 2–37).

The most accurate measurements of ocular deviation, however, use prisms in association with the covering of one eye (**cover tests**). There are three types of cover tests: the cover/uncover test, alternate cover test, and simultaneous prism cover test.

The monocular cover/uncover test is useful in diagnosing and differentiating between phorias and tropias. If movement occurs behind the covered eye, a phoria is present. With phorias, the eyes are straight both before and after the cover/uncover test. Only when sensory fusion is interrupted does the occluded eye deviate. On first placing the occluder and interrupting fusion, the phoric eye drifts; a refixation movement in the opposite direction occurs when the cover is removed (see Fig. 2–11). With tropias, however, one eye is already deviated prior to the test, and either the same eye (monocular strabismus) or the opposite eye (alternate strabismus) is deviated at the end of the test (see Fig. 2–12). If the patient has a nonalternating or monocular tropia, the deviation can be quantitated by introducing larger and larger prisms in front of the deviating eye until no refixation movement occurs on covering the initially fixating eye.

In the alternate cover (prism and cover) test, the cover is placed alternately in front of each eye, switching approximately every 2 seconds, to completely dissociate the eyes. Because simultaneous fixation by both eyes is not permitted, sensory fusion is eliminated, and any phoric component to the deviation is added to the tropic component. The total deviation, both latent and manifest, is obtained. Once the eyes are completely dissociated and the total deviation is manifest, larger and larger prisms are placed in front of one eye until no movement occurs as the cover is alternated from one eye to the other. The prism power necessary to completely eliminate any refixation movement by the nonoccluded eye is the amount of total deviation.

The simultaneous prism and cover test allows the examiner to quantitate the tropic component of a deviation that has a superimposed phoric component. This test does not dissociate the eyes; it allows sensory fusion to keep in abeyance the phoric component. The test is performed by simultaneously introducing a prism in front of the deviating eye and an occluder in front of the fixating eye. If movement occurs in the eye behind the prism, the end point has not been reached. Both cover and prism are removed, and larger prisms are chosen until no shift occurs in the deviated eye. The tropic component of the deviation is thus quantitated because sensory fusion is allowed at all times just prior to introducing the prism and cover.

Other Tests of Ocular Alignment

In addition to cover tests, other tests are available to quantitate ocular deviations. **Dissimilar image tests** create different images for the two eyes, which the examiner superimposes for the patient by using prisms. Examples include the red lens test and the single Maddox rod test. The red lens test requires the patient to view a penlight while a red lens is placed in front of the fixating eye. The fixating eye sees a red light, and the deviating eye a white light. The Maddox rod test uses a red Maddox rod instead of a red lens, and creates a line image in the fixating eye. With the red lens test, the patient is asked whether the two lights are superimposed. With the Maddox rod test, the patient is asked whether the line bisects the light (Fig. 2–38). If the answer to either question is no, prisms are used to align the images. Both tests are especially useful in detecting any incomitance in a deviation. As the eyes are rotated into different positions of gaze, the patient is asked to identify where the image separation becomes greater. Paresis or restriction of a specific extraocular muscle is identified if the separation is greater in the direction of action of the muscle. These tests are particularly useful in the work-up of diplopia (see Chapter 13).

Dissimilar target tests present different targets to the two eyes that the patient is asked to superimpose. The most frequently used dissimilar target tests are the major amblyoscope and Lee's, Hess's, and Lancaster's screen tests. Each of these tests requires specific equipment; they are useful, however, in determining the position of gaze in which the maximum deviation occurs.

The major amblyoscope (Fig. 2–39) presents separate test objects to each fovea, such as a bird and a cage (Fig. 2–40). The patient is asked to indicate when they are superimposed (the bird is inside the cage) as the examiner adjusts the arms of the instrument. Horizontal, vertical, and cyclorotational adjustments are possible;

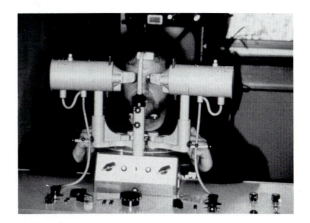

Figure 2–39. The major amblyoscope. *(From Nelson LB, Catalano RA: Atlas of Ocular Motility. Philadelphia, Saunders, 1989, p 81, with permission.)*

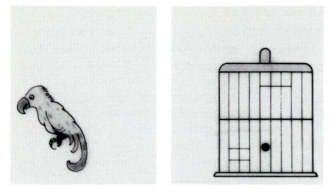

Figure 2–40. Test objects for the major amblyoscope. *(From Nelson LB, Catalano RA: Atlas of Ocular Motility. Philadelphia, Saunders, 1989, p 81, with permission.)*

the amounts of all of these rotations are read from graduated scales on the machine.

In each of the screen tests, the examiner projects or indicates a spot on a ruled screen that only one eye of the patient can see. The patient is then asked to project or indicate where a target seen by the other eye would lie if it were to superimpose the target of the first eye (Fig. 2–41). By repeating this in every position of gaze, the gaze position of maximum deviation can be identified. The results are recorded on miniaturized charts that replicate the screen, which are designed to identify an abnormally acting extraocular muscle (Fig. 2–42).

TESTS OF OCULAR MOTILITY

There are six extraocular muscles, which are named according to their location and the direction they traverse to insert on the globe (Figs. 2–43 and 2–44). Table 2–9

gives the different notations and abbreviations used to record ocular motility.

For each muscle, there is a singular position of the eye for which it acts as the primary mover (Fig. 2–45). The six positions corresponding to the six muscles are called the **cardinal positions of gaze.** In testing **ocular rotations,** the strength of each muscle is checked individually by sequentially rotating the eye through the cardinal positions. The reduced ability of an eye to rotate into a specific gaze suggests a congenital strabismus syndrome, a cranial nerve palsy, or an extraocular muscle restriction.

Ductions describe monocular movements. Adduction is movement of the eye nasally; abduction is a temporal movement. Versions and vergences describe binocular movements. **Versions** are movements of the two eyes in the same direction, at the same time, and of approximately the same magnitude. Versions are also called conjugate movements. Dextroversion describes movement of both eyes to the right; levoversion to the left. **Vergences** are binocular movements in which the eyes move in opposite directions, or disjugately. Convergence indicates that both eyes are rotated nasally; divergence indicates temporal rotation. Torsional movements are described as "cyclo" rotations (cyclovergences and cycloversions).

Oculocephalic (doll's-head) testing and **caloric testing** are used in patients with gaze palsies to determine if the palsy is of supranuclear origin. Both tests rely on the vestibular system's ability to drive the eyes in a particular direction. The doll's-head test is performed in conscious patients. While the patient fixates an object, the examiner rotates the patient's head horizontally or vertically. Caloric testing is performed on unconscious patients and those with potential neck in-

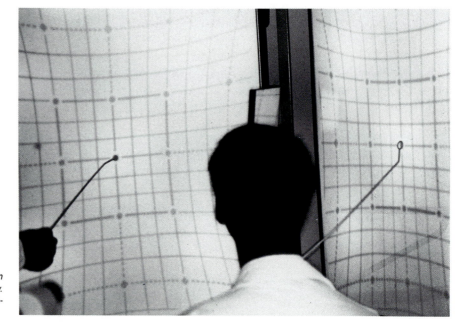

Figure 2–41. The Hess screen test. *(From Nelson LB, Catalano RA: Atlas of Ocular Motility. Philadelphia, Saunders, 1989, p 117, with permission.)*

DIAGNOSIS:
Weakness of left inferior rectus muscle No. # 1

Left Eye *picture c OD fixating*   Right Eye *picture c OS fixating*

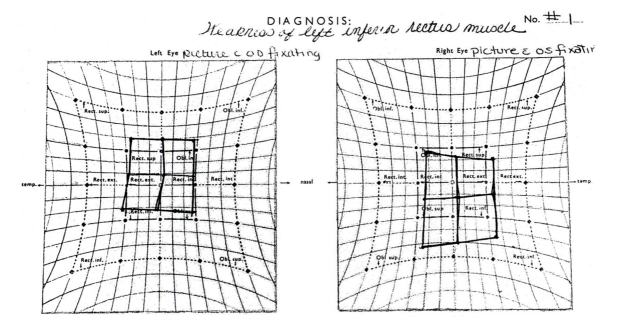

Figure 2–42. Recording of the Hess screen test. *(From Nelson LB, Catalano RA: Atlas of Ocular Motility. Philadelphia, Saunders, 1989, p 117, with permission.)*

juries. Cold or warm water is irrigated in an ear canal with the patient's head elevated 30 degrees above the horizontal. Cold water irrigation produces a nystagmus with the fast phase in the opposite direction of the irrigated ear; hot water produces the opposite (the fast phase is ipsilateral). The mnemonic COWS can be used to remember the direction of the fast phase (cold, opposite; warm, same). Bilateral cold water irrigation produces a nystagmus with the fast phase up; bilateral warm irrigation produces the opposite. If the eyes can be made to deviate in the direction of a gaze palsy, the disorder is of supranuclear origin (above the cranial nerve nucleus to extraocular muscle pathway).

Forced duction testing is used when an infranuclear gaze palsy exists, to differentiate a neurogenic from a restrictive ocular motor disorder. The test is performed by grasping the conjunctiva and episclera near the limbus with two forceps held 180 degrees apart (Fig. 2–46). The eye is moved into positions suspected of being restricted as a result of mechanical factors. Any resistance to passive movement is considered a positive result. In children, the test is performed under general anesthesia. Care is taken to not press the globe into the orbit, as this can give a false-negative result in the face of true restriction.

THREE-STEP TEST TO DIAGNOSE CYCLOVERTICAL MUSCLE PALSIES*

Patients with an acute palsy of one of the eight cyclovertical muscles will manifest a hypertropia. Parks (1958) described a method, based on Hofmann

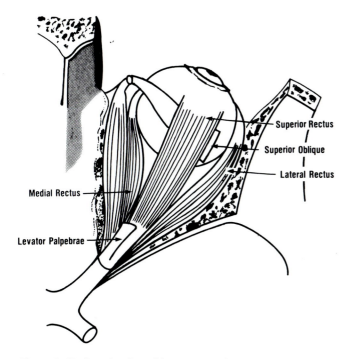

Figure 2–43. Superior view of the eye. *(From Nelson LB, Catalano RA: Atlas of Ocular Motility. Philadelphia, Saunders, 1989, p 3, with permission.)*

Superior Rectus
Superior Oblique
Lateral Rectus
Medial Rectus
Levator Palpebrae

*Reprinted from Nelson LB, Catalano RA: Atlas of ocular motility. Philadelphia, Saunders, 1989, pp 122–125, with permission.

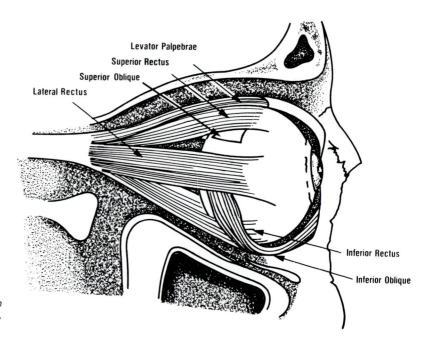

Figure 2–44. Lateral view of the eye. *(From Nelson LB, Catalano RA: Atlas of Ocular Motility. Philadelphia, Saunders, 1989, p 3, with permission.)*

and Bielschowsky's head tilt test of 1900, that uses three steps to identify which of the eight cyclovertical muscles is paretic in patients with an isolated, acute cyclovertical muscle palsy. This test is useful only if the following three conditions are met: the muscle involved is paretic, it is the only paretic muscle, and it is one of the muscles that have cyclovertical action. This test is not useful when more than one muscle is palsied, or when a restrictive disorder is present. The three-step test cannot be used to isolate paretic horizontally acting muscles.

Each step in the three-step test progressively halves the possible choices, so that at the end of the third step, only one muscle remains, which must be the paretic muscle. The first step reduces the possible choices from eight to four muscles simply by looking at which eye is higher. The second step reduces the possible choices to two by determining whether the deviation is worse in right or in left gaze. The second step is based on the fact that different muscles act in right and left gaze. The third step identifies the one paretic muscle. This step uses the utricular response that occurs on tilting the head (Fig. 2–47). This otolith response serves to keep the eyes vertically and cyclotorsionally aligned by rotating or torting the eyes in a direction opposite the head rotation. If the head is tilted to the right, the utricular reflex stimulates the right superior oblique and right superior rectus muscles to rotate the right eye in-

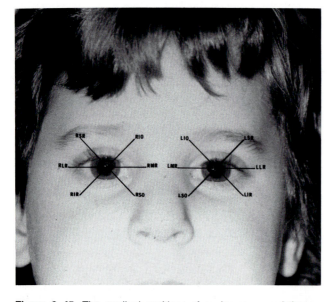

Figure 2–45. The cardinal positions of ocular gaze, and the extraocular muscle that acts in that position of gaze. (For abbreviations see Table 2–9.) *(From Nelson LB, Catalano RA: Atlas of Ocular Motility. Philadelphia, Saunders, 1989, p 25, with permission.)*

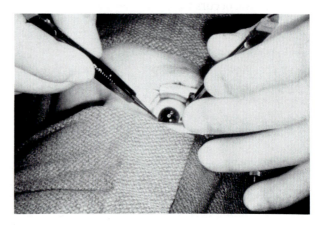

Figure 2–46. Forced duction testing.

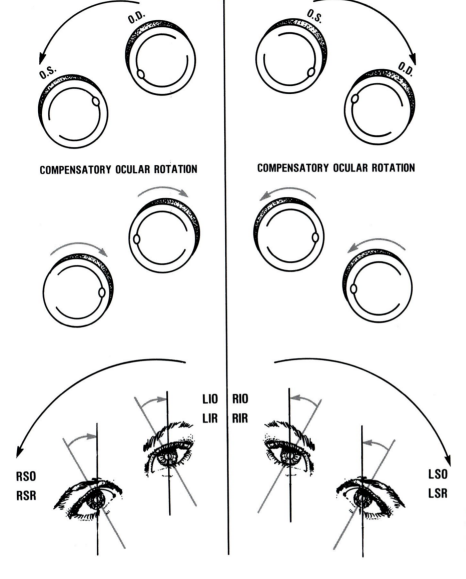

RIGHT HEAD TILT

O.D.

O.S.

COMPENSATORY OCULAR ROTATION

LEFT HEAD TILT

O.S.

O.D.

COMPENSATORY OCULAR ROTATION

LIO RIO
LIR RIR

RSO
RSR

LSO
LSR

Figure 2–47. Ocular movements upon tilting the head. *(From Nelson LB, Catalano RA: Atlas of Ocular Motility. Philadelphia, Saunders, 1989, p 123, with permission.)*

ward. The corresponding movement of the left eye is an outward rotation brought about by contracture of the left inferior oblique and left inferior rectus muscles. The opposite occurs with a left head tilt. In this manner the eyes remain vertically and cyclotorsionally aligned when the head is tilted.

Figure 2–48 demonstrates the three-step test for a patient with a right hypertropia. In the figure, below each set of eyes is a listing of the four cyclovertical muscles of each eye in an order that corresponds to the position of gaze for which each muscle acts as the prime mover of the eye. For instance, the elevators of the eye are the superior rectus and inferior oblique muscles. They are listed above the inferior rectus and superior oblique, which are depressors of the eye. The vertical rectus muscles are the prime movers in the abducted position, and the oblique muscles act when the eye is adducted. The rectus muscles are therefore listed

on the outside, and the oblique muscles are listed on the inside. Use of this notation to record the responses on the three-step test helps to isolate the one paretic muscle.

Three-step Test of Right Hypertropia

Step I

Refer to Figure 2–48. The first step involves determining which eye is higher. In this instance, the right eye is higher than the left. This means that the paretic muscle must be one that either depresses the right eye or elevates the left eye. Of the eight cyclovertical muscles, the muscles that depress the right eye are the right inferior rectus (RIR) and right superior oblique (RSO). The muscles that elevate the left eye are the left inferior oblique (LIO) and left superior rectus (LSR). One of

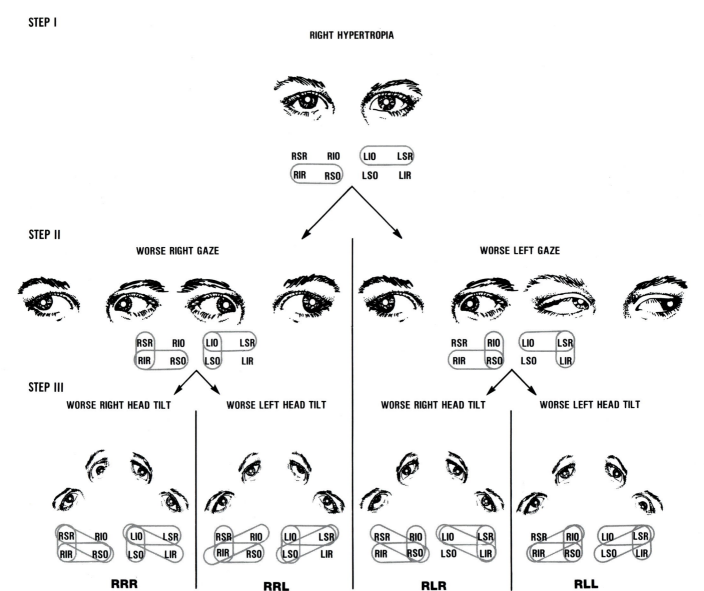

Figure 2–48. Three-step test for right hypertropia. *(From Nelson LB, Catalano RA: Atlas of Ocular Motility. Philadelphia, Saunders, 1989, p 125, with permission.)*

these four muscles must be paretic if the right eye is higher than the left eye. These muscles are circled on the diagram. This step reduces the possible paretic muscles from eight to four.

Step II
The second step determines whether the vertical deviation is greater in right or left gaze. If the deviation is worse in right gaze (Fig. 2–48, left), the paretic muscle must be one of the four that is used in right gaze. In the right eye these are the right superior rectus (RSR) and the RIR. For the left eye, the muscles that act in right gaze are the LIO and left superior oblique (LSO). These muscles are circled on the diagram. The same can be done if the deviation is worse in left gaze (Fig. 2–48, right). At the end of the second step, for any possible paresis, only two muscles have been circled twice, re-

ducing the possible choices for the paretic muscle from four to two.

Step III
The third step of the three-step test determines whether the vertical deviation is worse on right or left head tilt. As shown in Figure 2–47, on right head tilt the RSR and RSO contract to rotate the right eye inward, and the LIO and left inferior rectus (LIR) contract to rotate the left eye outward. On left head tilt the stimulated muscles are the RIR and RIO to rotate the right eye outward, and the LSR and LSO to rotate the left eye inward. Depending on whether the vertical misalignment is worse on right or left head tilt, the muscles that are used respectively are circled on the diagram. For every possibility only one muscle is circled three times. This muscle is the isolated paretic muscle. Below each

diagram are the abbreviated results. For example, a left inferior oblique palsy is present when a *Right* hypertropia is worse on *Right* gaze and *Right* head tilt (RRR).

A similar analysis can be performed for a patient with a left hypertropia. A patient with a left hypertropia worse on right gaze and right head tilt has a paretic RSR muscle. If the deviation is worse on right gaze and left head tilt, the LSO muscle is paretic. For patients with a left hypertropia worse on left gaze and right head tilt, the LIR is paretic. If it is worse on left gaze and left head tilt, the RIO must be paretic.

VISUAL FIELD EXAMINATION

Multiple tests are available to assess the field of vision. The majority of these are used to detect or monitor glaucoma, and are beyond the capabilities of young children. Examples include the Goldmann perimeter test and various automated visual field analyzers. In older children, a gross evaluation of the visual field can be accomplished via confrontational field testing.

Confrontational visual field testing requires only that the examiner have a normal visual field. Several different steps are useful in obtaining the maximum information. The examiner faces the patient from about 20 inches (50 cm) away and closes one eye; the facing eye of the patient is similarly occluded by paper tape or the patient's hand. Each individual fixates the other's nose. The patient is asked to count the number of fingers presented in the superior and inferior zones temporally and nasally. If the patient is successful, the examiner then presents fingers in more than one field. The ability to discern hand motion is used for patients unable to count fingers.

ANTERIOR SEGMENT EXAMINATION

The anterior segment examination is conducted using a slit lamp. A slit lamp is a binocular microscope positioned vertically on an adjustable table for examination of the eye (Fig. 2–49). The combination of superb illumination, magnification, and a stereoscopic view have made it the instrument of choice for examination of the anterior eye. Its name is derived from a special feature of the illumination system that projects the light beam as a slit, which can be varied in width, height, and angle of projection. Magnification is that of a simple microscope, with the optics designed such that the image is direct and virtual. Stereopsis is the appreciation of seeing an object in depth; it is achieved by viewing the object slightly disparately with each eye.

The slit lamp is used to detect inflammatory and red blood cells, or proteinaceous material (flare) in the anterior chamber of the eye. These are visualized by using a small, narrow slit of light, or a small cylindrical

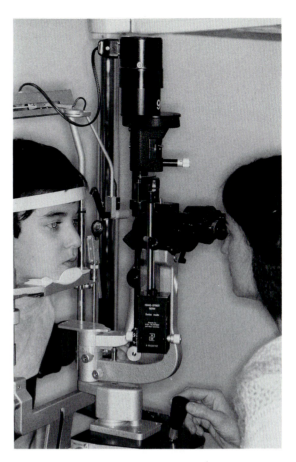

Figure 2–49. Slit-lamp examination.

dot of light in a darkened room. Two techniques are helpful in visualizing cells. The first involves keeping the illumination and observation arms steady and waiting for cells to pass through the light beam due to natural convection currents in the aqueous (cells will be illuminated as they pass through the light beam). The second technique involves gently oscillating the illumination beam from side to side while the observation arm is held steady. The slit lamp is also used to examine the iris for transillumination defects (Fig. 2–50). This is accomplished by directing the light beam indirectly into the pupil, and reflecting the light off the ocular lens (retroillumination).

Gonioscopy is a technique for examination of the anterior chamber angle. Because the opaque sclera and corneal limbus prevent direct inspection of this area, one of several different lenses is used to visualize the angle. Each lens has its own advantages. The Zeiss goniolens (Fig. 2–51) can be placed comfortably on the eye without the need for a gel-coupling medium. Zeiss lens gonioscopy places only minimum pressure on the eye and does not distort the cornea. Goldmann three-mirror gonioscopy requires a coupling agent, but has the advantage of also providing visualization of the peripheral and posterior retina (Fig. 2–20). Koeppe lens gonioscopy is performed with the patient in the recum-

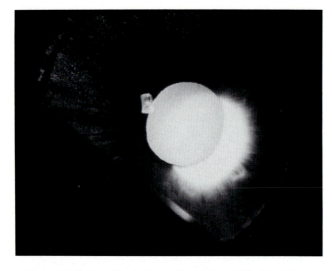

Figure 2–50. Transillumination of the iris in a child with albinism.

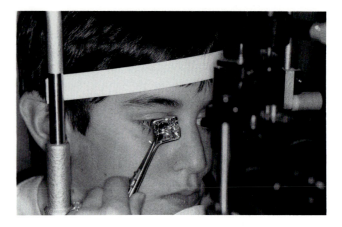

Figure 2–51. Zeiss lens gonioscopy.

bent position, without the use of a slit lamp. A dome-shaped Koeppe lens is placed on the eye, and the anterior chamber is visualized using a hand-held Barkan light and a binocular scope. Its advantage is that a lens can be placed on each eye, and rapid comparisons can be made between the two eyes. A Barkan lens is used in the performance of a goniotomy (Fig. 2–52).

The different notations and abbreviations used to record findings on the anterior segment examination are given in Table 2–10.

MEASUREMENT OF INTRAOCULAR PRESSURE (TONOMETRY)

A tonometer is an instrument used to measure intraocular pressure (IOP). Schiotz tonometry is based on indentation of the globe. A scale on the tonometer measures the amount of indentation for a given weight of the plunger (see Fig. 10–19). Charts are available for converting these scale readings to intraocular pressures based on the weight of the plunger (Table 2–11). The advantage of Schiotz tonometry is that it can be performed with minimal training and instrumentation. The patient should be recumbent and a topical anesthetic must be used. Care must be exercised not to apply pressure on the globe when spreading the eyelids, and to maintain a vertical alignment of the instrument.

Applanation tonometers do not indent the globe; rather, they measure the force necessary to flatten a given area (3.06 mm) of the cornea. The Goldmann applanation tonometer is standard equipment on both the Haag-Streit and Zeiss slit lamp (Fig. 2–53). It has the advantage of being less affected by gravity or scleral rigidity than the Schiotz tonometer. In cooperative infants, applanation tonometry can be performed with a hand-held Perkin's tonometer (Fig. 2–54). The proce-

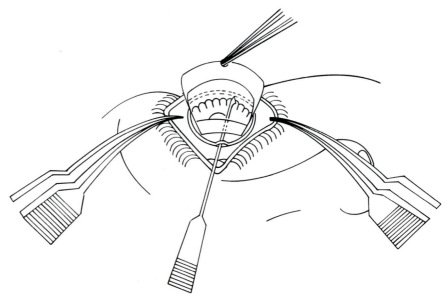

Figure 2–52. The performance of a goniotomy, demonstrating the view of the anterior chamber angle afforded by a Barkan lens.

TABLE 2–10. NOTATIONS AND ABBREVIATIONS USED TO RECORD FINDINGS ON THE ANTERIOR SEGMENT EXAMINATION

C,C,S	= cornea, conjunctiva, and sclera
AC	= anterior chamber
D + C	= deep and clear
Cells	= presence of red or white blood cells in the anterior chamber of the eye; graded on a scale of 0 to 4+
Flare	= presence of proteinaceous material in the anterior chamber
K	= keratometer reading (refractive power in the cornea)
KP	= keratic precipitates (accumulations of inflammatory cells on the posterior (endothelial) surface of the cornea
Hyphema	= layering of red blood cells in the anterior chamber (eight ball = complete filling of anterior chamber)
Hypopyon	= layering of inflammatory cells in the anterior chamber

From Catalano RA: Ocular emergencies. Philadelphia, Saunders, 1992, p 32, with permission.

TABLE 2–11. INTRAOCULAR PRESSURE (mm Hg) BY SCHIOTZ TONOMETRY

Tonometer Scale Reading	Plunger Weight (g)			
	5.5	7.5	10.0	15.0
0.0	41.4	59.1	81.7	127.5
0.5	37.8	54.2	75.1	117.9
1.0	34.5	49.8	69.3	109.3
1.5	31.6	45.8	64.0	101.4
2.0	29.0	42.1	59.1	94.3
2.5	26.6	38.8	54.7	88.0
3.0	24.4	35.8	50.6	81.8
3.5	22.4	33.0	46.9	76.2
4.0	20.6	30.4	43.4	71.0
4.5	18.9	28.0	40.2	66.2
5.0	17.3	25.8	37.2	61.8
5.5	15.9	23.8	34.4	57.6
6.0	14.6	21.9	31.8	53.6
6.5	13.4	20.1	29.4	49.9
7.0	12.2	18.5	27.2	46.5
7.5	11.2	17.0	25.1	43.2
8.0	10.2	15.6	23.1	40.2
8.5	9.4	14.3	21.3	38.1
9.0	8.5	13.1	19.6	34.6
9.5	7.8	12.0	18.0	32.0
10.0	7.1	10.9	16.5	29.6
10.5	6.5	10.0	15.1	27.4
11.0	5.9	9.1	13.8	25.3
11.5	5.3	8.3	12.6	23.3
12.0	4.9	7.5	11.5	21.4
12.5	4.4	6.8	10.5	19.7
13.0	4.0	6.2	9.5	18.1
13.5		5.6	8.6	16.5
14.0		5.0	7.8	15.1
14.5		4.5	7.1	13.7
15.0		4.1	6.4	12.6
15.5			5.8	11.4
16.0			5.2	10.4
16.5			4.7	9.4
17.0			4.2	8.5
17.5				7.7
18.0				6.9
18.5				6.2
19.0				5.6
19.5				4.9
20.0				4.5

From Catalano RA: Ocular emergencies. Philadelphia, Saunders, 1992, p 34, with permission.

dure for either involves instilling a topical anesthetic and fluorescein dye into the eye, and directing maximum illumination to the tonometer head. A prism incorporated within the head divides the produced image of a ring into an upper and lower half. The semicircles of the ring are aligned by adjusting a knob on the tonometer. This increases or decreases the force applied by the tonometer. The intraocular pressure in mm Hg is read from a scale on the tonometer when the inner margins of the two semicircles are juxtaposed (Fig. 2–55).

Digital tonometry is crude, but can give an approximation of intraocular pressure when the above instrumentation is unavailable. The technique simply involves palpating (ballotting) the globe with the eyelids closed. The patient should be looking down, and the examiner should use two fingers placed between the globe and superior orbit. A small amount of sponginess to the globe is normal. Firmness to the degree that indentation cannot be easily performed is consistent with elevated intraocular pressure. Molding of the

globe to the indenting finger, and movement of the internal structures of the eye, is consistent with a soft (hypotonic) eye.

The different notations and abbreviations used to record findings on tonometry are given in Table 2–12.

MEASUREMENT OF REFRACTIVE ERRORS

A refractive error refers to a mismatch in the focusing power and length of the eye. Nearsightedness, farsightedness, and astigmatism each describe specific refractive errors (see Chapter 5). An individual's refractive status can be determined objectively with minimal

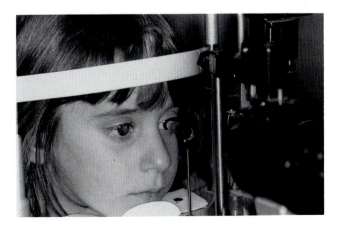

Figure 2–53. Applanation tonometry with a Goldmann tonometer at the slit lamp.

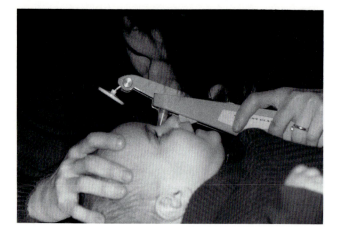

Figure 2–54. Applanation tonometry with a Perkin's tonometer in a cooperative infant.

TABLE 2–12. NOTATIONS AND ABBREVIATIONS USED TO RECORD FINDINGS ON TONOMETRY

T	=	tonometry
T$_{AP}$	=	applanation tonometry
T$_{SCH 5.5}$	=	Schiotz tonometry with a 5.5-g weight
FT	=	finger tension
TT	=	tactile tension (same as above)
IOP	=	intraocular pressure

▪ **EXAMPLE**

T$_{AP}$ ⟨ 12 / 13   Indicates that the intraocular pressure in the right eye measured by applanation tonometry was 12 mm Hg; in the left eye it was 13 mm Hg

Modified from Catalano RA: Ocular emergencies. Philadelphia, Saunders, 1992, p 36, with permission.

patient cooperation by streak retinoscopy. The streak retinoscope projects light into a patient's eye and illuminates an area of the retina. This light is reflected back in the patient's pupil as a red-orange band (reflex) with a slight shadow around it. If the child is hyperopic, the band moves with the movement of the retinoscope. If the child is myopic, the movement of the examiner's retinoscope creates a reflex light movement in the opposite direction. Lenses are interposed in the path of light to neutralize the refractive error (plus lenses for hyperopia, minus lenses for myopia). At the neutralization point of retinoscopy, the reflex appears as an on-off flash rather than a band of light.

Objective refraction by retinoscopy is the most useful method of detecting refractive errors in infants and developmentally delayed children. Automated refracting instruments (which use electronics and microcomputers) can be used with older, cooperative children (Fig. 2–56).

The refraction in older children can also be measured subjectively. A trial of various lenses, either loosely placed in a trial frame or within a phoropter (Fig. 2–57), is placed in front of the eyes. The refractive error is determined based on the child's responses to changes in the lenses.

Cycloplegics and Mydriatics

An individual's refractive error is neutralized for the resting state of the eye, focused at an infinite distance. Errors in the measurement can occur if the eye is fixating on a near object. Near fixation results in a change in the shape of the ocular lens to increase the power of the eye (accommodation). This introduces minus error into the refraction. To avoid this possibility, topical eyedrops that relax accommodation (cycloplegics) can be used during refraction. This is particularly indicated in infants and toddlers, children with a limited attention span, and farsighted patients. Retinoscopy and ophthalmoscopy are also facilitated by the use of mydriatic eyedrops, which dilate the pupil.

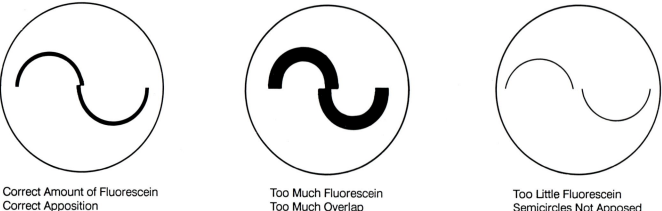

Correct Amount of Fluorescein
Correct Apposition

Too Much Fluorescein
Too Much Overlap

Too Little Fluorescein
Semicircles Not Apposed

Figure 2–55. Proper positioning of the semicircles for the measurement of intraocular pressure by applanation tonometry. *(From Catalano RA: Ocular Emergencies. Philadelphia, Saunders, 1992, p 35, with permission.)*

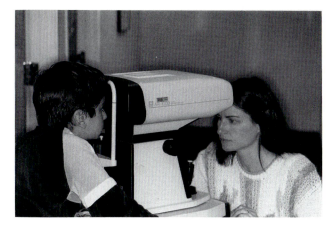

Figure 2–56. Automated refracting instrument.

TABLE 2–13. NOTATIONS AND ABBREVIATIONS USED TO RECORD FINDINGS ON FUNDUS EXAMINATION

D	= optic disc	C/D	= cup to disc ratio	HE	= hard exudate
M	= macula	DD	= disc diameters	SE	= soft exudate
V	= vessels	F	= fundus		

From Catalano RA: Ocular emergencies. Philadelphia, Saunders, 1992, p 40, with permission.

FUNDUS EXAMINATION

The method of direct ophthalmoscopy is described above. Indirect ophthalmoscopy is performed using a 14, 20, or 30-diopter lens. These give 4, 3, and 2X magnification, respectively, compared to the direct ophthalmoscope, which gives 15X magnification. The 20-diopter lens is most commonly used. It should be held with the convex side facing the observer; in the proper position, the two light reflexes formed on it are of the same size. Scleral depression is performed by indenting the posterior globe with a hand-held or thimble-like depressor. The patient is asked to look opposite the area to be examined as the depressor is situated on the eyelid over the area to be depressed. Placing the depressor above the tarsal plate of the eyelid reduces discomfort. The patient is then asked to look toward the depressor, as the globe is gently indented.

The optic disc is approximately 1.5 mm in diameter. Other structures in the fundus are often measured in terms of disc diameters (DD). The normal disc is pink in color with the exception of the physiologic cup, which appears as a white depression in the center of the disc. The cup-to-disc ratio refers to the relative size of the horizontal diameter of the cup to the disc diameter, and is given in terms of the nearest tenth (e.g., 0.1, 0.2). Other notations and abbreviations used to record findings on the fundus examination are given in Table 2–13.

For neonates, adequate cycloplegia and mydriasis without significant systemic side effects can be achieved by use of a solution containing cyclopentolate 0.5%, mydriacyl 1%, and phenylephrine 2.5%. Mydriasis occurs after 30 to 60 minutes. In very-low-birthweight infants, phenylephrine should be deleted from the solution. If adequate mydriasis is not achieved, a second instillation of drops may be necessary.

For children over one year of age, one instillation each of cyclopentolate 1% and phenylephrine 2.5% can be used to achieve adequate pupillary dilation and cycloplegia. Blacks and other darkly pigmented children may require a second instillation 5 to 10 minutes after the first to obtain a good effect. Maximum dilation occurs about 45 minutes after the initial instillation.

REFERENCES

American Academy of Ophthalmology. Preferred Practice Pattern: Comprehensive Pediatric Eye Evaluation. San Francisco, American Academy of Ophthalmology, 1992.

American Academy of Ophthalmology. Policy Statement: Infant and Children's Vision Screening. San Francisco, American Academy of Ophthalmology, 1991.

Catalano RA: Ocular Emergencies. Philadelphia, Saunders, 1992, pp 3–42, 91–96.

Freeman HM: Examination of the traumatized eye. In Miller D, Stegman R (eds): Treatment of Anterior Segment Ocular Trauma. Montreal, Medicopea, 1986, pp 95–119.

Friendly D: Examination techniques in pediatric ophthalmology. In Metz HS, Rosenbaum AL (eds): Pediatric Ophthalmology. New York, Medical Examination Publishing Co, 1982.

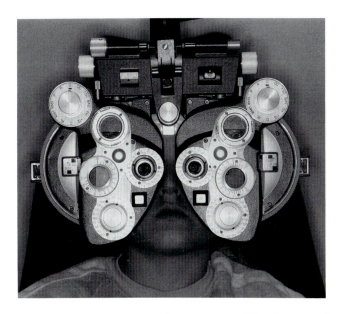

Figure 2–57. A phoropter, an instrument containing lenses and prisms, which can be combined and adjusted by manipulating various knobs.

Fulton A: Screening preschool children to detect visual and ocular disorders. Arch Ophthalmol 110:1553, 1992.

Hecht SD: Evaluation of the lacrimal drainage system. Ophthalmology 85:1250, 1978.

Isenberg SJ: Examination methods. In Isenberg SJ (ed): The Eye in Infancy. Chicago, Year Book, 1989.

Moody EA: Ophthalmic examinations of infants and children. In Harley RD (ed): Pediatric Ophthalmology, 2nd ed. Philadelphia, Saunders, 1983.

Nelson LB: Pediatric Ophthalmology. Philadelphia, Saunders, 1984.

Nelson LB, Catalano RA: Atlas of Ocular Motility. Philadelphia, Saunders, 1989, pp 2–43.

Parks MM: Isolated cyclovertical muscle palsy. Arch Ophthalmol 60:1027, 1958.

Richard JM (ed): A Manual for the Beginning Ophthalmology Resident, 3rd edition. San Francisco, American Academy of Ophthalmology, 1980.

Thompson HS, Corbett JJ, Cox TA: How to measure the relative afferent pupillary defect. Surv Ophthalmol 26:39, 1981.

VISUAL DEVELOPMENT, LEARNING DISABILITIES, AND FUNCTIONAL DISORDERS

ESSENTIAL INFORMATION FOR PRIMARY CARE PRACTITIONERS

Normal Visual Development

As in other areas of developmental biology, knowledge of "normal" behavior and function is essential to understanding abnormalities in visual development. Our appreciation of normal visual function in infants and young children continues to be revised as new methods and tests of visual activity are developed. In the past, the ability to elicit a fixation pattern, as well as the absence of an oculomotor disorder, was considered evidence that an infant's visual function was adequate. Although these clinical parameters remain useful, they do not provide a complete assessment of visual function.

Figure 3–1 is a time line representing the pattern by which visual activities normally develop. The human visual system is vulnerable to modification by external factors during both prenatal and postnatal development. The precise age range of the critical period, in which normal visual experience is necessary for full visual development, has yet to be defined. It appears, however, that complete visual development requires at least 5 or 6 years, and that the visual system remains very vulnerable until about 9 years of age.

Vision Screening

The previous chapter reviewed the American Academy of Ophthalmology's recommended schedule for preschool vision screening, and the fundamentals of the exam performed. To reiterate, ideally the red reflex test should be performed on all neonates, and this should be repeated along with a test of ocular alignment by 3 to 6 months of age. Visual acuity should be tested, and ocular alignment retested, at 3 and 5 years of age.

This rigid schedule attempts to detect amblyopia at an early age, when treatment is more likely to be efficacious. A review in 1983 demonstrated that only about 1 in 5 preschool children in the United States were screened for strabismus and amblyopia (Ehrlich et al. 1983). Despite much research during the past decade, progress toward a mass screening test has been slow. The reason is that the ideal test must fulfill stringent criteria. It must be sensitive, reliable, easy to administer, and cost effective. Although the ideal test has yet to be developed, techniques such as photoscreening and abbreviated preferential looking methods (described later in the chapter) offer promise.

Learning Disabilities

The process of acquiring knowledge is very visual; most learning involves looking at things. It is, there-

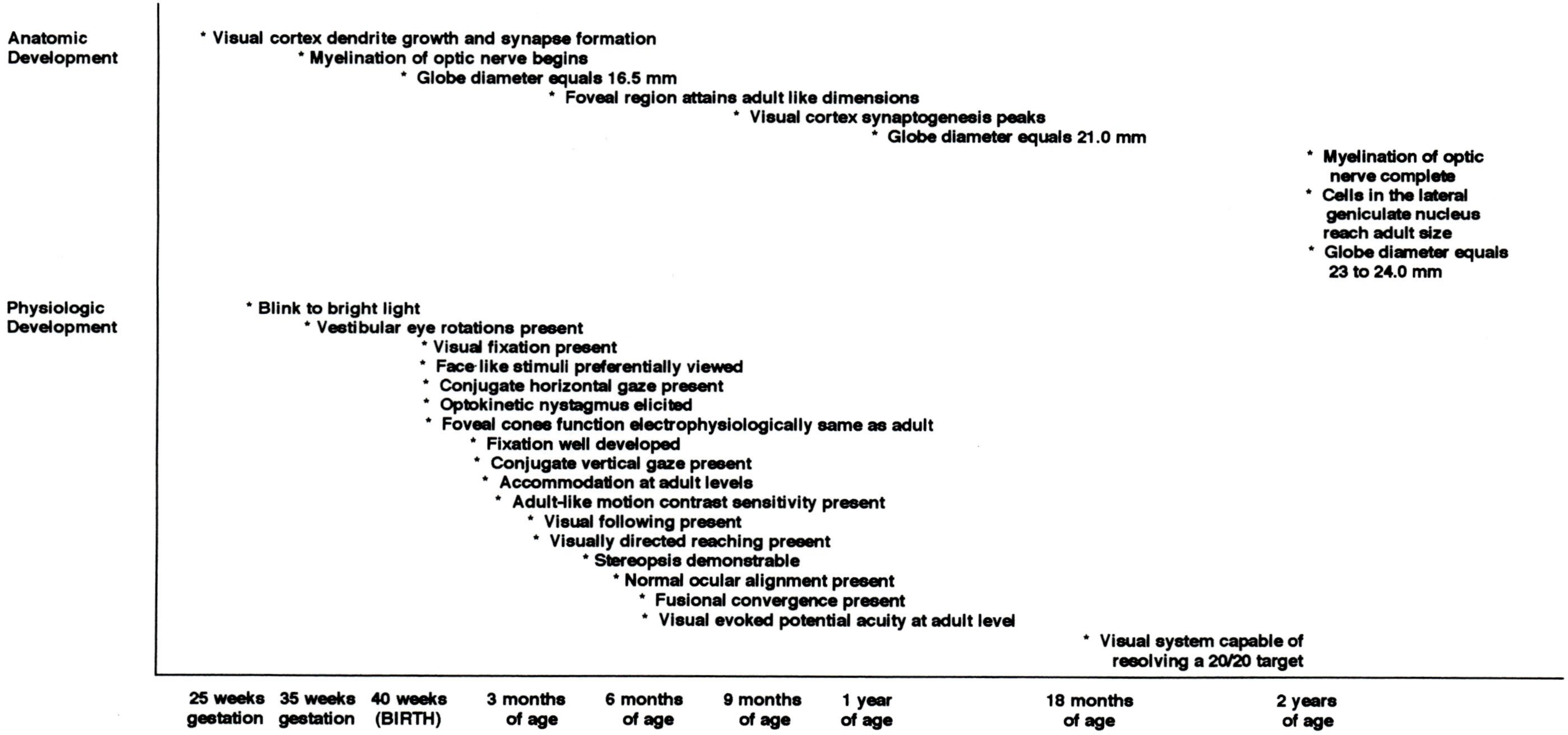

Anatomic Development

* Visual cortex dendrite growth and synapse formation
* Myelination of optic nerve begins
* Globe diameter equals 16.5 mm
* Foveal region attains adult like dimensions
* Visual cortex synaptogenesis peaks
* Globe diameter equals 21.0 mm
* Myelination of optic nerve complete
* Cells in the lateral geniculate nucleus reach adult size
* Globe diameter equals 23 to 24.0 mm

Physiologic Development

* Blink to bright light
* Vestibular eye rotations present
* Visual fixation present
* Face-like stimuli preferentially viewed
* Conjugate horizontal gaze present
* Optokinetic nystagmus elicited
* Foveal cones function electrophysiologically same as adult
* Fixation well developed
* Conjugate vertical gaze present
* Accommodation at adult levels
* Adult-like motion contrast sensitivity present
* Visual following present
* Visually directed reaching present
* Stereopsis demonstrable
* Normal ocular alignment present
* Fusional convergence present
* Visual evoked potential acuity at adult level
* Visual system capable of resolving a 20/20 target

25 weeks gestation	35 weeks gestation	40 weeks (BIRTH)	3 months of age	6 months of age	9 months of age	1 year of age	18 months of age	2 years of age

Figure 3–1. Time line of normal visual development.

fore, easy to think that the child who has difficulty learning has a visual problem. Actually, the eyes simply send information to the brain, which is responsible for interpreting this information. If the picture the eye sends is clear and focused (that is, there is no ocular abnormality that reduces vision), then the child who has difficulty interpreting this information has a learning, not a visual problem.

Several terms that describe learning disabilities are often misunderstood to imply ocular abnormalities. Dyslexia is a reading disability (generally 2 or more years behind one's age level) occurring in an individual of normal intelligence, with adequate sociocultural opportunities. A visual perception problem is an inability of the brain to interpret information that is received through the eyes. Use of this term is not inappropriate if one understands that "perception" is a function of the brain, not the eye. Unfortunately, to many individuals, the word "visual" insinuates an ocular abnormality. For this reason, the phrase "visual perception" should be avoided.

As many as 3 to 7 percent of school-aged children in the United States fulfill the criteria listed above, and are classified as dyslexic (Silver, 1986). Twin studies have suggested that there may be a genetic component to dyslexia, but no single major locus accounts for all of dyslexia (Pennington et al, 1991). As with many complex behavioral disorders, dyslexia is most likely multifactorial and polygenic, a concordance of multiple genes and the environment. Boys are three times more likely to have dyslexia than girls, the reason for which remains undetermined. There does not appear to be any relationship between birthweight or pre- or postnatal complications and dyslexia. Finally, hyperactive children are often classified as learning disabled. If successful management of their hyperactivity improves their learning, their problem was easy distractibility, not dyslexia.

Associated problems of dyslexic children are noted in Table 3–1. As is the case with most clinical syndromes, most dyslexics do not exhibit all these problems, and the presence of any of these alone does not diagnose dyslexia. It is also important to realize that many children omit, reverse, or substitute letters, or

TABLE 3–1. PROBLEMS OF DYSLEXIC CHILDREN

Reading dysfunction
Poor motor abilities
Poor spatial reasoning
Poor color naming
Poor object naming
Poor spelling
Poor motor speech (inability to utter smoothly sequenced sounds)
Poor phonemic sequencing (inability to repeat a sequence of sounds)
Poor writing skills (both form and content)

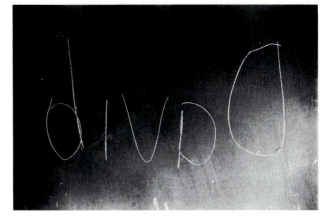

Figure 3–2. Mirror writing.

mirror write (Fig. 3–2) when learning how to read. The vast majority overcome this with practice. It is interesting that dyslexia is common in societies that speak languages such as English, in which certain letters (symbols) have as many as five different sounds. Dyslexia is very uncommon in societies which use languages such as Japanese, in which each symbol represents a unique sound.

Children with learning disabilities should have an eye examination to rule out a defect that prevents the brain from receiving a clear, focused image. Notably, eye muscle imbalance, "abnormal ocular dominance," and left-handedness do not cause learning disabilities. Reading ability appears to be more closely related to language problems than to visual–motor defects (Metzger & Werner, 1984; Vellutino, 1987). If a learning problem remains after correction of a structural defect of the eye, such as a refractive error, remedial education is indicated.

A great variety of techniques and devices have been promoted as efficacious in improving visual function, often under the pretense of "visual training." The individualized attention and education these involve usually account for the progress achieved. A conscientious school system should be able to achieve the same success, at much less cost. Visual training activities such as walking a balance beam, and video game techniques, may improve coordination and concentration, but have no direct effect on vision or depth perception.

Functional Ophthalmologic Disorders*

Several ophthalmologic abnormalities have a nonorganic or functional basis. The term "functional" implies that the disorder is one of function rather than structure. In this context, it means that the physical structure is undamaged and presumably capable of

*Modified from Catalano RA: Ocular emergencies. Philadelphia, Saunders, 1992, pp 441–456, with permission.

TABLE 3–2. OPHTHALMOLOGIC DISORDERS THAT CAN BE FUNCTIONAL

Loss of visual acuity or visual field
Spasm of the near reflex
Blinking
Eyelid pulling
Eyelash and eyebrow plucking
Voluntary nystagmus
Headache
Photophobia
Visual hallucinations
Pupillary abnormalities
Propulsion of the eyeballs

full function. Older terms that imply the same (such as hysteria, conversion reaction, and pithiatism) should be avoided, because their meaning and relationship to the psyche are even less lucid than "functional."

The term "functional" does not, in itself, indicate whether the apparent loss is feigned or fancied. Patients who deliberately and knowingly feign loss (malingerers), as well as highly suggestive individuals, without malicious intent, comprise the extremes of any functional disorder. Most patients fall between these extremes.

With every functional disorder, the challenge to the physician is to determine whether the alleged loss has an organic basis. Because the physician often sets out to disprove the child's claim of impairment, dealing with these children and the distorted physician–patient relationship is often frustrating. The most difficult child to examine and treat is the one with organic disease but with symptoms exaggerated out of proportion to the underlying pathology. A careful check of old records for existing disease is prudent when symptoms outweigh findings on examination. These patients are usually classified as having disease "with a functional overlay."

The most commonly encountered functional ophthalmologic disorder is loss of visual field or acuity. Less common disorders are visual hallucinations, photophobia, and headache (Table 3–2). A few disorders of ocular motility, including accommodative spasm and voluntary nystagmus, are almost always functional.

Disorders such as functional blinking and eyelid pulling occur predominantly in children. The distinguishing features of the latter are reviewed in Table 3–3.

Whether functional losses should be classified as psychiatric disorders is controversial. These children, or their caretakers, often report considerable situational stress, but generally they do not need psychiatric evaluation or treatment. This cannot be said of individuals who self-induce ocular injuries. Included in this group are adolescents with delusional psychoses. The latter need urgent psychiatric care.

COMPREHENSIVE INFORMATION ON VISUAL DEVELOPMENT, LEARNING DISABILITIES, AND FUNCTIONAL DISORDERS

Normal Visual Development

Morphological Considerations

The diameter of the normal globe increases from about 16.5 mm at birth to 24.5 mm in adulthood. More than half of this sagittal growth occurs during the first year of life. By approximately 18 months of age, a normal infant's visual system is capable of resolving a 20/20 target. Although the exact relationship between morphological change and visual function is still unclear, it is obvious that visual performance improves concurrently with the anatomic growth and development of the globe and the central visual system.

Although the retina is generally well developed at birth, structural and functional changes continue postnatally. The foveal region, including the cones, does not attain adult-like dimensions until approximately 4 months of age. However, electrophysiological and psychological studies suggest that the central retinal cones are functioning at an adult level at birth.

Although myelination of the anterior visual pathway was thought to be completed within the first month of life, recent studies contradict this thesis. By term, some fibers in the optic nerve near the globe begin to be myelinated, but the amount of myelin surrounding the individual nerves increases dramatically during the ensuing months, and may continue to in-

TABLE 3–3. FUNCTIONAL VISUAL DISORDERS OF CHILDREN

	Functional Visual Loss	Functional Blinking	Functional Eyelid Pulling
Associated stresses	Conflict at home or school, abuse	None usually identified	None usually identified
Other symptoms	Common	Rare	Rare
Affected sex	Female > male	Female = male	Female = male
Average age	9–12 years	3–7 years	5–9 years
Resolution with reassurance	Within 2 months in 75%	Usually rapid (days to weeks)	Usually rapid (days to weeks)
Recurrences	Rare	Rare	Rare

crease until 2 years of age. This extended period of my-elination most likely contributes to the normal delay of maturation of visual acuity.

Cortical neuronal dendritic growth and synaptic formation begin at 25 weeks of gestation. This growth is very active around the time of birth and continues into the first 2 postnatal years. In preterm infants of 25 to 33 weeks' gestational age, dendritic formation (as established with postmortem Golgi preparation) increases in correlation with an improvement in visual evoked potentials (Van Essen, 1984). Cells in the lateral geniculate nucleus increase in size rapidly during the first year of life, reaching adult size by 2 years of age. In animal studies, the onset of the critical period of visual development appears to coincide with the period of most rapid geniculate cell growth and the period of most rapid synapse formation in both the geniculate nucleus and the visual cortex. If this relationship is similar in humans, the most crucial period in visual development would be the first 24 months of life.

Form Perception

Newborns are able to discriminate curved shapes from straight ones as well as horizontal stripes from vertical ones. Face-like stimuli are preferentially viewed by newborns only a few minutes old. There seems to be a preprogrammed, genetically determined preference for the human face, which is undoubtedly related to infant maternal bonding.

Visually directed reaching can be demonstrated in infants less than 3 months old. It has been shown that infants as young as 2 weeks of age can differentiate between a "graspable" and a "nongraspable" display by reaching for one but not for the other. In a clinical setting, this phenomenon has not been useful, because the infant does not develop adequate postural tone and reflexes for testing until 6 months of age or older.

Accommodation

Accommodation is the process by which the refractive power of the anterior lens surface increases so that a near object may be imaged distinctly on the retina. The stimulus to accommodation is the maintenance of a clear retinal image. Assessments of infant visual function in the laboratory and clinical setting are routinely performed at relatively close range. Therefore, the role of accommodation is obvious.

Until recently, few objective data on infant accommodation were available. Early studies on infant accommodation concluded that infants from 6 days to 1 month of age exhibited no evidence of accommodation. It was believed that accommodation required several months to develop, and that adult-like function was not present until 4 months of age. More recent studies indicate that accommodative ability is present in the first weeks of life and reaches adult accuracy by 9 weeks of age (Banks, 1980).

Binocularity and the Ocular Motor System

The cortical integration of similar images from each eye into a unified perceptual whole is an acquired reflex called single binocular vision. To attain this, one needs two seeing eyes and alignment of the visual axes (that is, the visual axes of each eye must intersect the object of regard at the point of fixation). The slight horizontal displacement of the two eyes gives each one a slightly different view of the object and thus allows perception of the third dimension, depth. This is referred to as stereopsis.

Approximately 50 percent of all infants are born with their eyes aligned (Nixon et al, 1985). During the first month of life, alignment may vary from esotropia (turning toward the nose), to perfect alignment (orthophoria), to exotropia (eyes turning away from the nose). During this period, other transient deviations may occur. A misalignment in which one eye is higher than the other and varies with different positions of gaze is called skew deviation. Like transient horizontal misalignment, skew deviation may disappear if it is not due to a neuromuscular disorder. Flutter-like eye movements called opsoclonus may also be seen in the neonatal period. They must be differentiated from nystagmus, a rhythmic, periodic to-and-fro movement of the eyes. The latter requires a complete evaluation by an ophthalmologist when present at any age (see Chapter 7).

Although ocular deviations during the first months of life are not necessarily indicative of an abnormality, alignment is established in many infants by 4 weeks of age (Isenberg, 1990). The upper limits of normal for initial alignment ranges between 3 and 6 months of age. If constant misalignment is present at 3 months of age, however, referral to an ophthalmologist is indicated.

Animal experiments indicate that misalignment during the "critical period" (up to 9 years of age in humans) may result in neuroanatomic changes in the visual system. The lateral geniculate body is the area of the brain where the retinal ganglion cells synapse with cells projecting back to the visual cortex. When an eye of an otherwise normal macaque monkey is occluded or deviated during the "critical period," a reduction in the number and size of cells in the lateral geniculate body occurs (Crawford et al, 1975). In the visual cortex, two populations of cells are normally found: those receiving input predominantly from one of the two eyes and those receiving input from both eyes. Monkeys and kittens with strabismus or occlusion of one eye show a reduction in the number of cortical cells driven by the deviated or occluded eye, and a preponderance of cells driven by the nondeviated or nonoccluded eye (Baker et al, 1974).

Once alignment of two seeing eyes is attained, binocularly derived information is used to maintain this alignment throughout life. When the input for the binocular reflex is interrupted, alignment is often affected.

In early childhood, a pathologically affected eye often exhibits a misalignment, commonly a convergent deviation (esotropia). For this reason, all children with a misalignment after the age of 3 months require a complete ophthalmologic evaluation.

Proper alignment of the eyes allows an image to project onto the most sensitive part of the retina, the macula. This relationship must be continuously reinforced throughout the "critical period" for good visual acuity to be maintained. When the visual axes are misaligned or one is occluded during the critical period, the fixation reflex becomes altered and the visual acuity of the misaligned or occluded eye fails to develop or is reduced; this visual change is called amblyopia.

Neurobiologists have determined that the visual areas in the cerebral cortex in monkeys and humans are organized as two functionally distinct pathways, with each pathway processing a different kind of information (Tychsen & Lisberger, 1986; Van Essen, 1984). One area specializes in the analysis of visual motion, and is thought to be responsible for interpreting the direction, speed, and gross stereopsis of stimulus motion. This system may be responsible for ocular alignment, pursuit, fusion, and vergence. The second system is associated with the analysis of form (length, width, pattern, orientation) and color. This pathway likely controls visual acuity and fine stereopsis. Form vision appears to develop later, or more slowly (first 10 months of life), than motion vision (first 6 months of life). Although there is substantial evidence that these systems, in many respects, are functionally distinct, they are not totally independent. Many anatomic and physiological linkages between the areas have been demonstrated (Van Essen & Maunsell, 1983). Future developments of this research may lead to the biochemical manipulation of cortical plasticity, new treatment modalities for amblyopia and reduced depth perception, and the redevelopment of fusional pathways to improve the control of ocular alignment or reduce nystagmus.

Refractive Status

The human eye is a compound optical system that refracts or "bends" rays of light, focusing them on the retina. The refractive status of the eye is determined by the interaction of a number of factors, including the anterior-to-posterior length of the eye (axial length), the corneal curvature, and the power of the lens.

Emmetropia is the condition in which no refractive error exists. The refractive error (ametropia) that results when light is focused anterior to the retina is myopia or nearsightedness. This condition may occur because the eyeball is too long, the refractive components of the eye (the cornea and lens) have excessive power, or both. Hyperopia or farsightedness is the refractive error that occurs when light is focused behind the retina. This refractive error exists because the globe is too short, the refractive components of the eye are insufficient, or both. Astigmatism is the refractive error that is caused by an irregularity in the shape of the cornea or lens; it results in greater focusing power in one meridian than in another (see Chapter 5).

Variable myopic errors and astigmatism are common among premature infants, even without evidence of previous retinopathy of prematurity (Dobson et al, 1981; Kushner, 1982). The incidence of anisometropia (a difference in the refractive error of the two eyes) among premature infants was higher than that reported for full-term infants. Although early studies suggested that myopia in premature infants decreases with age, age-related changes in anisometropia and astigmatism have yet to be established for premature infants (Fledelius, 1976, 1982).

The refractive error of full-term infants has been determined to be moderately hyperopic (plus 2 diopters) with a bell-shaped curve distribution. In a study of 1000 newborns it was found that 75 percent were moderately hyperopic and 25 percent were myopic (Cook & Glasscock, 1951). Early studies suggested that hyperopia tends to increase until approximately age 7 years, and then it begins to decline (Brown, 1939). More recent studies have shown a steady decline in hyperopic refraction throughout childhood (Larsen, 1971).

The incidence of astigmatism in full-term infants is more common than in older children and adults (Friedburg & Sons, 1983; Sorsby & Leary, 1969). In one study, it was found that 19 percent of 1-week old infants had more than 1.0 diopter of astigmatism, which increased significantly at 3 months of age (Fulton et al, 1980). The incidence of astigmatism began to decrease after 6 months of age. Other investigators have confirmed the finding of large astigmatic errors during the first 6 months of life, which tended to decrease after that age (Abrahamsson et al, 1988; Atkinson et al, 1984). Whether the high incidence of transient astigmatic errors has any effect on the developing visual system has not been determined.

Myopia is not common in infants, although a congenital form, characterized by a high degree of myopia, can sometimes occur. Generally, children do not begin to show myopia until about the age of 8 years (Curtin, 1985). This childhood-onset myopia has been associated with high intellectual achievement (Rosner & Belkin, 1987) and high social class (Sperduto et al, 1983). These and other studies suggest the role of the environment in producing refractive errors; for example, the children of immigrants to more advanced societies are more myopic than their parents (Curtin, 1985). Nonetheless, it remains unclear as to whether myopia causes superior performance, or the intense reading and near work necessary for intellectual achievement cause myopia. It may be that the environment alters the expressivity of genes; myopia may be more likely to be expressed with intellectual nurturing. In advanced societies, this usually involves reading and near tasks, hence the stimulus toward prolonged accommodation and myopia (Angle & Wissmann, 1978; McBrien & Millodot, 1987; Rosner, 1989). In contrast, the desire to read and perform near tasks, by which advanced societies gauge intellectual achievement, may be nurtured by the clearer vision at near that myopes experience.

Normal and Abnormal Ocular Reflexes

Multiple developmental neurological reflexes (such as Moro's reflex) have been described in human infants. Each appears transiently, during a specific stage of development, and abates with the development of higher cortical functioning. In 1972, Perez described a neonatal reflex characterized by a pronounced widening of the palpebral fissures following an abrupt decrease of ambient illumination. He called this reflex "eye-popping" (Fig. 3–3). In association with the lid retraction, a downward rotation of the globe and marked eyelid retraction can occur. Loud noises and changes in position are capable of inducing the reflex, indicating that the

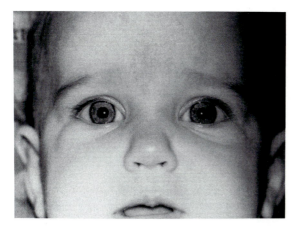

A

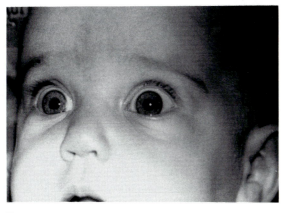

B

Figure 3–3. The eye-popping reflex. **A.** Photograph taken with the room lights on. **B.** Widening of the palpebral fissures immediately upon turning the room lights off.

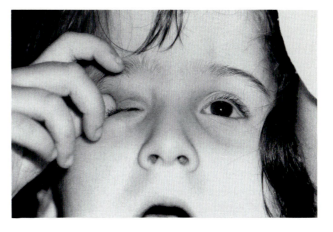

Figure 3–4. Blindism (eye pressing) in a visually impaired child.

optic nerve is not the only afferent pathway. Removal of light, however, is believed to be the most effective stimulus for the reflex (Victor, 1972).

The eye-popping reflex is present within the first 3 weeks of life in nearly 75 percent of infants with postconceptional ages of 28 to 42 weeks (Catalano, unpublished data). Prematurity, neonatal diseases, and maternal risk factors do not appear to affect the prevalence. As with other neonatal reflexes, the anatomic pathway of the eye-popping reflex is not known. The importance of the reflex may reside in demonstrating some function of the afferent arc of the visual system to at least the brainstem.

In contrast to eye-popping, visually impaired children may develop abnormal behavioral mannerisms, which have been called "blindisms" (Moller, 1992). The most frequently observed is eye pressing or gouging (Figs. 3–4 and 3–5). Other "blindisms" include light gazing, exaggerated finger play, and rocking. Early investigators believed these were done to provide self-stimulation (phosphenes from eye pressing). Eichel (1978), documented that non-sensory deprived chil-

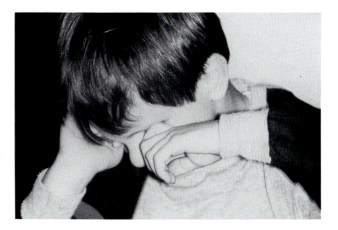

Figure 3–5. Another visually impaired child with eye pressing.

dren also exhibit these mannerisms. Behavior modification techniques are used to reduce or eliminate these acts.

Vision Screening

Amblyopia screening tests can be divided into two categories: direct and indirect. Direct tests attempt to assess visual acuity or function. Examples are tests of visual acuity, stereopsis, preferential looking, visual evoked potential, and fixation preference. Indirect tests are designed to detect factors known to cause amblyopia. Included are strabismus and media opacity screening, measurements of refractive error, and photoscreening (photorefraction).

De Becker and associates (1992) reported on the predictive value of a population-based preschool vision screening program, using the direct tests of visual acuity and stereopsis. Children 4 and 5 years old were screened for an acuity of 6/9–3 or worse in one or both eyes, or a stereoacuity worse than 200 seconds. The negative predictive value of the screening (the probability that children who passed the test did not have a potentially vision-threatening ocular condition) was 97.6 percent. The positive predictive value (indicating unnecessary referrals) was 50 percent. In addition to not detecting all children with disorders, this form of screening is labor intensive. Further, it does not address the findings of Ingram (1977, 1986), which suggest that, for optimum results, vision screening should take place before the age of 1 year.

A much investigated direct test, designed for younger patients, is preferential looking (PL), or a modification of this. These tests are based on the phenomenon that infants will preferentially fixate a patterned target over a blank gray target of equal space-average luminance. Children are presented a number of gratings of different spatial frequencies (stripe widths), in concert with a gray target. The right-left location of the grating is varied from one presentation to the next. Vision is estimated by determining the smallest stripe width that elicits preferential fixation (see Figs. 2–23 and 2–24). Most variants of PL are labor intensive, bulky, expensive, and/or in need of constant monitoring of alignment and calibration (Teller et al, 1986). Further, the percentage of 1- and 2-year-old children that can be successfully tested is low. Finally, although PL tests appear quite valuable in identifying and following deprivation amblyopia, they appear at this time to be less valuable in strabismic and anisometropic amblyopia (Stager, 1991). Visual evoked potential testing suffers the additional limitations of requiring expensive equipment and a technician, as well as the child's attention.

Clinical tests of stereopsis provide evidence of binocular function. Unfortunately, clinical measures of stereopsis in infants and young children often result in stereothresholds poorer than the criteria suggested to differentiate normal from anomalous binocular vision. In addition, most stereotests require the use of spectacles that incorporate polarizing filters to isolate the images presented to each eye. This further reduces their usefulness in young children. The Frisby and Lang stereotests do not require these filters, and are easier to administer to young children. Multiple studies, however, have demonstrated that neither test is appropriate to rule out, with certainty, the presence of amblyopia or anisometropia in the absence of strabismus (Cotter & Scharre, 1987; Lang & Lang, 1988; Manny et al, 1991). Stereopsis testing has also been advocated as a way to reduce the overreferral of children who obtain the minimum failing result on a visual acuity screening test. A recent study evaluated the use of the random dot E stereotest for this purpose (Ruttum & Nelson, 1991). These investigators found that stereopsis testing could reduce overreferrals, but at the expense of substantially increasing underreferrals. They concluded that the addition of stereopsis testing at its current sensitivity to a preschool vision screening program could not successfully modify current visual acuity referral criteria.

Because of the shortcomings of direct vision screening tests, many clinicians have advocated the use of indirect tests to screen for amblyogenic factors. In 1979, Ingram and associates suggested that identification of high hypermetropia at age 1 year could enable the prediction of most children who will subsequently develop amblyopia, strabismus, or both. Follow-up has shown that infants at 1 year of age with 3.5 D or more of hyperopia in any meridian have a 45 percent chance of developing strabismus by age 3.5 years, and a 48 percent chance of developing amblyopia (Ingram et al, 1986). Refraction, however, requires cycloplegia (eyedrops that inhibit accommodation), and the skill of retinoscopy. Conventional refraction techniques are, therefore, too skilled-labor-intense to be useful for mass screening.

A simpler test to perform is the Bruckner simultaneous red reflex test. This test has been advocated to screen for refractive errors, media opacities, and strabismus. It is performed using an ophthalmoscope (preferably with a halogen light source) set at the zero setting. The physician stands a few feet away from the child, who is seated in a parent's lap. As the child fixates the light source, the examiner views the pupils through the ophthalmoscope. Any inequality or interference with the red reflex (see Figs. 11–5 and 11–6) is considered a positive finding that requires further evaluation. The usefulness of this test, however, remains controversial, especially in young infants (Manny et al, 1991).

A promising technique for detecting anisometropia, astigmatism, high ametropia, and media opacities is photoscreening. The technique involves the use of a specially designed camera that records the image of the red reflex on instant (Polaroid) film. Two pictures are

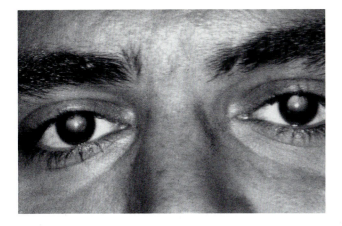

Figure 3–6. Photorefractive appearance of an individual with balanced high myopia (–6.0 D). The flash for this picture was horizontal; the white crescents are symmetrical.

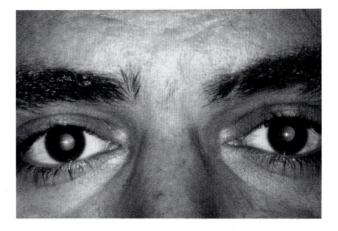

Figure 3–7. Photorefraction on same patient as Figure 3–6 with the flash directed vertically.

taken. The first is with the flash in the horizontal position, the second with it in the vertical position (Figs. 3–6 and 3–7). Analysis of the orientation, brightness, size, and symmetry of the red reflex, or crescent of light, enables an estimation of the refractive error, media opacities, or strabismus, all of which can lead to amblyopia. Photoscreening requires no head restraint and is easy to perform. Information for interpretation is immediately available through the use of Polaroid film. Improved methodology (Freedman & Preston, 1992) has resulted in a sensitivity rate of 87 percent and a specificity rate of 89 percent. It is also, however, not without limitations. Fixation is more difficult to obtain in children under age 6 months, and off-center fixation, which occurred in 29 percent of the children in the study, can cause false positive readings. Additionally, balanced high hyperopia can be missed if the child accommodates on the camera.

In summary, the importance of screening preschool children to detect visual and ocular problems has been widely recognized. No test is available, however, that meets all the criteria of being sensitive, reliable, easy to administer, and cost effective. Modalities such as photoscreening and shortened preferential looking methods show promise for rapid screening of large populations of small infants. Until they are fully developed and available, the American Academy of Ophthalmology's minimum guidelines for vision screening of infants and children (see Table 2–1) should be rigorously followed.

Learning Disabilities

Controversy as to the underlying deficit in dyslexia abounds. Sadun (1992) noted: "At different times during the last century, it has been fashionable to consider the basic problem variously as cognitive, psychological, chromosomal, biochemical, linguistic, visual, and the result of right/left brain confusion." An example of a recent hypothesis is that of Geiger and Lettvin (1987),

who proposed that dyslexics have an abnormal interaction between foveal and peripheral vision. They postulated that dyslexics have masking where normal readers have their best resolution (central or foveal vision), and that this degrades their ability to read in the foveal field. They suggested that their findings provide evidence that an alternative reading strategy can be learned. An accompanying editorial questioned their research technique (Shaywitz & Waxman, 1987). Another recently promoted hypothesis suggested that dyslexia is caused by poor control of eye movements (Pavlidis, 1983). Other investigators, however, have failed to corroborate this (Olson et al, 1983).

Very recently, a disorder called scotopic sensitivity syndrome has been promoted as the cause of reading disability in as many as 50 percent of dyslexics. Proponents propose that full spectral light produces overstimulation of the retinal photoreceptors, which in turn causes problems with vision. They advocate the use of colored spectacles or overlays to block specific wavelengths that an individual eye cannot handle. Whereas these filters may reduce glare, controlled studies have not found any benefit with this treatment (Cotton & Evans, 1990).

Older studies demonstrated a relationship of dyslexia to visual scanning deficits (Stein & Fowler, 1984), temporal order recall deficits (Bakker, 1972), and cross-modal integration deficits (Birch & Belmont, 1965). None of these theories has proven adequate to explain all cases or features of dyslexia. Furthermore, deficiencies of visual perception and visual-motor function are common findings in children with normal reading skills (Levine, 1984).

Numerous techniques and devices have been promoted to treat dyslexia. Controversy regarding the efficacy of many of these is common, as they are based on disputed hypotheses as to the cause of dyslexia. Some clinicians advocate physiological intervention, such as patterning (sensory stimulation techniques), optometric visual training, vestibular treatments, and megavitamins. Most ophthalmologists, however, are in accord with Silver (1986), who concluded that there is little or no empirical support for these therapies. Further, a joint policy statement of the American Academy of Ophthalmology, American Academy of Pediatrics, and American Association for Pediatric Ophthalmology and Strabismus (AAD, 1992) advocates for educational remediation of dyslexia, and against visual training and neurological organizational training (Table 3–4). This policy further notes that except for correcting refractive errors, glasses (with or without bifocals or prisms) have no value in the treatment of learning disabilities.

Remedial education involves teacher-intensive structured tutoring in skills specific to reading. A common approach is to have the child read a letter or word out loud, while tracing it with his or her finger. Over time letters are fused into words, and words into phrases. Other methods, such as using a ruler to keep one's place on the page, are used concomitantly.

Functional Ophthalmologic Disorders

Functional Visual Loss

Functional visual loss, also known as retinal anesthesia, ocular hysteria, hysterical amblyopia, visual conversion reaction, and the "ophthalmic flake syndrome," has been reported to comprise 1 to 5 percent of a typical ophthalmologist's practice. There is a 2:1 predominance of females and a clustering of children between ages 9 and 12 years. In children, the disorder is somewhat different than it is in adults, but the diagnostic techniques are the same.

The burden of proving normal visual function rests with the examiner. Suggested techniques to disprove visual loss are reviewed in Table 3–5. Disorders of childhood and adolescence that may be misdiagnosed as functional loss include mild amblyopia, keratoconus, retinitis pigmentosa without pigment, and early Stargardt's disease. It is also not uncommon for patients with organic disease to have a functional overlay. If a relative afferent pupillary defect is present (see Fig. 2–35), functional visual loss is at most only part of the diagnosis. Whenever there is reasonable doubt, or if good visual acuity cannot be confirmed with certainty, reexamination is prudent. The diagnosis of malingering is unusual in children. It should be made with great caution, because it implies that the child is consciously feigning disability for secondary gain.

Most children with functional visual loss have a moderate reduction in acuity, ranging from 20/30 to 20/100. The loss is more often bilateral than unilateral, and associated symptoms, including voluntary nystagmus, spasm of the near reflex, and even bitemporal hemianopsia, can often be elicited.

Several studies have demonstrated that many af-

TABLE 3–4. EXCERPTS FROM JOINT POLICY STATEMENT OF THE AAO, AAP, AND AAPO&S ON LEARNING DISABILITIES, DYSLEXIA, AND VISION (1992)

1. The issue of learning disorders, including dyslexia, has become a matter of increasing personal and public concern. . . . Concern for the welfare of children with dyslexia and learning disabilities has led to a proliferation of diagnostic and remedial treatment procedures, many of which are controversial. . . . Research has shown that the majority of children and adults with reading difficulties experience a variety of language defects that stem from complex, altered brain morphology and function, and that the reading difficulty is not due to altered visual function per se.
2. Learning disabilities, including dyslexia and other forms of reading or academic underachievement, require a multi-disciplinary approach to diagnosis and treatment. . . . Ocular defects should be identified as early as possible. . . . Treatable conditions include refractive errors, focusing deficiencies, eye muscle imbalances, and motor fusion deficiencies. . . . If no ocular defect is found, the child should be referred to a pediatrician to coordinate required multidisciplinary care.
3. Decoding of retinal images occurs in the brain after visual signals are transmitted from the retina via the visual pathways. Unfortunately, however, it has become common practice among some to attribute reading difficulties to one or more subtle ocular or visual abnormalities. Although the eyes are obviously necessary for vision, the brain interprets visual symbols. Therefore, correcting subtle visual defects cannot alter the brain's processing of visual stimuli. Children with dyslexia or related learning disabilities have the same ocular health statistically as children without such conditions. There is no peripheral eye defect that produces dyslexia or other learning disabilities, and there is no eye treatment that can cure dyslexia or associated learning disability. There is no peripheral eye defect which produces dyslexia.
4. Eye defects, subtle or severe, do not cause reversal of letters, words, or numbers. No scientific evidence supports claims that the academic abilities of dyslexic or learning disabled children can be improved with treatment based on (a) visual training, including muscle exercises, ocular pursuit, tracking exercises, or "training" glasses (with or without bifocals or prisms); (b) neurological organizational training (laterality training, crawling, balance board, perceptual training); or (c) tinted or colored lenses. Some controversial methods of treatment result in a false sense of security that may delay or prevent proper instruction or remediation. The expense of these procedures is unwarranted, and they cannot be substituted for appropriate remedial education measures. Claims of improved reading and learning after visual training or neurological organizational training, or use of tinted or colored lenses, are typically based upon poorly controlled studies that rely on anecdotal information or testimony. These studies are frequently carried out in combination with traditional educational remedial techniques.
5. The educator ultimately plays the key role in providing help for the learning disabled or dyslexic child or adult.

Reprinted from American Academy of Ophthalmology: Policy statement: Learning disabilities, dyslexia, and vision. San Francisco, AAO, 1992, with permission.

TABLE 3–5. TECHNIQUES TO DISPROVE VISUAL LOSS

- **IF THE VISUAL LOSS IS BINOCULAR**

  1. Test visual acuity binocularly starting with the 20/15 line. Express astonishment when the child cannot read this. Offer the 20/20 line as a major concession. If necessary, use the 20/25 line, calling it "huge."
  2. Make grimaces at the child and watch his or her reaction.
  3. Move a hand-held mirror in front of the child's face. It will be difficult for the child not to move the eyes (tracking his or her face) as the mirror moves.
  4. Rotate an O.K.N. drum in front of the child. Conscious inattention is necessary to avoid the development of optokinetic nystagmus.
  5. Check for saccadic accuracy. Quickly and innocuously ask child to "look here"; accuracy suggests good vision.

- **IF THE VISUAL LOSS IS MONOCULAR**

  1. Have the child read the eye chart while looking through a trial frame or phoropter. Slowly fog the "seeing eye" with high plus lenses.
  2. Test visual acuity with +2.00 and −2.00 diopter cylinders placed in front of each eye in a trial frame. Rotate them to neutralize each other in the "bad" eye, and add to each other in the "seeing" eye.
  3. While the child is reading, place a +10.00 diopter base-out prism in front of the "bad" eye. If it is being used, the eye will turn in.
  4. While the child is reading aloud, place a 10 diopter base-down prism in front of the "bad" eye. If the eye is being used, reading will immediately become difficult or impossible.
  5. Test for near stereovision using the Titmus or random dot E test. Excellent stereopsis is inconsistent with poor vision in one eye.
  6. Test visual acuity using the duochrome filter in the projector while the patient wears red-green glasses. The green lens

should be placed over the "seeing" eye because the red letters are more difficult to see.

  7. Have the child look at the Ishihara color plates while wearing red-green glasses, with the green lens over the "seeing" eye. If able to read the plates, the visual acuity in the "bad" eye is at least 10/200.

- **VISUAL FIELD ABNORMALITIES SUGGESTIVE OF A FUNCTIONAL DISORDER**

  Visual field testing for functional loss should be performed using a tangent screen or Goldmann perimeter. Automated perimetry, as currently practiced, may not be able to differentiate functional from organic disorders.

  1. Spiraling fields: Start the testing in one quadrant in the peripheral field. Mark a dot, and move to the next quadrant. Continue in a circular fashion; functional patients often constrict their visual field as the test progresses.
  2. Tubular fields: Test the child in front of a tangent screen at 1 m. Then move the child back to 2 m. The visual field should widen the farther the patient sits from the tangent screen. The field of the functional patient may constrict.
  3. Enlargement of field following pupillary dilation: Retest the visual field after dilating the pupils. The peripheral field may enlarge in suggestive patients.
  4. Monocular temporal hemianopsia: Recheck for the presence of a relative afferent pupillary defect, or the persistence of the hemianopsia on binocular testing. Rule out chiasmal compression; look for a junctional scotoma in the opposite eye.
  5. Loss of previously defined blind spot: The physiological blind spot should be consistently reproduced.
  6. Geometric fields: Suggestive patients may be talked into demonstrating triangular-, square-, or star-shaped visual fields. The use of pins on the tangent screen may be helpful.

---

fected children have significant family and/or school-related conflict (Catalano et al, 1986). Initial attempts to elicit this connection may be met with frank parental denial or disbelief. It is often only months after resolution that this is recognized. Many children are of above-average intelligence, and "previous to their visual loss" were "A" students. Stressful home situations are also common; several cases of physically or sexually abused children with this disorder have been reported.

The disorder is self-limited, but the duration of symptoms can be prolonged prior to diagnosis. Upon diagnosis and with reassurance to both the parents and child, symptoms resolve rapidly. Symptoms resolve in 25 percent of children within 1 day and 75 percent of affected children within 2 months (Catalano et al, 1986). There does not appear to be any correlation between the duration of symptoms prior to diagnosis and subsequent recovery time. Multiple anecdotal reports exist of resolution with hypnosis, plano glasses, placebo eyedrops or pills, and prayer meetings, but none has been proved more efficacious than reassurance

alone. Furthermore, reassurance and parental support may lead to a more rapid resolution than benign neglect or punishment.

There is substantial disagreement in the literature regarding the need for and efficacy of psychiatric intervention. Referral is usually indicated when the complex of symptoms is indicative of a severe psychiatric disturbance, but often reassurance by a concerned ophthalmologist and parent(s) is the only treatment necessary. Recurrence of symptoms or the late onset of other somatic complaints is rare.

Functional Blinking

Organic causes of excessive blinking include ocular conditions associated with pain or photophobia, systemic disorders (such as hypoparathyroidism, Gilles de la Tourette's syndrome, and tardive dyskinesia), and facial musculature syndromes (such as essential blepharospasm and hemifacial spasm).

Some clinicians use the term "functional blinking" to describe the benign episodic twitches of facial myokymia that are related to situational stress. Others reserve it for children who present with the isolated symptom of excessive blinking without other ocular or systemic signs or symptoms, and without baseline undulations of the orbicularis oculi muscle. Functional blinking is seen in young children, with an increased incidence in those age 3 to 7 years. Unlike functional visual loss, females are not predominantly affected. Furthermore, a temporally related stressful event can be identified in fewer than half of these children. In the majority of cases, the main secondary gain for the child is increased attention from the caretaker. Similar to functional visual loss and eyelid pulling, complete resolution of symptoms occurs within 1 day to 3 months in most children given reassurance only. Placebo treatments and psychiatric intervention are seldom, if ever, warranted. Recurrence of blinking or the development of other functional disorders is rare. The latter usually take the form of nose wrinkling, nose rubbing, or ear pulling (Vrabec, et al, 1989).

Functional Eyelid Pulling

Children can pull on their eyelids for several reasons. Usually they are trying to relieve ocular irritation secondary to misdirected eyelashes, a foreign body, or an inflammatory disorder of the eyelid. Occasionally, they are trying to create a stenopeic slit to reduce an uncorrected refractive error, or relieve diplopia related to a strabismic disorder. On rare occasions, children may pull on their eyelids in the absence of an underlying ocular or systemic disease (Figs. 3–8 and 3–9).

The mean age of children who do this is 7 years, and, like functional blinking, there is no female predominance (Catalano et al, 1990). Children appear to do this either to gain attention, or because their eyes were initially irritated and they developed a habit. When questioned, children may say they do this to "look funny" or because their "eyes are not opening

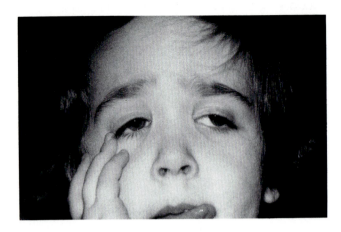
Figure 3–9. Functional eyelid pulling. This child pulls an eyelid outward from the lateral canthus.

enough." They often cite other children who do the same. Similar to functional blinking, but again unlike functional visual loss in children, there is usually no temporally related or recognized stressful event.

Resolution of symptoms occurs quickly (usually within 2 weeks) upon the physician's reassurance. Recurrences of this, as with other functional disorders in children, are rare.

Functional Eyelash and Eyebrow Plucking

Eyelash and eyebrow plucking is a common habit. Often it is done cosmetically, and commonly it occurs as a neurotic bad habit. It should be considered functional only when the patient is not consciously aware of the habit, or when the vigor with which it is done suggests a severe underlying systemic or emotional disorder (Figs. 3–10 and 3–11). Severely affected indi-

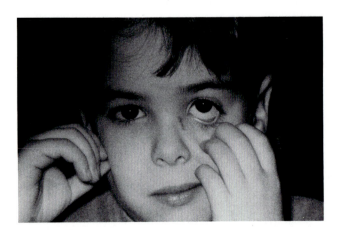
Figure 3–8. Functional eyelid pulling. This child pulls one eyelid straight down.

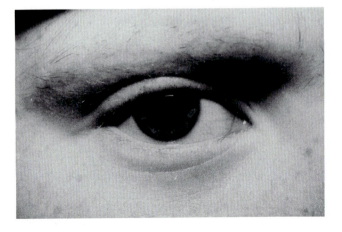
Figure 3–10. Functional eyelash and eyebrow plucking. Self-epilation of eyelashes and eyebrows. (Courtesy of Maury A. Marmor; from Catalano RA: Ocular emergencies. Philadelphia, Saunders, 1992, p 454, with permission.)

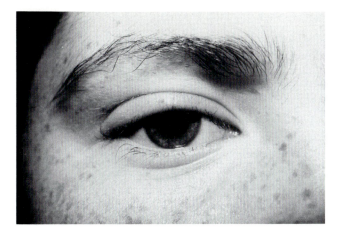

Figure 3–11. Functional eyelash and eyebrow plucking. Same patient as Figure 3–10, 3 months later after counseling. *(Courtesy of Maury A. Marmor; from Catalano RA: Ocular emergencies. Philadelphia, Saunders, 1992, p 454, with permission.)*

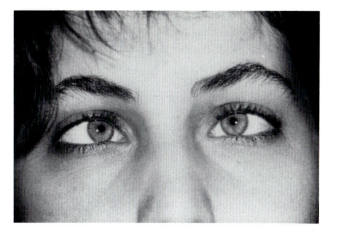

Figure 3–13. Spasm of the near reflex. Miosis and esotropia (inward turning of the eyes) during spasm. *(From Catalano RA: Ocular emergencies. Philadelphia, Saunders, 1992, p 447, with permission.)*

viduals also tend to pull out their scalp hair. Counseling may be required.

Spasm of the Near Reflex

The near-synkinetic response physiologically and unconsciously occurs to correct the otherwise blurred retinal image of near objects. It can also occur secondary to a conscious awareness of near. The response consists of the triad of convergence of the eyes, pupillary constriction, and accommodation of the ocular lens (an increase in the thickness and surface curvature of the lens to increase the focusing power of the eye).

Spasm of the near reflex, also known as accommodative spasm, consists of an excessive or inappropriate near response for the visual fixation distance. Characteristically, both pupils are miotic (small), the eyes are turned in as much as 50 degrees, and the accommoda-

tive power of the eye is increased up to 10 diopters (Figs. 3–12 and 3–13). The latter is confirmed by demonstrating less need for minus requirement (less myopia) on cycloplegic refraction (refraction using drops that paralyze the ability to accommodate) than on dry refraction. Invariably, it is difficult to maintain this spasm, and the typical patient presents with episodic or intermittent spasms lasting seconds to minutes. An occasional patient, however, may be able to maintain this for longer periods.

Patients with this disorder usually complain of headache, eyestrain, blurred vision, and/or diplopia. They may give a history of head trauma. On examination, the spasm can often be precipitated by having the patient fixate an interesting (accommodative) near object, manipulating the eyelids, or requesting that the patient gaze in a given direction. The most common misdiagnosis in these patients is bilateral sixth-nerve palsy. The intermittence of this condition, as well as the associated miosis and increased accommodation with these spasms, is suggestive against a sixth-nerve disorder.

Organic spasms of the near reflex have rarely been reported (Table 3–6). Usually patients with organic etiologies have associated neurological problems, or are unaware of their symptoms because of depressed con-

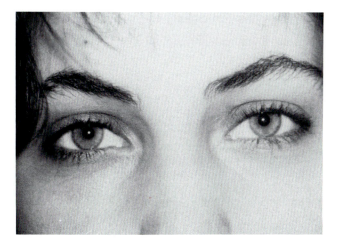

Figure 3–12. Spasm of the near reflex. Baseline state. *(From Catalano RA: Ocular emergencies. Philadelphia, Saunders, 1992, p 447, with permission.)*

TABLE 3–6. ORGANIC CAUSES OF SPASM OF THE NEAR REFLEX

Accommodative factor
Cerebellar tumor
Pituitary tumor
Vestibulopathy
Arnold-Chiari malformation
Previous head trauma

sciousness. Convergence spasm related to an accommodative factor can also rarely occur in children. Treatment for a latent hyperopia resolves this problem.

Voluntary Nystagmus

Voluntary nystagmus is a rapid, high-frequency, small-amplitude, difficult-to-maintain, horizontal oscillation of the eyes. It simulates a fine, rapid, pendular nystagmus, but actually consists of rapid right-to-left saccades. It can be recognized by its extreme rapidity (approximately 20 Hz) and the brevity of each episodic burst. Most subjects cannot sustain the oscillation for more than 10 seconds, and the maximum duration is estimated at less than 30 seconds. As many as 1 to 5 percent of the population may be able to generate these oscillations to some degree. There appears to be some hereditary influence, and it may be more common in individuals of British descent.

Unlike some of the other disorders discussed in this chapter, voluntary nystagmus is not a trait that develops or is seen in suggestive individuals. The subject has full appreciation of its occurrence and generates it either as a party trick or in a conscious effort to feign illness. Individuals with this ability were commonly seen in circus side shows of the past, and the medical literature cites many individuals who used this to be relieved from activities ranging from military duty to coal mining. It is now believed that "coal miner's nystagmus," a common affliction in England in the 18th and 19th centuries, was in fact voluntary nystagmus.

The disorder can usually be easily recognized by its rapidity and the inability of the individual to maintain the oscillation for longer than a few seconds. Individuals who appear to be able to maintain this for prolonged periods should be observed closely. Usually they turn away from the observer, grimace, or intermittently close their eyelids to rest their eyes between oscillatory bursts.

REFERENCES

Eye-popping Reflex

Perez RB: The eye-popping reflex of infants. Pediatrics 81:87, 1972.
Victor D: Eye-popping reflex in infants. Pediatrics 81:1223, 1972.

Functional Blinking

Jankovic J, Havins WE, Wilkins RB: Blinking and blepharospasm: Mechanism, diagnosis and management. JAMA 248:3160, 1982.
Miller NR, Gittinger JW, Keltner JL, et al: "Squeezing eyes": A clinical pathological conference. Surv Ophthalmol 26:97, 1982.
Vrabec TR, Levin AV, Nelson LB: Functional blinking in childhood. Pediatrics 83:967, 1989.

Functional Eyelid Pulling

Catalano RA, Trevisani MG, Simon JW: Functional eyelid pulling in children. Am J Ophthalmol 110:300, 1990.

Functional Visual Loss

Catalano RA, Simon JW, Krohel GB, Rosenberg PN: Functional visual loss in children. Ophthalmology 93:385, 1986.
Costenbader FD, Mousel DK: Functional amblyopia in early adolescence. Clin Proc Child Hosp 20:49, 1964.
Donin JF: The ophthalmic flake syndrome. In Smith JL (ed): Neuro-ophthalmology 1982. New York, Masson, 1981, pp 89–98.
Drews RC: Organic versus functional ocular problems. Int Ophthalmol Clin 7:666, 1967.
Gittinger JW Jr: Functional hemianopsia: A historical perspective. Surv Ophthalmol 32:427, 1988.
Gittinger JW Jr: Functional monocular temporal hemianopsia. Am J Ophthalmol 101:226, 1986.
Kathol RG, Cox TA, Corbett JJ, Thompson HS: Functional visual loss; follow-up of 42 cases. Arch Ophthalmol 101:729, 1983.
Keltner JL, May WN, Johnson CA, Post RB: The California syndrome: Functional visual complaints with potential economic impact. Ophthalmology 92:427, 1985.
Kramer KK, LaPiana FG, Appleton B: Ocular malingering and hysteria: Diagnosis and management. Surv Ophthalmol 24:89, 1979.
Miller BW: A review of practical tests for ocular malingering and hysteria. Surv Ophthalmol 17:241, 1973.
Rada RT, Meyer GG, Kellner R: Visual conversion reaction in children and adults. J Nerv Ment Dis 166:580, 1978.
Savir H, Segal M: A simple test for detection of monocular functional visual impairment. Am J Ophthalmol 106:500, 1988.
Smith TJ, Baker RS: Perimetric findings in functional disorders using automated techniques. Ophthalmology 94:1562, 1987.
Thompson HS: Functional visual loss. Am J Ophthalmol 100:209, 1985.
Weintraub MI: Hysterical Conversion Reactions. Jamaica, NY, Spectrum, 1983.

Learning Disabilities

American Academy of Ophthalmology. Policy statement: Learning Disabilities, Dyslexia, and Vision. San Francisco, AAO, 1992.
Bakker DJ: Temporal Order in Disturbed Reading. Rotterdam, University Press, 1972.
Birch HG, Belmont L: Auditory-visual integration, intelligence, and reading ability in school children. Percept Motor Skills 20:295, 1965.
Coles GS: The Learning Mystique: A Critical Look at "Learning Disabilities." New York, Pantheon, 1988.
Cotton MM, Evans KM: A review of the use of irlen (tinted) lenses. Aust NZ J Ophthalmol 18:307, 1990.
Council on Scientific Affairs: Dyslexia. JAMA 261:2236, 1989.
Duane DD, Gray DB (eds): The Reading Brain: The Biological Basis of Dyslexia. Parkton, ND, York Press, 1991.
Flax N: The contribution of visual problems to learning disability. J Am Optom Assoc 41:841, 1970.

Flax N, Solan HA, Suchoff IB: Optometry and dyslexia. J Am Optom Assoc 54:593, 1983.

Geiger G, Lettvin JY: Peripheral vision in persons with dyslexia. N Engl J Med 316:1238, 1987.

Helveston EM: Scotopic sensitivity syndrome. Arch Ophthalmol 108:1232, 1990.

Helveston EM: Management of dyslexia and related learning disabilities. Focal Points 1985: Clinical Modules for Ophthalmologists. San Francisco, American Academy of Ophthalmology, 1985.

Levine MD: Reading disability: Do the eyes have it? Pediatrics 73:869, 1984.

Lindgren SD, Richman L, Eliason M: Memory processes in reading disability subtypes. Dev Neuropsychol 2:173, 1986.

Metzger RL, Werner DB: Use of visual training for reading disabilities. A review. Pediatrics 73:824, 1984.

Olson RK, Kliegl R, Davidson BJ: Dyslexic and normal readers' eye movements. J Exp Psychol 9:816, 1983.

Pavlidis GT: The dyslexia syndrome and its objective diagnosis by erratic eye movements. In Rayner K (ed): Eye Movements in Reading. New York, Academic Press, 1983, pp 441–466.

Pennington BF, Gilger JW, Pauls D, et al: Evidence for major gene transmission of developmental dyslexia. JAMA 266:1527, 1991.

Sadun AA: Dyslexia at the *New York Times:* (Mis)understanding of parallel visual processing. Arch Ophthalmol 110:933, 1992.

Shaywitz BA, Waxman SG: Dyslexia. N Engl J Med 316:1268, 1987.

Shaywitz SE, Shaywitz BA, Fletcher JM, Escobar MD: Prevalence of reading disability in boys and girls. JAMA 264:998, 1990.

Silver LB: Controversial approaches to treating learning disabilities and attention deficit disorder. AJDC 140:1045, 1986.

Stein JF, Fowler S: A physiologic theory of visual dyslexia. Adv Neurol 42:233, 1984.

Vellutino FR: Dyslexia. Sci Am 256:34, 1987.

Vogel SA: Gender differences in intelligence, language, visual–motor abilities and academic achievement in males and females with learning disabilities: A review of the literature. J Learn Disabil 23:44, 1990.

Normal Visual Development

Abrahamsson M, Fabina G, Sjostrand J: Changes in astigmatism between the ages of 1 and 4 years: A longitudinal study. Br J Ophthalmol 72:145, 1988.

Angle J, Wissmann DA: Age, reading, and myopia. Am J Optom Physiol Opt 55:302, 1978.

Aslin RN, Dumais ST: Binocular vision in infants: A review and theoretical framework. Adv Child Dev Behav 15:54, 1980.

Baker FH, Grigg P, von Noorden GK: Effects of visual deprivation and strabismus on the response of neurons in the visual cortex of the monkey, including studies on the striate and prestriate cortex in the normal animal. Brain Res 66:185, 1974.

Banks MS: The development of visual accommodation during early infancy. Child Dev 51:646, 1980.

Braddick O, Atkinson J, French J, et al: A photorefractive study of infant accommodation. Vision Res 19:1319, 1979.

Brown EVL: Net average yearly changes in refraction of atropinized eyes from birth to middle life. Arch Ophthalmol 19:719, 1939.

Cook RC, Glasscock RE: Refractive and ocular findings in the newborn. Am J Ophthalmol 34:1407, 1951.

Crawford MLJ, Blake R, Cool SJ, von Noorden GK: Physiologic consequences of unilateral and bilateral eye closure in macaque monkeys. Some further observations. Brain Res 84:150, 1975.

Curtin BJ: The etiology of myopia. In Curtin BJ (ed): The Myopias: Basic Science and Clinical Management. Philadelphia, Harper & Row, 1985, pp 113–124.

Dobson V, Fulton AB, Manning K, et al: Cycloplegic refractions of premature infants. Am J Ophthalmol 91:490, 1981.

Eichel VL: Mannerisms of the blind: A review of the literature. J Vis Impairment Blindness 76:398, 1982.

Fledelius HC: Ophthalmic changes from age 10 to 18 years. A longitudinal study of sequels to low birth weight, IV. Ultrasound oculometry of vitreous and axial length. Acta Ophthalmol (Copenh) 60:403, 1978.

Fledelius HC: Prematurity and the eye. Ophthalmic 10-year follow-up of children of low and normal birth weight. Acta Ophthalmol (Copenh) (suppl)58:128, 1976.

Fox R, Aslin RN, Shea SL, et al: Stereopsis in human infants. Science 207:323, 1984.

Friedburg D, Sons S: Refraction during the first year of life and the development of astigmatism. Klin Mbl Augenheilk 182:309, 1983.

Fulton AB, Dobson V, Salem D, et al: Cycloplegic refractions in infants and young children. Am J Ophthalmol 90:239, 1980.

Isenberg SJ: Physical and refractive characteristics of the eye at birth and during infancy. In Isenberg SJ: The Eye in Infancy. Chicago, Year Book, 1990.

Kushner BJ: Strabismus and amblyopia associated with regressed retinopathy of prematurity. Arch Ophthalmol 100:256, 1982.

Larsen JS: The sagittal growth of the eye, I. Ultrasonic measurement of the anterior chamber from birth to puberty. Acta Ophthalmol (Copenh) 49:239, 1971.

McBrien NA, Millodot M: The relationship between tonic accommodation and refractive error. Invest Ophthalmol Vis Sci 28:997, 1987.

Mohindra I, Held R: Refractions in humans from birth to 5 years. Doc Ophthalmol 28:19, 1981.

Moller MA: The ophthalmologists role with visually impaired children. In Nelson LB, Calhoun JH, Harley RD (eds): Pediatric Ophthalmology, 3rd ed. Philadelphia, Saunders, 1992, pp 512–517.

Nelson, LB: Pediatric Ophthalmology. Philadelphia, Saunders, 1984.

Nelson LB, Rubin SE, Wagner, RS, Breton ME: Developmental aspects in the assessment of visual function in young children. Pediatrics 73:375, 1984.

Nixon RB, Helveston EM, Miller K, et al: Incidence of strabismus in neonates. Am J Ophthalmol 100:798, 1985.

Rosner M, Belkin M: Intelligence, education, and myopia in males. Arch Ophthalmol 105:1508, 1987.

Scharf J, Zonis S, Zeltner M: Refraction in premature babies: A prospective study. J Pediatr Ophthalmol Strabismus 15:48, 1978.

Slataper FJ: Age norms of refraction and vision. Arch Ophthalmol 43:466, 1950.

Sorsby A, Leary G: A longitudinal study of refraction and its components during growth. Medical Research Council, Special Report Series 309:1. London, Her Majesty's Stationery Office, 1969.

Sperduto RD, Seigel D, Roberts J, et al: Prevalence of myopia in the United States. Arch Ophthalmol 101:405, 1983.

Tychsen L, Lisberger SG: Visual motion processing for the initiation of smooth-pursuit eye movements in humans. J Neurophysiol 56:953, 1986.

Van Essen DC: Visual areas of the mammalian cerebral cortex. Ann Rev Neurosci Abstr 10:912, 1984.

Van Essen DC, Maunsell JHR: Hierarchical organization and functional streams in the visual cortex. Trends Neurosci 6:370, 1983.

Wiesel TN, Habel DH: Single-cell responses in striate cortex of kittens deprived of vision in one eye. J Neurophysiol 26:1003, 1963.

Spasm of the Near Reflex

Cogan DG, Freese CG Jr: Spasm of the near reflex. Arch Ophthalmol 54:752, 1955.

Dagi LR, Chrousos GA, Cogan DC: Spasm of the nerve reflex associated with organic disease. Am J Ophthalmol 103:582, 1987.

Guiloff RJ: Organic convergence spasm. Acta Neurol Scandinav 61:252, 1980.

Herman P: Convergence spasm. Mt Sinai J Med 44:501, 1977.

Jeanrot N: Convergence spasms in the adult. J Fr Ophthalmol 10:135, 1987.

Vision Screening

Abramov I, Hainline L, Duckman RH: Screening infant vision with paraxial photorefraction. Optom Vis Sci 67:538, 1990.

Angi MR, Cocchiglia A: The binocular infrared videorefractometer: An instrument for the screening of amblyogenic factors and the dynamic study of accommodation in children. Bollettina di Oculistica 69:305, 1990.

Atkinson J, Braddick OJ, Durden K, et al: Screening for refractive errors in 6–9 month old infants by photorefraction. Br J Ophthalmol 68:105, 1984.

Bobier WR: Quantitative photorefraction using an off-center flash source. Am J Optom Physiol Optics 65:962, 1988.

Cibis GW, Maino JH, Crandall MA: The Parsons visual acuity test for screening children 18 to 48 months old. Ann Ophthalmol 17:471, 1985.

Cotter SA, Scharre JE: The Lang stereotest: Performance by strabismic, amblyopic, and visually normal patients. Am J Optom Physiol Opt 64:68, 1987.

Day SH, Norcia AM: Photographic screening for factors leading to amblyopia. Am Orthopt J 38:51, 1988.

De Becker I, MacPherson HJ, LaRoche GR, et al: Negative predictive value of a population-based preschool vision screening program. Ophthalmology 99:998, 1992.

Ehrlich MI, Reinecke RD, Simmons K: Preschool vision screening for amblyopia and strabismus. Programs, methods, guidelines. Surv Ophthalmol 28:145, 1983.

Freedman HL, Preston KL: Polaroid photoscreening for amblyogenic factors: An improved methodology. Ophthalmology 99:1785, 1992.

Fulton A: Screening preschool children to detect visual and ocular disorders. Arch Ophthalmol 110:1553, 1992.

Helveston EM, Helveston BH, Ellis FD, et al: A performance test to accompany ophthalmic examination in the young school age child: The "draw a bicycle" test. J Pediatr Ophthalmol Strabismus 22:17, 1985.

Hsu-Winges C, Hamer RD, Norcia AM, et al: Polaroid photorefractive screening of infants. J Pediatr Ophthalmol Strabismus 26:254, 1989.

Ingram RM: Refraction as a basis for screening children for squint and amblyopia. Br J Ophthalmol 61:8, 1977.

Ingram RM, Traynar MJ, Walker C, Wilson JM: Screening for refractive errors at age 1 year: A pilot study. Br J Ophthalmol 63:243, 1979.

Ingram RM, Walker C, Wilson JM, et al: Prediction of amblyopia and squint by means of refraction at age 1 year. Br J Ophthalmol 70:12, 1986.

Lang JI, Lang TJ: Eye screening with the Lang stereotest. Am Orthoptic J 38:48, 1988.

Manny RE, Martinez AT, Fern KD: Testing stereopsis in the preschool child: Is it clinically useful? J Pediatr Ophthalmol Strabismus 28:223, 1991.

Reinecke RD: Screening 3-year-olds for visual problems: Are we gaining or falling behind? Arch Ophthalmol 105:1497, 1987.

Ruttum MS, Nelson DB: Stereopsis testing to reduce over-referral in preschool vision screening. J Pediatr Ophthalmol Strabismus 28:131, 1991.

Stager D: Preferential looking and recognition acuities in clinical amblyopia: Discussion. J Ped Ophthalmol Strabismus 28:326, 1991.

Taylor D: Screening for squint and poor vision. Arch Dis Child 62:982, 1987.

Taylor D: The assessment of visual function in young children: An overview. Clin Pediatr 17:226, 1978.

Teller DY, McDonald MA, Preston K, et al: Assessment of visual acuity in infants and children: The Teller acuity card procedure. Dev Med Child Neurol 28:779, 1986.

Tongue AC, Cibis GW: Bruckner test. Ophthalmology 88:1041, 1981.

Voluntary Nystagmus

Aschoff JC, Becker W, Rettelbach R: Voluntary nystagmus, saccadic suppression, and stabilization of the visual world. Vision Res 20:717, 1980.

Shults WT, Stark L, Hoyt WF, et al: Normal saccadic structure and voluntary nystagmus. Arch Ophthalmol 95:1399, 1977.

Zahn JR: Incidence and characteristics of voluntary nystagmus. J Neurol Neurosurg Psychiatry 41:617, 1978.

CHAPTER
4

ABNORMALITIES AFFECTING THE ENTIRE EYE AND THE PHAKOMATOSES

ESSENTIAL INFORMATION FOR PRIMARY CARE PRACTITIONERS

Abnormal Development of the Entire Eye

Several terms describe abnormal development of the entire eye. Each correlates with a different stage of arrest of embryogenesis. Anophthalmia means the congenital absence of the eye. It results from a failure of the optic vesicle or pit to develop. Microphthalmos means a small, deformed eye. It results from a retardation in growth that occurs once the optic pit has formed. Microphthalmos with cyst is a subcategory of the latter that results from defective closure of the embryonic fissure. Each of these abnormalities will be apparent at birth, and may be associated with other systemic findings (Table 4–1).

Systemic Syndromes that Affect the Entire Eye

Ocular abnormalities are a component of many systemic syndromes. We review most syndromes under the category where their principal ocular manifestations are found; for example, Marfan syndrome in Chapter 11 (*Disorders of the Lens*); cystinosis in Chapter 9 (*Disorders of the Cornea*). Two common disorders

that variably affect multiple structures of the eye are discussed in this chapter. These are Down syndrome and fetal alcohol syndrome.

Down Syndrome

Ocular and orbital abnormalities are nearly uniformly found in individuals with Down syndrome. With the exception of the vitreous, structural abnormalities have been documented in every ocular tissue. Despite this propensity to involve the eye, a specific phenotypic ocular expression of Down syndrome does not exist. No ocular finding is pathognomonic, as similar anomalies occur in otherwise normal individuals, or in persons with other mental or physical defects. No individual exhibits every abnormality, and subcategories of indi-

TABLE 4–1. ASSOCIATED FINDINGS IN INDIVIDUALS WITH ABNORMAL DEVELOPMENT OF THE EYE

Mental retardation
Skeletal anomalies
Craniofacial anomalies
Congenital heart disease
Seizures
Spastic diplegia
Cleft lip or palate

TABLE 4–2. MAJOR OCULAR FEATURES OF DOWN SYNDROME

Structure	Abnormality
Eyelids	Upward-slanting palpebral fissures Narrow interpupillary distance Prominent epicanthal folds Blepharitis Congenital eversion of the upper eyelid
Cornea	Keratoconus
Iris	Brushfield spots Iris hypoplasia
Lens	Congenital cataracts Flake-like cortical opacities
Retina	Increased number of vessels at the optic disc
Optic nerve	Idiopathic optic disc elevation
Strabismus	Esotropia (rarely exotropia)
Nystagmus	Horizontal, fine, rapid, pendular
Refractive	High myopia (> 8.00 diopters) High astigmatism (> 2.50 diopters)

TABLE 4–4. MAJOR OCULAR FEATURES OF THE PHAKOMATOSES

Disorder	Major Ocular Features
Neurofibromatosis	Neurofibromas of the eyelids, uvea, and orbits Thickened corneal nerves Iris nevi (Lisch nodules) Uveal nevi and melanomas Orbital and optic nerve meningiomas Optic nerve gliomas Retinal astrocytomas Infantile glaucoma
Tuberous sclerosis	Retinal astrocytomas
Ataxia telangiectasia	Telangiectasias of bulbar conjunctival venules
Von Hippel–Lindau syndrome	Retinal capillary hemangiomas
Sturge–Weber syndrome	Dilated episcleral and conjunctival vessels Diffuse choroidal hemangioma Infantile glaucoma
Wyburn–Mason syndrome	Ocular and orbital arteriovenous malformations

viduals with concordant constellations of findings do not exist. Although isolated reports of ocular features are numerous, only anomalies that occur frequently are discussed in this chapter (Table 4–2).

Fetal Alcohol Syndrome

Alcohol has been shown to freely cross the placental barrier. Infants born to mothers who imbibe can have a constellation of anomalies known as the fetal alcohol syndrome (FAS). Although not part of the criteria for diagnosis, as many as 90 percent of children with FAS have ocular abnormalities. These include eyelid anomalies, strabismus, and defects in intraocular structures. The ocular features of FAS are listed in Table 4–3, and are reviewed under "Comprehensive Information" later in the chapter.

TABLE 4–3. MAJOR OCULAR FEATURES OF THE FETAL ALCOHOL SYNDROME

Structure	Abnormality
Entire eye	Microphthalmos
Eyelids	Short horizontal palpebral fissures Ptosis
Cornea	Microcornea Peter's anomaly
Anterior segment	Axenfeld's anomaly
Retina	Tortuous vessels
Optic nerve	Hypoplasia
Strabismus	Esotropia (rarely exotropia)
Refractive	High myopia, hyperopia, and astigmatism

The Phakomatoses

In 1932, van der Hoeve collectively named several systemic syndromes characterized by tumors involving the eyes, skin, and central nervous system as phakomatoses (van der Hoeve, 1932). The term "phakomata" means "mother spot" or birthmark in Greek, and implies that the skin findings are markers for ocular and neurological tumors. These tumors are hamartomas; they arise from the faulty embryonal development of cells and tissues natural to an organ or site. The major phakomatoses include neurofibromatosis, tuberous sclerosis, ataxia telangiectasia, and the von Hippel–Lindau, Sturge–Weber, and Wyburn–Mason syndromes. The ocular features of each are listed in Table 4–4, and are reviewed under "Comprehensive Information" later in the chapter.

COMPREHENSIVE INFORMATION ON ABNORMALITIES AFFECTING THE ENTIRE EYE AND THE PHAKOMATOSES

Abnormal Development of the Eye

Anophthalmia

Anophthalmia is the congenital absence of the eye (Figs. 4–1 and 4–2). Three categories of the disorder have been described: (1) primary, due to isolated failure of optic vesicle or pit formation (the remainder of the neural tube is unaffected); (2) secondary, due to

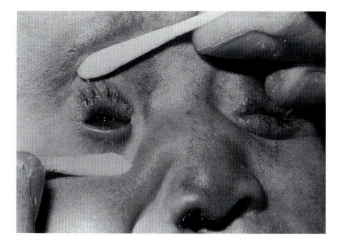

Figure 4–1. Bilateral anophthalmos. Note absence of the right globe. *(From Nelson LB, Brown GC, Arentsen JJ: Recognizing patterns of ocular childhood diseases. Thorofare, NJ, Slack, 1985, p 3, with permission.)*

complete suppression of forebrain development (the anophthalmia is a component of gross neural malformation); and (3) consecutive (degenerative), due to regression of a formed optic pit.

Anophthalmia can be difficult to distinguish clinically from profound microphthalmos. The diagnosis should be established by computed tomography, magnetic resonance imaging, or histological examination of the orbital contents.

Clinical anophthalmia has been reported in trisomy 13 syndrome and phenotype, various cerebral maldevelopments, and Klinefelter's syndrome. Most cases of anophthalmia occur sporadically, although autosomal dominant, autosomal recessive, and sex-linked recessive transmissions have been reported.

The causes for developmental failure of the optic vesicle or pit, or their regression, may include environ-

mental factors such as radiation, anoxia, or intrauterine infection. Animal models of anophthalmia suggest that suppression of the optic vesicles may result from the introduction of a variety of teratogenic factors, such as lithium, trypan blue, or actinomycin, at the time of optic vesicle development.

The orbit is concomitantly underdeveloped in anophthalmia. Expansion therapy should be initiated beginning the first month of life and continued until puberty. Progressively larger conformers are used to increase the size of the orbit until a suitable prosthesis can be worn.

Microphthalmos

Microphthalmic globes vary in size, and may be so small that they escape clinical detection. In addition to being abnormally small, many of these eyes have structural anomalies (see Figs. 9–8 and 9–9). Such eyes are often designated as having "complicated" microphthalmos (Table 4–5). Microphthalmos is also frequently accompanied by systemic abnormalities (see Table 4–1).

Microphthalmos represents a retardation in growth that occurs once the primary optic vesicle has formed and invaginated to form the optic pit. It has been caused in animal experiments by radiation, mechanical stimulation, and chemicals. Microphthalmos can also result from intrauterine toxoplasmosis or rubella, and it can occur as a component of a genetic syndrome such as Norrie's syndrome, oculodentodigital dysplasia, or Fanconi's syndrome.

Microphthalmos With Cyst

Microphthalmos with cyst results from a defective closure of the embryonic fissure. Proliferation of the neuroectoderm at the edge of a persistent embryonic fissure may form a cyst, the cavity of which is continuous with the interior of the microphthalmic globe. The cyst may be too small to detect clinically, or so large as to deform surrounding tissues. In the latter cases, the eye is often clinically undetectable (Figure 4–3).

The majority of cases are unilateral (Fig. 4–4). In rare cases, the anterior segment of the microphthalmic eye may appear normal. More commonly, the anterior eye displays marked disorganization and iridocorneal adhesions. The lens is frequently cataractous and dislocated, and the retina detached, disorganized, and gliotic.

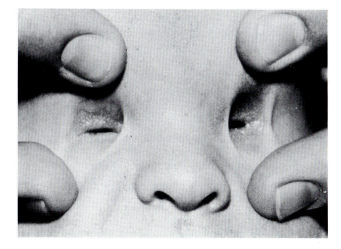

Figure 4–2. Bilateral anophthalmos. *(Courtesy of Robinson D. Harley; from Nelson LB: Pediatric ophthlamology. Philadelphia, Saunders, 1984, with permission.)*

TABLE 4–5. OCULAR FINDINGS OF COMPLICATED MICROPHTHALMOS

Corneal opacities
Cataract
Aniridia
Correctopia
Persistent pupillary membrane
Retinal abnormalities (gliosis, rosette formation)

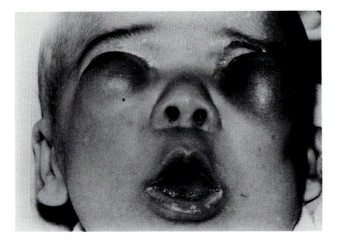

Figure 4–3. Bilateral microphthalmos with cyst. Note the discolored distension of both lower eyelids. The cysts were easily deformable and transmitted light. *(From Foxman S, Cameron JD: The clinical implications of bilateral microphthalmos with cyst. Am J Ophthalmol 97:632, 1984, with permission.)*

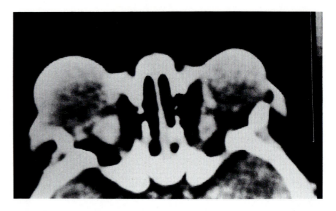

Figure 4–5. Axial CT of the orbits of patient in Figure 4–3 demonstrates large cystic cavities with a uniform fluid density. *(From Foxman S, Cameron JD: The clinical implications of bilateral microphthalmos with cyst. Am J Ophthalmol 97:632, 1984, with permission.)*

No consistent systemic anomalies have been documented in microphthalmos with cyst. In one series of 74 cases of the disorder, only 8 patients had systemic abnormalities (Natanson, 1908). These included cardiac, urogenital, facial, skeletal, and central nervous system (meningoencephalocele and hydrocephalus) defects.

The diagnosis of microphthalmos with cyst is facilitated by ultrasonography and neuroimaging. These tests usually demonstrate the cystic lesion adjacent to a microphthalmic eye (Figs. 4–5 and 9–32). Treatment consists of simple aspiration, excision of the cyst, or removal of both the cyst and microphthalmic eye, which usually necessitates orbital or eyelid reconstruction for prosthetic fitting.

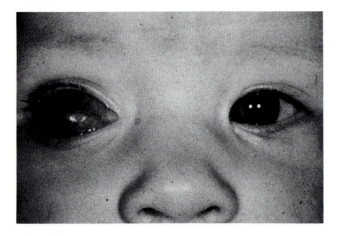

Figure 4–4. Microphthalmos with cyst in the right eye *(AFIP no. 22094 courtesy of Torrence A. Makley, Jr; from Nelson LB, Folberg R: Ocular developmental anomalies. In Duane T, Jaeger EA (eds): Biomedical Foundations of Ophthalmology. Philadelphia, Lippincott, 1984, with permission.)*

Down Syndrome

Down syndrome (DS) is the most common human chromosomal abnormality. It occurs in almost 1 in 600 live births. Although first described in 1866 (Down, 1866), it was only with the advent of karyotyping that

TABLE 4–6. MAJOR SYSTEMIC FEATURES OF DOWN SYNDROME

Structure	Abnormality
Central nervous system	Mental deficiency, near normal social skills Variable IQ (average 50)
Cranium	Small brachycephalic skull Flat occiput Sinus hypoplasia
Ears	Small, low-set, straight superior helix
Nose	Flat nasal bridge
Mouth	Dental hypoplasia Thickened, roughened, protruding tongue
Neck	Broad and short Redundant lax skin
Hands	Hypoplasia of middle phalanx of fifth finger Short, broad hands and feet
Feet	Wide space between 1st and 2nd toes
Dermatoglyphics	Simian crease Ulnar deviated loops on fingers
Musculoskeletal system	Diastasis recti abdominus Hypotonia, hyperextensibility
Heart	Atrial and ventricular defects Tetralogy of Fallot Patent ductus arteriosus
Gastrointestinal system	Duodenal atresia Imperforate anus Hirschsprung disease

From Catalano RA: Down syndrome. Surv Ophthalmology 34:388 (Table 1), with permission.

the cause of the syndrome, an extra chromosome 21, was determined (Lejeune et al, 1959).

The major systemic features of Down syndrome are summarized in Table 4–6; several are illustrated in Figure 4–6. The characteristic facies includes upward slanting palpebral fissures; an open mouth with a thick, roughened, protruding tongue; a flat nasal bridge; and small, low-set ears. Most individuals with DS have some degree of developmental deficiency. Congenital heart defects, typically endocardial cushion defects, occur in 30 to 50 percent of cases. Individuals with DS also have a 15 times greater risk of developing acute lymphoblastic leukemia, and an increased incidence of Alzheimer's disease, autoimmune thyroid disease, diabetes, and chronic active hepatitis. Infectious diseases also occur at an increased frequency; prior to antibiotics, DS children succumbed to pneumonia at 70 times the rate of other children. Finally, for unknown reasons, DS individuals are especially sensitive to the affects of atropine.

The ocular findings of DS are summarized in Table 4–2. External ocular findings include a narrowed interpupillary distance and epicanthus. Blepharitis occurs with an increased frequency, as does congenital eversion of the upper eyelids. Up to 8 percent of DS individuals develop keratoconus, and hydrops occurs much more frequently as a complication of keratoconus in DS (see Fig. 9–51). Congenital glaucoma has been reported in 12 DS children (see Fig. 10–47). White to light yellow, peripheral, 0.1- to 1.0-mm iris nodules, called Brushfield spots, associated with iris hypoplasia, occur in 80 to 90 percent of DS patients (Fig. 4–7). Flakelike "coronary-cerulean" lens opacities occur in 25 to 85 percent of subjects. Congenital cataracts occur at an increased frequency, and senile cataracts occur at a younger age.

An increased number of retinal vessels crossing the disc margin, often arranged in a spoke-like distribution, has also been described (Fig. 4–8). Remitting optic disc elevation, in the absence of papilledema and disc drusen, has been noted in some DS children. Strabismus, usually esotropia, occurs in 25 to 45 percent of DS

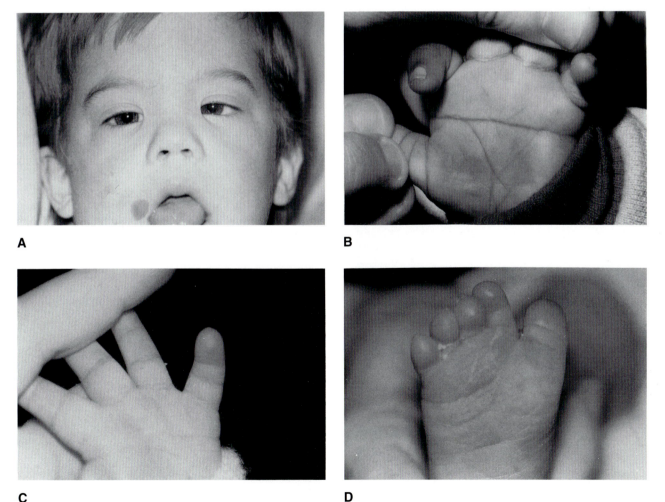

A　　　　　　　　　　　　　　　　　　　　**B**

C　　　　　　　　　　　　　　　　　　　　**D**

Figure 4–6. Systemic features of Down syndrome. **A.** Facies of Down syndrome. **B.** Simian crease. **C.** Hypoplasia of middle phalanx and incurving of fifth finger. **D.** Wide separation between first and second toes.

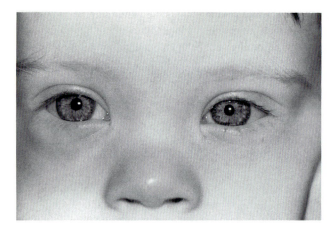

Figure 4–7. Brushfield spots in the iris in Down syndrome.

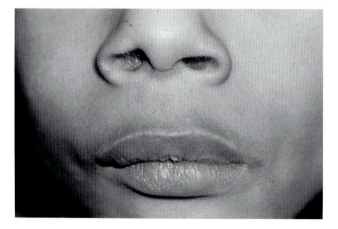

Figure 4–9. Facial dysmorphism in fetal alcoholism syndrome: poorly developed philtrum, and flat hypoplastic maxillary area.

patients (see Fig. 4–6), but amblyopia is surprisingly rarer, occurring in less than 10 percent of even the strabismic patients. Nystagmus, typically horizontal, fine, rapid, and pendular has been reported in 5 to 30 percent of DS individuals. It is especially prevalent in esotropic patients, and usually no ocular pathology contributing to poor retinal image formation is present. Finally, extremes in refractive errors have been well documented in DS. Thirty-five to 40 percent of individuals have high myopia (>8.00 diopters). Astigmatism of greater than 2.50 diopters has been reported in 18 to 25 percent.

Cataracts and keratoconus are the principle causes of visual loss in DS, but strabismus, blepharitis, and high refractive errors are additional treatable and common ocular conditions.

Fetal Alcohol Syndrome

The minimal criteria for the diagnosis of FAS are (1) prenatal and/or postnatal growth retardation at less than the 10th percentile; (2) central nervous system abnormalities (such as neurological abnormalities, developmental delay, and intellectual impairment); and (3) facial dysmorphism with two or more of the following: microcephaly, microphthalmia, short palpebral fissure, poorly developed philtrum, flat hypoplastic maxillary area, and thin upper lip (Fig. 4–9). Over 40 percent of children born to alcoholic mothers show the complete syndrome.

Other systemic anomalies include cardiovascular defects (atrial and ventricular septal defects, patent ductus arteriosus, peripheral pulmonary stenosis); metabolic abnormalities (hypoglycemia, hypocalcemia, and hyperbilirubinemia); and joint anomalies (limited motion at the elbow, interphalangeal, and metacarpalphalangeal joints); and decreased muscle tone.

Ocular anomalies include extremes in refractive er-

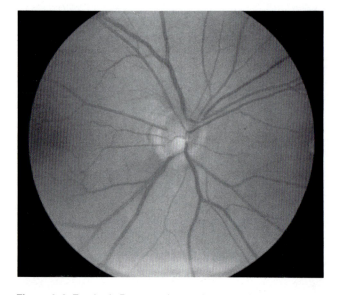

Figure 4–8. Fundus in Down syndrome, demonstrating an increased number of retinal vessels crossing the disc margin, arranged in a spoke-like pattern.

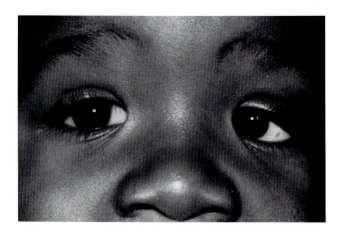

Figure 4–10. Eye changes in fetal alcohol syndrome: short horizontal palpebral fissures, ptosis, telecanthus, and esotropia.

rors, often causing poor vision. Outer eye changes include short horizontal palpebral fissures, ptosis, and telecanthus (increased distance between the medial canthi) (Fig. 4–10). Strabismus, most commonly esotropia, is found in almost half of the affected children. Anterior segment abnormalities include microcornea and Peter's and Axenfeld's anomalies. The fundus, however, is the most frequent site of intraocular anomaly. The most typical malformations are hypoplasia of the optic nerve head and increased tortuosity of the retinal vessels, especially the arteries. Optic nerve hypoplasia is associated with poor vision; there are no visual sequelae of tortuous retinal vessels.

The Phakomatoses

Neurofibromatosis (NF)

One in every 3000 to 4000 individuals is born with the neurofibromatosis (NF) gene. Half of these inherit the disorder from an affected parent; the others represent new mutations of a gene on chromosome 17 that has an unusually high spontaneous mutation rate (Barker et al, 1987). No racial, geographic, or ethnic predilection exists.

Four forms of NF have been described. The most common form, NF1 (peripheral NF), was first described in 1882 (von Recklinghausen, 1882). Bilateral acoustic neurofibromatosis (NF2, central NF) has only recently been recognized as a separate entity. Segmental neurofibromatosis (NF3) is a rare form in which hamartomas are limited to a circumscribed body part (usually the trunk). This disorder may result from a postzygotic somatic mutation, and as such may be less heritable. Cutaneous neurofibromatosis (NF4) has been described in only two families. Only café-au-lait spots are present in NF4; this disorder appears to be a forme fruste of NF1.

Von Recklinghausen Neurofibromatosis (NF1).

The criteria for diagnosing NF1, as adopted by a National Institutes of Health Consensus Conference, are listed in Table 4–7. Cutaneous, ocular, and neurological abnormalities occur in this disorder.

TABLE 4–7. DIAGNOSTIC CRITERIA FOR VON RECKLINGHAUSEN NEUROFIBROMATOSIS (NF1)

- **PRESENCE OF TWO OF THE FOLLOWING CRITIERA**
    1. Six café-au-lait spots
       >5 mm, if prepubertal
       >15 mm, if postpubertal
    2. Two or more neurofibromas of any type, or one plexiform neurofibroma
    3. Axillary or inguinal freckling
    4. A distinctive osseous lesion such as sphenoid dysplasia
    5. Optic nerve glioma
    6. Two or more iris Lisch nodules
    7. A first-degree relative with NF1

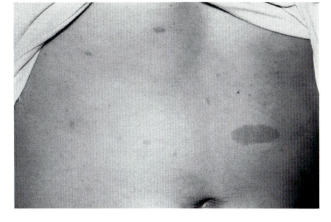

Figure 4–11. Café-au-lait spots on the abdomen in neurofibromatosis (NF1).

Flat, hyperpigmented skin lesions termed café-au-lait spots (Figs. 4–11 and 4–12), caused by an increased number of melanocytes in the basal epithelium, are present in over 99 percent of patients with NF1. Some may be present at birth. The number and size of these increase during the first decade, especially during the first 2 years of life. They are more commonly found on the trunk and extremities than on the face. Hyperpigmentation in intertriginous areas, particularly the axilla (axillary freckling, Fig. 4–13) is also common.

Neurofibromas are benign proliferations of Schwann cells and fibroblasts. Deeper peripheral and autonomic nerves of viscera and blood vessels may be involved, in addition to the usual tumors of the skin. Neurofibromas may be solitary, discrete, and nodular (Fig. 4–14), or diffuse and plexiform (Fig. 4–15). Plexiform neurofibromas of the upper eyelid are associated with a higher incidence of congenital glaucoma in the involved eye, as well as bony defects in the surrounding bones. Pregnancy and puberty are associated with an increase in the number and size of neurofibromas.

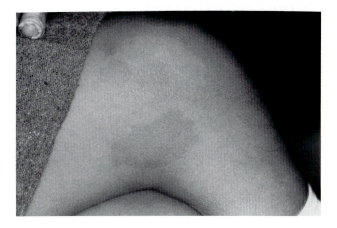

Figure 4–12. Café-au-lait spots on the leg of the same patient as Figure 4–11.

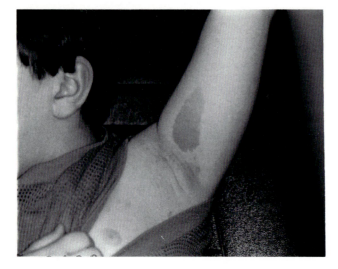

Figure 4–13. Axillary freckling in neurofibromatosis (NF1).

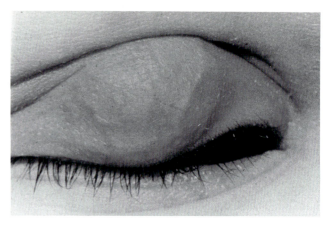

Figure 4–15. Neurofibroma of the upper eyelid. *(Courtesy of the Wills Eye Hospital slide collection.)*

The ocular findings of NF1 include Lisch nodules, uveal nevi, optic nerve gliomas, glial tumors of the retina, an increased incidence of meningiomas and congenital glaucoma, and thickened corneal nerves. Lisch nodules (Figs. 4–16 and 4–17) are present in 95 percent of patients with NF1, 6 years of age or older, and in about 30 percent of younger patients. They are comprised solely of melanocytic cells and do not interfere with vision. Uveal nevi (Fig. 4–18) may be present in up to 35 percent of patients with NF1, but do not appear to be associated with an increased risk of malignant melanoma.

Optic nerve and/or chiasmal gliomas occur in about 10 to 15 percent of children with NF1, and approximately 50 percent of children with optic nerve gliomas have NF1 (see Figs. 8–24 to 8–29). Differing from gliomas that arise in patients without NF, optic nerve gliomas associated with NF often proliferate in the subarachnoid space. This finding can be detected with magnetic resonance imaging. These tumors may be asymptomatic or associated with proptosis, nystagmus, strabismus, optic disc swelling, or optic atrophy; visual prognosis, however, is generally good. Meningiomas also occur more frequently in patients with NF1, producing slow loss of vision with only minimal proptosis. Glial hamartomas of the nerve fiber layer are rarely seen in NF1, being more common in patients with tuberous sclerosis (see below).

Infantile glaucoma is present in up to 50 percent of children with palpable plexiform neurofibromas of the upper eyelid. Glaucoma arises due to a developmental anomaly or tumor infiltration of the anterior chamber angle. Thickened corneal nerves are a rare finding in NF1.

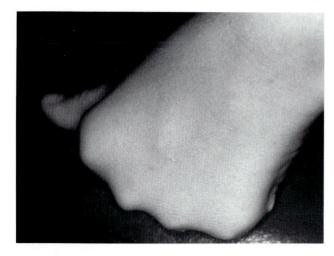

Figure 4–14. Solitary neurofibroma of a cutaneous nerve of the hand in neurofibromatosis (NF1).

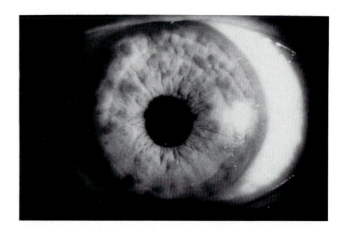

Figure 4–16. Lisch nodules of the iris in neurofibromatosis (NF1). *(Courtesy of the Albany Medical College slide collection.)*

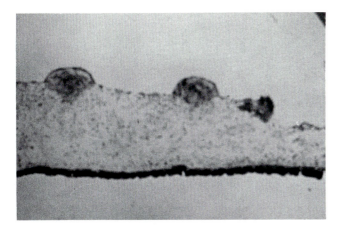

Figure 4–17. Histological section of Lisch nodules, demonstrating collections of benign melanocytic cells. *(Courtesy of the Albany Medical College slide collection.)*

TABLE 4–8. DIAGNOSTIC CRITERIA FOR BILATERAL ACOUSTIC NEUROFIBROMATOSIS (NF2)

■ *PRESENCE OF EITHER OF THE FOLLOWING CRITERIA*

1. CT or MRI evidence of bilateral internal auditory canal masses consistent with acoustic neuroma
2. A first-degree relative with NF2, and either:
   a. A unilateral internal auditory canal mass, or
   b. Two of the following:
      1. Neurofibroma
      2. Meningioma
      3. Optic nerve glioma
      4. Schwannoma
      5. Juvenile posterior subcapsular lenticular opacity

Bony abnormalities in NF1 include scoliosis; defects in the sphenoid, temporal, or frontal bones; and, rarely, spina bifida and syndactyly. Orbital asymmetry may be due to either unilateral orbital hypertrophy or hypoplasia. Congenital absence of the greater wing of the sphenoid bone, or its erosion by a plexiform neurofibroma, can result in an orbital encephalocele (see Figs. 8–64 and 8–65). A pulsating exophthalmos may be visible in affected individuals due to transmission of the systolic pulse of brain arterioles. Short stature and macrocephaly (head circumference greater than the 97th percentile) are common. The latter does not correlate with reduced intelligence, seizures, or headaches, all of which occur with greater incidence in patients with NF1.

Additional abnormalities that occur with some regularity in individuals with NF1 include hypertension, constipation, pruritus, and malignant neoplasms. The latter may also occur with increased incidence in first-degree female relatives. Ophthalmologists should also be aware that as many as 40 percent of children with NF1 have some form of learning disability.

Bilateral Acoustic Neurofibromatosis (NF2).

NF2 (central NF) affects only one in 50,000 individuals. It occurs secondary to a mutation of a gene on chromosome 22 (Rouleau et al, 1987). The criteria for diagnosing NF2 are listed in Table 4–8. The disorder is characterized by bilateral acoustic neuromas with a paucity of other findings. Only about one third of individuals with NF2 have six or more café-au-lait spots or cutaneous neurofibromas; 50 percent have neither.

Acoustic neuromas present in young adulthood with progressive hearing loss, imbalance, tinnitus, and headache. Multiple cranial nerves can become involved. Esotropia and diplopia can result from abducens paralysis; a central Bell's palsy from involvement of the seventh nerve; and facial dysesthesia from fifth cranial nerve enmeshment. Nearly 95 percent of affected individuals develop bilateral hearing loss with time. Surgery is the treatment of choice for rapidly progressing tumors, but may prematurely result in loss of hearing.

The principal ocular feature is the development of posterior subcapsular lens opacities (see Fig. 12–45) by young adulthood. Fibroglial proliferation anterior to the nerve fiber layer (epiretinal membrane), and combined hamartoma of the retina and retinal pigment epithelium (see Fig. 12–38), have also recently been described in NF2 (Sivalingam et al, 1991).

Tuberous Sclerosis

The constellation of mental retardation, epilepsy, and a vesiculopapular eruption that occurs over the cheeks and nasolabial folds in a butterfly distribution was first described by Bourneville (1880). The name "tuberous sclerosis" derives from the pathognomonic sclerotic

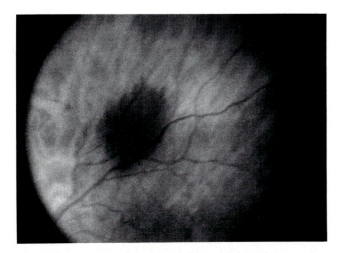

Figure 4–18. Uveal nevus in neurofibromatosis (NF1).

hamartomas (potato-like "tubers" or "brain stones") of the cerebral cortex. The complete diagnostic criteria for this disorder are listed in Table 4–9.

The abnormal gene is believed to be located on chromosome 9 and occurs with a prevalence of one in every 30,000 individuals. Although an autosomal dominant disorder, up to 80 percent of cases may occur as new mutations. There is no race or sex predilection.

Myoclonic spasms of the neck, trunk, and limbs, called infantile or salaam spasms, are the most common presenting sign, occurring in over 90 percent of affected infants. In childhood, these progress to grand mal seizures. Mental retardation is present in only 60 percent of patients, but progressive mental deterioration occurs in most cases. Neurological signs are related to the pale, hard, yellow-white proliferations of glial elements called "tubers" in the cerebral cortex and subependymal tissue (Fig. 4–19).

Cutaneous lesions include adenoma sebaceum, ash leaf spots, shagreen patches, subungual fibromas, and café-au-lait spots. **Adenoma sebaceum** is a misnomer, as these tumors are not adenomas, nor are they comprised of sebaceous tissue. Histologically they are angiofibromas. They present as early as 2 years of age, and will be present in 80 to 90 percent of affected individuals by age 6 years. In childhood, they appear as 1- to 2-mm reddish-brown papules on the malar region of the face; with time they increase in number and size (Fig. 4–20). **Ash leaf spots** are hypopigmented macules that are oval at one end and pointed at the other. They are usually greater than 1 cm in length, may be present at birth, and are best seen using a Wood's ultraviolet light. They occur in 15 to 50 percent of cases. **Shagreen patches** are thickened, slightly elevated patches of skin infiltrated with fibromatous tissue. They occur in the lumbar region in up to 20 percent of cases. **Subungual** or **periungual fibromas** are hamartomatous collections of blood vessels and connective tissue near the

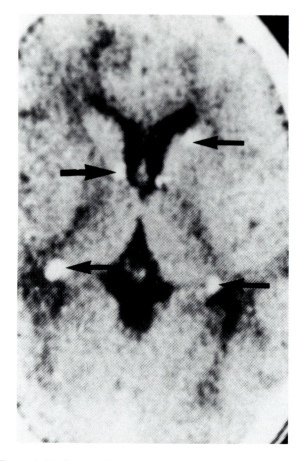

Figure 4–19. Computed tomography demonstrating "tubers" in the cerebral cortex in tuberous sclerosis (*arrows*). *(Courtesy of the Albany Medical College slide collection.)*

nail beds. Renal hamartomas occur in up to 80 percent of individuals; rhabdomyomas of the heart are a rarer finding.

The incidence of ocular findings has variably been reported as 3 to 100 percent. The most common abnor-

TABLE 4–9. DIAGNOSTIC CRITERIA FOR TUBEROUS SCLEROSIS

▪ *PRIMARY DIAGNOSTIC CRITERIA*

Unequivocal diagnosis when all three are present
1. Cortical tumors or subependymal hamartomas
2. Multiple retinal hamartomas
3. Adenoma sebaceum or periungual fibromas

▪ *SECONDARY DIAGNOSTIC CRITERIA*

Presumptive diagnosis when two or more of the following are present in a patient with two primary criteria
1. Infantile spasms
2. Ash leaf spots
3. Single retinal hamartoma
4. Multiple renal tumors
5. Cardiac rhabdomyoma
6. Affected first-degree relative

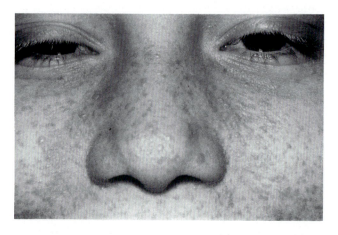

Figure 4–20. Angiofibromas (adenoma sebaceum) in tuberous sclerosis. *(Courtesy of John W. Simon.)*

mality is a flat, smooth, translucent to slightly gray angioglioma with ill-defined borders located in the superficial retina (Fig. 4–21). The classic **"mulberry"** or **"giant drusen"** lesion is less common (Fig. 4–22). This irregular, elevated, nodular white hamartoma of astrocytes can be as large as 3 disc diameters, and has a propensity to develop adjacent to or overlying the optic disc. It arises from the ganglion cell layer of the retina and usually does not significantly interfere with vision. Only rarely has vitreous hemorrhage or retinal detachment been associated with one of these tumors. They occur multiply or bilaterally in 15 to 30 percent of cases.

Angiomatosis of the Retina

Retinal capillary angiomas were first described by von Hippel (1904). Lindau subsequently established a relationship between these retinal tumors and hemangioblastomas of the cerebellum (1926). Today the term "von Hippel disease" is used for patients who have only retinal findings; "von Hippel–Lindau disease" is used for the 20 to 25 percent of patients with multisystem disease. Similar to the other phakomatoses, this disorder is transmitted as an autosomal dominant trait. This condition, however, is unusual in not becoming manifest until the second or third decade of life. Up to 80 percent of cases may be new mutations.

The actual vascular hamartoma of the cerebellum is often incorporated in the wall of a large solitary cyst. The lesion may also be multicystic (Fig. 4–23). Signs and symptoms of cerebellar dysfunction are frequent, but the initial symptoms are often secondary to increased intracranial pressure from expansion of the cystic lesion. Headache is the most common presenting symptom; other symptoms include vertigo and vomiting. Signs include papilledema and sixth cranial nerve

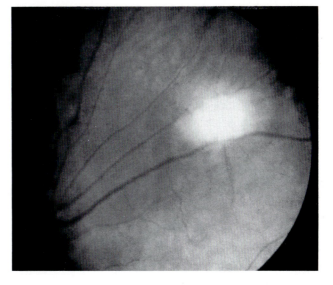

Figure 4–22. Mulberry or giant drusen in tuberous sclerosis. *(Courtesy of the Albany Medical College slide collection.)*

paresis. Polycythemia is associated in up to 20 percent of cases. Occasionally, hemangioblastomas develop in the brainstem, especially in the medulla. Up to 40 percent of individuals diagnosed with cerebellar hemangioblastomas will eventually be found to have von Hippel–Lindau disease. The cerebellar tumors in the latter individuals usually become symptomatic at a younger age (mean 28 years) than in patients with an isolated cerebellar lesion (mean 53 years).

Pheochromocytomas and renal carcinomas occur in 10 to 25 percent of individuals with the complete syndrome. Cysts of the pancreas, kidneys, and liver also occur.

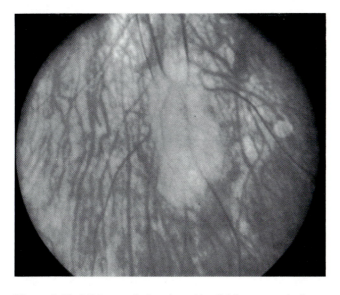

Figure 4–21. A flat, smooth, translucent to slightly gray angioglioma with ill-defined borders in tuberous sclerosis. *(Courtesy of the Albany Medical College slide collection.)*

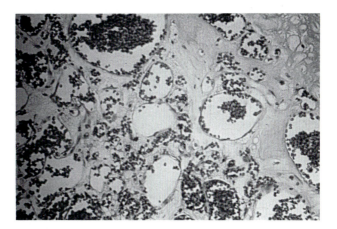

Figure 4–23. Multicystic cerebellar hemangioblastoma. *(Courtesy of the Albany Medical College slide collection.)*

The retinal tumors in von Hippel–Lindau disease are composed of thin-walled capillaries and solid masses of endothelial cells that often contain cystic cavities. Early tumors appear as minute, flat, reddish, superficial microvascular anomalies occurring in the capillary zone (stage I). These usually first appear in late childhood. Tumors slowly enlarge to form small pink nodules with prominent afferent and efferent feeder vessels (stage II, Fig. 4–24). As the angiomas enlarge, lipid can exudate from the abnormal capillary plexus into the surrounding retina (stage III, Fig. 4–25). Eventually an exudative retinal detachment or vitreous hemorrhage can occur (stage IV, Fig. 4–26). Secondary glaucoma and uveitis may ensue leading to visual loss (stage V). As many as 50 percent of eyes with angiomas eventually sustain visual loss.

Angiomas are bilateral or multiple in up to 60 percent of patients. The differential diagnosis includes Coats' disease (Table 4–10 and Fig. 4–27), toxocariasis, cavernous hemangioma, retinal macroaneurysm, and peripheral disciform degeneration of the retina. Discrete photocoagulation of the tumor can be useful for lesions < 2.5 cm; cryotherapy is recommended for larger tumors.

Encephalofacial Angiomatosis (Sturge–Weber Syndrome)

A syndrome characterized by a facial angioma present at birth, associated with ipsilateral infantile glaucoma and contralateral seizures, was first described by Sturge (1879). Weber (1929) elaborated on the clinical findings, and the syndrome came to be known as Sturge–Weber syndrome. Unlike the other phakomatoses, this disorder is not hereditary. There is no race or sex predilection.

Dilated capillaries in the dermis and subcutaneous tissue comprise the facial angioma, also called nevus flammeus or port wine stain (Fig. 4–28). These occur in

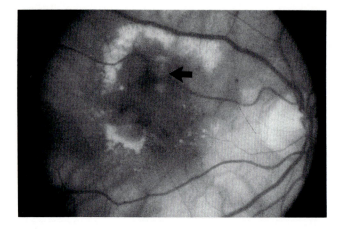

Figure 4–25. Stage III retinal capillary hemangioma (*arrow*). Note the lipid exudation. *(Courtesy of the Albany Medical College slide collection.)*

the distribution of the trigeminal nerve, particularly the first and second divisions. Although usually unilateral, bilateral involvement can occur (Fig. 4–29). Hypertrophy of the involved tissues is common, and occasionally the lips, palate, and tongue are involved. Laser therapy, using either the argon laser or the flashlamp-pumped pulsed-dye laser (at a wavelength of 577 or 585 nm and a pulse width of 450 microseconds) can be efficacious in lightening or eradicating the skin angiomas (Holy & Geronemus, 1992).

Dilated capillaries and venous channels in the ipsilateral meningeal sheaths are associated with cerebral dysfunction resulting in contralateral seizures. Nearly 50 percent of affected individuals develop seizures within the first 6 months of age. Calcium is deposited linearly in the affected cerebral cortex and is demonstrated radiographically by its "train track" appearance. As many as 25 percent of individuals are moderately to profoundly retarded.

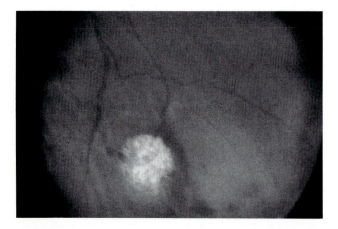

Figure 4–24. Stage II retinal capillary angioma. Note the afferent and efferent feeding vessels. *(Courtesy of the Albany Medical College slide collection.)*

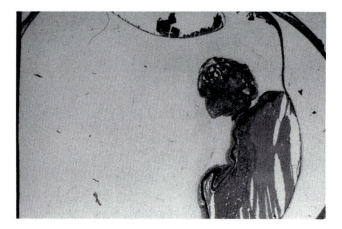

Figure 4–26. Histopathology of a stage IV retinal capillary angioma. Note the exudative retinal detachment. *(Courtesy of the Albany Medical College slide collection.)*

TABLE 4–10. DIFFERENTIAL DIAGNOSIS BETWEEN RETINAL ANGIOMATOSIS AND COATS' DISEASE

Feature	Retinal Angiomatosis	Coats' Disease
Pathology	Hemangioblastoma	Telangiectasia
Bilaterality	Often bilateral	Usually unilateral
Localization	Solitary tumors	Diffuse involvement
Sex predilection	Male = female	Usually male
Age of onset	Symptoms in adulthood	Symptoms in childhood
Systemic features	Some	None
Inheritance	Hereditary	Not hereditary

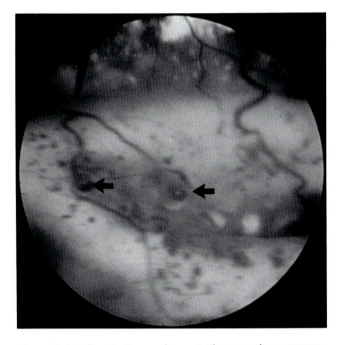

Figure 4–27. Coats' disease demonstrating saccular aneurysms (*arrows*). *(Courtesy of William Benson; from Nelson LB, Brown GC, Arentsen JJ: Recognizing patterns of ocular childhood diseases. Thorofare, NJ, Slack, 1985, p 97, with permission.)*

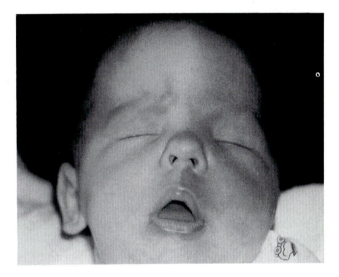

Figure 4–28. Nevus flammeus (port wine stain) in Sturge–Weber syndrome.

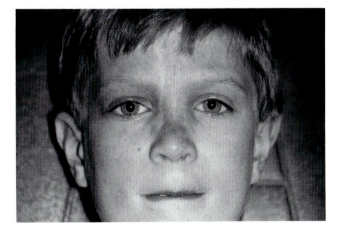

Figure 4–29. Bilateral nevus flammeus in Sturge–Weber syndrome.

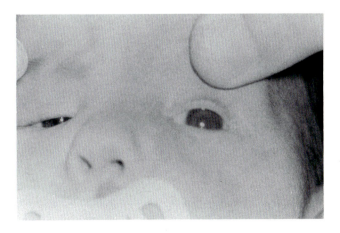

Figure 4–30. Congenital glaucoma in Sturge–Weber syndrome *(Courtesy of John W. Simon.)*

Infantile glaucoma occurs in up to 30 percent of cases; it is especially common if the angioma affects the upper eyelid. When present at an early age, it causes an enlarged eye (buphthalmos) (Fig. 4–30) and optic nerve cupping. The glaucoma results from either an anomalous anterior chamber angle, increased episcleral pressure, or a combination of both.

Thirty to 50 percent of affected patients also have choroidal hemangiomas in the ipsilateral eye. Most commonly these are flat, diffusely red, and velvety appearing. Their borders are feathery, and their presence obscures visualization of the choroidal vessels (Fig. 4–31). This appearance has been called "tomato catsup fundus." Histopathologically, they are cavernous hemangiomas. Usually they are asymptomatic, but occasionally a localized hemangioma can be associated with a secondary serous retinal detachment.

Klippel–Trenaunay–Weber syndrome is an unrelated autosomal dominant condition in which similar port wine stains occur on an extremity, associated with a local hypertrophy of the underlying bone and soft tissue (Fig. 4–32).

Wyburn-Mason Syndrome

Although arteriovenous malformations (AVMs) of retinal vessels have been described for over 100 years, Wyburn-Mason (1943) is credited with first associating these with ipsilateral AVMs of the midbrain and orbit. This rare disorder is not heritable. It is nearly always unilateral, present at birth, and is only minimally progressive. (See also Chapter 13.)

AVMs of the midbrain cause cranial nerve disturbances. Additional CNS findings include seizures, hydrocephalus, and spontaneous intracranial hemorrhage. Midbrain AVMs can extend through the optic

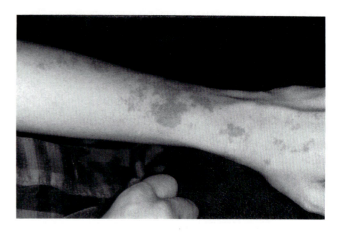

Figure 4–32. Klippel–Trenaunay–Weber syndrome (nevus flammeus) on an extremity.

tract to the orbit or retina. Signs of orbital involvement include proptosis, bruits, and dilation of conjunctival vessels (Fig. 4–33). Intracranial AVMs can also extend to the brainstem or maxilla.

Retinal AVMs, also known as racemose hemangiomas or cirsoid hemangiomas, appear as wormlike connections of arteries to veins. Arterialization of veins makes it difficult to differentiate these from arteries. Typically, the AVM involves the optic disc and one sector of the retina. Optic atrophy does not occur, and uninvolved retina demonstrates no electrophysiologic or visual field deficits. AVMs may be small and asymptomatic (see Fig. 13–16) or extensive, involving the entire posterior pole of the eye (see Fig. 13–17). The latter are associated with a higher incidence of central nervous system AVMs. Because the abnormal vessels are fully developed, retinal exudates and hemorrhages are

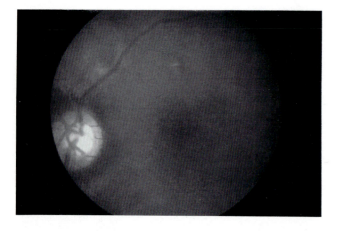

Figure 4–31. Choroidal hemangioma in Sturge–Weber syndrome, giving the eye a "tomato catsup" appearance. *(Courtesy of the Wills Eye Hospital slide collection.)*

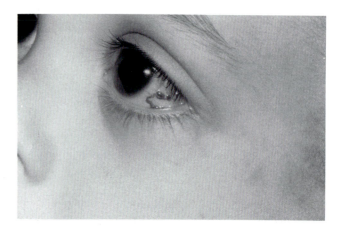

Figure 4–33. Dilated conjunctival vessels in a child with an orbital arteriovenous malformation.

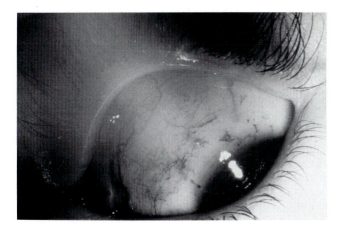

Figure 4–34. Telangiectasias of the venules in the bulbar conjunctiva in ataxia telangiectasia. *(Courtesy of the Albany Medical College slide collection.)*

extremely rare. The abnormal vessels also do not leak fluorescein dye. Occasionally a white glial tissue covers and parallels some of the vessels.

Ataxia Telangiectasia

Louis-Bar (1941) is credited with describing a syndrome characterized by cerebellar ataxia associated with skin and conjunctival telangiectasia. This syndrome differs from the other phakomatoses in being transmitted as an autosomal recessive disorder.

The ataxia is apparent as soon as the child begins to walk. Other cerebellar signs and mental and growth retardation subsequently become apparent. Ultimately, degenerative changes occur throughout the central nervous system.

Recurrent skin and respiratory infections occur secondary to an immune deficiency of both immunoglobulins and T-lymphocytes. The thymus is poorly developed, and there is an increased incidence of leukemia

and lymphoma. First-degree relatives also have an increased risk of cancer, especially breast cancer.

Ocular involvement is restricted to telangiectasias of venules occurring in the canthal region of the bulbar conjunctiva (Fig. 4–34). These are usually noted by 5 years of age and become more pronounced with age. Telangiectasias also occur in the skin of the face (Fig. 4–35), ears, and extremities, and on the palate. Ocular motor defects are also common. Initially, there is an inability to generate voluntary saccades; eventually, a total inability to move the eyes (ophthalmoplegia) can develop.

REFERENCES

Angiomatosis of the Retina

Annesley WH, Leonard BC, Shields JA, Tasman WS: Fifteen-year review of treated cases of retinal angiomatosis. Trans Am Acad Ophthalmol Otolaryngol 83:446, 1977.

Apple DJ, Goldberg MF, Wyhinny GJ: Argon laser treatment of von Hippel–Lindau retinal angiomas, II. Histopathology of treated lesions. Arch Ophthalmol 92:126, 1974.

Fill WL, Lamiell JM, Polk NO: The radiographic manifestations of von Hippel–Lindau disease. Radiology 133:289, 1979.

Goldberg MF, Duke JR: Von Hippel–Lindau disease. Am J Ophthalmol 66:693, 1968.

Hardwig P, Robertson DM: Von Hippel–Lindau disease: A familial, often lethal, multi-system phakomatosis. Ophthalmology 91:263, 1984.

Huson SM, Harper PS, Hourihan MD, et al: Cerebellar haemangioblastoma and von Hippel–Lindau disease. Brain 109:1297, 1986.

Lindau A: Studien über Kleinhirncysten. Bau Pathogenese und Beziehungen zur Angiomatosis retinae. Acta Pathol Microbiol Scand Suppl 1:1, 1926.

Von Hippel E: Über eine sehr seltene Erkrakung der Netzhaut: Klinische Beobachtungen. A von Graefes Arch Ophthalmol 59:83, 1904.

Watzke RC: Cryotherapy for retinal angiomatosis: A clinicopathologic report. Arch Ophthalmol 92:399, 1974.

Anophthalmia

Brunquel PJ, Papale JH, Horton JC, et al: Sex-linked hereditary bilateral anophthalmos. Pathologic and radiologic correlation. Arch Ophthalmol 102:108, 1984.

Frosini R, Papini M, Campana G, et al: Contribution of computerized tomography to the study of severe congenital ocular dysplasias. Study of a case of clinical anophthalmos. Ophthalmologica 183:72, 1978.

Kennedy RE: Growth retardation and volume determinations of the anophthalmic orbit. Trans Am Ophthalmol Soc 70:278, 1972.

Pearce WG, Nigam S, Rootman J: Primary anophthalmos: Histological and genetic features. Can J Ophthalmol 9:141, 1974.

Sassani JW, Yanoff M: Anophthalmos in an infant with multiple congenital anomalies. Am J Ophthalmol 83:43, 1977.

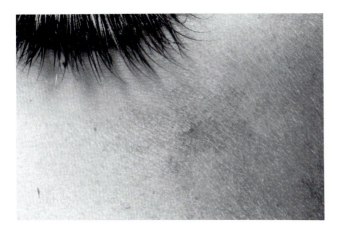

Figure 4–35. Facial telangiectasia in ataxia telangiectasia.

Ataxia Telangiectasia

Aguilar MJ, Kamoshita S, Landing BH, et al: Pathological observations in ataxia–telangiectasia: A report of five cases. J Neuropathol Exp Neurol 27:659, 1968.

Baloh RW, Yee RD, Boder E: Eye movements in ataxia–telangiectasia. Neurology 28:1099, 1978.

Centerwall WR, Miller MM: Ataxia, telangiectasia and sinopulmonary infection: A syndrome of slowly progressive deterioration in childhood. Am J Dis Child 95:385, 1958.

Hyams SW, Reisner SH, Neumann E: The eye signs in ataxia telangiectasia. Am J Ophthalmol 62:1118, 1966.

Louis-Bar D: Sur un syndrome progressif comprenant des telangiectasies capillaires cutanées et conjunctivales symetriques à disposition navoide de des troubles cérébelleux. Confin Neurol 4:32, 1941.

Perry TL, Kish SJ, Hinton D, et al: Neurochemical abnormalities in a patient with ataxia–telangiectasia. Neurology 34:187, 1984.

Sedgwick RP, Boder E: Progressive ataxia in childhood with particular reference to ataxia–telangiectasia. Neurology 10:705, 1960.

Swift M, Reitnauer PJ, Morrell D, Chase CL: Breast and other cancers in families with ataxia–telangiectasia. N Engl J Med 316:1289, 1987.

Waldmann TA, Misiti J, Nelson DL, et al: Ataxia–telangiectasia: A multisystem hereditary disease with immunodeficiency, impaired organ maturation, x-ray hypersensitivity, and a high incidence of neoplasia. Ann Intern Med 99:367, 1983.

Down Syndrome

Ahmad A, Pruett RC: The fundus in mongolism. Arch Ophthalmol 94:772, 1976.

Catalano RA: Down Syndrome. Surv Ophthalmol 34:385, 1990.

Catalano RA, Simon JW: Optic disc elevation in Down's syndrome. Am J Ophthalmol 110:28, 1990.

Culter AT, Benezra-Obeiter R, Brink SJ: Thyroid function in young children with Down syndrome. Am J Dis Child 140:479, 1986.

Down JL: Observations on ethnic classification of idiots. London Hospital Reports 3:259, 1866.

Gilbert HD, Smith RE, Barlow MH, Mohr D: Congenital upper eyelid eversion and Down's syndrome. Am J Ophthalmol 75:469, 1973.

Ginsberg J, Ballard ET, Buchind JJ, Kinkler AK: Further observations of ocular pathology in Down's syndrome. J Pediatr Ophthalmol 17:166, 1980.

Ginsberg J, Bofinger MK, Roush JR: Pathologic features of the eye in Down's syndrome with relationship to other chromosomal anomalies. Am J Ophthalmol 83:874, 1977.

Greenwood RD, Nadas AS: The clinical course of cardiac disease in Down's syndrome. Pediatrics 58:893, 1976.

Harris WS, Boodmann RM: Hypersensitivity to Atropine in Down's syndrome. N Engl J Med 279:407, 1968.

Hiles DA, Hoyme SH, McFarlane F: Down's syndrome and strabismus: Am Orthop J 24:63, 1974.

Jaeger EA: Ocular findings in Down's syndrome. Trans Am Ophthalmol Soc 158:808, 1980.

Kenyon KR, Kidwell EJ: Corneal hydrops and keratoconus associated with mongolism. Arch Ophthalmol 94:494, 1976.

Lejeune J, Gautier M, Turpin R: Les Chromosomes humains en culture de tissues. Comptes Rendus Seances Acad Sci 248:602, 1959.

Lott IT: Down's syndrome, aging and Alzheimer's disease: A clinical review. Ann NY Acad Sci 396:15, 1982.

Loudon MM, Day RE, Duke EMC: Thyroid dysfunction in Down's syndrome. Arch Dis Child 60:1149, 1985.

Mozar HN, Bal DG, Howard JT: Perspectives on the etiology of Alzheimer's disease. JAMA 257:1503, 1987.

Park SC, Mathews RA, Zuberbuhler JR, et al: Down's syndrome with congenital heart malformation. Am J Dis Child 131:29, 1977.

Robinson LL, Neglia JP: Epidemiology of Down's syndrome and childhood acute leukemia. In McCoy EE, Epstein CJ (eds): Oncology and Immunology of Down Syndrome. New York, Liss, 1987, pp 19–32.

Shapiro MB, France TD: The ocular features of Down's syndrome. Am J Ophthalmol 99:659, 1985.

Traboulsi EI, Levine E, Mets MB, et al: Infantile glaucoma in Down's syndrome (trisomy 21). Am J Ophthalmol 105:389, 1988.

Williams RDB: Brushfield spots and Wolfflin nodules in the iris: An appraisal in handicapped children. Dev Med Child Neurol 23:646, 1981.

Encephalofacial Angiomatosis

Barek L, Ledor S, Ledor K: The Klippel–Trenaunay syndrome: A case report and review of the literature. Mt Sinai J Med 49:66, 1982.

Holy A, Geronemus RG: Treatment of periorbital port-wine stains with the flash-lamp pumped pulsed dye laser. Arch Ophthalmol 110:793, 1992.

Morgan G: Pathology of the Sturge–Weber syndrome. Proc R Soc Med 56:422, 1963.

Phelps CD: The pathogenesis of glaucoma in Sturge–Weber syndrome. Ophthalmology 85:276, 1978.

Ratz JL, Bailin PL: The case for use of the carbon dioxide laser in the treatment of port-wine stains. Arch Dermatol 123:74, 1987.

Sturge WA: A case of partial epilepsy apparently due to a lesion of one of the vasomotor centers of the brain. Trans Clin Soc Lond 12:162, 1879.

Susac JO, Smith JL, Scelfo RJ: The "tomato-catsup" fundus in Sturge–Weber syndrome. Arch Ophthalmol 92:69, 1974.

Weber FP: Notes on association of extensive haemangiomatous naevus of the skin with cerebral (meningeal) hemangioma, especially cases of facial vascular naevus with contralateral hemiplegia. Proc R Soc Med (Sect Neurol) 22:25, 1929.

Fetal Alcohol Syndrome

Altman B: Fetal alcohol syndrome. J Pediatr Ophthalmol 13:255, 1976.

Jones KL, Smith DW: Recognition of the fetal alcohol syndrome in early infancy. Lancet 2:999, 1973.

Jones KL, Smith DW, Ulleland CN: Pattern of malformation in offspring of chronic alcoholic mothers. Lancet 1:1267, 1973.

Little R: Maternal alcohol use during breast feeding. N Engl J Med 321:425, 1989.

Miller MT, Epstein RJ, Sugar J, et al: Anterior segment anomalies associated with the fetal alcohol syndrome. J Pediatr Ophthalmol Strabismus 21:8, 1984.

Stormland K: Ocular involvement in the fetal alcohol syndrome. Surv Ophthalmol 31:277, 1987.

Microphthalmos

Cross HE, Yoder F: Familial nanophthalmos. Am J Ophthalmol 81:300, 1976.

Gorlin RS, Meskin LM, Geme JW: Oculodentodigital dysplasia. J Pediatr 63:69, 1963.

Kung HW: Hypoplastic anemia with multiple congenital defects. Pediatrics 10:286, 1952.

Mann I: Developmental Abnormalities of the eye, ed 2. Philadelphia, Lippincott, 1957.

Silver HK, Blair WC, Kempe CH: Fanconi syndrome. Am J Dis Child 83:14, 1952.

Sugar MS, Thompson JP, David JD: The oculodentodigital dysplasia syndrome. Am J Ophthalmol 61:1448, 1966.

Warburg M: Norrie's disease. A congenital progressive oculoacousticocerebral degeneration. Acta Ophthalmol 89:1, 1966.

Microphthalmos With Cyst

Arstikaitis M: A case report of bilateral microphthalmos with cysts. Arch Ophthalmol 82:480, 1969.

Foxman S, Cameron JD: The clinical implications of bilateral microphthalmos with cyst. Am J Ophthalmol 97:632, 1984.

Markley TA, Battles M: Microphthalmos with cyst. Report of two cases in the same family. Surv Ophthalmol 13:200, 1969.

Natanson L: Über Mikrophthalmus und Anopthalmus congenitus mit Serosen. Orbitopolpelbralcysten. Albrecht von Graefes Arch Ophthalmol 67:185, 1908.

Porges Y, Gershoni-Baruch R, Leibu R, et al: Hereditary microphthalmia with colobomatous cyst. Am J Ophthalmol 114:30, 1992.

Waring GO, Roth AM, Rodigues MM: Clinicopathologic correlation of microphthalmos with cyst. Am J Ophthalmol 82:714, 1976.

Weiss A, Greenwald M, Martinez C: Microphthalmos with cyst: Clinical presentations and computed tomographic findings. J Pediatr Ophthalmol Strabismus 22:6, 1985.

Neurofibromatosis

Barker D, Wright E, Nguyen K, et al: Gene for von Recklinghausen neurofibromatosis is in the pericentromeric region of chromosome 17. Science 236:1100, 1987.

Blatt J, Jaffe R, Deutsch M, Adkins JC: Neurofibromatosis and childhood tumors. Cancer 57:1225, 1986.

Charles SJ, Moore AT, Yates JRW, et al: Lisch nodules in NF type 2. Arch Ophthalmol 107:1571, 1989.

Destro M, D'Amico DJ, Gragoudas ES: Retinal manifestations of neurofibromatosis. Diagnosis and management. Arch Ophthalmol 109:662, 1991.

Dossetor FM, Landau K, Hoyt WF: Optic disc glioma in neurofibromatosis type 2. Am J Ophthalmol 108:602, 1989.

Freeman AG: Proptosis and neurofibromatosis. Lancet 1:1032, 1987.

Kaiser-Kupfer MI, Friedlin V, Datiles MB, et al: The association of PSC lens opacities with bilateral acoustic neuroma in patients with NF type 2. Arch Ophthalmol 107:541, 1989.

Listernick R, Charrow J, Greenwald MJ, et al: Optic gliomas in children with neurofibromatosis type 1. J Pediatr 114:788, 1989.

Martuza RL, Eldridge R: Neurofibromatosis 2. N Engl J Med 318:684, 1988.

Politi F, Sachs R, Barishak R: Neurofibromatosis and congenital glaucoma. Ophthalmologica 176:155, 1978.

Riccardi VM: Neurofibromatosis: The importance of localized or otherwise atypical forms. Arch Dermatol 123:882, 1987.

Riccardi VM, Eichner J: Neurofibromatosis: Phenotype, natural history and pathogenesis. Baltimore, Johns Hopkins University Press, 1986.

Rouleau SA, Wertelecki W, Haines JL, et al: Genetic linkage of bilateral acoustic neurofibromatosis to a DNA marker on chromosome 22. Nature 329:246, 1987.

Sivalingam A, Augsburger J, Perilongo G, et al: Combined hamartoma of the retina and retinal pigment epithelium in a patient with neurofibromatosis type 2. J Pediatr Ophthalmol Strabismus 28:320, 1991.

Specht CS, Smith TW: Uveal malignant melanoma and von Recklinghausen's neurofibromatosis. Cancer 62:812, 1988.

Von Recklinghausen FD: Über die Multiplen Fibrome der Hau: Ihre Beziehung zu den Multiplen Neuromem. Berlin, A Hirschwald, 1882.

Phakomatoses (General)

Beck RW, Hanno R: The phakomatoses. Int Ophthalmol Clin 25:97, 1985.

Font RL, Ferry AP: The phakomatoses. Int Ophthalmol Clin 12:1, 1972.

Miller N (ed): Walsh and Hoyt's Clinical Neuroophthalmology, ed 4. Baltimore, Williams & Wilkins, 1988, vol 3, p 1747.

Riccardi VM: The phakomatoses. In Emergy AEH, Rimoin, DL (eds): Principles and Practice of Medical Genetics. Edinburgh, Churchill Livingstone, 1983, vol 1, pp 313–320.

Van der Hoeve J: Eye symptoms in phakomatoses. Trans Ophthalmol Soc UK 52:380, 1932.

Tuberous Sclerosis

Boesel CP, Paulson GW, Kosnik EJ, Earle KM: Brain hamartomas and tumors associated with tuberous sclerosis. Neurosurgery 4:410, 1979.

Bourneville DM: Contribution a l'étude de l'idiotie: Sclerose tuberose des circonvolutions cérébrale: Idiotie et épilepsie hémiplégique. Arch Neurol 1:81, 1880.

Curatolo P, Cusmai R, Pruna D: Tuberous sclerosis: Diagnostic and prognostic problems. Pediatr Neurosci 12:123, 1985.

Dulac O, Lemaitre A, Plouin P: Bourneville syndrome: Clinical and EEG features of epilepsy in the first year of life. Bol Lega Ital Epil 45:39, 1984.

Frerebeau PH, Benezech J, Segnarbieux F, et al: Intraventricular tumors in tuberous sclerosis. Childs Nerv Syst 1:45, 1985.

Fryer AE, Chalmers A, Connor JM, et al: Evidence that the gene for tuberous sclerosis is on chromosome 9. Lancet 1:659, 1987.

Gutman I, Dunn D, Behrens M, et al: Hypopigmented iris spot: An early sign of tuberous sclerosis. Ophthalmology 89:1155, 1982.

Kingsley DPE, Kendall BE, Fitz CR: Tuberous sclerosis: A clinico-radiological evaluation of 110 cases with particular reference to atypical presentation. Neuroradiology 28:38, 1986.

McLaurin RL, Towbin RB: Tuberous sclerosis: Diagnostic and surgical considerations. Pediatr Neurosci 12:43, 1985.

Pampiglione G, Pugh E: Infantile spasms and subsequent appearance of tuberous sclerosis syndrome. Lancet 2:1046, 1975.

Williams R, Taylor D: Tuberous sclerosis. Surv Ophthalmol 30:143, 1985.

Wyburn-Mason Syndrome

Bernth-Petersen P: Racemose haemangioma of the retina: Report of three cases with long term follow-up. Acta Ophthalmol 57:669, 1979.

Hopen G, Smith JL, Hoff JT, Quencer R: The Wyburn–Mason syndrome. Concomitant chiasmal and fundus vascular malformations. J Clin Neuro-ophthalmol 3:53, 1983.

Lakhanpal V, Krishna Rao CVG, Schocket SS, Salcman M: Wyburn–Mason syndrome. Ann Ophthalmol 12:694, 1980.

Wyburn-Mason R: Arteriovenous aneurysm of mid-brain and retina, facial naevi and mental changes. Brain 66:163, 1943.

CHAPTER

5

REFRACTIVE ERRORS AND EYEGLASSES FOR INFANTS AND CHILDREN

ESSENTIAL INFORMATION FOR PRIMARY CARE PRACTITIONERS

The lens of a camera focuses light rays to a single sharp image at the film plane. Similar to a camera, the cornea and lens of the eye focus light rays to form a sharp image on the retina. The term used to describe the bending of light rays as they pass through the eye is **refraction.** An eye that bends or refracts light rays too much, too little, or irregularly is said to have a **refractive error.** In eyes with refractive errors, the image is blurred, similar to the image formed by an unfocused camera.

Light rays are refracted when they pass between transparent mediums that differ in density. The greater the difference in density between two mediums, the more the light rays are bent. For the eye, the greatest difference in density occurs at the air–cornea interface. The cornea, therefore, is the principle refractive surface of the eye, responsbile for approximately two thirds of its refractive power. This power is given in terms of the diopter (D), which is defined as the inverse of the focal length (in meters) of a refractive surface.

The ocular lens does not bend light rays with as much power as the cornea. Unlike the cornea, however, it can readily change its shape, and thereby its power. The flexible addition of power accomplished by changing the curvature of the lens surface is called **accommodation.** This increase in power is used to bring objects closer than infinity to a focus on the retina. The ability to accommodate is greatest during infancy, and gradually diminishes throughout life. By 45 years of age, most individuals need reading glasses or bifocals to resolve near visual objects. The term used to describe the loss of accommodative ability with age is **presbyopia.**

Refractive States of the Eye

In the perfect eye, the refractive power of the cornea and resting lens is just enough to focus light rays from a distant object onto the retinal plane. In order to do this, the length of the eye (actually the distance between the lens and the retina) has to exactly match the distance from which light rays passing from the lens are focused. The condition whereby the length of the eye precisely matches the power of the cornea and lens is called **emmetropia** (Fig. 5–1). When the refractive power of the anterior segment of the eye is disproportionate to the length of the eye, a refractive error, or **ametropia,** exists. If the plane of the retina lies in front of the plane where light rays are focused, **hyperopia** occurs (Fig. 5–2). If the plane of the retina lies behind the plane where the cornea and lens bring an object to a focus, **myopia** occurs (Fig. 5–3).

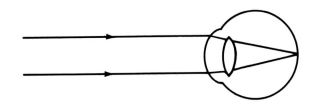

Figure 5–1. Emmetropia. Light rays are precisely focused on the retina.

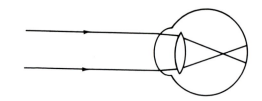

Figure 5–3. Myopia. Light rays come to a focus in front of the retina.

Signs and Symptoms of a Refractive Error

Myopia. Myopic children have blurred distant vision. They may be able to read printed material easily, but not the blackboard or street signs. They often are not cognizant that this is abnormal. Once learned, the myopic child will squint to see distant objects clearly.

Hyperopia. Most hyperopic children are asymptomatic. Some, however, may have crossed eyes (accommodative esotropia; see Chapter 6), or complain of ocular discomfort or fatigue (asthenopia) after prolonged reading or other near visual tasks. Children with high hyperopic errors are more likely to develop amblyopia than highly myopic children. This is especially true when one eye is more hyperopic than the other (**anisometropia**).

Astigmatism. A child with astigmatism will have blurred vision at all distances. Children with moderate astigmatism may be more symptomatic (fatigue, headaches, discomfort) than those with greater astigmatism. This is because the former make more of an effort to focus their eyes to see clearly. Similar to children with high hyperopia, children with large astigmatic errors may develop refractive amblyopia.

Age of Onset of Refractive Errors

The average newborn is hyperopic (farsighted), and may also have astigmatism. Hyperopia generally increases until age 7, at which time it gradually resolves and myopia may begin (see Chapter 3). Physiological myopia most commonly arises in grammar or middle school. Small astigmatic errors fluctuate with age, but high astigmatism is generally present at birth, and unchanging through life.

A mass on the eyelid or in the orbit may distort the shape of the eye and induce an astigmatism. A droopy eyelid (ptosis) may do the same. In young children, the astigmatism may resolve with resolution of the mass.

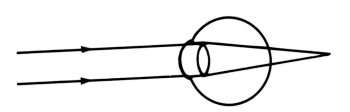

Figure 5–2. Hyperopia. Light rays come to a focus behind the retina.

Referral Criteria for a Potential Refractive Error

Vision screening is most commonly performed by the child's primary care provider, or school nurse, prior to the child's start of school. Preschool children who are unable to achieve 20/40 or better visual acuity (20/30 by first grade) in either eye, should be referred to an ophthalmologist or optometrist, unless the cause of their impairment has been medically confirmed by prior examination, and their visual acuity is stabilized. Some practitioners suggest that schools and primary care physicians also screen children for hyperopia using the **plus sphere test.** This test is performed by placing hyperopic lenses in front of the child's eyes as they read the visual acuity chart. These practitioners suggest that children who can still read the 20/20 line using +1.50 spheres be referred to an eye care professional. Visual acuity standards for referral, however,

TABLE 5–1. RISK FACTORS FOR THE DEVELOPMENT OF REFRACTIVE ERROR

- Prematurity (high myopia)
- Developmental abnormality
  - Down syndrome
  - Albinism
  - Fetal alcohol syndrome
  - Cornelia de Lange syndrome
  - Chromosome 18 partial deletion
  - Ehlers–Danlos syndrome
  - Marfan syndrome
  - Rubinstein–Taybi syndrome
  - Stickler/Wagner syndrome
- Mass pressing on the eye
  - Capillary hemangioma
  - Eyelid infection (chalazion)
  - Epibulbar or orbital dermoid
  - Mass in the lacrimal sac (dacryocele)
- Congenital lid droop (ptosis)
- Family history
  - Hyperopia (The onset of refractive accommodative esotropia, characterized by hyperopia and crossed eyes, is usually between ages 1 and 4)
  - Childhood myopia (onset between ages 5 and 9)
  - Astigmatism (high astigmatism is present at birth and changes minimally with age)
  - Ocular trauma or surgery

are usually sufficient and less likely to result in over-referral.

Premature infants and those with a chromosomal abnormality should be examined for refractive error within the first year of life (Table 5–1). Infants and children with a mass on the eyelid, in the orbit, or with a droopy eyelid (ptosis) should be examined for the presence of an induced astigmatism. Additional signs of a potential refractive error include misaligned eyes (particularly inward deviating eyes), squinting, and vague ocular discomfort (asthenopia) following prolonged near visual work.

Glasses prescriptions can change rapidly in children. Any child with a refractive error significant enough to warrant correction should be reexamined yearly.

Treatment of Refractive Errors

Refractive errors in children are treated with spectacles, and rarely with contact lenses (both are described later in the chapter). Surgical correction for refractive errors is inappropriate in childhood. Numerous studies exist that purportedly demonstrate a beneficial effect of various modalities in retarding the natural progression of refractive error (particularly myopia). These modalities include cycloplegic agents (atropine), bifocal glasses, and glasses that under- or overcorrect

---

TABLE 5–2. FACTS AND MISCONCEPTIONS REGARDING REFRACTIVE ERRORS AND GLASSES

- *THE CAUSE OF REFRACTIVE ERRORS*
    1. Refractive errors are strongly, but probably not exclusively, influenced by hereditary factors.
    2. There is no conclusive evidence that bad reading habits, poor illumination, excessive illumination, or dietary deficiency cause refractive errors.
    3. Sitting close to the television is usually not due to, and will not cause, refractive errors.
    4. "Eye exercises" cannot reduce refractive errors, or improve vision or depth perception.
    5. Glasses do not cause the eyes to become "weaker" (i.e., to have an increase in refractive error).

- *THE BENEFITS/DISADVANTAGES OF GLASSES*
    1. Wearing glasses at a young age will not prevent the need for "stronger" glasses in the future.
    2. Weak "reading glasses" or bifocals do not improve a child's ability to read.
    3. The full-time use of glasses will not cause a child to "become dependent upon them."
    4. Limiting the use of glasses will not "strengthen the eyes."

- *THE USE OF GLASSES*
    1. Children younger than 5 years of age with a refractive error significant enough to warrant correction should wear their glasses at all times.
    2. Older children without misalignment (strabismus) or amblyopia do not need to wear their glasses at all times.
    3. Children with hyperopia (farsightedness) combined with a tendency for their eyes to turn in may see just as well with as without their glasses. For these children, glasses are prescribed to treat the misalignment of the eyes, not reduced vision, and should be worn at all times.

- *CHILDREN'S ADAPTATION TO GLASSES*
    1. Children adapt to new glasses much more quickly than adults adapt to a change in their glasses. Properly prescribed and fit glasses for myopia should be accepted within hours; those for hyperopia and astigmatism within days.
    2. If glasses are not accepted, the child should be reexamined. If the prescription and fit are proper, the child's and/or parents' adjustment to the glasses should be explored.
    3. Unlike adults, children readily adapt to bifocals.

- *QUALITY OF GLASSES AND REFRACTION*
    1. A small error in the prescription and/or the grinding of spectacle lenses is usually well tolerated by children, without harm.
    2. The quality of both lenses and frames does vary by dispenser.
    3. Minor scratches on spectacles are usually well tolerated by children, and do not substantially reduce vision.
    4. Glasses that slide down the nose, or are tilted on the face, do not "harm the eyes." Unless the prescription is very strong, vision through poorly fit glasses is not appreciably reduced.
    5. Bifocals in children should be set so that the top line of the bifocal bisects the pupils (see Fig. 5–8).

- *FREQUENCY OF EYE EXAMINATIONS AND GLASSES CHANGES*
    1. Children who wear glasses should be refracted yearly, but small changes do not warrant a change in glasses.
    2. Some children with farsightedness and astigmatism may "outgrow" the need for glasses, but myopic children usually do not.

- *CONTACT LENSES*
    1. Contact lens wear requires high motivation and maturity.

the refractive error. None of these studies, however, have sufficient control populations to corroborate these claims.

Atropine paralyzes the eye's ability to accommodate, which some clinicians believe is related to myopic progression. The ideal dose of this drug, the number of years it should be used, and its efficacy upon withdrawal have not been conclusively demonstrated. Side effects of pupillary dilation (causing photophobia), and blurred reading vision (requiring the use of bifocals), reduce compliance. In place of atropine, some optometrists advocate bifocals to inhibit accommodation. Most ophthalmologists, however, do not believe that adequate scientific studies have been conducted to support this treatment. Even more controversial than the use of bifocals is the use of contact lenses, exercises, hormones, and diets to retard myopic progression.

Certain myths regarding refractive errors and the use of glasses are extant in Western societies. Principles to guide the general practitioner are listed in Table 5–2.

Spectacles for Children

Spectacle lenses are available in safety glass, plastic, and polycarbonate. The latter two are lighter than glass, but less scratch resistant. Scratch-resistant coatings are available at additional cost, but do not prevent scratches from inappropriate care. Children should be taught to remove their glasses using both hands, and to never lay their glasses face down. Dry cloths and paper towels will scratch plastic lenses; water or liquid soap should also be used when cleaning these lenses.

Standards for resistance to breakage of spectacle lenses are mandated by Federal law. Polycarbonate lenses are especially strong and should be prescribed for functionally one-eyed children; polycarbonate is also used in sports goggles. Protective lenses should be 3 mm thick, and sports goggles should meet the Z87 American National Safety Institute (ANSI) Standards.

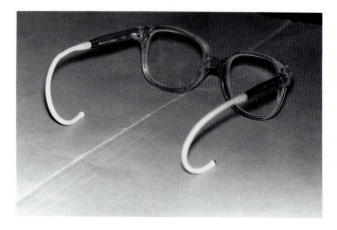

Figure 5–5. Wraparound (cable) temples used for infant glasses.

Eyeglass frames are much more likely to break than lenses, especially at the hinge of the earpiece and bridge of the nose. Spring-loaded flexible hinges allow some outward bending of the earpieces, but are more expensive (Fig. 5–4). Missing screws should not be replaced by paper clips or wires, as trauma may result in their penetration into the eye.

The nasal bridge of children less than 4 years old is flat. To prevent slippage of glasses, earpieces that wrap around the ears (cable temples) should be used in this age group (Fig. 5–5). Special harnesses are also available for young infants. When a harness is used, care must be taken to ensure that the elastic bands are not too tight. Rolled or flared nosepads, or silicone pads with nonskid surfaces, are available to help secure the glasses of older children. Alternately, a strap can be worn behind the ears (Fig. 5–6). A child has outgrown his or her frames when the bend in the earpiece occurs anterior to the ear (Fig. 5–7).

The thick appearance of strong lenses can be minimized by choosing small frame sizes, and by tinting,

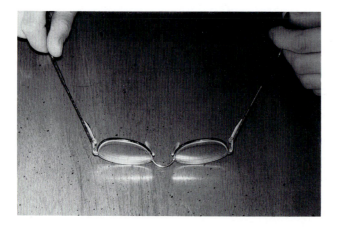

Figure 5–4. Spring-loaded, flexible hinges on the earpieces of spectacles allow some outward bending at the temple.

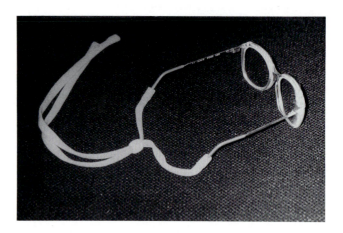

Figure 5–6. One of a multitude of straps available to hold a child's glasses in place.

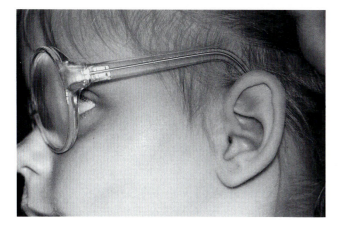

Figure 5–7. A child has outgrown a pair of glasses when the bend in the earpiece is no longer flush with the ear.

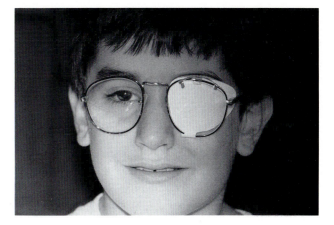

Figure 5–9. Clip-on occluder for the treatment of amblyopia.

grinding, or beveling the edges of the lens. Tinted lenses and lenses that darken in bright illumination (such as Photogray and Photosun) are not generally prescribed for children.

Special Glasses and Occluders for Children

Bifocals in children should be set so that the top line of the bifocal bisects the pupils (Fig 5–8). "No-line" bifocals can be used when indicated, but are more expensive.

For the treatment of amblyopia, several different types of lens occluders are available. These attach to the glasses with either metal clips (Fig. 5–9) or a suction cup (Fig. 5–10).

Prisms in Glasses

Prisms are used when there is a small deviation in the alignment of the eyes, and the possibility exists for bet-

ter binocularity if the eyes can be optically aligned. Prisms are also used in some older children to eliminate double vision (diplopia). A large misalignment of the eyes cannot be treated with prisms; the glasses will be too heavy, and cosmetically unacceptable. Fresnel prisms (press-on plastic prisms) are lightweight and easily interchangeable (Fig. 5–11 and 5–12). The lines on the Fresnel prism, however, can reduce visual acuity.

Contact Lenses for Children

Although most refractive errors in children are correctable with contact lenses, contacts should not be prescribed until an individual is mature enough to independently care for them. The insertion of contact lenses can cause corneal abrasions, and ocular infections are more common with the use of contacts. It is not wise to prescribe contacts if only the parents are motivated.

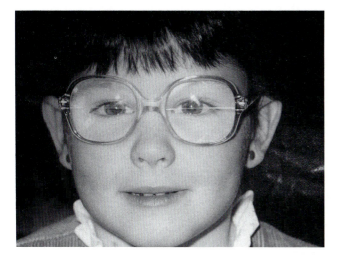

Figure 5–8. Proper fitting of a bifocal for a child. Note that the top line of the bifocal bisects the pupil.

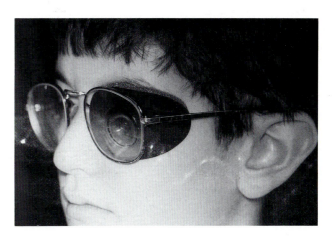

Figure 5–10. Occluder fastened to glasses by suction cup.

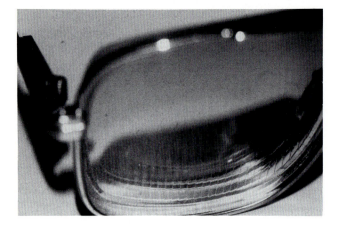

Figure 5–11. Fresnel prism applied to spectacle lens.

Frequency of Use of Spectacles

Guidelines for the frequency of use of glasses are based on the child's refractive error, age, and visual needs. Older children with minimal myopia may only need to wear their glasses to view the blackboard, movies, or television. They may be content with blurred distant vision for other tasks, and should not be forced to use their glasses at all times. Similarly, full-time use is not required of older hyperopic children unless the eyes also have a tendency to turn in (esodeviation), or amblyopia is present.

Full-time use is required for preschool-age children with hyperopia or astigmatism sufficient to warrant spectacle correction. It is also required for any child with astigmatism or other refractive error large enough to interfere with normal visual development (amblyogenic).

Children should never be prevented from wearing their glasses with the mistaken notion that this will cause them to become dependent upon them. An increase in refractive error cannot be prevented by denying glasses. Children who want to wear their glasses

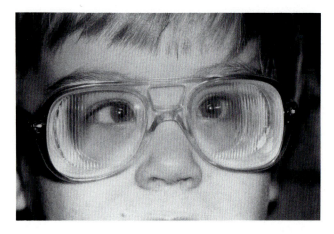

Figure 5–12. Child wearing Fresnel prisms.

more frequently than they did at a younger age have either developed an increased refractive error, or have come to realize that the world can be viewed more clearly and comfortably with their glasses.

To ease the burden on teachers, any child prescribed glasses should wear them full time in school, except for swimming. For contact sports, sports goggles that fit over the glasses (and the appropriate face mask or helmet) should be used.

COMPREHENSIVE INFORMATION ON REFRACTIVE ERRORS

Definitions

Accommodation: The ability of the eye to increase its refractive power through increasing the curvature of the lens surface. Accommodative ability decreases with age.

Ametropia: The condition that exists when the refractive power of the cornea and the lens does not match the length of the eye. Light rays are brought to a focus in front of or behind the retina; a blurred image is formed on the retina (see Fig. 5–2 and 5–3).

Aniseikonia: A difference in the shape or the size of the images presented by the two eyes to the visual cortex. An asymmetry of the power of the two eyes leads to an asymmetry in retinal image size even if the images on both retinas are focused (see Fig. 5–13).

Anisometropia: A difference between the refractive power of the two eyes. When this occurs, a focused image in both eyes cannot be simultaneously formed without the assistance of glasses or contact lenses.

Astigmatism: A lack of uniformity in the curvature of the cornea or lens such that the refractive power of the eye differs from one meridian to the next. Rays of light do not come to a single sharp focus; rather, they form a complicated image referred to as the conoid of Sturm, when the astigmatism is regular (see Fig. 5–22 and 5–23).

Diopter (D): A measure of the refractive power of any lens system such as the eye. It is equivalent to the inverse of the focal length of the lens measured in meters.

Emmetropia: The absence of a refractive error. The refractive power of the cornea and resting lens correlates to the length of the eye. Light rays infinitely far away are brought to a focus on the retina (see Fig. 5–1).

Hyperopia: The condition whereby the power of the eye is too weak for the length of the eye. Distant light rays come to a focus behind the retina when the eye is at rest. Objects are seen clearly only if the eye can increase its power through accommodation of the lens (see Fig. 5–21). The eye needs to accommodate even more for near objects, hence distant objects are more easily resolved (farsighted).

Myopia: The condition whereby the power of the eye is too strong for the length of the eye. Distant light rays come to a focus in front of the retina (see Fig. 5–14). Only objects closer than the myopic far point are seen clearly (near-sighted).

Presbyopia: The decrease in ability to change the curvature of the lens (accommodate) with age.

Refraction: The bending of light rays as they travel between mediums of different density.

Aniseikonia

It is an oversimplification to state that myopic eyes are too long and hyperopic eyes are too short. Rather, the refractive power of the anterior segment is too great for the length of the eye in myopia and insufficient in hyperopia. Although the average eye is 24 mm in length, smaller and longer eyes can still be emmetropic if the power of the anterior segment is correlated with the length of the eye. Figure 5–13 shows two different sized eyes, both of which are emmetropic. For each eye, the refractive power of the cornea and lens is proportionate to the length of the eye. The refracting power of the smaller eye must be greater because it brings light rays to a focus at a shorter distance. The only difference between the two eyes is that the image formed in the larger eye is larger than that formed in the smaller eye.

In Figure 5–13, each eye creates a perfectly focused image of the fixated object. If this represents the two eyes of a given individual, the images presented by each eye to the visual cortex will differ in size. This difference in image size, due to the difference in refractive power of the two eyes, is called **aniseikonia.**

Myopia

Myopia describes the condition in which the cornea and lens of the nonaccommodating eye focus parallel rays of light, entering the eye from infinity, in front of the retina (Fig. 5–14). Myopia occurs when the refractive power of the eye is too strong for the length of the eye. Light rays from objects closer than infinity do not enter the eye in parallel; rather, they enter the eye with some divergence. At the myopic far point, the divergence of light rays emanating from a near object matches the greater refractive (converging) strength of the myopic eye. Objects at this distance are focused precisely on the retina with the eye at rest. Accommodation allows objects closer than the myopic far point, which emanate light rays with even greater divergence, to be focused on the retina. Any object beyond the far point is brought to a focus in front of the retina. The myopic individual, who can only focus objects at or closer than his far point, is said to be **nearsighted.**

Twenty to forty percent of the US population has myopia. The most common type, **physiological myopia,** occurs when both the refractive power and the length of the eye fall within normal distribution curves but are mismatched such that the power of the eye is too great for its length. This type of myopia gradually begins during grade school and slowly progresses until the eye is fully grown at puberty. During adolescence the change can be rapid, requiring frequent prescription changes; occasionally progression can continue or become manifest again during the early twenties.

Pathological Myopia

Pathological changes occur in eyes that are much longer than average. A refractive error greater than −6.0 to −8.0 D usually signifies pathological myopia. The greater the myopia, the more frequent and severe are degenerative changes. The optic nerve may enter the scleral canal obliquely, giving it a vertically **tilted**

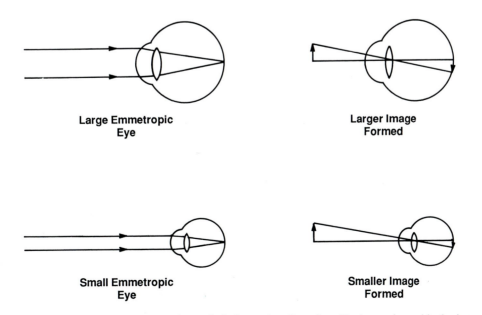

Large Emmetropic Eye

Larger Image Formed

Small Emmetropic Eye

Smaller Image Formed

Figure 5–13. Aniseikonia. In each eye the image is precisely focused on the retina. The image formed in the larger eye (top), however, is larger than that formed in the smaller eye (bottom).

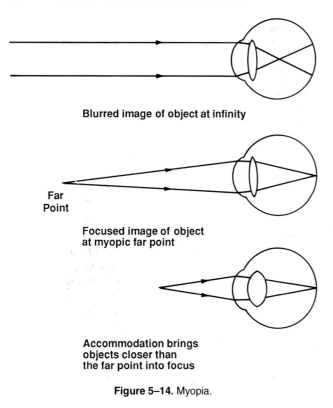

Blurred image of object at infinity

Far Point

Focused image of object at myopic far point

Accommodation brings objects closer than the far point into focus

Figure 5–14. Myopia.

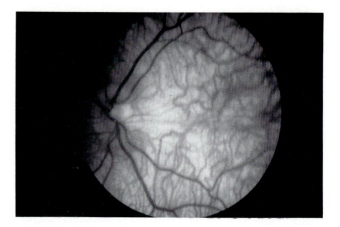

Figure 5–16. Tigroid appearance of the retina due to thinning and atrophy of the retinal pigment epithelium and choriocapillaris in a myopic eye. The optic nerve in this eye is also tilted.

appearance, and the choroid and retina may terminate some distance from the nerve at its temporal border, creating a **myopic crescent** (Fig. 5–15). Thinning and atrophy of the retinal pigment epithelium and choriocapillaris can give the retina a tigroid appearance due to the prominence of the large underlying choroidal vessels (Fig. 5–16). A **staphyloma,** or outpouching of the optic nerve, can also occur (Fig. 5–17). Ruptures in Bruch's membrane between the choroid and retina can allow new vessels to grow under the sensory retina. These fragile new vessels rupture easily, resulting in subretinal hemorrhages and loss of vision (Fig. 5–18). Pigment accumulation in the macula,

called a **Fuch's spot,** can occasionally be seen in eyes greater than 12 D myopic (Fig. 5–19). Retinal breaks occur at an increased incidence and at an earlier age in pathological myopia. Over one third of nontraumatic retinal detachments occur in myopic eyes. Full or partial thickness macular holes can also occur (Fig. 5–20). Liquefaction of the vitreous leads to the development of floaters and early vitreous detachment. Finally, primary (open-angle) glaucoma occurs with a greater incidence in high myopia.

Like all refractive errors, myopia is strongly influenced by hereditary factors; it may, however, be the product of multiple genes. High myopia in some families appears to follow an autosomal recessive inheritance pattern. Most investigators believe that external factors such as excessive near work, dim lighting, excessive use of the eyes, and nutritional factors do not influence the progression of myopia. Myopia has been associated, however, with prematurity, mental retardation, and various ocular syndromes (see Table 5–2).

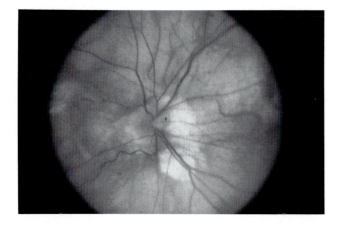

Figure 5–15. Tilted optic nerve, with myopic crescent in a myopic eye.

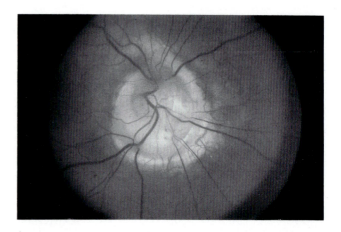

Figure 5–17. Optic nerve staphyloma (outpouching) in high myopia.

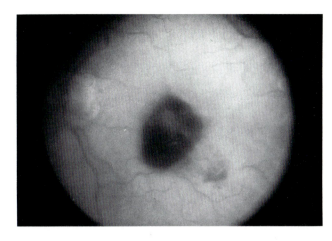

Figure 5–18. Macular hemorrhage subsequent to bleeding from a subretinal neovascular membrane in pathological myopia.

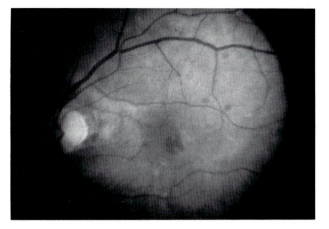

Figure 5–20. Macular hole in high myopia.

Hyperopia

Hyperopia describes the condition in which the cornea and lens of the nonaccommodating eye focus parallel rays of light, entering the eye from infinity, behind the plane of the retina (Fig. 5–21). It occurs when the refractive power of the eye is too weak for the length of the eye. If the lens is able to accommodate, additional power can be introduced to further converge light rays toward the retina. Because light rays from distant objects approach the eye with less divergence, less converging or accommodative power is required to focus these rays on the retina. The lesser accommodation necessary to focus distant objects makes them easier to resolve (**farsightedness**). Farsighted individuals have to accommodate to see objects at any distance clearly, but accommodate less for distant objects.

A multitude of terms are used to describe hyperopia. **Total hyperopia** is the total amount of hyperopia elicited by paralyzing accommodation with cycloplegic agents. Total hyperopia consists of **manifest hyperopia**, which is the amount elicited without cyclo-

plegia, and **latent hyperopia**, which is the residual hyperopia uncovered only with cycloplegia. Of an individual's manifest hyperopia, **absolute hyperopia** is the amount that cannot be overcome by accommodation, whereas **facultative hyperopia** is the amount that can be compensated for by accommodation.

Three out of every four infants are hyperopic, the majority being between 1 to 4 D hyperopic. Hyperopia increases until age 7 years, after which it decreases. Hyperopic children usually see well at all distances be-

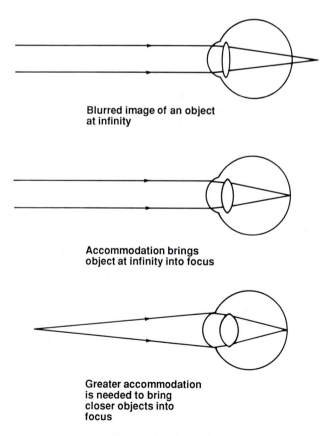

Blurred image of an object at infinity

Accommodation brings object at infinity into focus

Greater accommodation is needed to bring closer objects into focus

Figure 5–21. Hyperopia.

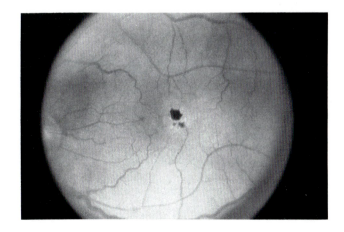

Figure 5–19. Fuch's spot in a myopic eye.

cause the accommodating ability of the lens is very great in childhood. With high levels of hyperopia, however, nonvisual symptoms such as ocular discomfort (**asthenopia**), headaches, and lack of interest in reading may occur. In some children, high hyperopia is related to an inward turning, or esotropia, of the visual axes of the eyes. Called **accommodative esotropia,** this misalignment is brought on by the relationship between accommodation and convergence. A blurred retinal image stimulates accommodation, which is accompanied by convergence. Individuals with small to moderate amounts of hyperopia counter the convergence elicited by accommodation with fusional divergence. With high hyperopia, the convergence elicited by accommodation exceeds fusional divergence and esotropia results. The typical child with accommodative esotropia often has a hyperopia of between 4 and 5 D.

Astigmatism

Astigmatism describes the condition in which the curvature of the cornea or lens is not uniform. The refractive power of the eye differs from one meridian to the next, preventing rays of light from coming to a single sharp focus. The astigmatism is said to be **regular** when the meridians of maximal and minimal power are aligned at right angles to each other. **Irregular** astigmatism signifies that these meridians are not at right angles or that the curvature varies in the same meridian. Irregular astigmatism is most frequently caused by corneal scars or keratoconus.

Instead of converging rays to a point focus, an eye with regular astigmatism focuses parallel rays of light to two separate focal lines at right angles to each other (Fig. 5–22). Light passing through the steeper meridian is brought to a linear focus in front of and at 90 degrees to light passing through the flatter meridian. The complicated image that results from refracting a point source of light is called the **conoid of Sturm.** The distance between the two focal lines within this is called the **interval of Sturm.** Lying between the focal lines is a region where the diverging tendency of rays in one meridian equals the converging tendency of rays in the opposed meridian. This zone is called the **circle of least confusion,** and the uncorrected visual acuity of an individual with astigmatism is best when the circle of least confusion is brought to lie on the retina by accommodation.

Classification of Astigmatism

Several terms are used to describe different types of astigmatism. In most astigmatic eyes, the vertical meridian is steeper than the horizontal meridian. This is called **"with the rule"** astigmatism (Fig. 5–23). **"Against the rule"** describes the opposite condition. Other terms are used to describe where the focal planes lie in an astigmatic eye. **Simple myopic astigmatism** denotes that one focal plane lies on the retina and the other falls anterior to it. **Simple hyperopic astigmatism** denotes that one meridian is focused posterior to the retina. **Compound myopic** and **compound hyperopic astigmatism** denote that both meridians are focused on the same side of the retina; **mixed astigmatism** denotes that one meridian is focused in front and the other behind the retina.

Most astigmatism is due to a lack of uniformity in the steepness of the cornea, rather than the lens. The percentage of infants with an astigmatism greater than 1 D is at least twice that of adults, and is perhaps as high as 50 percent. The majority of infants have against the rule astigmatism. Infantile astigmatism disappears during the childhood years. Small degrees of astigmatism (< 1.50 D) may cause no symptoms. With greater amounts of astigmatism, however, asthenopia and reduced visual acuity occur.

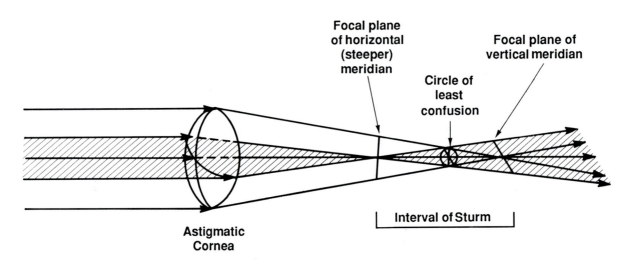

Figure 5–22. Regular astigmatism (the conoid of Sturm). Instead of converging light to a point focus, light rays are focused to two separate focal lines.

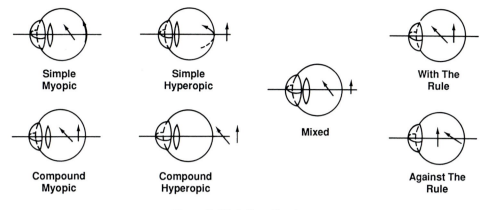

Figure 5–23. Astigmatism types.

Correction of Refractive Errors

Myopia is corrected with a concave (minus) lens, which diverges the light entering the eye (Fig. 5–24). This divergence counterbalances the excess converging power of the eye, allowing the image to be focused on the retina. The minus lens can also be thought of as focusing objects to the plane of the myopic far point. Hyperopia is treated with a convex (plus) lens, which adds convergence to the light entering the eye (Fig. 5–25). The correct plus lens will converge rays from infinity to the hyperopic far point, which the eye can then focus onto the retina.

Guidelines for the prescription of glasses are based on the child's refractive error, age, and visual needs. A child's world of interest is at close range, and minimally myopic children may not complain as long as their vision is clear. Repka (1991) noted that 6-year-old myopic children may be content with distance vision of 20/100. Tolerance for blurred vision decreases with age to 20/70 by 8 years, and 20/40 by 12 years. Spectacles for minimally myopic children should be mandated for school use, and made optional for other activities, such as viewing television or movies.

Despite the great ability of children to accommodate, a hyperopic child with ill-defined ocular discomfort from extended use of the eyes (**asthenopia**) will

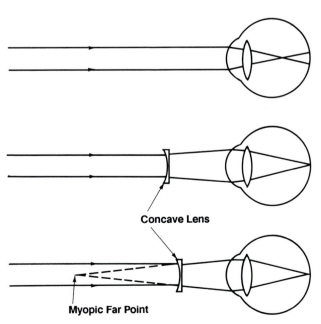

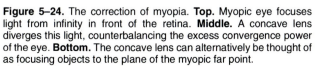

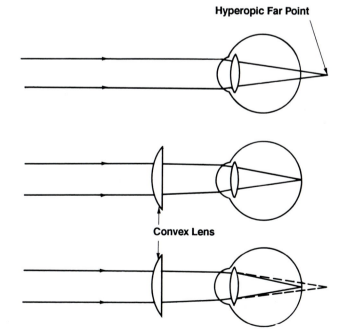

Figure 5–24. The correction of myopia. **Top.** Myopic eye focuses light from infinity in front of the retina. **Middle.** A concave lens diverges this light, counterbalancing the excess convergence power of the eye. **Bottom.** The concave lens can alternatively be thought of as focusing objects to the plane of the myopic far point.

Figure 5–25. The correction of hyperopia. **Top.** Hyperopic eye focuses light from infinity behind the retina. **Middle.** A convex lens adds convergence to focus light rays on the retina. **Bottom.** The convex lens can alternatively be thought of as converging light rays from infinity to the plane of the hyperopic far point.

likely appreciate spectacle correction. Repka found that 6-year-old children are content to wear, at least some of the time, glasses to correct a hyperopia of 4.0 D. With the exception of those with esotropia, it is better to undercorrect hyperopia as long as some accommodative ability exists. Most hyperopic children accommodate to a certain degree at all times (physiological or latent hyperopia). Correcting for the total hyperopia (determined by paralyzing accommodation with the use of a cycloplegic agent) may result in overcorrection and intolerance of glasses. Prescribing for the manifest hyperopia (without cycloplegia) is, therefore, recommended. The exception is hyperopic children with esotropia (inward deviation of the eyes). These children should be given their full correction to eliminate any convergence of the eyes related to accommodation (see Chapter 6). One to two weeks may be required for these children to adapt to their glasses; they should be instructed to wear them at all times.

Astigmatism causes blurred vision at all distances, and amblyopia can occur with an astigmatism of greater than 1.5 D. Visual acuity with this amount of astigmatism is generally 20/40 or worse, and affected children usually appreciate the improvement afforded by correction. The full astigmatic correction is recommended for these children. A child with less than 1.5 D of astigmatism should also receive the full astigmatic correction when spectacles are being prescribed to correct a concomitant myopia or hyperopia. Children who have glasses prescribed for astigmatism should wear their spectacles at all times.

Some eye care practitioners prescribe bifocals for children with physiological myopia. They believe that by reducing the need for the eye to accommodate, the progression of myopia can be retarded. Less controversial is the use of bifocals for children with an esotropia that is greater at near than distant fixation. As noted above, in order to view near objects, the eyes must turn in as well as accommodate. Children whose eyes converge excessively with accommodation are said to have a **high accommodative convergence to accommodation ratio.** Bifocals reduce the need for accommodation at near and thereby reduce accommodative convergence. They may be indicated if they eliminate the esotropia at near, or reduce it to less than 8 to 10 prism diopters, provided that their eyes are straight at distant fixation (see Chapter 6). Children also wear bifocals after the removal of a congenital or traumatic cataract. Bifocals in children are set higher than those for adults.

The executive style is most often used, but other styles may be satisfactory if the bifocal is set to bisect the pupil with the child's fixation directed straight ahead (see Fig. 5–8).

REFERENCES

American Academy of Ophthalmology, Eye Care for the American People Committee. Eye Care for the American People. *Ophthalmology* 94 (suppl):44, 1987.

Bogan S, Simon JW, Krohel G, Nelson LB: Astigmatism associated with adnexal masses in infancy. Arch Ophthalmol 105:1368, 1987.

Cook RC, Glasscock RE: Refractive and ocular findings in the newborn. Am J Ophthalmol 34:1407, 1951.

Curtin BJ: The Myopias. Philadelphia, Harper & Row, 1985.

Fuchs E: Der centrale schwarzen Flecke bei Myope. Z Augenheilkd 5:171, 1905.

Fulton AB: Optical properties of children's eyes. In Spaeth GL: Modern Concepts of Eye Care in Children. Thorofare, NJ, Slack, 1986, p 37–45.

Gordon RA, Donzis PB: Myopia associated with retinopathy of prematurity. Ophthalmology 93:1593, 1986.

Guyton DL: Prescribing cylinders: The problem of distortion. Surv Ophthalmol 22:177, 1977.

Hirsch MJ: The refraction of children. Am J Optom 41:395, 1964.

Larsen JS: The sagittal growth of the eye, I. Ultrasonic measurements of the anterior chamber from birth to puberty. Acta Ophthalmol 49:239, 1971.

Michaels DD: Visual Optics and Refraction. St. Louis, Mosby, 1980.

Milder B, Rubin ML: The Fine Art of Prescribing Glasses Without Making a Spectacle of Yourself. Gainesville, FL, Triad Scientific Publishers, 1978.

Raab EL: Etiologic factors in accommodative esodeviation. Trans Am Ophthalmol Soc 80:657, 1982.

Repka MX: Refraction in infants and children. In Nelson LB, Calhoun JH, Harley RD: Pediatric Ophthalmology, ed 3. Philadelphia, Saunders, 1991, pp 94–106.

Rubin ML: Optics for Clinicians, ed 2. Gainesville, FL, Triad Scientific Publishers, 1977.

Safir A: Refraction and Clinical Optics. New York, Harper & Row, 1980.

Schepens CL, Marden BA: Data on the natural history of retinal detachment. Am J Ophthalmol 61:213, 1966.

Slataper FJ: Age norms of refraction and vision. Arch Ophthalmol 43:466, 1950.

Weinstein GW: Correction of ametropia with spectacle lenses. In Duane TD, Jaeger EA: Clinical Ophthalmology. Philadelphia, Lippincott, 1978.

AMBLYOPIA AND STRABISMUS

ESSENTIAL INFORMATION FOR PRIMARY CARE PRACTITIONERS

Amblyopia

Amblyopia is defined as poor vision in an eye, despite the correction of any refractive error with glasses, and in the absence of any ophthalmoscopically visible lesion of the retina, especially of the macular region. The poor vision is also not due to a definable lesion elsewhere in the visual pathways, or the central nervous system.

The development of normal visual acuity requires a clear and focused image on the retina. If both retinas do not receive a clearly defined image, bilateral amblyopia can result. More commonly, one image is distorted or misaligned, causing unilateral amblyopia. Regardless of the cause, amblyopia develops in early childhood. The reversibility of the condition is dependent on the duration of impairment and the age at which appropriate treatment is begun.

The frequency of amblyopia ranges from 1.3 to 3 percent in preschool- and school-age children. Between 2 and 2.5 percent of the general population have amblyopia. In a population of 200 million, this would mean that approximately 4 million have amblyopia.

A child with unilateral amblyopia functions adequately in most everyday situations through the use of monocular clues to judge depth. The major functional defect in amblyopia is central visual acuity reduction. The amblyopic eye will have normal peripheral vision, but a child with amblyopia will have difficulty performing tasks requiring accurate close-range depth perception. The amblyopic child also lacks the "back-up" capability of a second eye, if the healthy eye suffers visual reduction or loss.

Strabismus

Strabismus (Greek, "to squint or look obliquely at") is a general term meaning dissociated or misaligned eyes. The misalignment may be manifest in any field of gaze, may be constant or intermittent, and may occur at distance fixation, near fixation, or both. Strabismus affects between 2 and 5 percent of the preschool population, and is an important cause of visual and psychological disability.

Orthophoria is the ideal condition of ocular balance. It implies that both eyes are simultaneously directed at the object of regard even when a cover is placed in front of one eye. **Heterophoria** is a latent tendency toward misalignment; the eye deviates only under certain conditions, such as fatigue, illness, stress, or tests that interfere with the maintenance of normal fusion (such as covering one eye) (Fig. 6–1). If the amount of heterophoria is large, it may give rise to

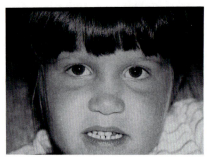
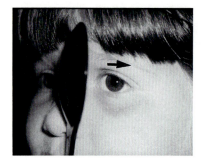

Figure 6–1. Exophoria, left eye. Upon covering the eye with an occluder, it turns outward. *(From Nelson LB, Catalano RA: Atlas of ocular motility. Philadelphia, Saunders, 1989, p 85, with permission.)*

bothersome symptoms, such as transient diplopia or asthenopia. A sign of intermittent strabismus is the closure of one eye (Fig. 6–2). This is most commonly noted in children whose eyes have a tendency to turn outward (particularly when exposed to bright sunlight). Monocular eye closure can occur, however, with any ocular deviation. It may be a mechanism to reduce photophobia, more so than diplopia (Wiggins & von Noorden, 1990).

Heterotropia is a misalignment of the eyes that is manifest at all times. Different prefixes describe the direction the deviated eye is turned. **Eso**tropia (Fig. 6–3) means that the visual axis of the deviated eye is directed inward. **Exo**tropia (Fig. 6–4) describes a divergent position of the deviated eye. **Hyper**tropia (Fig. 6–5) means that the deviated eye is turned upward, and **hypo**tropia (Fig. 6–6) downward. Esophoria, exophoria, hyperphoria, and hypophoria describe the respective latent counterparts. Strabismus is categorized with respect to the nonfixating eye. This is useful in identifying the deviating eye in vertical strabismus. A left hypotropia appropriately identifies the deviating eye in Figure 6–6, as opposed to describing this patient as having a right hypertropia.

Congenital describes any strabismus present by 6 months of age, regardless of whether it was noted at birth. All other deviations are considered **acquired.** The modifier **monocular** is used when there is a defi-

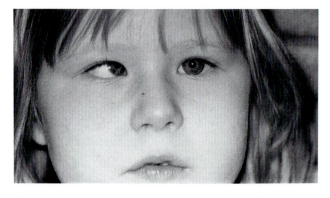

Figure 6–3. Esotropia (inward turning) of the right eye.

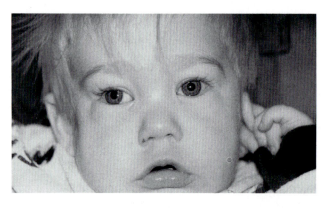

Figure 6–4. Exotropia (outward turning) of the right eye.

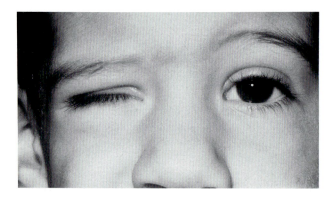

Figure 6–2. Unilateral eyelid closure in a child with an intermittent turning outward of the right eye (exotropia).

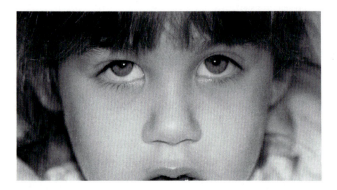

Figure 6–5. Hypertropia (upward turning) of the right eye.

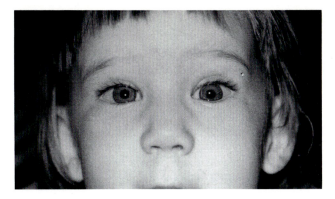

Figure 6–6. Hypotropia (downward turning) of the left eye.

TABLE 6–1. AMBLYOPIA

- *CHARACTERISTICS*

1. May be unilateral or bilateral
2. Visual acuity worse when reading a row as opposed to individual symbols (the crowding phenomenon)
3. Less degradation in vision with reduced room illumination than in eyes with organic disease
4. Less reduction of visual acuity when looking through a neutral-density filter than in eyes with organic macular disease
5. Relative afferent pupillary defect not usually seen unless the amblyopia is very dense; and even then is subtle (see Fig. 2–35)
6. Fixation with the amblyopic eye may be eccentric (nonfoveal)

- *CATEGORIES*

Strabismic	Usually unilateral; results from prolonged and continual fixation by one eye, and suppression of images from the other eye.
Refractive	Associated with large hyperopic, myopic, or astigmatic errors.
Anisometropic	Subtype of above when amblyopia occurs only in the more ametropic eye.
Deprivation	(Amblyopia ex anopsia) Occurs when a focused retinal image cannot be formed on the retina because of an obstruction in the visual axis.

nite preference to use one eye; **alternating** strabismus is used when there is no ocular preference. In the patient with monocular strabismus, the nondominant eye is often amblyopic. Strabismus can also be **comitant,** the same in any direction of gaze, or **incomitant,** varying with the direction of gaze. If the deviation is the same at distance and near fixation a normal accommodative convergence to accommodation ratio (AC/A) exists. A **high AC/A** ratio indicates that there is excessive convergence with accommodation; a **low AC/A** ratio indicates deficient convergence with accommodation.

COMPREHENSIVE INFORMATION ON AMBLYOPIA AND STRABISMUS

Amblyopia

Classification of Amblyopia

The development of amblyopia results from impairment at different levels of the retinocortical pathway during the sensitive period of visual development. Clinical and basic research has indicated that the essential mechanisms operative in the different forms of amblyopia are similar, and result from abnormal binocular interaction or foveal deprivation. For convenience and clarity, however, amblyopia is classified according to the different clinical settings in which it is found (Table 6–1).

Strabismic Amblyopia. Proper alignment of the eyes permits bifoveal fixation, which is necessary for the development of normal binocular single vision. Misalignment of one eye results in lack of central fixation, and to some extent the loss of capacity for form discrimination in the deviated eye.

It has been shown that the duration of strabismus correlates more closely with the eventual development of amblyopia than does the child's age at the time the deviation appeared. Children with strabismus who strongly favor one eye are more likely to develop amblyopia than are those who alternate fixation. Further, children with esotropia had an approximately four times greater incidence of amblyopia than those with exotropia (Costenbader et al, 1948).

Refractive Amblyopia. Amblyopia can occur in eyes with hyperopic, myopic, or astigmatic errors, if the error is so large as to blur or distort the retinal image. Refractive errors of more than 4.5 diopter of hyperopia, or 2.5 diopter of astigmatism, induce the greatest risk for developing amblyopia (AAO, 1992). Very hyperopic eyes are more likely to develop profound amblyopia than highly myopic eyes. This is because the hyperopic eyes will not be at focus for any distance, whereas the myopic eyes may be at focus at near range. Disorders that cause refractive amblyopia by inducing astigmatism and distorting the retinal image include ptosis, orbital tumors, and dislocated lenses.

Anisometropic Amblyopia. Anisometropia (unequal refractive error in the two eyes) can cause unilateral amblyopia. A difference of more than 1.5 D of hyperopia or astigmatism, or 3.0 D of myopia, can be amblyogenic (AAO, 1992). Unilateral high hyperopia is more amblyogenic than unilateral high myopia.

In anisohyperopia, the retina of the better eye receives a clearly defined image; however, no stimulus is provided for further accommodative effort in the more hyperopic eye. The retinal image in the latter eye remains unfocused, resulting in amblyopia. In anisomyopia, the more myopic eye is likely to be used for near work, and the less myopic eye for distance. Unless the myopia is severe, both retinas receive clear images, and amblyopia does not occur. Uniocular astigmatism can also result in amblyopia. As the astigmatic difference increases, the degree of amblyopia tends to increase as well.

Visual Deprivation Amblyopia.
Any ocular abnormality that occludes the visual axis and prevents the formation of a clear, focused retinal image during the critical period of visual development will result in deprivation amblyopia. Examples include corneal opacities, congenital cataracts, and vitreous hemorrhage. Deprivation amblyopia that occurs and is untreated during the first 2 to 3 months of life can be irreversible. Bilateral occurrence during this period also results in the development of nystagmus.

Theoretical Considerations in Amblyopia
Wiesel and Hubel (1963) demonstrated the effects of visual deprivation induced by eyelid closure or strabismus in visually immature kittens. They showed that the cell size in a lateral geniculate nucleus (LGN) receiving input from a deprived eye was significantly smaller than in a LGN receiving input from a nondeprived eye. Also, the number of cortical neurons that could be stimulated via a deprived eye was significantly reduced.

Other investigators have demonstrated that there is a sensitive period of visual development in each animal, following which structural and functional recovery does not occur. The precise age range during which the human visual system is vulnerable has yet to be defined. By clinical observation, it appears that the visual system is most sensitive during the early months of life. Humans remain quite vulnerable until age 5 or 6 years, and somewhat vulnerable until about 9 years of age.

Detection of Amblyopia
In strabismic children, spontaneous alternation of fixation suggests that neither eye is amblyopic (Fig. 6–7). Amblyopia can also be detected by covering the eye that appears straight, and observing the fixation pattern of the other eye. If the uncovered eye has wandering fixation, or the child shows a lack of visual interest, amblyopia is present (Fig. 6–8).

In the absence of ocular misalignment, close observation of visual alertness, and the maintenance of fixation on an object is important. A child who objects to occlusion of one eye, but not the other, is likely to have amblyopia in the second eye.

Subjective testing of visual acuity can be attempted in children older than 3 years of age. Although any difference in acuity between the two eyes may be designated as amblyopia, a two-line difference is usually used for diagnostic purposes. With amblyopia, the visual acuity for isolated symbols is usually better than for groups of symbols. This observation is referred to as the crowding phenomenon. Several signs that are useful in differentiating eyes with amblyopia from those with an organic loss of vision are reviewed in Table 6–1.

Treatment of Amblyopia
The goal of amblyopia treatment is to obtain normal and equal vision in each eye. This goal, unfortunately,

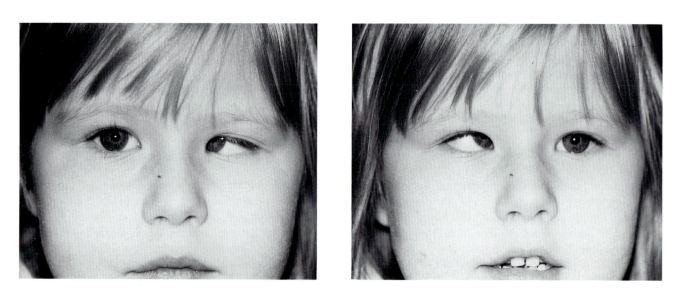

Figure 6–7. The detection of amblyopia: Spontaneous alternation of fixation suggests that there is probably no amblyopia.

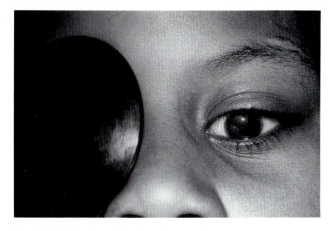

Figure 6–8. The detection of amblyopia: If an eye wanders, and fails to fixate, when its fellow eye is covered, it likely has poor vision.

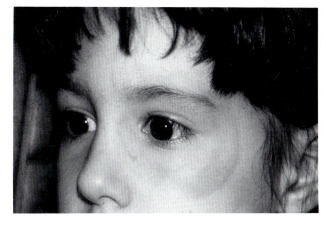

Figure 6–10. Contact dermatitis from the glue of an eye patch.

is not always reached. The younger the age at which treatment is instituted, the more likely it is to be successful.

The first step in the treatment of amblyopia is optical correction of any significant refractive error. In the presence of anisometropia, or high hyperopia, without strabismus, glasses alone should be tried prior to occlusion therapy. In these cases, occlusion can induce strabismus from the interruption of peripheral fusion. This can sometimes, but not always, be avoided if the maximum vision obtainable through correcting the refractive error is achieved, prior to initiating occlusion therapy for any residual amblyopia.

When occlusion therapy is needed, an opaque adhesive patch is used (Fig. 6–9). A complication is the development of a contact dermatitis (Fig. 6–10). Clip-on or press-on occluders can be used by children with glasses (Figs. 6–11 and 6–12). Occlusion therapy should

be initiated full time (every waking hour). Some clinicians, however, allow the patch to be removed 1 hour each day to prevent occlusion amblyopia in the previously sound eye. Patching is initially prescribed at 1 week for every year of age. Children less than 1 year of age should be reexamined in less than 1 week. Reexamination in the compliant patient age 1 to 2 years is biweekly, and in those age 3 to 5 years, monthly. Occlusion is continued until the acuity plateaus, and is maintained for 3 to 6 months or until the fixation preference switches to the previously amblyopic eye. If the vision does not improve after 3 to 6 months of full-time occlusion, further occlusion is unlikely to be beneficial.

An improvement in acuity must be maintained until the child reaches visual maturity, generally considered to be age 9 years. Maintenance therapy involves part-time patching or the use of a neutral-density filter on the glasses (Figs. 6–13 and 6–14). The

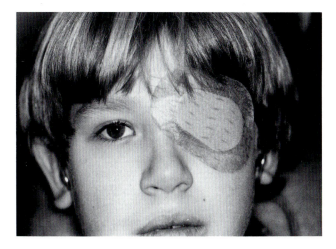

Figure 6–9. Occlusion therapy using a patch that adheres to the skin and completely occludes the eye.

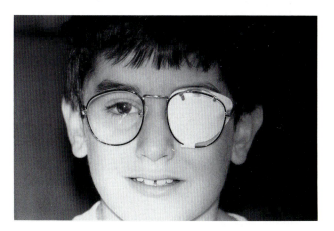

Figure 6–11. Clip-on eyeglass occluder.

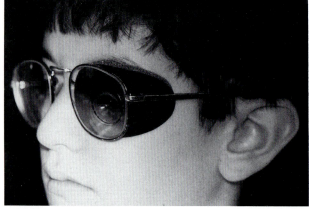

Figure 6–12. Press-on eyeglass occluder. Note how the clip-on and press-on occluders wrap around the eye to prevent "peeking."

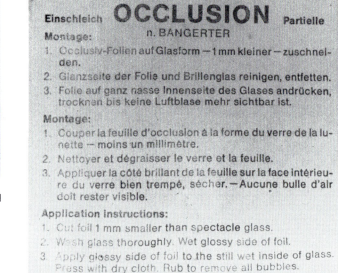

Figure 6–14. Instructions for placement of neutral density filter.

regimen is tailored to gradually reduce the amount of patching, or the density of the filter.

Occlusion therapy can sometimes be difficult to institute or continue. In children with very poor vision in an eye, it may be helpful to progressively increase patching over the first week of treatment. A restraint to prevent the child from pulling off the patch also may be needed. Examples include mittens taped to the arms (Fig. 6–15) and devices that prohibit elbow flexion (Fig. 6–16). The latter allows children to use their hands but prevents their hands from reaching their face.

An alternative to occlusion is the use of cycloplegic agents (such as atropine 0.5 or 1.0 percent) in the fixating eye. If the vision in the sound eye is reduced to a level worse than the amblyopic eye, the fixation pattern will shift. This therapy does not work well with profound amblyopia. Atropine can also be absorbed systemically, causing hyperactivity and high fevers; this can be decreased by placing pressure over the na-

solacrimal canaliculi at the time of eyedrop administration. Other techniques include the use of opaque contact lenses, phospholine iodide drops, and blurring by optical means. According to the American Academy of Ophthalmology (1992), "Eye movement exercises, 'passive' occlusion, or methods designed to stimulate or suppress vision using flashing lights or high-contrast rotating patterns have not been validated to be clinically effective [in treating amblyopia] in controlled studies."

A pilot study undertaken to investigate the efficacy of levodopa in the treatment of amblyopia in children ages 7 to 12 years noted an improvement in visual

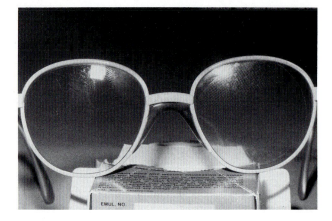

Figure 6–13. Neutral-density filter placed on the back surface of the left lens.

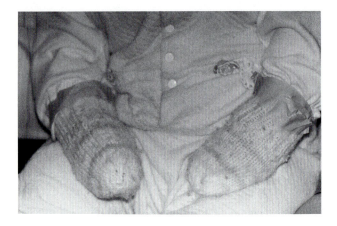

Figure 6–15. Mittens taped to the arms to prevent removal of eye patches.

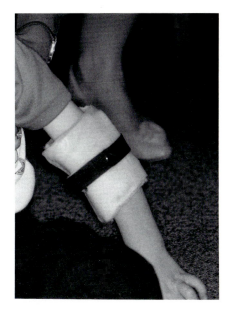

Figure 6–16. Homemade device used to prevent elbow flexion, and thus the removal of eye patches.

function (acuity, contrast sensitivity, and pattern visual evoked responses), lasting up to 5 hours (Leguire et al, 1992). It remains undetermined, however, whether this can be maintained with chronic dosing.

Strabismus

Congenital (Infantile or Early-Onset) Esotropia

Congenital esotropia is the most common form of strabismus, occurring in 1 to 2 percent of the population (Nelson et al, 1987). The sex distribution is equal. Transmission in many families is as an irregular auto-

somal dominant trait; in others it may be recessive. It is very common to find a history of strabismus in the parents or siblings of affected patients.

As many as 40 to 50 percent of infants with congenital esotropia have amblyopia (Costenbader, 1961). Some infants "cross-fixate," using alternate eyes in the opposite field of gaze (Fig. 6–17). This protects against the development of amblyopia, but not absolutely. A better assessment of visual acuity can be obtained by noting the point at which alternation of fixation occurs with the movement of a target along the horizontal plane. If no amblyopia exists, fixation will spontaneously alternate as the object crosses the midline. With amblyopia, the sound eye continues to follow the target beyond the midline, into the abducted position (Dickey et al, 1991).

Typically, the deviation in congenital esotropia is 50 prism diopters or more. The misalignment tends to be similar at distance and near fixation. It is difficult to perform the prism cover test with most young infants. The Hirschberg and Krimsky methods are, therefore, often substituted. In a commonly used adaptation of the Krimsky technique, two base-out prisms are used, apex to apex, to center the pupillary light reflexes in infants with large angles of deviation (Fig. 6–18).

Children with congenital esotropia tend to have cycloplegic refractions similar to those of normal children of the same age. This finding contrasts markedly with the characteristic hyperopia associated with refractive accommodative esotropia.

Associated Findings in Congenital Esotropia

DISSOCIATED VERTICAL DEVIATION. A dissociated vertical deviation (DVD) consists of a slow upward deviation of one or alternate eyes (Fig. 6–19). Occasionally, ex-

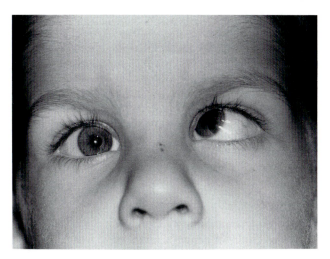

A

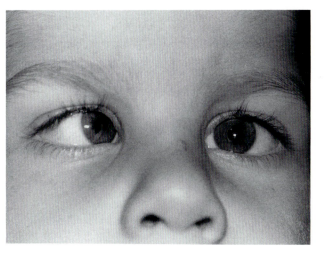

B

Figure 6–17. Cross-fixation in congenital esotropia. **A.** Fixation with the right eye for the left visual field. **B.** Fixation with the left eye for the right visual field.

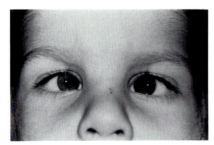

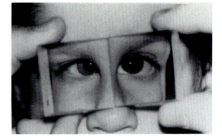

Figure 6–18. Modified Krimsky test used to measure the angle of deviation in congenital esotropia.

cyclotorsion can be demonstrated on upward drifting of the eye and incyclotorsion on downward movement. DVD may be latent, detected only when the involved eye is covered, or manifest, occurring intermittently or constantly. It is differentiated from a true vertical deviation because no corresponding hypotropia occurs in the other eye on cover testing. Bielschowsky's phenomenon is another feature of DVD, characterized by downward movement of the occluded eye when filters of increasing density are placed before the fixating eye.

The incidence of DVD in patients with congenital esotropia is high, ranging from 46 to 90 percent (Nelson, 1992). Early horizontal alignment does not decrease the incidence, suggesting that DVD is a time-related phenomenon, not significantly modified by the achievement of binocular vision.

DVD can be estimated using a base-down prism in front of the involved eye. The strength of the prism is adjusted until no movement occurs as the cover is shifted from the involved to the fixating eye. Because this technique is difficult, and may be inaccurate, some observers prefer to estimate a DVD on a semiquantitative grading scale of 1 to 4+.

INFERIOR OBLIQUE OVERACTION (IOOA). The incidence of inferior oblique overaction (IOOA) of one or both inferior oblique muscles in patients with congenital esotropia has been reported to be as high as 78 percent (Hiles et al, 1980). Similar to DVD, IOOA can be classified as grades 1 to 4+. Grade 1 means 1 mm of higher elevation of the adducting eye in gaze up and to the side. Grade 4 indicates 4 mm of higher elevation. It is best to measure the difference in elevation between the two eyes by comparing the 6-o'clock position of each limbus.

IOOA and DVD are both conditions that can cause excessive elevation of an eye in adduction. The differentiating features of these two conditions are listed in Table 6–2. IOOA results in elevation of the involved eye as it moves nasally (Fig. 6–20). The vertical misalignment in DVD, however, also occurs in abduction, and in the primar position. When the adducting eye in IOOA fixates, there is a corresponding hypotropia in the contralateral abducting eye. In DVD, contralateral hypotropia does not occur.

NYSTAGMUS. Rotatory nystagmus may occur in children with congenital esotropia, and tends to decrease during the first decade of life. Latent nystagmus can also occur. The latter is a predominantly horizontal, jerk nystagmus, elicited by occluding either eye. The slow phase is toward the side of the occluded eye. This type of nystagmus also tends to diminish with time. To measure visual acuity in the presence of latent nystagmus, a method that retains a relative binocular state by partially blurring the image in the nonviewing eye should be used. Techniques include the use of fogging lenses, or viewing polarized or duochrome slides through polarizing or green lenses, respectively.

Differential Diagnosis of Congenital Esotropia.
During the first year of life, a number of conditions can simulate congenital esotropia and cause diagnostic difficulty (Table 6–3). Because the management of these conditions may differ from the treatment of congenital esotropia, their recognition is important.

Pseudoesotropia is one of the most common reasons an ophthalmologist is asked to evaluate infants. Costenbader (1961) found that of 753 patients sus-

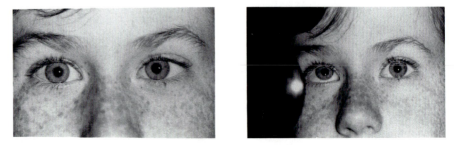

Figure 6–19. Dissociated vertical deviation. Interruption of fusion causes the occluded eye to drift upward.

TABLE 6–2. DISTINGUISHING FEATURES OF DISSOCIATED VERTICAL DEVIATION AND INFERIOR OBLIQUE OVERACTION

Feature	Dissociated Vertical Deviation	Inferior Oblique Overaction
Elevation	In adduction and abduction	In adduction only
Hypotropia	No corresponding hypotropia in opposite eye	Corresponding hypotropia in opposite eye
Comitancy	Usually comitant (same in adduction, primary position, and abduction)	Incomitant (greater in field of action of inferior oblique muscle)
Variability	Variable hyperdeviation	Hyperdeviation not variable
Strabismus pattern	Not associated with "A" or "V" pattern	Commonly associated with "V" pattern
Upward versus downward gaze	Same amount of hyperdeviation in upward as downward gaze	More hyperdeviation in upward than downward gaze
Associated ocular movements	Hyperdeviation can be associated with torsional movement and abduction	Hyperdeviation not associated with torsional movement

From Scott WE, Sutton VJ, Thalacker JA: Superior rectus recessions for dissociated vertical deviation. Ophthalmology 89:317, 1982.

pected by their parents of having esotropia, 47 percent had pseudoesotropia. This condition is characterized by the false appearance of esotropia when the visual axes are accurately aligned. The appearance may be caused by a flat, broad nasal bridge, prominent epicanthal folds, and/or a narrow interpupillary distance (Figs. 6–21 and 2–32). The observer sees less sclera nasally than would be expected, which creates the impression that the eyes are turned in toward the nose. This appearance is especially marked when the child looks to the side (Fig. 6–22). A more symmetric appearance of the sclera can be demonstrated to parents by retracting the excessive skin covering the nasal sclera.

It is important to realize that esotropia can also occur in children with wide nasal bridges and prominent epicanthal folds (Fig. 6–23). A true manifest deviation should be ruled out by the use of the corneal light reflex (see Fig. 2–10) and the cover/uncover test (see Fig. 2–12), when possible. Once pseudoesotropia has been confirmed, parents can be reassured that the child will "outgrow" the appearance of esotropia. As the child grows, the bridge of the nose becomes more prominent and displaces the epicanthal folds, so that the sclera visible medially becomes proportional to the amount visible laterally. Because true esotropia can yet develop in children with pseudoesotropia, parents and pediatricians should, however, be cautioned that reassessment is required if the apparent deviation does not improve.

Treatment of Congenital Esotropia. The primary goal of treatment in congenital esotropia is to reduce the deviation at distance and near to orthophoria, or as close to it as possible. Ideally, this results in normal sight in each eye, straight-looking eyes, and the development of at least a rudimentary form of sensory fusion that will maintain motor alignment.

Patients with congenital esotropia never become bifixators (that is, do not develop stereoscopic acuity of 40 seconds of arc), regardless of their age at surgical alignment. Clinical evidence suggests, however, that alignment within 10 prism diopters of orthophoria before 2 years of age is associated with the attainment of some degree of binocular vision and stereopsis.

Early and vigorous amblyopia therapy is an important component in the treatment of congenital esotropia. Once alternate fixation can be demonstrated, each eye is assumed to have equal vision, and patching is discontinued. Surgery is performed after the treatment of amblyopia has reached a plateau. It is easier to adjust occlusion intensity before surgery, as a fixation preference may be difficult to ascertain after successful alignment. In addition, both amblyopia and full-time patching present impediments to the development of binocular vision during the postoperative period. Fortunately, the amblyopia associated with congenital esotropia is amenable to treatment. Continued monitoring for amblyopia, after surgical correction and through early childhood, however, remains necessary.

Various surgical techniques have been used for the

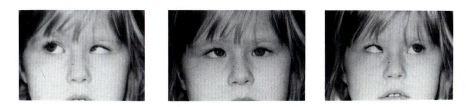

Figure 6–20. Overaction of both inferior oblique muscles. Note how each eye elevates in the adducted position.

TABLE 6–3. DIFFERENTIAL DIAGNOSIS OF CONGENITAL ESOTROPIA

Pseudoesotropia
Duane's retraction syndrome
Möbius syndrome
Nystagmus blockage syndrome
Congenital sixth-nerve palsy
Early-onset accommodative esotropia
Sensory esotropia
Esotropia in the neurologically impaired

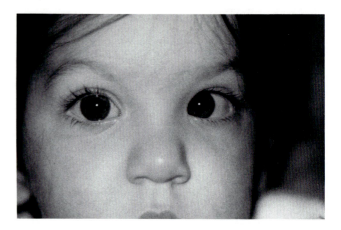

Figure 6–22. Pseudoesotropia in another child with a wide nasal bridge. The "crossed eyes" appearance is accentuated by gaze to the side.

correction of congenital esotropia. Proponents of two-muscle surgery advocate either symmetric recession of both medial rectus muscles, or monocular medial rectus recession combined with lateral rectus resection, regardless of the size of the preoperative deviation (Figs. 6–24 and 6–25). Both procedures are graded, with more millimeters of surgery performed for larger deviations. If a second procedure is required, symmetric resections of both lateral rectus muscles or a recess–resect procedure in the fellow eye are performed. Because of an unacceptable incidence of undercorrections in large-angle congenital esotropia, some surgeons have instituted three and four horizontal rectus muscle surgery as an initial procedure.

Accommodative Esotropia

Accommodative esotropia is defined as a "convergent deviation of the eyes" associated with activation of the accommodative reflex. Esotropia that is related to accommodative effort may be divided into three major categories: (1) refractive, (2) nonrefractive, and (3) partial or decompensated.

Refractive Accommodative Esotropia.

Refractive accommodative esotropia usually presents at 2 to 3 years of age. The typical history is that of a sudden

onset of esotropia, or progressively more frequent intermittent esotropia. Occasionally, children 1 year of age or younger will present with all the clinical features of accommodative esotropia. The American Academy of Ophthalmology's preferred practice pattern on esotropia (1992) notes that consideration should be given to prescribing glasses to infants under age 1 year with a hyperopia of 3.0 D or greater, to reduce the incidence of esotropia. Baker and Parks (1980) reported on 21 patients with an onset of accommodative esotropia prior to age 1 year. Approximately 50 percent of their patients whose esodeviation was initially controlled with glasses decompensated into nonaccommodative esotropia. Additionally, as many as 65 percent of corrected congenital esotropes will require spectacle correction of hypermetropia to control esotropia at some time postoperatively (Hiles et al, 1980).

The refraction of patients with refractive accommodative esotropia averages +4.75 D, with a range of

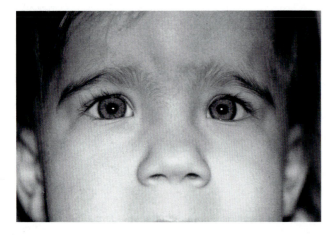

Figure 6–21. Pseudoesotropia. This child has a wide nasal bridge allowing more sclera to be visible temporally than nasally, giving the appearance of crossed eyes.

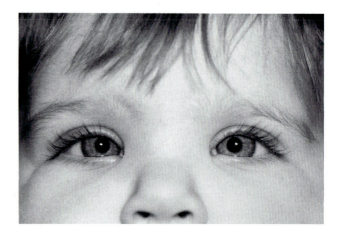

Figure 6–23. A child with a wide nasal bridge, prominent epicanthal folds and esotropia. Note that the light reflex is not centered in the pupils.

The initial treatment of refractive accommodative esotropia is to give the full hyperopic correction, determined by cycloplegic refraction (Fig. 6–26). Glasses alone will be successful in realigning the eyes 75 percent of the time (AAO, 1992). Beginning around age 4 to 5 years, an attempt can be made to reduce the strength of the hyperopic correction to enhance fusional divergence and to maximize visual acuity. Close monitoring of the child with a reduced correction is necessary to ensure that the alignment continues to be controlled.

It is important to warn parents that the esodeviation will appear to increase without glasses, after the initial correction is worn. Parents frequently state that before wearing glasses their child had a small, or very intermittent esodeviation. After wearing glasses for a few weeks, however, the deviation that occurs when the child removes the glasses has become quite large and frequent. Parents often blame this on their child becoming dependent on the glasses. This situation can best be explained on the basis of the child learning and wanting to use the appropriate amount of accommodative effort to see objects clearly, with the glasses. When the child removes the glasses, he or she will exert accommodative effort because of a desire to again bring objects into proper focus, resulting in a rapid development of esodeviation.

Nonrefractive Accommodative Esotropia. Children with nonrefractive accommodative esotropia usually present between 2 and 3 years of age with an esodeviation that is greater at near than at distance fixation. The refractive error in this condition may be hyperopia or myopia, but the average refraction is +2.25 D. Notably, many patients have combined refractive and nonrefractive accommodative esotropia (Fig. 6–27).

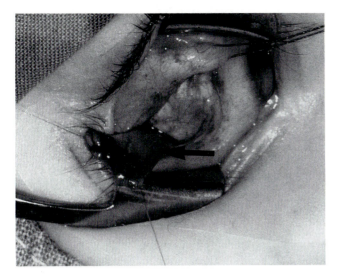

Figure 6–24. Strabismus surgery, demonstrating in this case the lateral rectus muscle, with a suture placed through it (*arrow*).

+3.00 to +10.00 D. The angle of esodeviation is the same when measured at distance and near fixation, and is usually moderate in magnitude, ranging between 20 to 40 prism D. Amblyopia is common, especially when the esodeviation has become constant.

The mechanism of refractive accommodative esotropia involves uncorrected hyperopia and insufficient fusional divergence. When an individual exerts a given amount of accommodation, a specific amount of convergence (accommodative convergence) is associated with it. An uncorrected hyperope must exert excessive accommodation to clear a blurred retinal image. This in turn will stimulate excessive convergence. If the amplitude of fusional divergence is inadequate, or sensory fusion is impeded by an obstruction in the visual axis, esotropia will result.

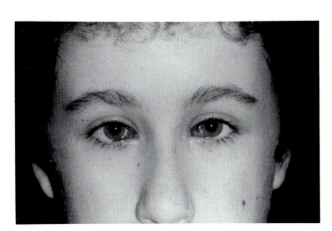

Figure 6–25. Postoperative appearance one day after recession of both medial rectus muscles to correct an esotropia.

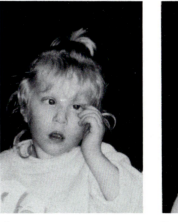 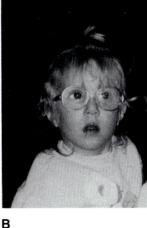

A   **B**

Figure 6–26. Refractive accommodative esotropia. **A.** Without glasses there was an esotropia of 30 prism diopters at both distance and near fixation. **B.** With the appropriate hyperopic glasses, the eyes are straight.

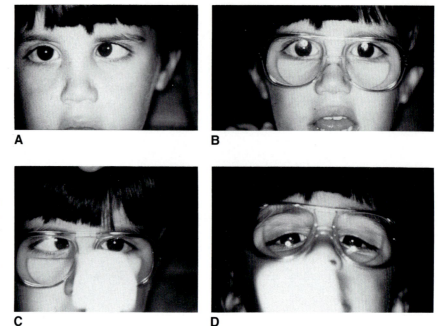

Figure 6–27. Child with both refractive and nonrefractive accommodative esotropia. **A.** Esodeviation at distance fixation. **B.** Reduction of esodeviation at distance fixation with hyperopic glasses. **C.** Nonrefractive esodeviation at near fixation due to a high AC/A ratio. **D.** Through the bifocals, the esotropia at near fixation is reduced. *(From Nelson LB, Catalano RA: Atlas of ocular motility. Philadelphia, Saunders, 1989, p 145, with permission.)*

In nonrefractive accommodative esotropia, there is a high accommodative convergence to accommodation (AC/A) ratio; the effort to accommodate elicits an abnormally high accommodative convergence response. To elicit this response, the examiner should have the patient fixate an accommodative target, such as small letters or a detailed picture. A large deviation at near fixation may be entirely missed if the patient fixates on a light source, as opposed to fixating on a descriptive accommodative target (Fig. 6–28).

There are a number of methods to measure the AC/A ratio: the heterophoria method, fixation disparity method, gradient method, and the clinical evaluation of distance and near deviation. Most clinicians prefer to assess the AC/A ratio using the distance–near comparison. This method allows the AC/A ratio to be evaluated more easily and quickly because it employs conventional examination techniques and requires no calculations. The AC/A relationship is derived by simply comparing the distance and near deviation. If the near measurement is greater than 10 prism diopters more esotropic than the distance measurement, the AC/A ratio is considered to be abnormally high.

The management of nonrefractive accommodative esotropia may involve a variety of modalities. Many pediatric ophthalmologists attempt to correct the esodeviation at near with bifocals, provided the distance deviation is less than 10 prism diopters. Initially, a +2.50 executive-type bifocal with the top of the lower segment bisecting the pupil is given (Fig. 6–29). It is important to communicate clearly with the optician as to how the bifocal should be placed, to prevent an inappropriate pair of glasses being dispensed (Figs. 6–30 and 6–31). In follow-up, the child should wear the least amount of hyperopic bifocal correction that is necessary to maintain straight eyes at near fixation.

Miotics have also been used successfully in patients with a high AC/A ratio. Their use, however, has been associated with the development of pupillary cysts, and in adults, with retinal detachment and cataract. In addition, miotics can result in prolonged apnea after anesthesia if succinylcholine is used. They are, therefore, not recommended for long-term use. Several investigators have performed surgery for a high AC/A ratio when the esodeviation at near fixation is no longer controlled with bifocals, with variable results.

Figure 6–28. Child with a high AC/A ratio. Note that the esodeviation is not elicited when the child fixates a light source (**A**), but is manifest upon fixating a small accommodative target (**B**).

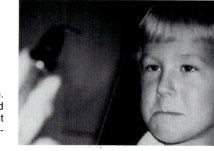

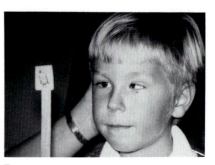

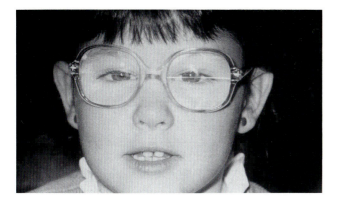

Figure 6–29. Proper positioning of bifocal segment in a child. Note how the bifocal bisects the pupil.

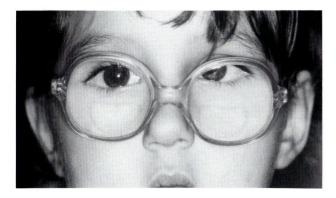

Figure 6–30. Improper bifocal for a child, set at an adult level.

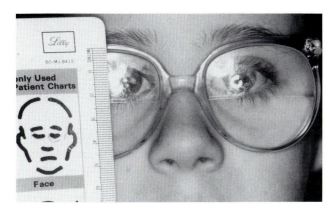

Figure 6–31. Improper bifocal for a child. Instead of bisecting the pupil, the bifocal bisects the glasses frame.

Partial or Decompensated Accommodative Esotropia. Refractive and nonrefractive accommodative esotropias do not always present in their "pure" forms. If these patients have a significant reduction in their esodeviation with full hyperopic correction, but a residual esodeviation persists, they are said to have partial accommodative esotropia (Fig. 6–32). This condition commonly occurs where there is a delay of months between the onset of accommodative esotropia and antiaccommodative treatment. Sometimes the esotropia may initially be eliminated with glasses; but slowly, a nonaccommodative portion becomes evident, in spite of the patient's wearing the maximum amount of hyperopic correction consistent with good vision. This is called decompensated accommodative esotropia.

It is not uncommon to encounter children who were prescribed inappropriate glasses to treat partial or decompensated esotropia nonsurgically. Examples include glasses upon which large Fresnel prisms have been ground or applied (Fig. 6–33), and glasses upon which occluders have been placed over the nasal part of the lens (Figs. 6–34 and 6–35). Large Fresnel prisms are usually not tolerated because they blur the vision and are cosmetically unacceptable. Occluders covering the nasal aspect of the lens do not prevent the eyes from crossing. The child still fixates with only one eye; the other is simply buried behind the occluder.

The indications for surgery for partial or decompensated accommodative esotropia remain controversial. Some ophthalmologists believe that all esotropias should be reduced to less than 10 prism diopters to enhance the development of peripheral sensory fusion and motor alignment. Other ophthalmologists feel that surgery should be performed only if the deviation is cosmetically significant. In either case, surgery is performed only on the nonaccommodative portion of the deviation. Orthoptic therapy, such as training to recognize diplopia and increase vergence amplitudes, has not been shown to be an effective treatment.

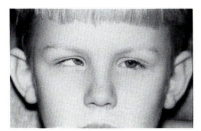
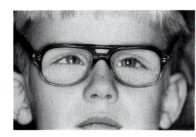

Figure 6–32. Partial accommodative esotropia. The appropriate hyperopic glasses did not completely reduce the deviation.

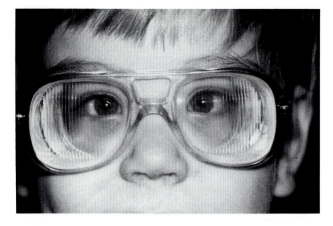

Figure 6–33. Inappropriate glasses for decompensated esotropia. Fresnel prisms have been ground on the posterior surface of the lens, but are of such high power that they blur vision.

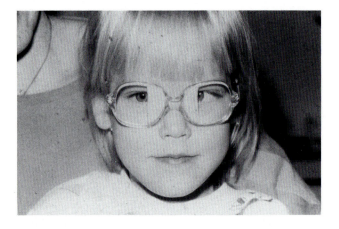

Figure 6–34. Inappropriate glasses for partial accommodative esotropia. The occluder placed on the nasal half of each lens does not prevent the eyes from turning in.

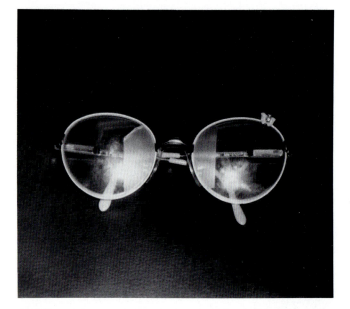

Figure 6–35. Same inappropriate use of an occluder on the nasal half of each lens as in Figure 6–34. In this case scotch tape was used.

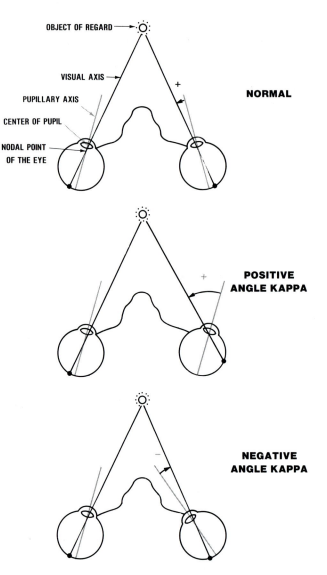
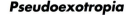

Figure 6–36. The angle kappa. *(From Nelson LB, Catalano RA: Atlas of ocular motility. Philadelphia, Saunders, 1989, p 97, with permission.)*

Pseudoexotropia

Pseudoexotropia is the appearance of divergent eyes, when they are in fact aligned. This appearance results from a positive angle kappa, or a wide interpupillary distance.

The angle kappa is the angle formed between the visual axis and the pupillary axis (Fig. 6–36). The visual axis is directed from the object of regard through the nodal point of the eye. The pupillary axis connects the center of the pupil, perpendicular to the cornea, with the nodal point. Normally, the two do not correspond because the fovea is slightly temporally displaced. The corneal light reflex will normally be slightly nasal to the pupillary center. By definition, a nasally displaced corneal light reflex is termed a **positive angle kappa.** A small positive angle of up to 5 degrees is physiological.

A larger nasal displacement of the corneal light reflex (positive angle kappa) mimics exotropia (Figs. 6–37 and 6–38). A temporal displacement of the light reflex,

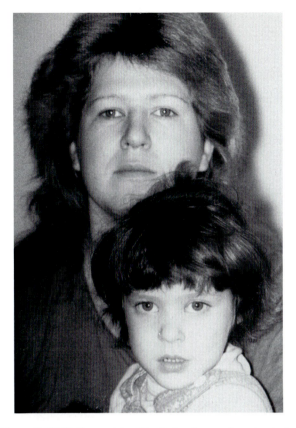

Figure 6–37. Mother and daughter both with pseudoexotropia due to a positive angle kappa.

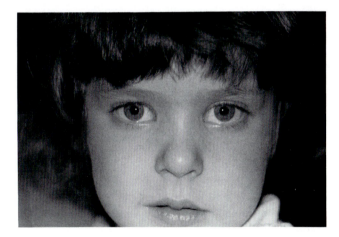

Figure 6–38. Close-up of child in Figure 6–37, demonstrating the divergent appearance of the eyes.

termed a **negative angle kappa,** mimics esotropia. Conversely, a large positive angle kappa may mask an esodeviation, and a negative angle kappa may mask an exodeviation.

A common cause of a large positive angle kappa and pseudoexotropia is dragged (temporally displaced) maculas associated with retinopathy of prematurity. A child with this condition is shown in Figure 6–39. Clinically, covering either eye will not result in any ocular movement. The diagnosis is confirmed by the ophthalmoscopic appearance of ectopic maculas (Fig. 6–40).

Congenital Exotropia

Exotropia occurring by 6 months of age in an otherwise healthy child is rare. In a review of 150 patients in whom an exotropia was noted prior to age one, Moore and Cohen (1985) could find only 10 with the criteria of true congenital exotropia. Eliminated were those patients with craniofacial abnormalities, neurological disease, restrictive syndromes, or any vision-impairing ocular defect.

Although congenital exotropia can initially be intermittent, most cases progress quickly to a constant alternating exotropia (Fig. 6–41). Amblyopia is not common, because of this alternation. The exotropia is often quite large, averaging 35 prism diopters or greater. Those children with an exotropia of 50 prism diopters or greater often appear to have decreased adduction on side gaze. With gaze right or left, the abducting eye fixates while the opposite eye approaches the midline and stops (Fig. 6–42). This is similar to the cross-fixation phenomenon seen in congenital esotropes. Occlusion or the doll's-head maneuver usually demonstrates that good adduction is possible.

Patients with congenital constant exotropia are operated on as early as 6 months of age, similar to the way in which patients with congenital esotropia are managed.

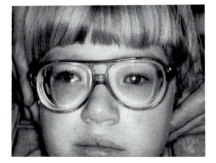 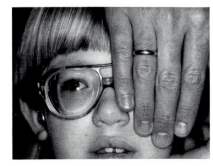

Figure 6–39. Pseudoexotropia in a child with dragged maculas and high myopia secondary to retinopathy of prematurity. Note that covering an eye does not elicit any movement in the opposite eye, which continues to appear divergent.

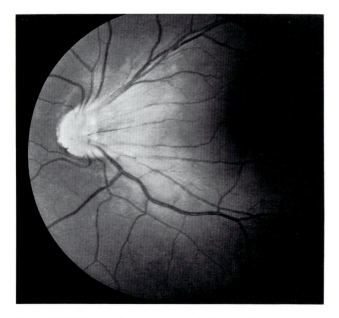

Figure 6–40. Temporally dragged macula due to retinopathy of prematurity. Note also the straightening of the posterior pole vessels. *(From Nelson LB, et al: Recognizing patterns of ocular childhood diseases. Thorofare, NJ, Slack, 1985, p 121, with permission.)*

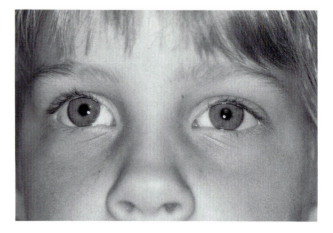

Figure 6–43. Phase II exodeviation: Exotropia at distance fixation.

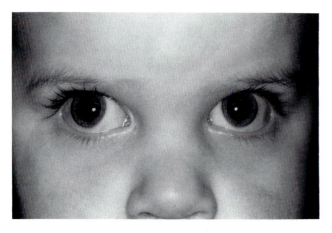

Figure 6–41. Congenital exotropia.

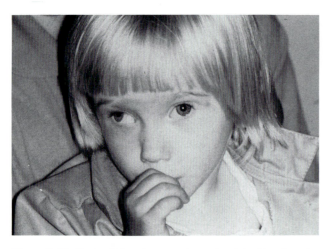

Figure 6–42. Congenital exotrope gazing to the right. Note how the left eye approaches the midline and stops.

Exodeviations in Childhood

Although the natural history of untreated exodeviations in childhood is not well-delineated, many pediatric ophthalmologists believe that they tend to follow a typical course. The age of onset varies, but is often between age 6 months and 4 years. In nearly all cases, initially the deviation is greater at distance fixation, and intermittent. In the early stages, no deviation is usually present at near fixation (Figs. 6–43 and 6–44). With time, the frequency, but not the size, of the exodeviation increases. The four phases that this entity can be thought of as evolving through are as follows (Calhoun et al, 1987):

Phase I   Exophoria at distance, orthophoria at near
Phase II   Intermittent exotropia at distance, orthophoria or exophoria at near
Phase III   Exotropia at distance, exophoria or intermittent exotropia at near
Phase IV   Exotropia at distance and near

Children in phase I are asymptomatic, and often remain undetected. In phase II, an intermittent exotropia is noticed by the family when the child views at distance during periods of fatigue or inattentiveness. During this phase, there is no suppression scotoma, and the child may report diplopia, or infer it by closing one eye, especially in bright sunlight. When examining a child in phase II, the exotropia is easily elicited by the cover test, but the deviating eye returns quickly with a blink or a change of fixation. In phase III, a suppression scotoma develops to avoid diplopia when fixating at distance. Instead of making a correcting fusional con-

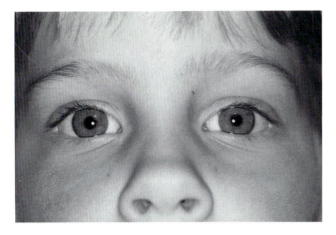

Figure 6–44. Phase II exodeviation: Orthophoria at near fixation.

vergent movement, an eye which turns out upon occlusion remains deviated when the occluder is removed. In phase III, some degree of binocular function can still be demonstrated at near. By phase IV, however, no binocularity is present, and a constant exotropia is present, even at near (Fig. 6–45). Not all children progress through each stage; some remain in phase II into adulthood.

Although most pediatric ophthalmologists agree that the treatment for intermittent exotropia is surgical, opinions vary widely regarding the timing of surgical intervention and the preoperative use of nonsurgical treatments. The latter include the use of base-in prisms, overcorrecting minus lenses, and orthoptic exercises. Indications for surgery are based on indirect evidence that a suppression scotoma is developing. Retaining some innate binocular function increases the likelihood that, postoperatively, the eyes will stay aligned indefinitely.

When the deviation is intermittent, is eliminated with a blink, and occurs only with fatigue, observation is warranted. If the condition is progressing from phase II to III (that is, it occurs during periods when the child is alert, and lasts through a blink or change in fixation), surgery is indicated to prevent further development of a suppression scotoma (Calhoun et al, 1987). If the child shows signs of diplopia (covers one eye for distance viewing), surgery is also indicated. An older child who does not have diplopia in the presence of an obvious exodeviation at distance fixation is in phase III. Although the ideal time for surgery has passed, surgery still should be urged to try to maintain whatever binocular function remains at near fixation. By phase IV, the suppression scotoma is firmly set. The surgical indication for this stage is cosmesis.

It is generally well accepted that the best long-term results in surgery for childhood-onset exodeviations occur when there is an initial overcorrection to produce esotropia (Fig. 6–46). The best opportunity for satisfactory alignment occurs with an overcorrection of 11 to 20 diopters at 2 to 10 days after surgery (Raab & Parks, 1969). Parents should, therefore, be advised that transient esotropia, sometimes with diplopia, is expected and desired after surgery for exotropia.

"A" and "V" Pattern Strabismus

An ocular misalignment is classified as comitant if the same deviation occurs in each of the cardinal positions of gaze (Fig. 6–47). Strabismus is classified as having an "A" or "V" pattern if a horizontal change of alignment occurs as the eyes move from straight up, to straight ahead, to straight down gaze. These patterns must be considered if strabismus surgery is planned, especially if a compensatory chin up or chin down position exists (Fig. 6–48). The latter results from an individual's innate desire for fusion, which an A or V pattern often allows.

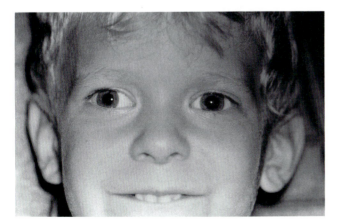

Figure 6–45. Phase IV exodeviation: Exotropia at near fixation.

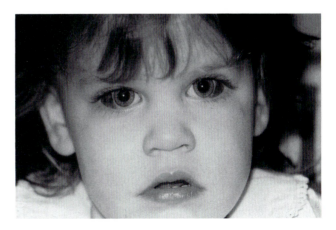

Figure 6–46. Consecutive esotropia 2 days after surgery for childhood-onset exotropia.

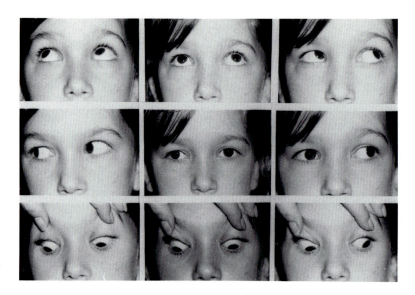

Figure 6–47. Comitant exotropia. The deviation is the same in each of the cardinal positions of gaze.

A and V patterns are demonstrated by measuring a deviation in the primary position, and with the eyes directed approximately 25 degrees in upward and downward gaze, while the patient fixates on a distant object. Between upward gaze and downward gaze, a difference of 10 prism diopters in the horizontal alignment is usually sufficient to diagnose an A pattern; a difference of 15 prism diopters diagnoses a V pattern.

A Patterns. With an A pattern, the eyes turn in more (or turn out less) in straight upward gaze and turn in less in straight downward gaze (Fig. 6–49 and 6–50).

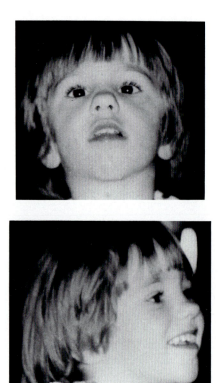

Figure 6–48. A child with a V-pattern exotropia, who maintains a chin up head position. This is done to achieve fusion, which is possible in downward gaze.

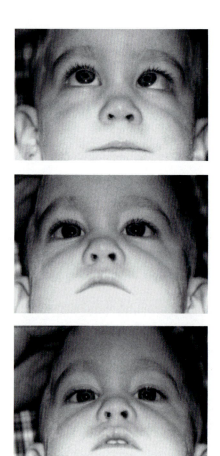

Figure 6–49. "A"-pattern esotropia.

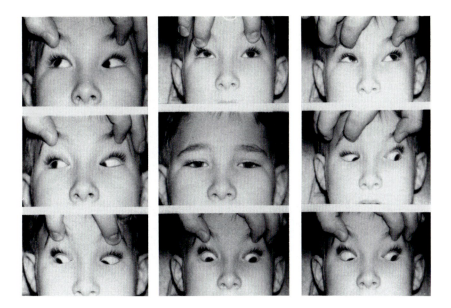

Figure 6–50. "A"-pattern exotropia.

Often, the inferior oblique muscles underact, which causes decreased abduction in upward gaze. Overaction of the superior oblique muscles increases abduction in downward gaze.

V Patterns. With a V pattern, the eyes turn out more (or turn in less) in straight upward gaze and turn out less in straight downward gaze (Figs. 6–51 and 6–52). Often, the inferior oblique muscles overact, which causes increased abduction in upward gaze. Underaction of the superior oblique muscles decreases abduction in downward gaze.

A and V patterns can be surgically corrected in one of several ways: moving the insertions of the horizontal rectus muscles up or down, weakening either the inferior or superior oblique muscles, or moving the insertions of the vertical rectus muscles laterally or medially. The latter is seldom performed.

Moving a horizontal rectus muscle insertion up or down (offsetting) weakens the action of that muscle only when the eye is moved in the direction of the offsetting. For example, if the medial rectus muscle is moved up one-half tendon width, in primary position its action will not be substantially altered. On straight-upward gaze, however, the new insertion of the medial rectus, now one-half tendon width higher, will be rotated closer to its origin, or in effect recessed. Its action in upward gaze will thus be reduced. It follows that moving the medial rectus muscle toward the apex of an A or V pattern, regardless of whether the medial rectus

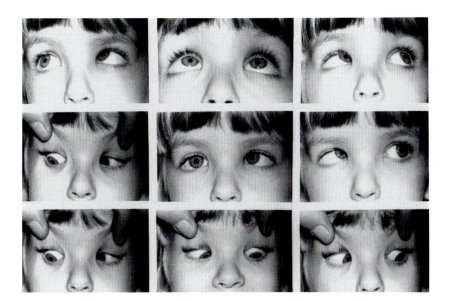

Figure 6–51. "V"-pattern esotropia.

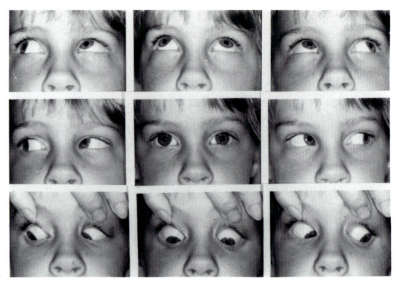

Figure 6–52. "V"-pattern exotropia.

is recessed or resected, is appropriate for correcting the A or V syndrome. Conversely, moving the lateral rectus muscle toward the open end of the A or V is appropriate for surgery performed on that muscle. It is generally accepted that offsetting two horizontal rectus muscles one-half tendon width will correct approximately 15 prism diopters of the A or V pattern (Metz & Schwartz, 1977). Offsetting larger amounts gives unpredictable results.

The oblique muscles should be weakened only if they are overacting, and only if there is some degree of underaction of the opposing oblique muscles. If this advice is ignored, an opposite pattern, with the unoperated oblique muscles overacting, will likely develop postoperatively. Additionally, if there is fusion in any gaze, far or near, even if intermittent, the superior oblique muscles should not be weakened. The weakening effect is likely to be unequal, resulting in signs and symptoms of unilateral or bilateral superior

oblique palsy. Weakening of the inferior oblique muscles, however, does not create a similar problem.

Weakening two overacting inferior oblique muscles causes about 15 prism diopters of eso shift in upward gaze (for example, a lessening of exotropia, or an increase in esotropia). This procedure has no effect on horizontal alignment in primary position or downward gaze. Weakening both overacting superior oblique muscles causes much more convergence in downward gaze, about 25 to 45 prism diopters, with up to 10 prism diopters of convergence in primary position, and no effect, or an exo shift, in upward gaze (Calhoun et al, 1987).

A pattern described as "X" is commonly seen in patients with a large exotropia. All four oblique muscles overact, as detected on lateral gaze, with some additional exotropia or divergence in upward and downward gaze. For an X pattern, appropriate surgery for the exotropia alone should be performed, which usu-

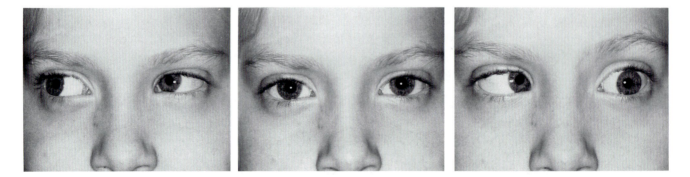

Figure 6–53. Type I DRS, left eye. Note the limitation of abduction, slight restriction of adduction, narrowing of the palpebral fissure on adduction, and widening of the fissure on attempted abduction.

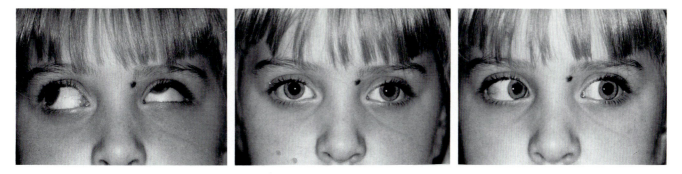

Figure 6–54. Type II DRS, left eye. Note the exotropia of the affected eye, limitation and upshooting of the eye on attempted adduction, and slightly limited abduction.

ally corrects the appearance of overaction of the oblique muscles.

Strabismus Syndromes

Duane's Retraction Syndrome (DRS). In 1905,
Duane summarized the clinical findings, and offered theories on the pathogenesis and treatment of an unusual ocular motility disorder that came to bear his name. It is now recognized that approximately 1 percent of all individuals with strabismus have this syndrome (Kirkham, 1970).

The clinical findings of Duane's retraction syndrome (DRS) include a unilateral or bilateral abnormality of horizontal gaze, retraction of the globe on attempted adduction, and an upward or downward displacement of the globe in adduction. Huber (1974), using electromyography, classified DRS into three types:

- **Type I** is characterized by a marked limitation or complete absence of abduction, normal or only slightly restricted adduction, narrowing of the palpebral fissure and retraction of the globe on adduction, and widening of the palpebral fissure on attempted abduction (Fig. 6–53). Electromyography demonstrates an absence of electrical activity in the lateral rectus muscle on abduction, and paradoxical activity on adduction.
- **Type II** is characterized by limitation or absence of adduction, and exotropia of the affected eye. Abduction can be normal, or slightly limited, and there is retraction of the globe on attempted adduction (Fig. 6–54). Electromyography reveals electrical activity of the lateral rectus muscle on both abduction and adduction.
- **Type III** is characterized by severe restriction of both abduction and adduction, with retraction of the globe and narrowing of the palpebral fissure on attempted adduction (Fig. 6–55). Electromyography demonstrates electrical activity of both horizontal rectus muscles on both adduction and abduction.

DRS more frequently occurs in the left eye than the right eye, and in females more than males. Most cases are unilateral, but bilateral and asymmetric involvement is possible. In several large series, the ratio of left eye versus right eye was 3:1, the prevalence of bilaterality was 20 percent and there was a slight preponderance of females over males (54 versus 46 percent) (Isenberg & Urist, 1977; Maruo et al, 1979).

Type I is the most common form of DRS, followed in order by types II and III. Most patients with types I and II DRS have straight eyes in the primary position during infancy and childhood. Some children with type I DRS develop an esodeviation in the primary position, and adopt a compensatory head turn toward the side of the involved eye to maintain binocular vision. With type II DRS, an exotropia can develop, in which case the head turn is away from the involved eye (Fig. 6–56).

In two large series the incidence of amblyopia in DRS patients was 10 and 14 percent, respectively (Isenberg & Urist, 1977; O'Malley et al, 1982). In an-

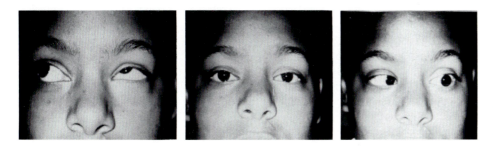

Figure 6–55. Type III DRS, left eye. Note the restriction of both abduction and adduction.

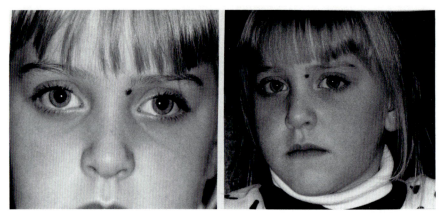

Figure 6–56. Compensatory face turn away from the involved eye in a patient with type II DRS (same patient as Fig. 6–54).

other study, a 3 percent incidence of amblyopia was noted in 72 patients, and the authors commented that this incidence is similar to that in the general population (Tredici & von Noorden, 1985).

A number of ocular and systemic anomalies have been associated with DRS. Ocular anomalies include cataracts, iris anomalies, Marcus Gunn jaw-winking, crocodile tears, and microphthalmos. Systemic associations include Goldenhar's syndrome (corneal dermoids, preauricular skin tags, misshapen ears, and deafness) and Klippel–Feil syndrome (cervical spina bifida, cleft palate, facial anomalies, perceptive deafness, and malformations of the ears, feet, and hands).

Data from autopsy studies provide evidence that DRS involves an abnormality of the sixth cranial nerve. In an autopsy case of bilateral type III DRS, both abducens nuclei and nerves were absent, and both lateral rectus muscles were innervated by a branch from the inferior division of the oculomotor nerve. The same findings, limited to the involved side, have been demonstrated in a second patient with unilateral DRS (Miller et al, 1982).

Indications for surgery for patients with DRS are a significant deviation in primary position, an anomalous head position, or a large upward or downward displacement on adduction that is cosmetically unacceptable. In most patients with type I DRS and esotropia, an ipsilateral medial rectus recession can significantly improve the esodeviation and the face turn. Resection of the lateral rectus should never be performed, as this will increase retraction of the globe in adduction. Patients who have type II DRS with exotropia in the primary position and a face turn away from the involved eye, require a recession of the ipsilateral lateral rectus muscle. An up- or down-shooting can be reduced by splitting the lateral rectus muscle into a Y configuration, to reduce its leash effect. This has been shown to be effective without inducing strabismus in the primary position (Rogers & Bremer, 1984). Inferior oblique weakening alone has not been effective in eliminating upshooting (von Noorden & Murray, 1986).

Nystagmus Blockage Syndrome. The nystagmus blockage syndrome is characterized by nystagmus that begins in early infancy, and is associated with esotropia (Fig. 6–57). The nystagmus is reduced or absent with the fixating eye in adduction. As the fixating eye follows a target moving laterally (towards the primary position and then into abduction), the nystagmus amplitude increases and the esotropia decreases. When the fellow eye is occluded a head turn develops in the direction of the uncovered eye (Fig. 6–58). This abnormal head posture allows the uncovered eye to persist in an adducted position.

Cuppers (1971) noted the nystagmus blockage syndrome in 139 (10.2 percent) of 1352 esotropic patients. Von Noorden (1985) encountered this syndrome in 12 percent of 789 consecutive patients with congenital esotropia. An increased incidence of hydrocephalus during infancy has been reported in patients with this condition.

A number of features distinguish primary infantile esotropia from the nystagmus blockage syndrome. Although nystagmus can be noted in primary infantile esotropia, in the latter condition the nystagmus amplitude does not change with gaze position. Children

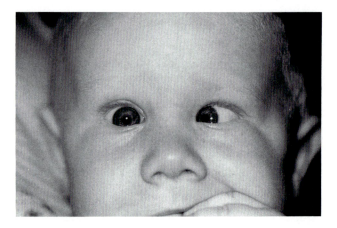

Figure 6–57. Nystagmus blockage syndrome with esotropia in the primary position.

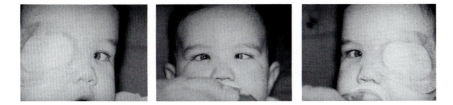

Figure 6–58. Nystagmus blockage syndrome. Note that when either eye is covered, the child turns his face in the direction of the uncovered eye in order to fixate in adduction.

with congenital esotropia frequently cross-fixate in side gaze and do not have amblyopia. Children with the nystagmus blockage syndrome are more likely to have amblyopia. When a patch is placed on one eye of a child with congenital esotropia, there is no compensatory head turn, as there is in nystagmus blockage syndrome. Finally, when a base-out prism is placed before the fixating eye in a child with the nystagmus blockage syndrome, the fellow eye will remain in adduction and the esotropia may increase. In children with congenital esotropia, the fellow eye turns out and the esotropia is reduced.

Cyclic Strabismus. Cyclic strabismus is a relatively rare disorder of ocular motility that occurs in approximately one in 3000 to 5000 cases of strabismus. It was first mentioned at the Strabismus Ophthalmic Symposium II in 1958 (Burian, 1958), and was first described in a publication by Costenbader and Mousel (1964). Since then, approximately 50 cases have been reported. A thorough history and repeated examinations are often necessary to elicit the cyclical nature of the deviation. An awareness of the typical characteristics of cyclic strabismus may enable one to make the diagnosis more readily.

Cyclic strabismus is usually an acquired condition with an onset at 3 to 4 years of age. Rarely, cases with an onset at birth or in adult life have been reported. Miotics have converted some children with constant esotropia to cyclic esotropia, and accidental or surgical trauma has been associated with cyclic strabismus in a few cases. Two cases of cyclic esotropia following surgery for intermittent exotropia have also been reported (Nelson, 1992).

The deviation in cyclic strabismus is typically a large-angle esotropia alternating every 48 hours with orthophoria or a small-angle esodeviation (Fig. 6–59). Variations include vertical deviations, incomitance that may be manifest as a mild V pattern, and exotropia. Cycles of 1, 3, 4, and 5 days have also been reported, as well as cycles of 48 hours of esotropia alternating with 24 hours of orthophoria. The duration of cycling may be as short as 2 weeks, in which case the diagnosis may be missed, or it may persist for several years, before the deviation becomes constant.

Patients with cyclic strabismus often have a family history of strabismus. There is no sexual predilection or relationship to refractive error or visual acuity. The fact that most cases occur between the ages of 3 and 5

years may explain the frequently found mild hyperopic error. The patients reported with a myopic refractive error have been postsurgical cases.

Fusion and binocular vision are usually absent or defective on the strabismic day, with marked improvement on the straight day. Diplopia on strabismic days is unusual; it is a prominent symptom only in those patients who developed cyclic strabismus after the age of 5 or 6 years. Younger children avoid diplopia through suppressing the image from one eye.

Cyclic esotropia is noted for its unpredictable response to various forms of therapy, with the exception of surgery, which is usually curative. Surgical correction of the total esodeviation with either a bimedial recession or a monocular medial rectus recession and lateral rectus resection has been the most successful mode of therapy.

Brown's Syndrome. An ocular motility disorder characterized by an inability to actively or passively elevate the adducted eye, Brown's syndrome can be congenital or acquired. It can also be permanent or transient. The distinguishing feature is an almost linear improvement in elevation of the eye from the adducted to the abducted position (Fig. 6–60). The palpebral fissure occasionally widens on attempted elevation in adduction, and the involved eye may depress in adduction. No overaction of the superior oblique muscle, however, is found on duction testing. Exodeviation (V pattern) often occurs when the eyes move upward from a midline position. Most children will be orthophoric in the primary position. With time, however, hypotropia can develop, often with a compensatory face turn toward the opposite eye. Some children note discomfort on attempted elevation in adduction; they may also feel or even hear a click under the same circumstances, or notice a palpable mass or tenderness in the trochlear region.

When present from birth, the etiology of the syndrome is believed to be a tight superior oblique tendon. Normal upward saccades in adduction have confirmed the restrictive nature of the condition. Acquired Brown's syndrome can be secondary to superior oblique surgery, scleral buckling bands, trauma, focal metastases to the superior oblique, and inflammation of the trochlea following sinus surgery. An identical motility pattern can occur in individuals with juvenile or adult rheumatoid arthritis, for unknown reasons.

If patients with Brown's syndrome are orthophoric

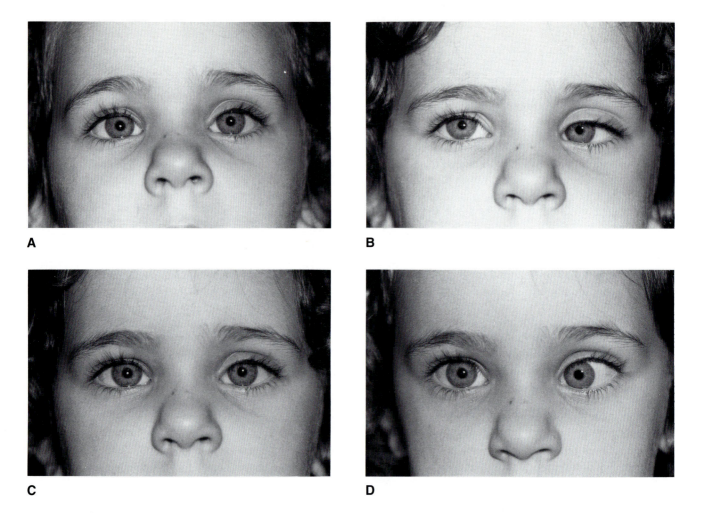

A **B** **C** **D**

Figure 6–59. Cyclic left esotropia and hypotropia. The photographs were taken on 4 consecutive days. Note the deviation on alternating days. **A.** Day one. **B.** Day two. **C.** Day three. **D.** Day four.

in primary position, and without an anomalous head posture, surgery is not necessary. Such patients may experience diplopia when elevating the involved eye in adduction, but will learn to avoid this position of gaze. If the eye is hypotropic in primary position, or if a head turn is cosmetically significant, surgery should be considered to try to restore binocular function in the primary position.

Tenotomy or tenectomy of the superior oblique will eliminate the restriction of elevation in Brown's syndrome. However, these weakening procedures result in superior oblique palsy in 54 to 85 percent of cases. In view of the high incidence of superior oblique palsy following surgery for Brown's syndrome, simulta-

neous superior oblique tenotomy and inferior oblique recession should be performed (Fig. 6–61).

Double Elevator Palsy. Double elevator palsy is a condition whereby an eye cannot elevate in any field of gaze (Fig. 6–62). It results from a weakness of both elevator muscles of the eye (the superior rectus and inferior oblique muscles), or a mechanical obstruction to elevation of the eye.

The affected eye is often hypotropic in the primary position, and a true or pseudoptosis is also usually concomitant. When fixating with the paretic eye, a hypertropia of the nonparetic eye occurs (Fig. 6–63). Affected patients often maintain a chin-up position to

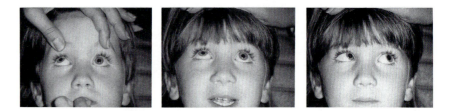

Figure 6–60. Brown's syndrome, left eye.

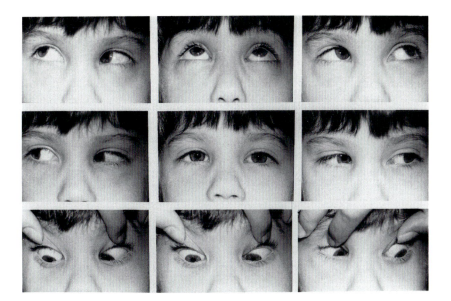

Figure 6–61. Surgical result following bilateral superior oblique tenotomies and inferior oblique recessions for Brown's syndrome. Note the underaction of all of the oblique muscles.

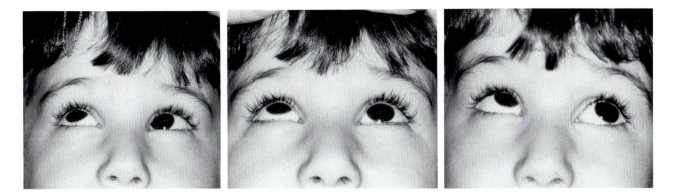

Figure 6–62. Double elevator palsy, left eye.

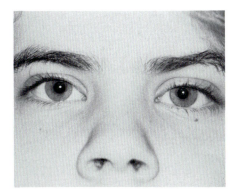

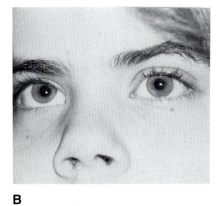

A   **B**

Figure 6–63. Double elevator palsy, left eye. **A.** When fixating with the right eye, the left eye is hypotropic and a pseudoptosis is present. **B.** When fixating with the left eye, hypertropia of the right eye occurs.

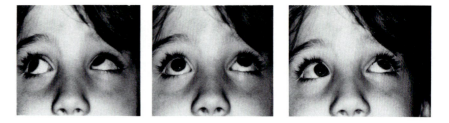

Figure 6–64. Acquired double elevator palsy, right eye, following an orbital floor fracture.

achieve binocular vision. Rarely, patients with double elevator palsy will have reduced elevation in all positions of gaze, but no hypotropia in primary position.

Scott and Jackson (1977) found that 73 percent of their patients with congenital double elevator palsy had restriction of the ipsilateral inferior rectus muscle, as determined by forced duction testing. They also noted that affected patients had an accentuated lower eyelid fold that became more prominent with attempted upward gaze.

Acquired double elevator palsies may be secondary to blowout fractures with entrapment of the inferior rectus muscle (Fig. 6–64), or may be innervational. The latter are frequently associated with pupillary anomalies and weakness of convergence, suggesting a lesion in the pretectum of the brainstem. These cases most likely result from small vascular infarcts.

If a patient with double elevator palsy is orthophoric in primary position, surgery is not indicated. If there is a vertical deviation in primary position and the forced duction test is positive, an inferior rectus recession is indicated. When the forced duction test is negative, a Knapp procedure (transposing the medial and lateral recti to the corners of the insertion of the superior rectus) should be performed (Knapp, 1969). As much as 35 prism diopters of hypotropia can be corrected with this procedure, but only a modest increase

in elevation results. If the hypotropia is less than 30 prism diopters and the forced duction is negative, a graded resection of the superior rectus and recession of the inferior rectus may also be successful.

Ptosis surgery should be avoided until the hypotropia is corrected. The lowered eyelid position may be secondary to the globe's hypotropic position (pseudoptosis), intrinsic levator weakness (true ptosis), or both. Once the eye alignment is improved, the ptosis can be reevaluated.

Möbius Syndrome. Möbius syndrome is a rare congenital disturbance consisting of varying abnormalities of the fifth through the twelfth cranial nerves, as well as limb abnormalities. Möbius (1888, 1892) first suggested that this congenital, bilateral, abducens-facial paralysis might be an independent pathological entity, thus gaining eponymic distinction.

The etiology of Möbius syndrome is presently unknown. Two theories to explain the condition implicate either mesodermal or ectodermal dysplasia. Neither theory is proven, and it is likely that Möbius syndrome arises from a variety of disorders that can affect the brainstem, cranial nerve nuclei, peripheral nerves, or muscles. Inheritance is usually sporadic, but isolated cases of autosomal dominant transmission have been reported.

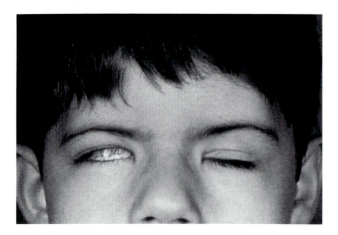

Figure 6–65. Möbius syndrome demonstrating seventh-nerve palsy with intact Bell's phenomenon, right eye. *(From Nelson LB et al: Recognizing Patterns of Ocular Childhood Diseases. Thorofare, NJ, Slack, 1985, p 187, with permission.)*

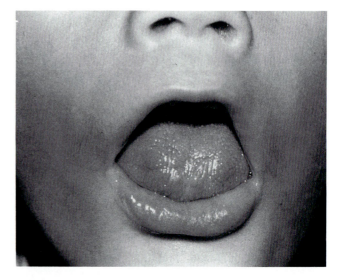

Figure 6–66. Möbius syndrome demonstrating inability to protrude the tongue beyond the lips. *(From Nelson LB, Catalano RA: Atlas of Ocular Motility. Philadelphia, Saunders, 1989, p 199, with permission.)*

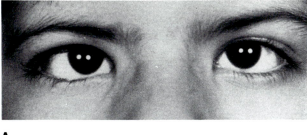

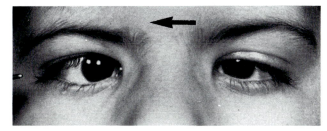

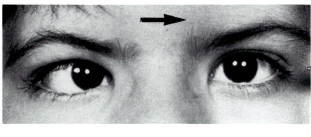

Figure 6–67. Möbius syndrome. **A.** Esotropia in the primary position. **B.** Right abducens palsy on right gaze. **C.** Left abducens palsy on left gaze. *(From Nelson LB et al: Recognizing Patterns of Ocular Childhood Diseases. Thorofare, NJ, Slack, 1985, p 187, with permission.)*

Möbius syndrome is usually detected within the first few weeks of life. Affected infants have difficulty sucking and feeding due to a unilateral or bilateral facial palsy (Fig. 6–65). The palsy can be complete or incomplete. Affected infants also incompletely close their

eyelids during sleep, and typically have a mask-like facies. They are unable to grin or wrinkle their forehead.

Paresis of other muscles supplied by cranial nerves also occurs. Often there is partial atrophy of the tongue, and an inability to protrude the tongue beyond the lips (Fig. 6–66). Paralysis of the soft palate and muscles of mastication may occur as well. Various skeletal and muscle defects are common, and include absence or hypoplasia of the pectoral muscles, syndactyly, club feet, and congenital limb amputations.

The ocular findings of Möbius syndrome include a unilateral or bilateral inability to abduct the eyes, with a resultant esotropia (Fig. 6–67). Although horizontal movements are usually lacking, vertical movements and convergence are intact. Pupillary constriction, vision, and the retina are also normal.

The forced duction test and the character of the muscles, when encountered at surgery, are abnormal. Horizontal, but not vertical, forced ductions are usually positive. The horizontal muscles are also often thickened, taut, and fibrotic. Electromyographic studies have shown that the electrical activity of affected horizontal muscles waxes and wanes, suggesting an underlying supranuclear lesion. Saccadic velocities are also extremely slow, both toward abduction and adduction, indicating significant weakness of both lateral and medial rectus function. Even after recession of the taut medial rectus muscles to treat an associated esotropia, there is usually little horizontal eye movement, because of the concomitant bilateral gaze palsy.

Congenital Ocular Motor Apraxia (OMA).
Congenital ocular motor apraxia (OMA) is characterized by a defect in the generation of voluntary horizontal saccades. Conspicuous head thrusts on attempted gaze to the side are considered a compensatory and pathognomonic sign (Fig. 6–68). The head thrust is toward and beyond the target. With it there is a rapid contraversive deviation of the eyes, followed by a slow movement of the eyes and head back toward the mid-

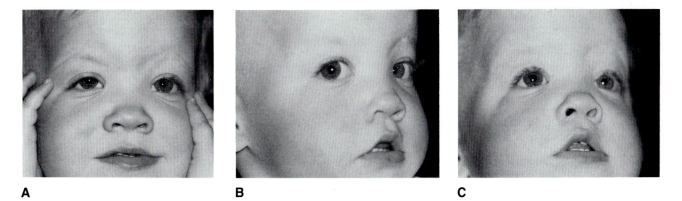

Figure 6–68. Ocular motor apraxia. **A.** Child gazing straight ahead. **B.** When the child's attention is directed toward a toy to her left, her head thrusts far to the left, and her eyes make a rapid contraversive movement to the right. **C.** Her head and eyes slowly move back toward midline to pick up fixation of the toy on her left side.

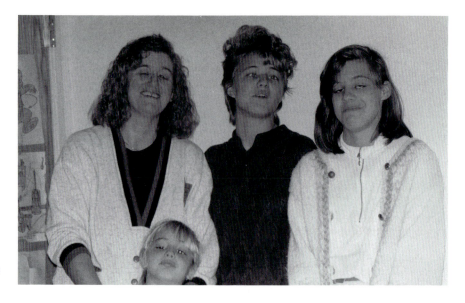

Figure 6–69. Mother and three daughters with congenital fibrosis syndrome.

line. The eye movement is believed to be initiated by the vestibuloocular reflex elicited by the head thrust. Random eye movements, oculocephalic reflexes, and vertical saccades are normal. The saccadic phase of the optokinetic reflex, however, is also abnormal or absent.

Ocular motor apraxia may be asymmetric in up to one third of affected children (Catalano et al, 1988). Asymmetric involvement is characterized by the absence of voluntary saccades and the presence of a head thrust only on gaze to one side.

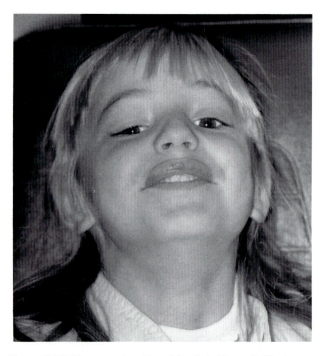

Figure 6–70. Youngest daughter of family in Figure 6–69, demonstrating ptosis and chin-up head position.

Although the origin of OMA remains unknown, it has been postulated that the responsible lesion lies in the cortical or subcortical region of the frontal lobes, the brainstem, the cerebellum, or the corpus callosum. Familial cases have been reported, and some cases are associated with Gaucher's disease. There is no known surgical treatment, but the disorder becomes less noticeable with time. The affected individual learns to compensate by slowly turning the head, rather than the eyes, in the horizontal direction of interest.

Generalized Fibrosis Syndrome. Generalized fibrosis syndrome is characterized by the presence of fibrous tissue in place of muscle fibers in the extraocular muscles. The various clinical presentations depend on the number of muscles affected, degree of fibrosis, and whether the involvement is unilateral or bilateral (Figs. 6–69 to 6–71). Although the condition has been known since the 19th century, it was Brown (1950) who coined the term "general fibrosis syndrome" after evaluating and treating three sporadic cases. The condition is congenital, and males and females are equally affected. Although Waardenburg (1924) suggested that an autosomal recessive mode occurs, several large pedigrees have indicated that autosomal dominant inheritance is more common.

Common findings in generalized fibrosis syndrome include the following:

1. Fibrosis of the extraocular muscles.
2. Fibrosis of Tenon's capsule.
3. Adhesions between muscles, Tenon's capsule, and the globe.
4. Inelasticity and fragility of the conjunctiva.
5. Absence of elevation or depression of the eyes.
6. Little or no horizontal movement of the eyes.

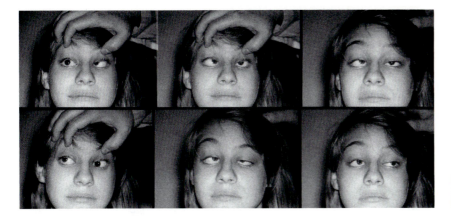

Figure 6–71. Middle daughter of family in Figure 6–69, demonstrating attempted ocular rotations.

7. Ocular fixation 20 to 30 degrees below the horizontal.
8. Blepharoptosis.
9. Chin elevation.

Other ocular findings include convergence on attempted upward gaze and divergence on attempted downward gaze. Amblyopia is common, which may partly be due to the difficulty of wearing an optical correction due to the chin-up head position, when there is associated significant refractive errors.

Less common ocular anomalies include Marcus Gunn jaw-winking, choroidal coloboma, pendular nystagmus, and bilateral optic nerve hypoplasia. Associated systemic anomalies include ventricular septal defects, talipes equinovalgus, unilateral facial palsy, and facial asymmetry.

Congenital fibrosis of the inferior rectus muscle is probably a variant of the generalized fibrosis syndrome (Harley et al, 1978). The inferior rectus alone, or together with the levator muscle, may be involved with little or no involvement of the other extraocular muscles. The condition may be unilateral or bilateral and is commonly asymmetrical. Because patients cannot elevate their eyes even to the midline, they adapt a compensatory chin-up head position (Fig. 6–72).

Another variant of the generalized fibrosis syndrome is strabismus fixus, in which the eyes are so firmly fixed that they cannot be actively or passively moved. Horizontal movement is particularly affected; some vertical movement may be possible. Affected individuals may have straight eyes (Fig. 6–73), but often the eyes are fixed in a marked esotropic or exotropic position.

The goal of surgical management in the generalized fibrosis syndrome is to center the eyes and improve any compensatory head posture. In patients with significant hypotropia, maximal recession or disinsertion of the inferior rectus muscles is indicated. Elevation of the hypotropic eye, however, accentuates the ptosis. Bilateral frontalis suspension is accordingly required soon after the strabismus surgery. Because these patients often do not have a Bell's phenomenon, corneal drying may occur after ptosis surgery. The lid should, therefore, be elevated only to the upper pupillary border.

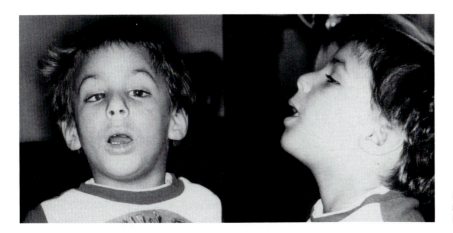

Figure 6–72. Another child with congenital fibrosis syndrome, demonstrating ptosis and chin-up head position.

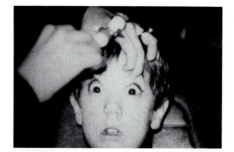

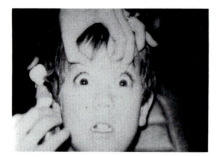
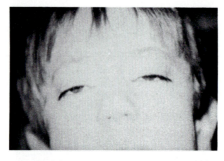
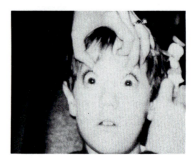

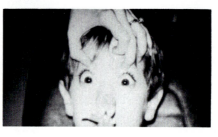

Figure 6–73. Strabismus fixus. The eyes are so firmly fixed that they can not be actively or passively moved in any direction. There is also an associated ptosis.

REFERENCES

"A" and "V" Pattern Strabismus

Albert DG: In Parks MM (ed): Annual review: Strabismus. Arch Ophthalmol 58:152, 1957.

Breinin GM: Vertically incomitant horizontal strabismus. The A-V patterns. NY State J Med 61:2243, 1961.

Calhoun JC, Nelson LB, Harley RD: Atlas of Pediatric Ophthalmology Surgery. Philadelphia: Saunders, 1987, pp 17–19.

Diamond GR, Parks MM: The effect of superior oblique weakening procedures on primary position horizontal alignment. J Pediatr Ophthalmol Strabismus 18:35, 1981.

Duane A: Isolated paralyses of the ocular muscles. Arch Ophthalmol 26:317, 1897.

Fierson WN, Boger WP, Diorio PC, et al: The effect of bilateral superior oblique tenotomy on horizontal deviation in A-pattern strabismus. J Pediatr Ophthalmol Strabismus 17:364, 1980.

Goldstein JH: Monocular vertical displacement of the horizontal rectus muscles in the A and V patterns. Am J Ophthalmol 64:265, 1967.

Knapp P: A and V pattern: Symposium on strabismus. Trans New Orleans Acad Ophthalmol. St. Louis, Mosby, 1972, pp 242–254.

Knapp P: Vertically incomitant horizontal strabismus: The so-called A and V syndrome. Trans Am Ophthalmol Soc 57:666, 1959.

Metz HS, Schwartz L: The treatment of A and V patterns by monocular surgery. Arch Ophthalmol 95:251, 1977.

Miller JE: Vertical recti transplantation in the A and V syndromes. Arch Ophthalmol 64:175, 1960.

Parks MM, Mitchell PR: A and V patterns. In Duane, TD, Jaeger EA (eds): Clinical Ophthalmology. Philadelphia, Lippincott, 1987.

Rubin SE, Nelson LB, Harley RD: A complication of weakening the superior oblique in A pattern esotropia. Ophthalmic Surg 15:134, 1984.

Scott AB: V pattern exotropia. Electromyographic study of an unusual case. Invest Ophthalmol 12:232, 1961.

Stager DR, Parks MM: Inferior oblique weakening procedures. Arch Ophthalmol 90:15, 1973.

Urets-Zavalia A, Solares-Zamora J, Olmos HR: Anthropological studies on the nature of cyclovertical squint. Br J Ophthalmol 45:578, 1961.

Urets-Zavalia A: Abduccion en la elevaccion. Arch Ophthalmol 22:1, 1948.

Urets-Zavalia A: Paralysis bilateral congenital del muscle lucius inferior. Arch Ophthalmol 23:172, 1948.

Urist JJ: Surgical treatment of esotropia with bilateral elevation in adduction. Arch Ophthalmol 47:220, 1952.

Urist JJ: Horizontal squint with secondary vertical deviation. Arch Ophthalmol 46:245, 1951.

Accommodative Esotropia

American Academy of Ophthalmology: Preferred Practice Pattern. San Francisco: AAO, 1992.

Baker JD, Parks MM: Early onset accommodative esotropia. Am J Ophthalmol 90:11, 1980.

Cassin B, Beecham B, Friedberg K: Stereo-acuity, fusional amplitudes and AC/A ratio in accommodative esotropia. Am Orthopt J 26:60, 1976.

Mary E, Freeman D, Peltman P, et al: Visual acuity development in human infants. Evoked potential measurement. Invest Ophthalmol Vis Sci 15:150, 1976.

Parks MM: Abnormal accommodative convergence in squint. Arch Ophthalmol 59:364, 1958.

Parks MM, Wheeler MD: Concomitant esodeviations. In Duane TD, Jaeger EA (eds): Clinical Ophthalmolgy. Philadelphia, Lippincott, 1985.

Pollard ZF: Accommodative esotropia during the first year of life. Arch Ophthalmol 94:1912, 1976.

Preslan MW, Beauchamp GR: Accommodative esotropia: Review of current practices and controversies. Ophthalmic Surg 18:68, 1987.

Amblyopia

American Academy of Ophthalmology: Amblyopia, Preferred Practice Pattern. San Francisco, AAO, 1992.

Costenbader FD, Bair D, McPhail A: Vision in strabismus. A preliminary report. Arch Ophthalmol 40:438, 1948.

Crawford MLJ: The visual deprivation syndrome. Ophthalmology 84:465, 1978.

Dickey CF, Metz HS, Stewart SA, et al: The diagnosis of amblyopia in cross-fixation. J Pediatr Ophthalmol Strabismus 28:171, 1991.

Flynn JT: Amblyopia revisited. J Pediatr Ophthalmol Strabismus 28:183, 1991.

Hubel DH, Wiesel TN: The period of susceptibility to the physiological effects of unilateral eye closure in kittens. J Physiol 206:419, 1970.

Ingram RM, Walker C, Wilson JM, et al: Prediction of amblyopia and squint by means of refraction at age 1 year. Br J Ophthalmol 70:12, 1986.

Kushner BJ: Amblyopia. In Nelson LB, Calhoun JC, Harley RD (eds): Pediatric Ophthalmology, ed 3. Philadelphia, Saunders, 1991.

Leguire LE, Rogers GL, Bremer DL: Levodopa and childhood amblyopia. J Pediatr Ophthalmol Strabismus 29:290, 1992.

Mandava N, Simon JW, Jenkins PL: Preferential looking and recognition acuities in clinical amblyopia. J Pediatr Ophthalmol Strabismus 28:323, 1991.

Tanlanai T, Goss DA: Prevalence of monocular amblyopia among anisometropes. Am J Optomet Physiol Opt 56:704, 1979.

Von Noorden GK: Amblyopia: A multidisciplinary approach. Invest Ophthalmol Vis Sci 26:1704, 1985.

Von Noorden GK: Mechanisms of amblyopia. Doc Ophthalmol 34:93, 1977.

Von Noorden GK: Classification of amblyopia. Am J Ophthalmol 63:238, 1967.

Wiesel TN, Hubel DM: Effects of visual deprivation on morphology and physiology of cells in the cat's lateral geniculate body. J Neurophysiol 26:978, 1963.

Brown's Syndrome

Baker RS, Conkin JD: Acquired Brown's syndrome from blunt orbital trauma. J Pediatr Ophthalmol Strabismus 24:17, 1987.

Brown HW: True and simulated superior oblique tendon sheath syndromes. Doc Ophthalmol 34:123, 1973.

Brown HW: Isolated inferior oblique paralysis: An analysis of 97 cases. Trans Am Ophthalmol Soc 55:415, 1957.

Brown HW: Congenital structural anomalies. In Allen JH (ed): Strabismus Ophthalmic Symposium I. St. Louis, Mosby, 1950.

Hamed LM: Bilateral Brown syndrome in three siblings. J Pediatr Ophthalmol Strabismus 28:306, 1991.

Hermann JS: Acquired Brown's syndrome of inflammatory origin. Arch Ophthalmol 96:1228, 1978.

Parks MM, Eustis HS: Simultaneous superior oblique tenotomy and inferior oblique recession in Brown's syndrome. Ophthalmology 94:1043, 1987.

Slavin ML, Goodstein S: Acquired Brown's syndrome caused by focal metastasis to the superior oblique muscle. Am J Ophthalmol 103:598, 1987.

Von Noorden GK, Olivier R: Superior oblique tenectomy in Brown's syndrome. Ophthalmology 90:303, 1982.

Wang FM, Weitenbaker C, Behrens MM, et al: Acquired Brown's syndrome in children with juvenile rheumatoid arthritis. Ophthalmology 91:23, 1984.

Wilson ME, Eustis HS, Parks MM: Brown's syndrome. Surv Ophthalmol 34:3, 1989.

Wright KW, Silverstein D, Marrone AC, et al: Acquired inflammatory superior oblique tendon sheath syndrome. A clinicopathologic study. Arch Ophthalmol 100:1725, 1982.

Childhood Onset Exodeviations

Burke MJ: Intermittent exotropia. In Nelson LB, Wagner RS, (eds): Strabismus Surgery. Boston, Little, Brown, 1985.

Calhoun JC, Nelson LB, Harley RD: Atlas of Pediatric Ophthalmic Surgery. Philadelphia, Saunders, 1987, pp 8–10.

Hiles DA, Davies GT, Costenbader FD: Long-term observation on unoperated intermittent exotropia. Arch Ophthalmol 80:336, 1968.

Parks MM, Mitchell PR: Concomitant exodeviation. In Duane TD, Jaeger EA (eds): Clinical Ophthalmology. Philadelphia, Lippincott, 1987.

Pratt-Johnson JA, Barlow JM, Tillson G: Early surgery in intermittent exotropia. Am J Ophthalmol 84:689, 1977.

Raab EL, Parks MM: Recession of the lateral recti: Early and late post operative alignments. Arch Ophthalmol 82:203, 1969.

Richard JM, Parks MM: Intermittent exotropia. Surgical results in different age groups. Ophthalmology 90:1172, 1983.

Wiggins RE, von Noorden GK: Monocular eye closure in sunlight. J Pediatr Ophthalmol Strabismus 27:16, 1990.

Congenital Esotropia

Birch EE, Stager DR: Monocular acuity and stereopsis in infantile esotropia. Invest Ophthalmol Vis Sci 26:1624, 1985.

Costenbader FD: Infantile esotropia. Trans Am Ophthalmol Soc 59:397, 1961.

Foster RS, Paul OT, Jampolsky A: Management of infantile esotropia. Am J Ophthalmol 82:291, 1976.

Friendly DS: Management of infantile esotropia. In Nelson LB, Wagner RS (eds): Strabismus Surgery, Int Ophthalmol Clin 25. Boston, Little, Brown, 1985, pp 37–52.

Greenwald MJ: A randomized comparison of surgical procedures for infantile esotropia. Am J Ophthalmol 98:642, 1984.

Harcourt B, Mein J, Johnson F: Natural history and associations of dissociated vertical deviation. Trans Ophthalmol Soc UK 100:495, 1980.

Helveston E: Origins of congenital esotropia. Am Orthoptic J 36:40, 1986.

Hiles DA, Watson A, Biglan AW: Characteristics of infantile esotropia following early bimedial rectus recession. Arch Ophthalmol 98:697, 1980.

Ing MR: Early surgical alignment for congenital esotropia. J Pediatr Ophthalmol Strabismus 20:11, 1983.

Nelson LB: Strabismic disorders. In Nelson LB, Calhoun JH, Harley RD: Pediatric Ophthalmology, ed 3. Philadelphia, Saunders, 1992, pp 128–175.

Nelson LB, Wagner RS, Simon JW, Harley RD: Congenital esotropia. Surv Ophthalmol 31:363, 1987.

Noel LP, Parks MM: Dissociated vertical deviation associated findings and results of surgical treatment. Can J Ophthalmol 17:10, 1982.

Raab EL: Dissociated vertical deviation. In Nelson LB, Wagner RS (eds): Strabismus Surgery, Int Ophthalmol Clin 25. Boston, Little, Brown, 1985, pp 119–131.

Taylor DM: Is congenital esotropia functionally curable? Trans Am Ophthalmol Soc 70:259, 1972.

Tolchin JG, Lederman ME: Congenital (infantile) esotropia: Psychiatric aspects. J Pediatr Ophthalmol Strabismus 15:160, 1978.

Von Noorden GK: Infantile esotropia: A continuing riddle. Am Orthoptic J 34:52, 1984.

Congenital Exotropia

Hiles DA, Biglan AW: Early surgery of infantile exotropia. Trans Penn Acad Ophthalmol 36:161, 1983.

Moore S, Cohen RL: Congenital exotropia. Am Orthoptic J 35:68, 1985.

Parks MM, Mitchell PR: Concomitant exodeviation. In Duane TD, Jaeger EA (eds): Clinical Ophthalmology. Philadelphia, Lippincott, 1990.

Rubin SE, Nelson, LB, Wagner RS, et al: Infantile exotropia in healthy children. Ophthalmic Surg 19:792, 1988.

Congenital Ocular Motor Apraxia

Catalano RA, Calhoun JA, Reinecke RD, Cogan DG: Asymmetry in congenital ocular motor apraxia. Can J Ophthalmol 23:318, 1988.

Cogan DG: Congenital ocular motor apraxia. Can J Ophthalmol 1:253, 1966.

Cogan DG: A type of congenital motor apraxia presenting jerky head movements. Trans Am Acad Ophthalmol Otolaryngol 56:853, 1952.

Rendle-Short J, Appleton B, Pearn J: Congenital ocular motor apraxia. Aust Paediatr J 9:263, 1973.

Summers CG, MacDonald JT, Wirtschafter JD: Ocular motor apraxia associated with intracranial lipoma. J Pediatr Ophthalmol Strabismus 24:267, 1987.

Zee DS, Yee RD, Singer HS: Congenital ocular motor apraxia. Brain 100:581, 1977.

Cyclic Strabismus

Burian HM: Round table discussion. In Allen JH (ed): Strabismus Symposium II. St. Louis, Mosby, 1958.

Caputo AR, Greenfield PS: Cyclic esotropia. Ann Ophthalmol 10:775, 1978.

Chamberlain W: Cyclic esotropia. Am J Ophthalmol 18:31, 1968.

Costenbader FD, Mousel DK: Cyclic esotropia. Arch Ophthalmol 71:180, 1964.

Costenbader FD, O'Neill JF: Cyclic strabismus. In Bellows JD (ed): Contemporary Ophthalmology Honoring Sir Steward Duke-Elder. Baltimore, Williams & Wilkins, 1972.

Friendly DS, Manson RA, Albert DG: Cyclic strabismus. A case study. Doc Ophthalmol 34:189, 1973.

Gadoth N, Dickerman, Z, Lerman M, et al: Cyclic esotropia with minimal brain dysfunction. J Pediatr Ophthalmol Strabismus 18:14, 1981.

Helveston EM: Cyclic strabismus. Am J Ophthalmol 23:48, 1973.

Muchnick RS, Sanfilippo S, Dunlap EA: Cyclic esotropia developing after strabismus surgery. Arch Ophthalmol 94:459, 1976.

Parlato CJ, Nelson LB, Harley RD: Cyclic strabismus. Ann Ophthalmol 15:1126, 1983.

Richter CP: Clock-mechanism esotropia in children: Alternate-day squint. Johns Hopkins Med J 122:218, 1968.

Troost BT, Abel L, Noreika J, et al: Acquired cyclic esotropia in an adult. Am J Ophthalmol 91:8, 1981.

Vemura Y, Tomita M, Tanaka Y: Consecutive cyclic esotropia. J Pediatr Ophthalmol Strabismus 14:278, 1977.

Windsor CE, Berg EF: Circadian heterotropia. Am J Ophthalmol 67:565, 1969.

Double Elevator Palsy

Callahan M: Surgically mismanaged ptosis associated with double elevator palsy. Arch Ophthalmol 99:108, 1981.

Hoyt CS: Acquired "double elevator" palsy and polycythemia vera. J Pediatr Ophthalmol Strabismus 15:362, 1978.

Jampel RS, Fells P: Monocular elevation paresis caused by a central nervous system lesion. Arch Ophthalmol 80:45, 1968.

Kirkham TH, Kline LB: Monocular elevation paresis, Argyll Robertson pupils and sarcoidosis. Can J Ophthalmol 11:330, 1976.

Knapp P: The surgical treatment of double elevator paralysis. Trans Am Ophthalmol Soc 67:304, 1969.

Lessell S: Supranuclear paralysis of monocular elevation. Neurology 25:1134, 1975.

Malbran E, Norris AL: Unilateral paralysis of the elevators of supranuclear origin. Br J Ophthalmol 39:73, 1955.

Mather TR, Saunders RA: Congenital absence of the superior rectus muscle: A case report. J Pediatr Ophthalmol Strabismus 24:291, 1987.

Metz HS: Double elevator palsy. Arch Ophthalmol 97:901, 1979.

Rosner S: Double elevator paralysis. Am J Ophthalmol 55:87, 1963.

Scott WE, Jackson OB: Double elevator palsy: The significance of inferior rectus restriction. Am Orthopt J 27:5, 1977.

White JW: Paralysis of the superior rectus and the inferior oblique muscle of the same eye. Arch Ophthalmol 27:366, 1942.

Duane's Retraction Syndrome

Blodi FC, Van Allen MW, Yarbrough JC: Duane's syndrome: A brain stem lesion. Arch Ophthalmol 72:171, 1964.

Breinin GM: Electromyography: A tool in ocular and neurologic diagnosis, II. Muscle palsies. Arch Ophthalmol 57:165, 1957.

Duane A: Congenital deficiency of abduction, associated with impairment of adduction, retraction movements, contraction of the palpebral fissure and oblique movements of the eye. Arch Ophthalmol 34:133, 1905.

Gourdeau A, Miller N, Zee D, et al: Central ocular motor abnormalities in Duane's retraction syndrome. Arch Ophthalmol 99:1809, 1981.

Hotchkiss MG, Muller NR, Clark AW, et al: Bilateral Duane's retraction syndrome. A clinical-pathologic case report. Arch Ophthalmol 98:870, 1970.

Hoyt WF, Nachtigaller H: Anomalies of ocular nerves: Neuroanatomic correlates of paradoxical innervation in Duane's syndrome and related congenital ocular motor disorder. Am J Ophthalmol 60:443, 1965.

Huber A: Electrophysiology of the retraction syndrome. Br J Ophthalmol 59:293, 1974.

Isenberg S, Urist MJ: Clinical observations in 101 consecutive patients with Duane's retraction syndrome. Am J Ophthalmol 84:419, 1977.

Jay WM, Hoyt CS: Abnormal brain stem auditory-evoked potentials in Stilling–Turk–Duane retraction syndrome. Am J Ophthalmol 89:814, 1980.

Kirkham TH: Anisometropia and amblyopia in Duane's syndrome. Am J Ophthalmol 69:774, 1970.

Maruo T, Kusota N, Arimoto H, et al: Duane's syndrome. Jpn J Ophthalmol 23:453, 1979.

Miller NR, Kiel SM, Green WR, et al: Unilateral Duane's retraction syndrome (type 1). Arch Ophthalmol 100:1468, 1982.

O'Malley ER, Helveston EM, Ellis FD: Duane's retraction syndrome—plus. J Pediatr Ophthalmol Strabismus 19:161, 1982.

Pfaffenbach DD, Cross HH, Kearns TP: Congenital anomalies in Duane's retraction syndrome. Arch Ophthalmol 88:635, 1972.

Pressman SH, Scott WE: Surgical treatment of Duane's syndrome. Ophthalmology 93:29, 1986.

Rogers GL, Bremer DL: Surgical treatment of the upshoot and downshoot in Duane's retraction syndrome. Ophthalmology 91:1380, 1984.

Scott AB, Wong GY: Duane's syndrome: An electromyographic study. Arch Ophthalmol 87:140, 1972.

Tredici TD, von Noorden GK: Are anisometropia and amblyopia common in Duane's syndrome? J Pediatr Ophthalmol Strabismus 22:23, 1985.

Von Noorden GK, Murray E: Up- and down-shooting in Duane's retraction syndrome. J Pediatr Ophthalmol Strabismus 23:212, 1986.

Generalized Fibrosis Syndrome

Apt L, Axelrod RN: Generalized fibrosis of the extraocular muscles. Am J Ophthalmol 85:822, 1978.

Brodsky MC, Pollock SC, Buckley EG: Neuron misdirection in congenital ocular fibrosis syndrome: Implications and pathogenesis. J Pediatr Ophthalmol Strabismus 26:159, 1989.

Brown HW: Congenital structural anomalies. In Allen JH (ed): Strabismus Ophthalmic Symposium I. St. Louis, Mosby, 1950.

Crawford JS: Congenital fibrosis syndrome. Can J Ophthalmol 5:331, 1970.

Harley RD, Rodrigues MM, Crawford JS: Congenital fibrosis of the extraocular muscles. Trans Am Ophthalmol Soc 76:197, 1978.

Hiatt RL, Halle AA: General fibrosis syndrome. Ann Ophthalmol 15:1103, 1983.

Laughlin RC: Congenital fibrosis of the extraocular muscles. Am J Ophthalmol 41:432, 1956.

Letson RD: Surgical management of the ocular congenital fibrosis syndrome. Am Orthopt J 30:97, 1980.

Martinez L: A case of fixed strabismus. Am J Ophthalmol 31:80, 1948.

Villasecca A: Strabismus fixus. Am J Ophthalmol 48:51, 1959.

Von Noorden GK: Congenital hereditary ptosis with inferior rectus fibrosis. Arch Ophthalmol 83:378, 1970.

Waardenburg PJ: Ueber eine recessive Form angeborenener Ophthalmoplegia. Genetica 6:487, 1924.

Möbius Syndrome

Abbott RL, Metz HS, Weber AA: Saccadic velocity studies in Möbius syndrome. Ann Ophthalmol 10:619, 1978.

Gadoth N, Biedner B, Torok G: Möbius syndrome and Poland anomaly: Case report and review of the literature. J Pediatr Ophthalmol Strabismus 16:374, 1978.

Gilles FH: Selective symmetrical neuronal necroses of certain brain stem tegmental nuclei in temporary cardiac standstill. J Neuropathol Exp Neurol 22:318, 1963.

Graham PJ: Congenital flaccid bulbar palsy. Br Med J 2:26, 1964.

Henderson JC: The congenital facial diplegia syndrome: clinical features, pathology and aetiology. A review of sixty-one cases. Brain 62:381, 1939.

Merz M, Wojtowicz S: The Möbius syndrome. Report of electromyographic examinations in two cases. Am J Ophthalmol 63:837, 1967.

Metz HS: Saccadic velocity measurements in strabismus. Trans Am Ophthalmol Soc 81:630, 1983.

Möbius PJ: Ueber infantilen Kernschwund. Munch Med Wschr 39:17, 1892.

Möbius PJ: Ueber angeborenen doppelseitig Abducens-Facialis- Lahmung. Munch Med Wschr 35:91, 1888.

Parks MM: Ophthalmoplegic syndromes and trauma. In Duane TD, Jaeger EA (eds): Clinical Ophthalmology. Philadelphia, Lippincott, 1985.

Phillips WH, Dirion JK, Graves GO: Congenital bilateral palsy of the abducens. Arch Ophthalmol 8:355, 1932.

Pitner SE, Edwards JE, McCormick WF: Observations on the pathology of the Möbius syndrome. J Neurol Neurosurg Psychiatr 28:362, 1965.

Reed H, Grant W: Möbius syndrome. Br J Ophthalmol 41:731, 1957.

Richards RN: The Möbius syndrome. J Bone Jt Surg 35:437, 1953.

Rogers GL, Hatch GF, Gray I: Möbius syndrome and limb abnormalities. J Pediatr Ophthalmol Strabismus 14:134, 1977.

Thakkar N, O'Neil W, Duvally J, et al: Möbius syndrome due to brain stem tegmental necrosis. Arch Neurol 34:124, 1977.

Van Allen MW, Blodi FC: Neurologic aspects of the Möbius syndrome. Neurology 10:249, 1960.

Wallis PG: Creatinuria in Möbius syndrome. Arch Dis Child 35:393, 1960.

Wishnick MM, Nelson LB, Huppert L, et al: Möbius syndrome and limb abnormalities with dominant inheritance. Ophthalmic Pediatr Genet 2:77, 1983.

Yasuna H, Schlezinger NS: Congenital bilateral abducens: Facial paralysis (Möbius syndrome). Arch Ophthalmol 54:137, 1955.

Nystagmus Blockage Syndrome

Adelstrin F, Cuppers C: Zum Problem der echten und scheinbaren Abducenslahmung (das sogenannte "blockierungs-Syndrome"). Augenmuskellshmungen, Buch d Augenarzt 46:271, 1966.

Cuppers C: Probleme der operativen Therapie des okularen Nystagmus. Klin Monatsbl Augenheilkd 195:145, 1971.

Dell'Osso LF, Ellenberger C, Abel AL, et al: The nystagmus blockage syndrome. Congenital nystagmus, manifest latent nystagmus or both? Invest Ophthalmol Vis Sci 24:1580, 1983.

Frank JW: Diagnostic signs in the nystagmus compensation syndrome. J Pediatr Ophthalmol Strabismus 16:317, 1979.

Von Noorden GK: Binocular vision and ocular motility: Theory and Management of Strabismus, ed 3. St. Louis, Mosby, 1985.

Von Noorden GK: The nystagmus compensation (blockage) syndrome. Am J Ophthalmol 82:283, 1976.

Von Noorden GK, Wong SY: Surgical results in nystagmus blockage syndrome. Ophthalmology 93:1028, 1986.

ESSENTIAL INFORMATION FOR PRIMARY CARE PRACTITIONERS

Nystagmus is a rhythmic, "to-and-fro" oscillation of the eyes. It can be elicited in all persons by stimulating the vestibular system, and a few individuals can volitionally produce it. When nystagmus arises spontaneously and involuntarily, a visual or central nervous system disorder should be suspected. Associated abnormalities include developmental defects of the eye; ischemic, toxic, or compressive neurological afflictions; and chromosomal and metabolic disorders. The challenge for the physician is to identify those individuals in whom the nystagmus is a sign of a treatable neurological condition.

In actuality, nystagmus in children rarely indicates a significant central nervous system disorder. Over 90 percent of infants presenting with nystagmus have a disorder confined to their eyes or anterior visual pathways (Gelbart & Hoyt, 1988; Lambert et al, 1989). A stepwise, methodical approach can reveal these abnormalities in most cases, and direct the appropriate neuroradiological or electrophysiological workup in the remainder.

The approach to the child with nystagmus involves distinguishing physiological from pathological movements of the eyes. For the latter, it is helpful to establish whether there is an associated afferent (sensory) visual defect. Additional information regarding the child's future development and visual prognosis can be ascertained by determining whether the nystagmus is congenital or acquired; localizing or nonlocalizing; and constant, changing, or progressive. The suggested clinical approach to the infant who presents with nystagmus is reviewed in this chapter.

Nomenclature

The parent of an affected infant describes nystagmus as "jiggling," "wiggling," "dancing," or "jumping" eyes. The physician should describe the nystagmus according to the type, speed, and amplitude of movement.

In the past, three principal morphological types of nystagmus were distinguished. It was believed that afferent visual disorders were characterized by a pendular movement of the eyes in which the oscillations were of similar speed in either direction; this was called sensory or pendular nystagmus (Fig. 7–1). This type of nystagmus is usually horizontal and remains horizontal and pendular on upward and downward gaze. On lateral gaze, however, it converts to a jerk nystagmus in the direction of gaze. It typically decreases in the position of rest, and can be elicited by attempts at fixation. In contrast, efferent disorders were believed to be characterized by a nystagmus with biphasic rhythm. The

121

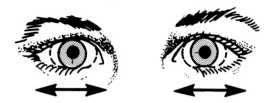

Figure 7–1. Pendular nystagmus. Both eyes move pendularly to the right and then to the left.

first phase is a fast movement of both eyes in one direction; the second a slow drift back in the opposite direction. Jerk nystagmus was considered characteristic of efferent (motor) disorders (Fig. 7–2). A third type, searching nystagmus, was described in blind and nearly blind individuals. Searching nystagmus is characterized by slow, roving, or drifting ocular movements, without fixation. The eyes typically meander aimlessly in all directions, but the principal movement is horizontal. Two more unusual forms of nystagmus were also described. The first was rotatory nystagmus, in which the eyes appear to rotate around the anterior–posterior axis of the eye (Fig. 7–3); the second was elliptical, in which the ocular movement tracks an oval pattern.

Although electronystagmography has not found a consistent relationship between waveforms and afferent and efferent disorders (Yee et al, 1976), it remains clinically useful to think of nystagmus associated with afferent conditions as being either searching or pendular, and nystagmus related to efferent disorders as being jerk. This distinction should only be made after the first birthday, because nystagmus waveforms change during the first year of life (Jan et al, 1986).

Nystagmus is further described according to its plane, amplitude, and rate. Oscillations may be principally horizontal, vertical, or rotary (torsional). A conscious effort should be made to describe the amplitude of nystagmus in degrees and the speed of movement in cycles per second (Hertz, abbreviated Hz). The amplitude may be fine (less than 5 degrees), moderate (5 to 15 degrees), or large (greater than 15 degrees). The rate may be slow (1 to 2 Hz), medium (3 to 4 Hz) or fast (≥ 5 Hz). Lenses can be used to magnify the ocular movements. Slit-lamp examination of the anterior eye

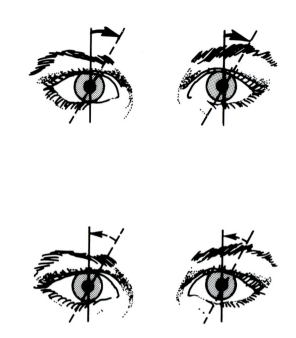

Figure 7–3. Rotatory nystagmus to the left. A rapid rotation of both eyes to the left is followed by a slow rotation back.

and ophthalmoscopic examination of the retina are also useful in evaluating rhythmic movements. Electronystagmography allows a more exact and permanent objective recording.

Family History

The most common heritable transmission of nystagmus is X-linked (McKusick, 1968). The family history should, therefore, particularly address whether any maternal uncle or the maternal grandfather has nystagmus. If a parent has nystagmus, autosomal dominant transmission is likely; autosomal recessive patterns of inheritance are more difficult to identify. A family history of nystagmus and good vision is consistent with hereditary congenital motor nystagmus. A family history of night blindness or color deficiency suggests congenital stationary night blindness or achromatopsia. This history is especially important for achromatopsia, because not every child with this disorder is photophobic (light sensitive) in the first few months of life (Hoyt, 1986). The family's ethnic background may suggest one of the infantile amaurotic conditions, such as Tay–Sachs disease, or a lipofuscinosis.

Perinatal History

The prenatal and developmental history of an infant with nystagmus is reviewed to determine the possibility of an intrauterine infection, especially toxoplasmosis or rubella. A maternal history of anticonvulsant or psychotropic drug use, gestational diabetes, or alcohol abuse suggests an optic nerve abnormality (such as hypoplasia). The birth history reviews the possibility of

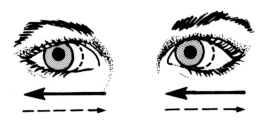

Figure 7–2. Jerk nystagmus to the right. A fast movement of both eyes to the right is followed by a slow drift back to the left.

neonatal asphyxia. A history of apnea at birth and the need for artificial respiration suggests cerebral hypoxia. A skull ultrasound in the nursery demonstrating intraventricular hemorrhage suggests cerebral injury.

History of Current Illness

Parents should be questioned about any signs that might suggest increased intracranial pressure. These include irritability, nausea, vomiting, bulging fontanelles, and increased head size. Any symptoms of posterior fossa disease (such as ataxia, seizures, or strabismus) should also be elicited. A child with delayed growth and nystagmus should be suspected of having a bilateral optic nerve disorder (particularly optic nerve hypoplasia) and deMorsier's syndrome.

Nystagmus History

The nystagmus history should detail when the nystagmus was first noted. It is not unusual for nystagmus to manifest after the child becomes 2 to 3 months of age, because the neonatal visual and motor systems are immature. This question is also of importance because nystagmus that presents within the first few months of life is less likely to be associated with a central nervous system tumor than one that is first noticed at 6 or more months of age (Lavery et al, 1984). Parents should also be queried whether the nystagmus is constant and symmetric between the eyes. Asymmetric, intermittent nystagmus is characteristic of spasmus nutans. Nystagmus patterns change during the first year of life, and these changes should be noted. Congenital nystagmus tends to decrease in amplitude with time, whereas the amplitude in some acquired types of nystagmus tends to increase as the process evolves (Buckley, 1990). It is also well known that the amplitude and fre-

quency of congenital motor nystagmus increases when a child is stressed or ill. The same occurs with periodic alternating nystagmus. Parents are also asked about any associated head movement or face turn. Head bobbing and torticollis is suggestive of spasmus nutans. A face turn is common in congenital motor nystagmus, but is not pathognomonic for this etiology. Face or head turns are more common in jerk nystagmus than pendular nystagmus (Cogan, 1967). Suggested disorders based on historical findings are summarized in Table 7–1.

Physical Examination

Identification of facial asymmetry, malposition of the ears, dental anomalies, skin tags, and digital abnormalities (such as supernumerary, missing, or fused digits) suggests a developmental syndrome (Fig. 7–4 and Table 7–2). Diminished pigmentation, and a history of poor tanning, is suggestive of albinism. Global retardation suggests a diffuse central nervous system (CNS) abnormality. The latter is corroborated by a history of seizures or meningitis, or the presence of an abnormal head circumference. Children with developmental delay should undergo a neurological workup.

Examining and Recording Nystagmus Patterns

An infant with nystagmus should be observed for an extended period to determine whether the nystagmus regularly changes in direction over time. This is called periodic alternating nystagmus (PAN) and is described later in the chapter. Notation should also be made as to whether both eyes are moving similarly, whether the pattern changes with eye position, and whether the frequency or amplitude of the nystagmus varies. An oscil-

---

TABLE 7–1. APPROACH TO THE INFANT WITH NYSTAGMUS: HISTORICAL FINDINGS

Finding	Suggested Disorder
Family history of nystagmus	Congenital motor nystagmus
Family history of night blindness or color deficiency	Congenital stationary night blindness or achromatopsia
Ashkenazi Jewish descent	Tay–Sachs disease
Maternal anticonvulsant or psychotropic drug use	Optic nerve abnormality (e.g., hypoplasia)
Maternal (gestational) diabetes	Optic nerve hypoplasia
Maternal alcohol abuse	Optic nerve hypoplasia
Intrauterine infection	Toxoplasmosis, Rubella
Neonatal asphyxia	Cerebral atrophy
Neonatal seizures, meningitis	Cerebral injury
Intraventricular hemorrhage	Cerebral injury
Irritability, vomiting, bulging fontanelles	Increased intracranial pressure
Ataxia, seizures, strabismus	Posterior fossa disease
Short stature, delayed growth	DeMorsier's syndrome
Fair skin that does not tan	Albinism
Marked photophobia	Achromatopsia
Presentation after 6 months of age	Increased incidence of central nervous system tumor
Nystagmus worse when child is ill, fatigued, or stressed	Congenital motor nystagmus, periodic alternating nystagmus
Asymmetric nystagmus/head bobbing	Spasmus nutans

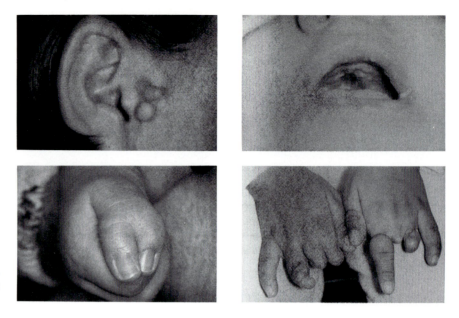

Figure 7–4. Signs of chromosomal or multisystem developmental anomaly: Anomalies of the ears, mouth, and hands.

latory movement that remains horizontal on vertical gaze is consistent with congenital motor efferent nystagmus, latent nystagmus, PAN, or peripheral vestibular nystagmus (Walsh & Hoyt, 1969). Pendular nystagmus usually becomes jerk on side gaze. The fast phase of jerk nystagmus may change directions depending on the position of gaze. For completeness, the nystagmus direction, frequency, and amplitude should be recorded for each of the cardinal positions of gaze as well as straight ahead, straight up, and straight down (Fig. 7–5). Figure 7–6 demonstrates a useful worksheet to record the nystagmus pattern.

Throughout the examination the clinician should be attuned to several characteristics regarding the nystagmus. These are summarized in Table 7–3 along with etiologic considerations.

TABLE 7–2. APPROACH TO THE INFANT WITH NYSTAGMUS: PHYSICAL EXAMINATION FINDINGS

Finding	Suggestion
Low-set ears, skin tags, dental anomalies, supernumerary digits	Chromosomal or other multisystem developmental anomaly
Fair skin, blond hair, absent tan	Albinism
Global developmental delay, abnormal head circumference	Diffuse central nervous system abnormality
Head bobbing, rapid, asymmetric nystagmus	Spasmus nutans

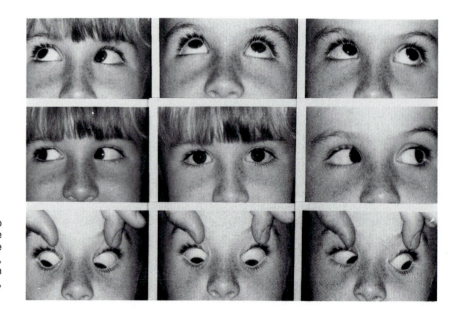

Figure 7–5. The positions of gaze used to record nystagmus amplitude and speed: the cardinal positions of gaze (up and to the right, far to the right, down and to the right, up and to the left, far to the left, and down and to the left); as well as straight up, straight ahead, and straight down.

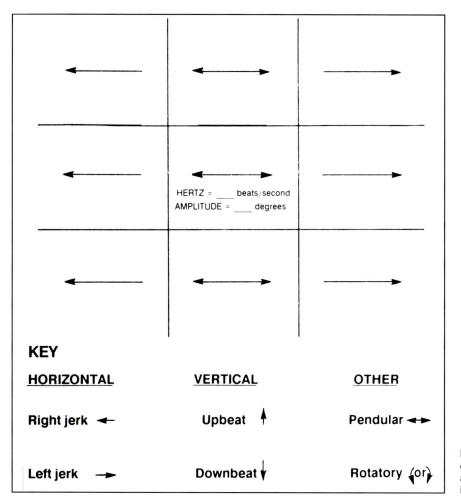

KEY

HORIZONTAL	VERTICAL	OTHER
Right jerk ←	Upbeat ↑	Pendular ←→
Left jerk →	Downbeat ↓	Rotatory (or)

HERTZ = ____ beats/second
AMPLITUDE = ____ degrees

Figure 7–6. Nystagmus recording sheet indicating a pendular nystagmus in straight ahead gaze which becomes jerk nystagmus in right and left gaze.

Visual Acuity Determination

Parents should be asked about their child's visual development. Questions such as whether their child recognizes them by sight, visually searches for toys, or fixates on faces are helpful in guiding the parent's

TABLE 7–3. APPROACH TO THE INFANT WITH NYSTAGMUS: NYSTAGMUS CHARACTERISTICS

Characteristic	Possible Etiology
Variable amplitude	Congenital motor nystagmus Periodic alternating nystagmus
Variable pattern	Cerebellar disorder
Regular change in direction over fixed time period	Periodic alternating nystagmus
Asymmetry between eyes	Spasmus nutans
Associated head movement	Spasmus nutans
Associated head position	Congenital motor nystagmus > other jerk nystagmus > pendular nystagmus
Nystagmus that remains horizontal on vertical gaze	Congenital motor nystagmus Periodic alternating nystagmus Peripheral vestibular nystagmus

assessment. The average child should fixate on faces and objects by 3 to 4 months of age; children with albinism have delayed visual maturation, and children with severe visual handicaps may respond only to bright lights. The child who can fixate and follow faces or toys has a much better visual prognosis than the child who appears visually inattentive.

In the physician's office, an infant's vision can be grossly tested by assessing their ability to fixate and follow moving objects, or attend to visual stimuli. The examiner's face is often the best object to use to test the child's ability to fixate and follow. Preferential looking techniques allow a more quantitative measurement of visual function (Fig. 7–7; see also Chapter 2). The ability to optically elicit ocular movements, such as the superimposition of a vertical optokinetic response in a child with horizontal nystagmus, is also noted (Fig. 7–8). If the latter is absent, there is a high likelihood that vision is grossly defective.

The visual acuity of children is tested binocularly and monocularly, at distant and near fixation. Children with an idiosyncratic head position should be tested with the head in the anomalous as well as normal position.

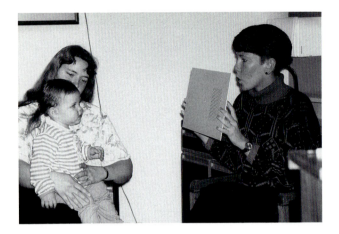

Figure 7–7. Preferential looking determination of spatial acuity using Teller acuity cards.

Pupillary Reactions

The pupillary responses in all children with nystagmus should be tested for the briskness of response and for the presence of an afferent pupillary defect or a paradoxical pupillary reaction. Brisk pupillary constriction to bright light is a favorable prognostic indicator for visual function. A sluggish response suggests a retinal, optic nerve, or third-nerve disorder. Many children with cortical visual impairment retain brisk pupillary responses. A relative afferent pupillary defect (RAPD) will be detected if there is asymmetry between the afferent paths of the eyes. This response is characterized by bilateral pupillary dilation with continuous light stimulation to an injured or abnormally developed eye. The "swinging flashlight test," used to detect a RAPD, is performed in a dim room by alternately illuminating the eyes. A penlight is directed obliquely in one eye and then the other from below. Constriction of the iris in the illuminated eye is a "direct response." Constriction of the opposite iris is a "consensual response." In the absence of a RAPD, pupillary constriction does not

vary in either eye when they are alternately illuminated. With a RAPD, however, both pupils constrict when light is directed into the unaffected eye, and dilate when directed into the affected eye (see Fig. 2–35). A relative afferent pupillary defect is an atypical finding in the infant with nystagmus; nystagmus usually develops only when both eyes are involved in the pathologic process.

A paradoxical pupillary response is also rare, but when present, is highly suggestive of congenital stationary night blindness, achromatopsia, or optic nerve hypoplasia. It has also been reported in some patients with Leber's congenital amaurosis (LCA), Best's disease, albinism, or retinitis pigmentosa (Hoyt, 1986; Walsh & Hoyt, 1969). To test for this response the eyes are adapted to ambient room illumination, so that the pupils are moderately constricted (about 4 mm in diameter). The normal reaction upon turning off the room lights is a slow steady dilation of the pupils (Fig. 7–9). A paradoxical reaction is characterized by an immediate constriction during the first 20 seconds, followed by a slow dilation after 1 minute. The important response to assess is the immediate reaction of the pupil upon decreasing illumination.

Ocular Examination

Any severe bilateral ocular malformation or tumor can impair vision and be associated with either searching or pendular nystagmus. Detection of an obvious bilateral anterior segment malformation (such as mesodermal dysgenesis, congenital cataracts, or congenital glaucoma) is seldom difficult. More subtle abnormalities of the iris, retina, and optic nerve require greater skill to detect.

Iris transillumination occurs in albinism. To detect this a penlight can be directed onto the lower eyelid while the observer looks at the iris in a darkened room. Subtle transillumination is difficult to appreciate by this technique, but in older children this can be detected at the slit lamp. A coloboma of the iris in association with nystagmus suggests the coloboma also involves the macula or optic nerve, with a poor visual prognosis. A near total absence of the iris is called aniridia. This is also associated with macular hypoplasia and nystagmus.

In infants without obvious anterior ocular abnormalities, examination of the posterior eye is of great importance. Most abnormalities of the posterior eye can be screened by using the red reflex test. This test is performed by looking through the ophthalmoscope at the patient's eyes from a distance of about 2 feet (Fig. 7–10). The room lights should be dimmed. In the absence of abnormality, the examiner should appreciate homogeneous red reflexes emanating from the child's pupils. Leukocoria (a white pupil) suggests that the child has a cataract, retinoblastoma, coloboma, or other defect (Fig. 7–11).

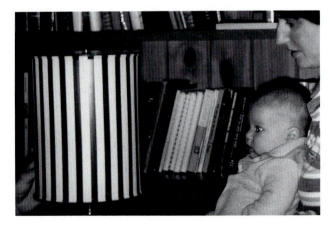

Figure 7–8. Elicitation of optokinetic nystagmus in an infant using an optokinetic drum.

ILLUMINATION	**NORMAL REACTION**	**PARADOXICAL REACTION**
Lights on	4 mm	4 mm
Lights off < 20 seconds	6 mm	2 mm
Lights off > 60 seconds	6 mm	6 mm

Figure 7–9. Paradoxical pupillary reaction.

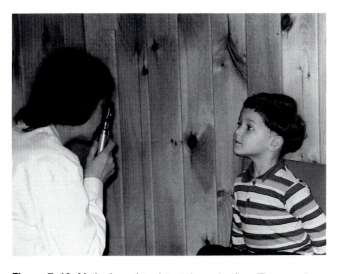

Figure 7–10. Method used to detect the red reflex. The examiner looks through the ophthalmoscope at the child's pupils, from a distance of about 2 feet.

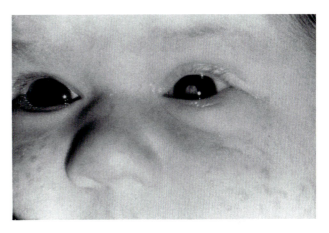

Figure 7–11. Leukocoria in the left eye in a child with a retinoblastoma.

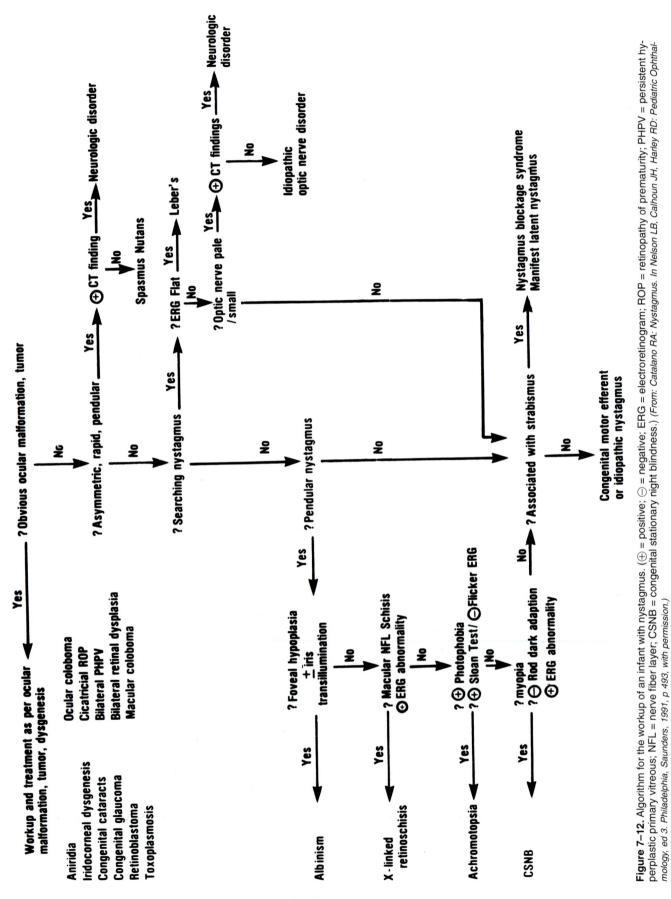

Figure 7–12. Algorithm for the workup of an infant with nystagmus. (⊕ = positive; ⊖ = negative; ERG = electroretinogram; ROP = retinopathy of prematurity; PHPV = persistent hyperplastic primary vitreous; NFL = nerve fiber layer; CSNB = congenital stationary night blindness.) *(From: Catalano RA: Nystagmus. In Nelson LB, Calhoun JH, Harley RD: Pediatric Ophthalmology, ed 3. Philadelphia, Saunders, 1991, p 493, with permission.)*

Experienced practitioners can gain valuable information from direct examination of the optic nerve and macula. Obvious abnormalities (such as cicatricial retinopathy of prematurity, retinoblastoma, and coloboma) are easily recognized with the ophthalmoscope. The clinician should also attempt to assess the optic nerve size and color, status of the retinal vasculature, and crispness of the macular reflex. Optic nerve hypoplasia, pallor, atrophy, or congenital anomaly suggests a neuro-ophthalmologic disorder. Retinal vasculature attenuation is a sign of significant retinal abnormality. A blunted macular reflex is consistent with albinism or aniridia. It should be remembered, however, that the macula does not fully develop until several months after birth. Finally, refraction should be performed by those trained in this procedure. The presence of myopia greater than 3.00 diopters in early infancy is suggestive of poor retinal functioning (Hoyt, 1986).

Nystagmus is often associated with strabismus, particularly an inward turning of the eyes (esotropia). This often occurs because poor visual development in infancy is associated with esotropia as well as nystagmus. In some children, however, the esotropia serves to dampen the nystagmus. The so-called nystagmus blockage syndrome is discussed below.

Whereas most of the ocular disorders associated with nystagmus are easy to diagnose, certain conditions are difficult or impossible to detect on clinical examination alone. These include Leber's congenital amaurosis, achromatopsia, congenital stationary night blindness, hereditary optic atrophy, mild optic nerve hypoplasia, and ocular albinism. Figure 7–12 was developed to assist the clinician in this situation. This figure is an algorithm for examining the child or infant with nystagmus, which relies on the nature of the nystagmus. If the nystagmus is asymmetric, rapid, and pendular, the workup is that for spasmus nutans; if symmetric and searching, the workup is directed toward severe retina and optic nerve disorders; if symmetric and pendular and not periodic and alternating, albinism or an isolated cone dysfunction or macular abnormalities should be ruled out. Congenital motor nystagmus becomes a diagnosis of exclusion, with resultant reasonably good visual prognosis.

COMPREHENSIVE INFORMATION ON NYSTAGMUS

Nystagmus Associated With Ocular Conditions

Bilateral visual loss, or the lack of development of vision, within the first 2 years of life is usually associated with bilateral nystagmus. Between 2 and 6 years of age the association is variable; after 6 years, visual loss rarely results in nystagmus. Acquired monocular vi-

sual loss, due to an anterior visual pathway abnormality, can result in a fine, rapid, monocular nystagmus (Donin, 1967; Zee et al, 1974).

Table 7–4 lists the ocular conditions associated with nystagmus according to the presence or absence of strabismus. The latter disorders are subdivided into spasmus nutans and nystagmus due to afferent abnormalities. The major focus of this section will be the afferent abnormalities that occur in the absence of an obvious ocular abnormality. By their nature, these disorders are usually diagnosed in infancy or early childhood.

Nonstrabismic Ocular Conditions

Afferent Conditions With Obvious Ocular Malformation, Dysgenesis, or Tumor. Any congenital or perinatal condition that results in occlusion of the visual axis, distortion of the retinal image, or malformation of the sensory retina or the optic nerve can result in nystagmus. Although electronystagmography

TABLE 7–4. OCULAR CONDITIONS ASSOCIATED WITH NYSTAGMUS

I. Nonstrabismic ocular conditions associated with nystagmus
  A. Spasmus nutans
  B. Afferent conditions with obvious bilateral malformation, dysgenesis, or tumor
    1. Ocular coloboma
    2. Congenital cataract
    3. Congenital glaucoma
    4. Retinoblastoma
    5. Cicatricial retinopathy or prematurity
    6. Iridocorneal dysgenesis
    7. Aniridia
    8. Persistent hyperplastic primary vitreous
    9. Retinal dysplasia
    10. Congenital toxoplasmosis
    11. Congenital "macular coloboma"
  C. Afferent conditions without obvious ocular malformation, dysgenesis, or tumor
    1. Conditions typically associated with searching nystagmus
      a. Leber's congenital amaurosis
      b. Bilateral optic nerve hypoplasia/atrophy
    2. Conditions typically associated with pendular nystagmus
      a. Albinism
        1. Ocular albinism
        2. Oculocutaneous albinism
      b. Achromatopsia
      c. Congenital stationary night blindness
      d. Macular disorder
        1. Congenital retinoschisis
II. Strabismus associated with nystagmus
  A. Nystagmus blockage syndrome
  B. Latent nystagmus
  C. Manifest latent nystagmus

Modified from Catalano RA: Nystagmus. In Nelson LB, Calhoun JH, Harley RD: Pediatric Ophthalmology, ed 3. Philadelphia, Saunders, 1991, p 491, with permission.

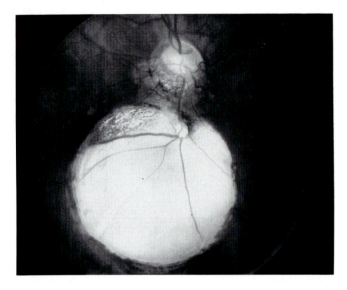

Figure 7–13. Retinal coloboma.

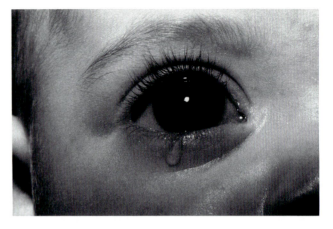

Figure 7–15. Congenital glaucoma characterized by an enlarged cloudy cornea and tearing.

may show complex or varied waveforms, the type of nystagmus is often related to the severity of the visual impairment. A moderate disruption in vision often results in pendular nystagmus, whereas a more severe form of the same disorder may produce a searching nystagmus. Although this may be helpful prognostically, ocular malformations usually are readily recognized and do not present diagnostic dilemmas. Excellent reviews already exist for many of the disorders to be mentioned. These are listed below with the more common ocular malformations associated with nystagmus: bilateral colobomas (Fig. 7–13; Pagon, 1981); congenital cataracts (Fig. 7–14; Calhoun, 1991); congenital glaucoma (Fig. 7–15; DeLuise & Anderson, 1983); retinoblastoma (Fig. 7–16; Ellsworth, 1988); aniridia (Fig. 7–17; Nelson et al, 1984); congenital toxoplasmosis with macular involvement (Fig. 7–18; Schlaegel, 1988;

bilateral cicatricial retinopathy of prematurity (Flynn, 1985); iridocorneal dysgenesis (Figs. 10–31 to 10–36; Townsend, 1974); persistent hyperplastic primary vitreous (Fig. 11–25; Haddad et al, 1974); bilateral retinal dysplasia (François, 1984); and congenital macular colobomas (Moore et al, 1985).

The first question asked in our flowchart (Fig. 7–12) is whether an obvious ocular malformation coexists. When severe ocular malformation is present bilaterally, the nystagmus almost invariably can be consid-

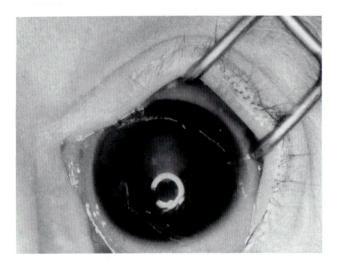

Figure 7–14. Congenital cataract.

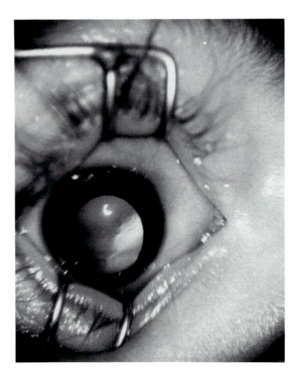

Figure 7–16. Retinoblastoma.

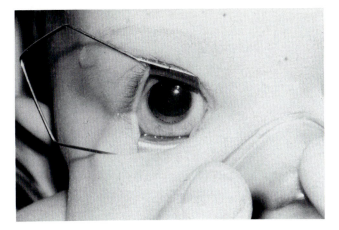

Figure 7–17. Aniridia. *(Courtesy of John W. Simon; from Catalano RA: Ocular Emergencies. Philadelphia, Saunders, 1992, p. 253, with permission.)*

ered a manifestation of poor visual input due to the malformation. In the absence of obvious ocular malformation, other causes of infantile nystagmus must be considered. At this juncture the nature of the nystagmus becomes important diagnostically. The next consideration is whether the nystagmus is consistent with that seen in spasmus nutans.

Spasmus Nutans. The classic triad of signs in spasmus nutans includes (1) monocular or dissociated, small-amplitude, rapid nystagmus; (2) head bobbing; and (3) an anomalous head position. The latter two are not always present (Weissman et al, 1986). The nystagmus usually develops between 4 and 8 months of age, and ceases spontaneously by age 3 to 4 years. It can, however, be variable in its onset and duration. A similar clinical presentation has been noted in children with chiasmatic gliomas (Albright et al, 1984) and sub-

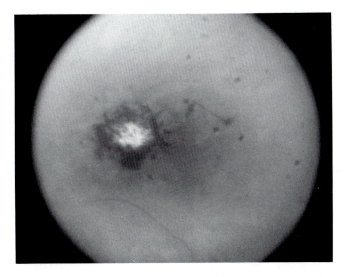

Figure 7–18. Congenital toxoplasmosis with macular involvement.

acute necrotizing encephalomyopathy (Sedwick et al, 1984). Distinguishing clinical features of these latter disorders include optic atrophy, poor feeding (due to diencephalic abnormality), and irritability, vomiting, and bulging fontanelles (due to increased intracranial pressure). Even in the absence of these signs, spasmus nutans should only be considered after these other conditions have been excluded.

Until more distinguishing characteristics of spasmus nutans are elucidated (such as waveform on electronystagmography, clinical findings, or history), it is usually prudent to obtain computed tomography (CT) with intravenous contrast, or magnetic resonance imaging (MRI) to rule out an intracranial process in an infant presenting with acquired, asymmetric, rapid, and pendular nystagmus.

Afferent Conditions Without Obvious Ocular Malformation, Dysgenesis, or Tumor. Although exceptions occur, the character of the nystagmus in infants with afferent disorders typically reflects the severity of the visual loss. Searching nystagmus is usually observed in children whose vision is less than 20/200. Pendular nystagmus is seen when the visual acuity of at least one eye is better than 20/200 (Jan et al, 1986). It is useful clinically to employ these distinctions to categorize the nystagmus, realizing that exceptions occur.

Leber's congenital amaurosis (LCA) is characterized by diminished vision in the perinatal period. Visual acuity is less than 20/200 in up to 95 percent of affected individuals, and a searching nystagmus is present in 75 percent (Noble & Carr, 1978). A markedly reduced or absent response to the ERG is noted in virtually all patients (Fig. 7–19). One third or more may have psychomotor retardation, mental retardation, or associated renal and skeletal abnormalities (Roizenblatt & Cunha, 1980). The latter disorders are usually not present in those children with greater than 5 diopters of hyperopia. This finding is useful in planning the educational program for affected children (Wagner et al, 1985).

A variety of ocular conditions, including keratoconus, keratoglobus, macular colobomas, disc edema, cataract, and strabismus, have also been associated with LCA. The fundus appearance may be normal, especially in infancy, or there may be optic pallor with a granular, bone spicule pigmentation and arteriolar narrowing. The latter findings often become more prominent with age. Histopathological studies have shown the outer retinal layers to be almost completely replaced by gliosis, with sparing of the bipolar and ganglion cells (Sears et al, 1977).

Optic nerve disorders, either atrophy or hypoplasia, are likely if there is searching nystagmus and the ERG is normal. If the optic nerves are pale, or if CNS abnormalities are present, the infant should be evalu-

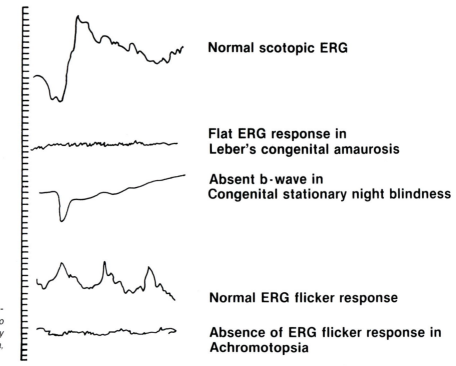

Normal scotopic ERG

Flat ERG response in
Leber's congenital amaurosis

Absent b-wave in
Congenital stationary night blindness

Normal ERG flicker response

Absence of ERG flicker response in
Achromotopsia

Figure 7–19. Normal and abnormal electroretinographic (ERG) findings. *(From Catalano RA: Nystagmus. In Nelson LB, Calhoun JH, Harley RD: Pediatric Ophthalmology, ed 3. Philadelphia, Saunders, 1991, p 495, with permission.)*

ated neuroradiologically to rule out an intracranial process such as hydrocephalus or chiasmatic glioma. **Optic nerve hypoplasia (ONH)** is a congenital, nonprogressive condition characterized by a paucity of axons within the optic nerve and a diminished ganglion cell layer of the retina (Lloyd & Buncic, 1980). Ophthalmoscopically, hypoplasia of the optic nerve is recognized as a small, pale nervehead, within a normal-sized opening in the sclera for the optic canal (Fig. 7–20). If the optic canal is surrounded by pigmentation,

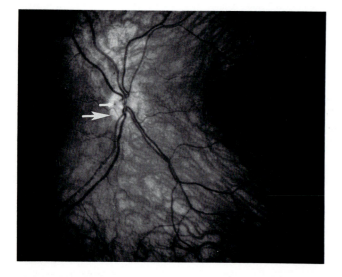

Figure 7–20. Optic nerve hypoplasia. The small arrow indicates the edge of the optic nerve; the large arrow, the edge of the opening in the sclera for the optic canal.

two "rings" may be appreciated (the "double-ring sign"). The first ring is the scleral opening, and the second the pigmented rim surrounding this. The retinal vessels usually appear relatively normal, but the retina may be deeply red in color because of the thinness of the nerve fiber layer of the retina.

Severe bilateral ONH results in a searching nystagmus, but mild, unilateral ONH may be asymptomatic. In one study, 78 percent of those with bilateral involvement, poor vision, and nystagmus had additional ocular abnormalities, compared with 21 percent of patients with unilateral ONH (Skarf & Hoyt, 1984). Delayed development is the most frequent nonvisual associated problem, followed by hypopituitarism, cerebral palsy, and epilepsy (Margalith et al, 1984).

In 1956, deMorsier noted an association of bilateral ONH with absence of the septum pellucidum and dysplasia of the anterior third ventricle and corpus callosum. Subsequent investigators have associated hypopituitarism with this disorder (Hoyt et al, 1970). Rarer systemic associations include midline facial defects and abnormalities of the cerebral cortex, brainstem, and cerebellum (Frisen & Holmegaard, 1978). Associated ocular malformations include microphthalmos, coloboma, aniridia, and strabismus.

ONH is believed to result from a defect in the differentiation of retinal ganglion cell axons. It has been associated with embryonic insults at or after 6 weeks of gestation, and with maternal ingestion of quinidine (McKinna, 1966) or anticonvulsants (Hoyt & Billson, 1978). It is more common in children of severely diabetic and of adolescent mothers (Margalith et al, 1984).

Reports of a few bilateral cases have suggested that in some families an autosomal dominant or recessive gene may be causative (Hackenbruch et al, 1975).

ONH is also a common finding in fetal alcohol syndrome. This syndrome is characterized by short palpebral fissures, a thin frenulum of the upper lip, ptosis, and prominent epicanthal folds (Fig. 7–21). Mental retardation may be mild to severe, and there may be associated abnormalities of the cardiovascular and skeletal systems. Additional findings include high myopia, microphthalmia, strabismus, and tortuosity of the retinal vessels (Stromland, 1987).

Albinism is a genetically determined disturbance in melanogenesis. Various subtypes exist, including oculocutaneous albinism (Fig. 7–22), ocular albinism, and several syndromes in which albinism is associated. The major ophthalmologic findings are minimal to marked iris transillumination from decreased pigmentation (Figs. 7–23 and 7–24), macular hypoplasia (Fig. 7–25), and a paucity of retinal pigmentation (Fig. 7–26). Additional findings include nystagmus, photophobia (light sensitivity), high refractive errors, and reduced visual acuity.

Multiple inheritance patterns have been noted for albinism (Kinnear et al, 1985, O'Donnell & Green, 1988). It is apparent that multiple alleles are responsible for melanogenesis. The hairbulb incubation test can demonstrate the presence or absence of tyrosinase activity and provide biochemical evidence for heteroge-

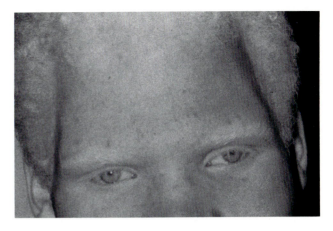

Figure 7–22. Oculocutaneous albinism.

neity, but alone cannot separate the various forms of albinism known to exist. Clinical, biochemical, and ultrastructural criteria are now used for this purpose (Witkop, 1985). A precise diagnosis is essential for counseling the family about the implications of the disease and the heritable pattern. Prenatal diagnosis of oculocutaneous albinism by electron microscopic study of desquamated skin cells is also possible (Eady et al, 1983).

The clinical management of children with albinism involves protecting the skin and maximizing vision. Albinos often have delayed visual maturation; they gradually become more visually attentive after 2 to 3 months of age. They also often have high refractive errors and may benefit significantly from spectacle correction. Near acuity is relatively better than far, and most albinos can read small print without low-vision aids. They can, therefore, be educated through the normal school system. Adequate protection of the skin by

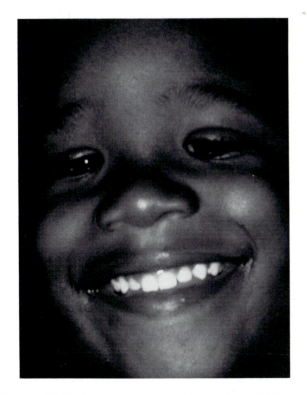

Figure 7–21. Fetal alcohol syndrome. Note the ptosis, short palpebral folds, prominent epicanthal folds, strabismus, and short frenulum of the upper lip.

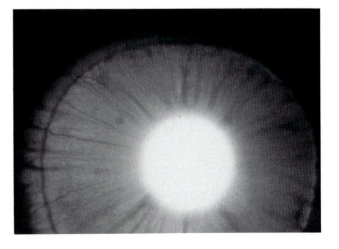

Figure 7–23. Marked iris transillumination in oculocutaneous albinism. *(From Catalano RA: Nystagmus. In Nelson LB, Calhoun JH, Harley RD: Pediatric Ophthalmology, ed 3. Philadelphia, Saunders, 1991, p 496, with permission.)*

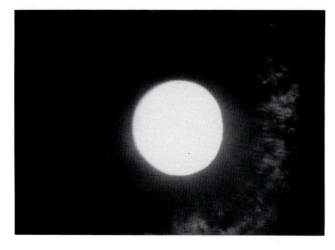

Figure 7–24. Minimal iris transillumination in ocular albinism.

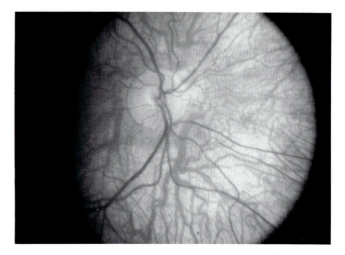

Figure 7–26. Paucity of pigmentation in the fundus of a child with albinism.

ultraviolet barriers and clothing is necessary because of the increased risk of skin cancer.

It is important to recognize two special subtypes of albinism because they may have life-threatening complications. The Chekiak–Higashi syndrome is a lethal condition in which albinism is associated with a defect in cellular immunity (T cells) as well as leukocytes. The neutrophils of these patients show reduced migration and deficient chemotaxis and bactericidal capacity. Affected children have an increased susceptibility to gram-positive infections. Those surviving childhood infections often die of malignant lymphoreticular infiltration of the tissues (Blume & Wolff, 1972; Brahmi, 1983). The Hermansky–Pudlak syndrome is an association of oculocutaneous albinism with hemorrhagic diathesis and a ceroid-like accumulation in the reticuloendothelial cells; it is unusually prevalent in Puerto

Ricans. The bleeding tendency is low, but deaths from hemorrhage following minor surgical or dental procedures have been reported. These patients have a qualitative defect in their platelets. Aspirin and cyclooxygenase inhibitors should be avoided because they may convert the mild bleeding disorder into a severe one. Additional associations include the development of restrictive lung disease, ulcerative colitis, kidney disease, and cardiomyopathy (Hermansky & Pudlak, 1959; Schinella et al, 1983).

Congenital stationary night blindness (CSNB) is a heritable disorder in which the predominant symptom is night blindness. It is characterized by a normal fundus appearance, normal daylight visual fields, the absence of rod dark adaptation, and lack of progression. A defect in neural transmission at the bipolar level, rather than a disorder of rhodopsin, is believed causative (Carr, 1983; Krill, 1977).

Multiple inheritance patterns have been identified in CSNB; autosomal dominant, autosomal recessive, and X-linked. The phenotypic expression is specifically related to inheritance. X-linked CSNB is associated with diminished visual acuity, nystagmus, and myopia ranging from 3.50 to 11.0 diopters. These findings occur in only a few families with autosomal recessive inheritance patterns, and never in patients with autosomal dominant CSNB (Carr, 1974; Hittner et al, 1981).

The visual acuity in X-linked CSNB ranges between 20/30 and 20/100. Patients with acuities worse than 20/60 have an obvious pendular nystagmus, but electronystagmography can occasionally detect nystagmus when the acuity is better (Krill, 1977). Color vision is normal or, at worst, only mildly abnormal, differentiating this disorder from achromatopsia. The diagnosis is made in infants by electrophysiological findings. A reduction or absence of the positive (b-wave) response to scotopic testing is characteristic (see Fig. 7–19). In addi-

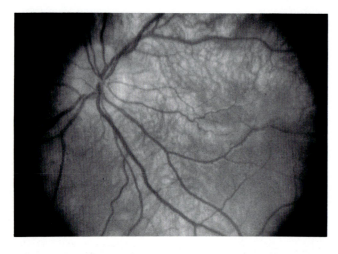

Figure 7–25. Macular hypoplasia in albinism. *(From Catalano RA: Nystagmus. In Nelson LB, Calhoun JH, Harley RD: Pediatric Ophthalmology, ed 3. Philadelphia, Saunders, 1991, p 496, with permission.)*

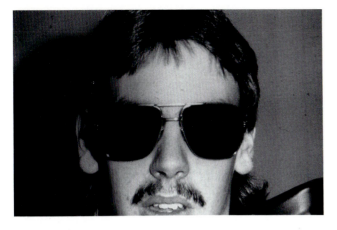

Figure 7–27. Highly occlusive sunglasses used by a patient with achromatopsia and severe photophobia. *(From Catalano RA: Nystagmus. In Nelson LB, Calhoun JH, Harley RD: Pediatric Ophthalmology, ed 3. Philadelphia, Saunders, 1991, p 497, with permission.)*

tion, a paradoxical pupillary reaction (see Fig. 7–9) occurs in some young patients with X-linked CSNB (Barricks et al, 1977).

Oguchi's disease is a related autosomal recessive congenital stationary disorder with diminished night vision. Unlike CSNB, there is a peculiar homogeneous yellow to grayish-white discoloration of the fundus, and only occasionally mildly abnormal vision in the range of 20/25 to 20/50. The abnormal coloration usually disappears after 2 to 3 hours of dark adaptation and begins to reappear after about 10 minutes of light exposure. This phenomenon suggests a disorder of retinal pigment kinetics, but normal rhodopsin kinetics

have been reported in at least one affected patient. ERG findings in Oguchi's disease are similar to those of CSNB; an absent b-wave is characteristic. In Oguchi's disease, however, the ERG may become less abnormal after prolonged dark adaptation (Carr, 1974; Wilder, 1953).

Achromatopsia (rod monochromatism) is a rare congenital disorder with a prevalence of only 3 in 100,000 (Verriest, 1969). It is characterized by a complete loss of color vision, diminished visual acuity to 20/400, photophobia (Fig. 7–27), and typically a pendular nystagmus in the primary position. A striking characteristic of the nystagmus is its low amplitude, of usually less than 3 degrees. This makes clinical detection of the nystagmus difficult, but differentiates this disorder from albinism, in which the amplitude of nystagmus is larger (Yee et al, 1981). The photophobia and nystagmus may diminish and even disappear beyond 15 years of age, but the visual acuity does not improve (Carr, 1983; Krill, 1977).

Histopathology has demonstrated that the cone photoreceptors in achromatopsia are either missing or severely maldeveloped. Because of severe photophobia, children with this disorder may prefer to play outside at dusk and may have better vision in dim illumination (hemeralopia) (Krill, 1977). In older children, findings on two tests can be helpful diagnostically. The Sloan achromatopsia test[*] (Fig. 7–28) uses six test

---

[*] Available from Macbeth Color and Photometry Co., 2441 North Calvert Street, Baltimore, MD 21218.

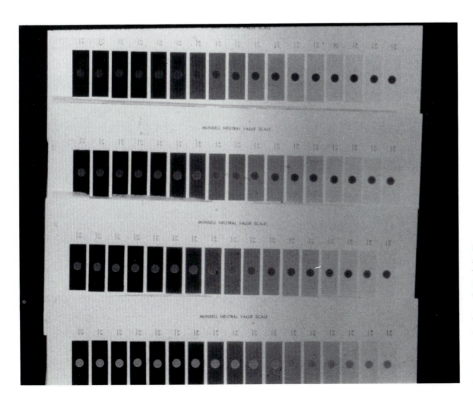

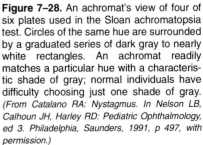

Figure 7–28. An achromat's view of four of six plates used in the Sloan achromatopsia test. Circles of the same hue are surrounded by a graduated series of dark gray to nearly white rectangles. An achromat readily matches a particular hue with a characteristic shade of gray; normal individuals have difficulty choosing just one shade of gray. *(From Catalano RA: Nystagmus. In Nelson LB, Calhoun JH, Harley RD: Pediatric Ophthalmology, ed 3. Philadelphia, Saunders, 1991, p 497, with permission.)*

plates. On each of these is a graduated series of 17 rectangular strips that vary in color from almost white to almost black. In the center of each rectangle is a circle of known hue. Achromats have no difficulty matching each of six different hues to a particular shade of gray. Because of the qualitative difference between a color and gray, normal subjects have difficulty identifying a "perfect" match (Sloan, 1954). Findings on the anomaloscope test, in which affected individuals find red lights to be dim and green lights bright, are also unique. These tests are useful only in older individuals. In infants one must rely on electrophysiological findings. In achromatopsia the ERG flicker response is absent (see Fig. 7–19), and the photopic single-flash response is reduced. The scotopic response is normal.

A form of incomplete rod monochromatism also exists. This incomplete form has been called blue cone monochromatism, because blue cones are involved minimally or not at all. The inheritance of this disorder appears to be X-linked. Visual acuity is in the 20/60 range, nystagmus is minimal, and photophobia is absent. Unlike achromatopsia, this condition appears to be slowly progressive; the finding of macular scarring is not uncommon in older affected individuals (Fig. 7–29). Blue cone monochromatism is distinguished from achromatopsia by color plate discrepancies. On color vision testing blue cone monochromats distinguish between blue-green and purple-blue, but achromats do not. Differences in the eye movement response to optokinetic stimuli moving from the nasal to the temporal field can also be used to differentiate these two conditions (achromats respond poorly). Because blue cones probably represent only a small portion of all retinal cones, the ERG is just as abnormal in this disorder as in complete achromatopsia. Patients with blue

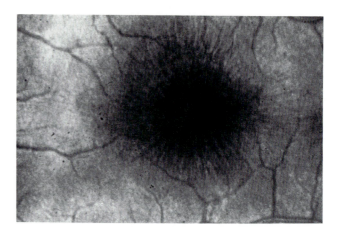

Figure 7–30. Macula in X-linked retinoschisis.

cone monochromatism, however, show a peak illumination sensitivity near 440 nm, whereas patients with rod monochromatism demonstrate a peak sensitivity near 504 nm (Berson et al, 1983; Yee et al, 1985).

X-linked juvenile retinoschisis is an autosomal recessive disorder characterized by vitreous degeneration and cleavage of the retina at the level of the nerve fiber layer. Macular involvement is the most frequent finding, and is recognized as numerous folds that radiate in a spokewheel configuration (Fig. 7–30). Peripheral retinoschisis occurs in 50 percent of affected boys (Fig. 7–31). Expressivity of the disorder is variable; it is not unusual to find nearly normal visual acuity in some members of an affected family and light perception in others. Typically, the visual acuity is reduced to between 20/50 and 20/100. With increasing age, this gradually diminishes to about 20/200 (Krill, 1977). Nystagmus is also a variable accompaniment. Only

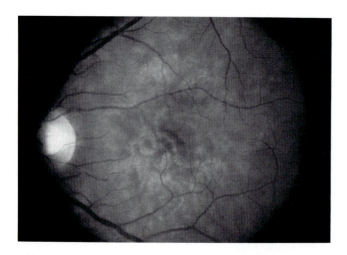

Figure 7–29. Macular scarring in an older individual with blue cone monochromatism.

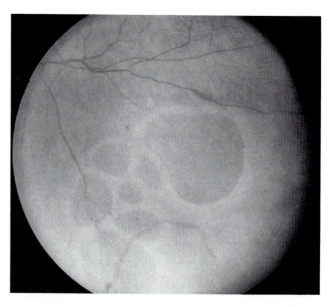

Figure 7–31. Peripheral retinoschisis in X-linked retinoschisis.

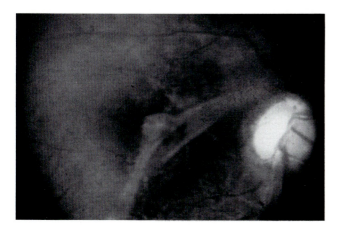

Figure 7–32. Vitreous veil in X-linked retinoschisis.

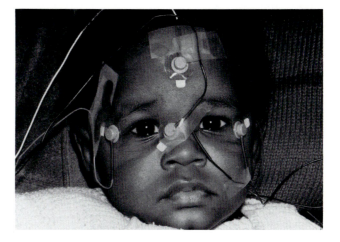

Figure 7–34. Setup to perform electronystagmography (recording of the eye movements to quantitatively determine the nystagmus type). *(From Nelson LB, Catalano RA: Atlas of Ocular Motility. Philadelphia, Saunders, 1989, p. 121, with permission.)*

two of 14 patients who presented to Wills Eye Hospital with X-linked retinoschisis had nystagmus (J. Augsberger, personal communication).

Vitreous strands and veils may also be present (Fig. 7–32). If retinal vessels are pulled off with these veils, vitreous hemorrhage can result. This is frequently the presenting sign of the disorder (Balian & Falls, 1960). Macular pseudocysts are a late finding in about half of the affected individuals. In the absence of these findings the ERG is useful diagnostically. The characteristic ERG finding is an intact a-wave but reduced scotopic and photopic b-waves. The a-wave is preserved because it arises from the photoreceptors, which do not detach.

Strabismus Associated With Nystagmus

Nystagmus Blockage Syndrome (NBS). The nystagmus blockage syndrome (NBS) is a variant of congenital nystagmus in which a sustained adduction effort, resulting in esotropia, occurs to dampen the nystagmus. The incidence of NBS in esotropic patients has been variably reported as between 4 and 10 percent. The syndrome is characterized by an inverse relationship between the angle of esotropia and the amplitude of nystagmus. Nystagmus increases when the eye is abducted. The desire to maintain adduction is evidenced when one eye is occluded. Instead of the un-

occluded eye rotating to the straight-ahead position, it continues to turn in. The infant continues to fixate in this position, and will usually turn the face or head to the ipsilateral side to look straight ahead (Fig. 7–33). Two other findings distinguish this disorder. The angle of esotropia increases when a base out prism is placed before the fixating eye, and the pupil does not constrict when the eye assumes its adducted position (demonstrating that no accommodative mechanisms are at play).

Nystagmus blockage syndrome is usually apparent early in infancy. Overaction of the inferior oblique muscles and dissociated vertical deviations occur less frequently in NBS than in essential infantile esotropia (Dell'Osso et al, 1983; von Noorden & Wong, 1986).

Latent or Manifest Latent Nystagmus. Latent nystagmus (LN) describes a conjugate congenital jerk nystagmus evoked by occlusion of one eye. The fast phase is always toward the viewing (nonoccluded) eye. Alternate occlusion of the eyes results in reversal of the nystagmus direction. The amplitude increases with gaze directed to the side of the fixating eye. All patients with LN have strabismus, usually an esotropia and/or a dissociated vertical deviation, but this alone does not cause the nystagmus.

Manifest latent nystagmus (MLN) is a condition in which abnormal visual input from one eye, usually due to amblyopia, causes a latent nystagmus to be-

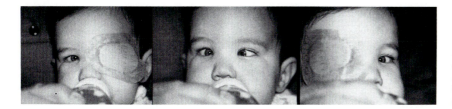

Figure 7–33. The nystagmus blockage syndrome. With occlusion of either eye, the infant maintains an adducted position of gaze, and turns her head to the ipsilateral side to fixate straight ahead.

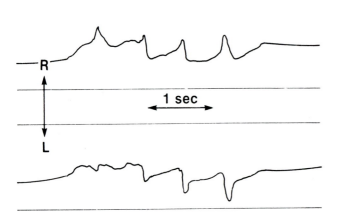

Figure 7–35. Electronystagmography recording.

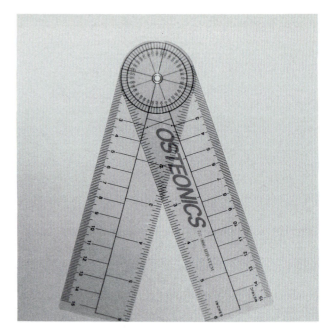

Figure 7–37. Protractor used to measure face turns.

come manifest. As with LN, the fast phase is always in the direction of the fixating eye. Quantitative electronystagmography is useful in distinguishing NBS from MLN with esotropia (Figs. 7–34 and 7–35). The latter is much more common (Dell'Osso et al, 1979).

Congenital Motor, Efferent, or Idiopathic Nystagmus. Congenital nystagmus (CN) is characterized by a conjugate, principally jerk nystagmus that becomes apparent in the perinatal period. Occasionally, a pendular and/or rotary component is present. The nystagmus may be minimized in a particular position of gaze. This position, called the null point, is frequently straight ahead, but can be in any direction causing a compensatory face turn or abnormal head position (Fig. 7–36). This face turn can be measured with a protractor (Figs. 7–37 and 7–38). Away from the null zone, and with fixation attempts, the nystagmus amplitude increases. Abnormal head posturing is not

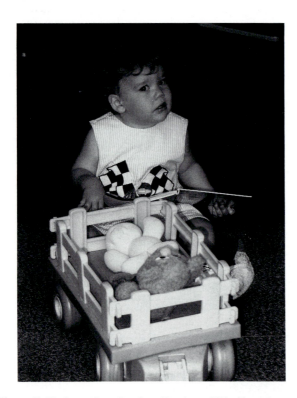

Figure 7–36. Anomalous head position in a child with nystagmus. The amplitude of the nystagmus is dampened in some children when their eyes are placed in an eccentric position. In order to gaze straight ahead these children turn their heads and face to the opposite side.

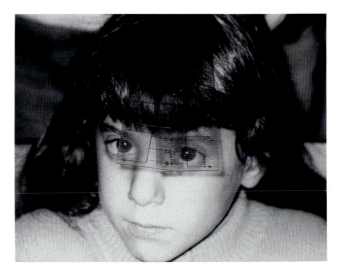

Figure 7–38. Method of measuring face turns. One side of the protractor is aligned with the patient's gaze, the other with her nose. The angle of the face turn is read directly from the protractor.

pathognomonic of congenital nystagmus; it can occur in periodic alternating nystagmus and other forms of jerk nystagmus. Face turns are less frequently noted with pendular nystagmus.

Several other features are also characteristic but not pathognomonic of congenital nystagmus. The amplitude of the nystagmus increases with illness, anxiety, and stress. When this occurs, the patient's vision is proportionately decreased. Convergence dampens the nystagmus, and horizontal CN remains horizontal in vertical gaze. Away from the null zone, the fast phase of the nystagmus is in the direction of gaze (Alexander's law). Finally, the nystagmus is abolished during sleep (Dell'Osso et al, 1988).

The visual acuity of affected patients is relatively good; 20/20 to 20/70 acuity is typical. Additional features include the absence of oscillopsia, an inversion of the optokinetic reflex, and occasionally a positive family history. The diagnosis is much easier to make in children who are old enough for acuity and color vision testing. Acuity better than 20/100 excludes Leber's congenital amaurosis and achromatopsia, the absence of myopia excludes congenital stationary night blindness, a normal fundus examination excludes macular and optic nerve disorders, and the absence of iris transillumination and a normal fovea exclude all the types of albinism. It is important to make this diagnosis as early as possible, because its implication for reasonably good vision can assuage parental anxiety.

Physiological, Optokinetic, and Voluntary Nystagmus

Rhythmic oscillations of the eyes can be induced in most individuals on extreme lateral gaze, stimulation of the vestibular system, or optokinetic stimulation. A few individuals can rhythmically move their eyes voluntarily.

End-point Nystagmus

End-point nystagmus is an unsustained "jerk" nystagmus of fine amplitude that occurs on extreme lateral gaze. The fast phase is always in the direction of gaze, and the amplitude may be greater in the abducting (turning out) eye (Abel et al, 1978b).

Vestibular Nystagmus

A jerk nystagmus can be evoked by altering the equilibrium of the endolymph in the semicircular canals. It can be elicited by rapidly accelerating or rotating the head, or by irrigating the ear canal with cold or warm water. When either of these occur, the vestibular nuclei initiate a slow drift of the eyes in the direction of flow of the endolymph. Brainstem and frontomesencephalic pathways return the eyes to the original position with a fast corrective movement.

Cold temperature inhibits the flow of endolymph,

and heat stimulates it. Cold water irrigation of an ear canal thus causes the endolymph to flow toward the irrigated ear and a slow drift of the eyes to the same side. The fast phase, for which the nystagmus is always described, is to the opposite side. Pure horizontal or vertical nystagmus can be induced by rotating the body with the head held in a specific orientation. Rotatory nystagmus, however, can only be produced by a pathological vestibular condition (Baloh & Honrubia, 1979; Paige, 1984).

Optokinetic Nystagmus (OKN)

Optokinetic nystagmus (OKN) is an induced jerk nystagmus elicited by moving repetitive visual stimuli across the visual field (see Fig. 7–8). The slow phase occurs as the eyes pursue a moving target; the fast phase is a saccade in the opposite direction to fixate a subsequent target in the series. The parieto-occipital lobe controls the slow pursuit movement, and the frontal lobes control the fast corrective phase. The presence of OKN in a visually immature infant demonstrates that some visual input is present. A defect in the OKN response in a hemianopic patient localizes the lesion to the parieto-occipital lobe (Smith, 1963). A dissociated response is seen in internuclear ophthalmoplegia. The latter disorder is characterized by an impaired ability of an eye to turn inward (adduct) on contralateral gaze, with horizontal nystagmus in the opposite (abducting) eye (Fig. 7–39). With optokinetic stimulation, the nystagmus of the abducting eye is increased. Additional findings include vertical nystagmus on attempted upward gaze, and normal convergence (Fig. 7–40).

An inversion of the OKN response can occur in congenital motor nystagmus. In a patient with a left-beating nystagmus, the slow movement of an OKN stimulus to the right would be expected to enhance the fast phase movement to the left. In congenital motor nystagmus, however, the fast phase inverts to the right, the direction the stimulus is moving (Halmazzi et al, 1980a).

Voluntary Nystagmus

A few individuals can voluntarily move their eyes in a rapid pendular fashion. Voluntary nystagmus is usually very rapid (20 Hz) and horizontal. Convergence and pupillary constriction are often associated, and the nystagmus can rarely be sustained for more than 30 seconds at a time (Aschoff et al, 1976; Nagle et al, 1980).

Nystagmus Associated With Neurological Disorders

Gaze Paretic Nystagmus

Parieto-occipital, cerebellar, and brainstem lesions that affect the conjugate gaze mechanism cause gaze paretic nystagmus. This disorder is similar to endpoint nystagmus, but it occurs in a less extreme position of gaze and

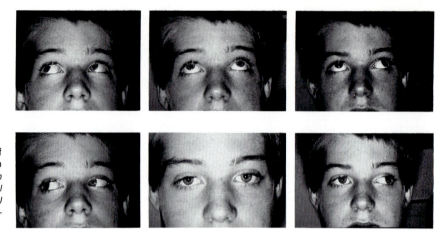

Figure 7–39. Internuclear ophthalmoplegia of the right eye. Note the inability of the right eye to turn inward on left gaze. *(Reprinted with permission from Catalano RA, Sax RD, Krohel GB: Unilateral internuclear ophthalmoplegia after head trauma. Am J Ophthalmol 101:492, 1986; copyright by The Ophthalmic Publishing Company.)*

is of greater amplitude. In addition, patients recovering from a gaze palsy often go through a phase characterized by gaze paretic nystagmus. During this period, they cannot maintain an eccentric gaze and their eyes drift slowly back to the primary position on attempted lateral gaze. A corrective saccade repositions the eyes eccentrically. The fast phase of the nystagmus is in the direction of gaze. Barbiturates and phenytoin (Dilantin) cause a similar nystagmus (Abel et al, 1978a).

Convergence–Retraction Nystagmus (Nystagmus Retractorius)

Variable bursts of sustained retraction and convergence of the eyes on attempted upward gaze suggests a midbrain disorder. Co-contraction of all the extraocular muscles causes retraction. Convergence occurs because of the greater strength of the medial rectus muscles. Infants with this disorder should be evaluated for the presence of congenital aqueductal stenosis. In chil-

dren, this finding suggests a pinealoma or hydrocephalus; in adults, a vascular accident in the tectal or pretectal area is usually responsible. Convergence-retraction nystagmus usually occurs in association with paralysis of upward gaze, defective convergence, pupillary abnormalities (light–near dissociation of pupillary constriction), lid retraction, and accommodative spasm (Huber, 1971; Smith et al, 1959). This constellation of findings constitutes Parinuad's syndrome.

Periodic Alternating Nystagmus (PAN)

Periodic alternating nystagmus (PAN) is a horizontal jerk nystagmus in which the direction of the nystagmus changes spontaneously at a regular interval. A typical cycle lasts several minutes, and is characterized by a sequence of fast beats in one direction, interrupted by a short neutral period, and followed by fast beats in the opposite direction (Fig. 7–41). PAN usually remains horizontal in upward gaze. It may prevail during sleep and may coexist with downbeat nystagmus, both of which suggest an abnormality in the caudal medulla (Baloh et al, 1976). Children with PAN will occasionally demonstrate spontaneous, alternate face turning, confirming an alternating null position of the eyes. The site of the lesion in congenital PAN is unknown, but in acquired cases an abnormality in the vestibulocerebellar pathway is likely. PAN has also been reported in a handful of patients with chronic otitis or albinism (Duke-Elder & Scott, 1971). Neurosurgical intervention can be efficacious in patients with cerebellar compression. Baclofen is useful in other symptomatic patients (Halmazzi et al, 1980).

Downbeat Nystagmus

Downbeat nystagmus is characterized by repetitive cycles in which the eyes rapidly jerk downward, followed by a slow return upward. It is believed that a deficit in downward pursuit causes the eyes to drift upward, and a corrective saccade jerks the eyes downward. Downbeat nystagmus is maximized when the

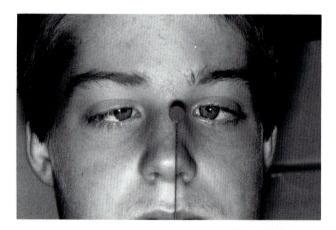

Figure 7–40. Retention of convergence of the right eye in the same child with internuclear ophthalmoplegia. *(Reprinted with permission from Catalano RA, Sax RD, Krohel GB: Unilateral internuclear ophthalmoplegia after head trauma. Am J Ophthalmol 101:492, 1986; copyright by The Ophthalmic Publishing Company.)*

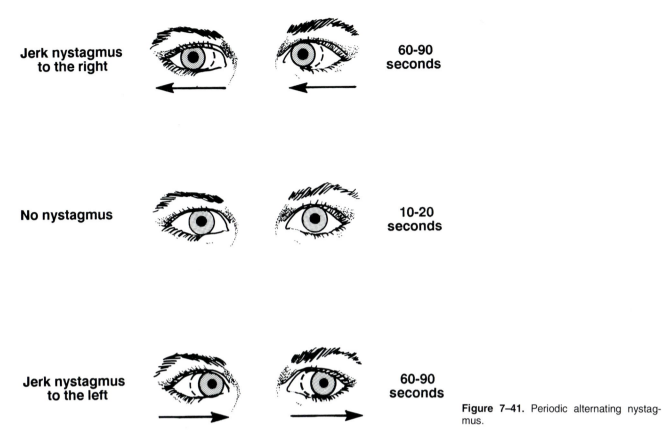

Jerk nystagmus to the right — 60-90 seconds

No nystagmus — 10-20 seconds

Jerk nystagmus to the left — 60-90 seconds

Figure 7–41. Periodic alternating nystagmus.

eyes are deviated laterally and slightly below the midline, with the head erect or hyperextended. It suggests a structural lesion at the cervicomedullary junction, and is usually accompanied by oscillopsia (the perception that the world is spinning). Toxins such as alcohol and anticonvulsants can also elicit this condition (Burde & Henkind, 1981; Halmazzi et al, 1983).

Upbeat Nystagmus
A pursuit deficit similar in type but opposite in direction to downbeat nystagmus is thought to cause upbeat nystagmus. Of interest, upbeat nystagmus can increase or convert to downbeat nystagmus with convergence. It may occur with congenital lesions of the cerebellar vermis or medulla, or after meningitis (Daroff, 1973; Fischer et al, 1983).

See-Saw Nystagmus
See-saw nystagmus describes a torsional oscillation of both eyes in which one eye rises and intorts as the fellow eye falls and extorts (Fig. 7–42). The nystagmoid movement is pendular and the torsional movement of the eyes alternates to provide the see-saw effect. This disorder may be congenital, but most affected patients have large parasellar tumors expanding within the third ventricle. An associated finding is bitemporal hemianopsia (Daroff, 1965; Fein & Williams, 1969). Magnetic resonance imaging should be performed to rule out an intracranial mass. Management of the nys-

tagmus involves treating the inciting cause. If it persists after neurosurgical intervention, oral clonazepam or baclofen may be helpful.

Central Vestibular Nystagmus
A lesion of the vestibular nuclei, or its pathways, produces a horizontal and rotatory jerk nystagmus on lateral gaze, usually to the side opposite the lesion. It may

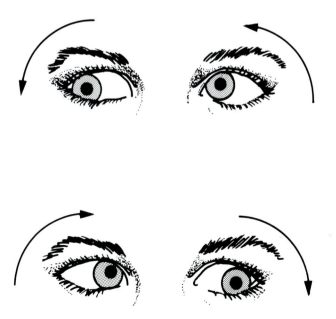

Figure 7–42. See-saw nystagmus.

be bidirectional, beating to the left on left gaze and to the right on right gaze, and it may become vertical on vertical gaze. In contrast to peripheral vestibular nystagmus, vertigo, tinnitus, and deafness are not usually associated. The nystagmus is usually a sign of demyelinating disease, vascular accident, encephalitis, or tumor. It may become chronic if the underlying cause cannot be corrected (Brandt & Daroff, 1980; Leigh & Zee, 1983).

Peripheral Vestibular Nystagmus

Lesions of the labyrinth or eighth cranial nerve cause a horizontal and rotatory jerk nystagmus on lateral gaze, with the fast phase on the side opposite the lesion. Vertigo may be marked, and tinnitus and deafness occur in concert. Peripheral vestibular nystagmus can be intermittent and can last minutes, days, or weeks. Visual fixation can decrease the intensity of the nystagmus and vertigo. Central pathways eventually compensate, even if the underlying cause remains. Common etiologies include Meniere's disease, infectious and vascular disorders, and trauma (Recker, 1980; Zee et al, 1982).

Cortical Visual Impairment

Nystagmus does not usually occur in patients with cortical blindness, because visual input to the brain is retained via the extrageniculostriate visual system (Perenin et al, 1980). In the absence of this, nystagmus will develop.

Acquired Fixation Nystagmus

Posterior fossa disease may bring about a jerk or pendular, horizontal or vertical nystagmus, and oscillopsia on attempted fixation. Fixation nystagmus is usually associated with demyelinating disease of the brainstem (Walsh & Hoyt, 1969). Rarely, it can occur congenitally, in association with an afferent or efferent visual pathway disorder. It diminishes when fixation is abolished.

SUMMARY

Nystagmus is a nonspecific sign that may occur physiologically or pathologically. The approach to diagnosing and managing infants presenting with nystagmus, as outlined, includes obtaining a family, perinatal, and nystagmus history; performing an ophthalmologic examination; and when appropriate, obtaining electrophysiological and neuroradiological studies.

If an ocular abnormality severe enough to impair visual function is present, the management is as per the disorder. In the absence of obvious ocular malformation, the workup is governed by the nature of the predominant ocular oscillation. If the nystagmus is asymmetric, rapid, and pendular, CT or MRI may be indicated to rule out an intracranial process. If a CNS

disorder is not present, the presumptive diagnosis of asymmetric, rapid nystagmus is spasmus nutans. Searching nystagmus in an infant usually implies a severe retinal or optic nerve disorder. These infants should undergo ERG testing to rule out LCA, and their optic nerves should be carefully inspected. If their nerves appear pale or other CNS signs are present, neurological examination and neuroradiological imaging are performed. If the nystagmus is symmetric and pendular, a careful search is made for foveal hypoplasia and iris transillumination, which suggest albinism. In the absence of these, electrophysiological studies and careful ophthalmoscopy may detect an isolated cone or macular abnormality. Congenital motor (efferent) nystagmus is essentially a diagnosis of exclusion with a relatively good visual prognosis.

REFERENCES

Achromatopsia

Berson, EL, Sandberg MA, Rosner B, Sullivan PL: Color plates to help identify patients with blue cone monochromatism. Am J Ophthalmol 95:741, 1983.

Fleischman JA, O'Donnell FE: Congenital X-linked incomplete achromatopsia. Arch Ophthalmol 99:468, 1981.

Glickstein M, Heath GG: Receptors in the monochromat eye. Vis Res 15:633, 1975.

Sloan LL: Congenital achromatopsia: A report of 19 cases. J Opt Soc Am 44:117, 1954.

Verriest G: Les défiencies de la vision des couleurs. Bull Soc Ophthalmol Fr 69:901, 1969.

Yee RD, Baloh RW, Honrubia V: Eye movement abnormalities in rod monochromacy. Ophthalmology 88:1010, 1981.

Yee RD, Farley MK, Bateman JB, Martin DA: Eye movement abnormalities in rod monochromatism and blue cone monochromatism. Graefes Arch Clin Exp Ophthalmol 223:55, 1985.

Albinism

Abo T, Roder J, Abo W, et al: Natural Killer (HNK-1+) cells in Chediak–Higashi patients are presented in normal numbers but are abnormal in function and morphology. J Clin Invest 70:193, 1982.

Blume RS, Wolff SW: The Chediak–Higashi syndrome: studies in four patients and a review of the literature. Medicine 51:247, 1972.

Brahmi Z: Nature of the natural killer cell hyporesponsiveness in the Chediak–Higashi syndrome. Hum Immunol 6:81, 1983.

Davies BH, Tuddenham EGD: Familial pulmonary fibrosis associated with oculocutaneous albinism and platelet function defect. A new syndrome. Q J Med 45:219, 1976.

Eady RAJ, Gunner DB, Garner A, Rodeek CH: Prenatal diagnosis of oculocutaneous albinism by electron microscopy of fetal skin. J Invest Dermatol 80:210, 1983.

Fonda G, Thomas H, Gore GV: Educational and vocational

placement and low vision corrections in albinism. Sight Sav Rev 41:29, 1971.

Hermansky R, Pudlak P: Albinism associated with hemorrhagic diathesis and unusual pigmented reticular cells in the bone marrow. Blood 14:162, 1959.

Keeler CE: Albinism, xeroderma pigmentosa and skin cancer. Natl Cancer Inst Monogr 10:349, 1963.

King RA: Autosomal dominant oculocutaneous albinism with a mild phenotype. Am J Hum Genet 31:75, 1979.

Kinnear PE, Jay B, Witkop CJ: Albinism. Surv Ophthalmol 30:75, 1985.

Kugelman TP, VanScott EJ: Tyrosinase activity in melanocytes of human albinos. J Invest Dermatol 37:73, 1961.

O'Donnell FE, Green WR: The eye in albinism. In Duane TD, Jaeger EA (eds): Clinical Ophthalmology. Philadelphia, Harper & Row, 1988.

O'Donnell FE, Hambrick GW, Green WR, et al: X-linked ocular albinism. Arch Ophthalmol 94:1883, 1976.

O'Donnell FE, King RA, Green WR, Witkop CJ: Autosomally recessively inherited ocular albinism. Arch Ophthalmol 96:1621, 1978.

Padgett GA, Reiquam CW, Henson JB, et al: Comparative studies of susceptibility to infection in the Chediak–Higashi syndrome. J Pathol Bacteriol 95:509, 1968.

Schinella RA, Greco MA, Barton LC, et al: Hermansky–Pudlak syndrome with granulomatous colitis. Ann Intern Med 92:20, 1983.

Witkop CJ: Inherited disorders of pigmentation, Clin Dermatol 4:70, 1985.

Witkop CJ: Epidemiology of skin cancer in man: Genetic factors. In Laerum OD, Iverson OH (eds): Biology of Skin Cancer. VICC Technical Report Series, vol. 63. Geneva, International Union Against Cancer, 1981, pp 67–72.

Witkop CJ, Hill CW, Desnick S, et al: Ophthalmologic, biochemical, platelet, and ultrastructural defects in the various types of oculocutaneous albinism. J Invest Dermatol 60:433, 1973.

Witkop CJ, Nance WE, Rawls RF, White JG: Autosomal recessive oculocutaneous albinism in man: Evidence for genetic heterogeneity. Am J Hum Genet 22:55, 1970.

Yegin O, Sanal O, Yeralan O, et al: Defective lymphocyte locomotion in Chediak–Higashi syndrome. Am J Dis Child 137:771, 1983.

Congenital Motor Nystagmus

Cogan DG: Congenital nystagmus. Can J Ophthalmol 2:4, 1967.

Dell'Osso LF, Daroff RB: Congenital nystagmus waveforms and foveation strategy. Doc Ophthalmol 39:155, 1975.

Gelbart SS, Hoyt CS: Congenital nystagmus; a clinical perspective in infancy. Graefes Arch Clin Exp Ophthalmol 226:178, 1988.

Halmazzi GM, Giesty MA, Leech J: Reversed optokinetic nystagmus (OKN): Mechanisms and clinical significance. Arch Neurol 7:429, 1980a.

Leigh RJ, Zee DS: The neurology of eye movements. Philadelphia, Davis, 1983, p 225.

Yee RD, Wong EK, Baloh RW, Honrubia V: A study of congenital nystagmus: Waveforms. Neurology 26:326, 1976.

Congenital Stationary Night Blindness

Barricks MF, Flynn JT, Kushner BJ: Paradoxical pupillary responses in congenital stationary night blindness. Arch Ophthalmol 95:1800, 1977.

Carr RE: Congenital stationary night blindness. Trans Am Ophthalmol Soc 72:448, 1974.

Carr RE, Ripps, H: Rhodopsin kinetics and rod adaptation in Oguchi's disease. Invest Ophthalmol 5:508, 1966.

Carr RE, Ripps H, Siegel IM, Weale RA: Rhodopsin and the electrical activity of the retina in congenital night blindness. Invest Ophthalmol 5:497, 1966.

Carroll FD, Haig C: Congenital stationary night blindness without ophthalmoscope or other abnormalities. Arch Ophthalmol 50:35, 1953.

Hittner HM, Borda RP, Justice J: X-linked recessive congenital stationary night blindness, myopia, and tilted discs. J Pediatr Ophthalmol Strabismus 18:15, 1981.

Klien BA: A case of so-called Oguchi's disease in the U.S.A. Am J Ophthalmol 22:953, 1939.

Krill AE, Martin D: Photopic abnormalities in congenital stationary night blindness. Invest Ophthalmol 10:625, 1971.

Nettleship E: A pedigree of congenital night blindness with myopia. Trans Ophthalmol Soc UK 32:21, 1912.

Nettleship E: A new pedigree of hereditary night blindness. Ophthalmol Rev 30:377, 1911.

Nettleship E: A history of congenital stationary night blindness in nine consecutive generations. Trans Ophthalmol Soc UK 27:269, 1910.

Ten Doesschate J, Alpern M, Lee GB, Heyner F: Some visual characteristics of Oguchi's disease. Doc Ophthalmol 20:406, 1966.

Wilder H: Oguchi's disease. Am J Ophthalmol 36:718, 1953.

Leber's Congenital Amaurosis

Carr RE: Electrodiagnostic tests of the retina and higher centers. In Harley RD (ed): Pediatric Ophthalmology, ed 2. Philadelphia, Saunders, 1983, pp 189–206.

Flanders M, Lapointe ML, Brownstein S, Little JM: Keratoconus and Leber's congenital amaurosis: A clinicopathologic correlation. Can J Ophthalmol 19:310, 1984.

Flynn JT, Cullen RF: Disc oedema in congenital amaurosis of Leber. Br J Ophthalmol 59:497, 1975.

Foxman SG, Heckenlively JR, Bateemant JB, Wirtschafter JD: Classification of congenital and early onset retinitis pigmentosa. Arch Ophthalmol 103:1052, 1985.

Francois J: Leber's congenital tapetoretinal degeneration. Int Ophthalmol Clin 8:929, 1968.

Hoyt CS: The apparently blind infant. Trans New Orleans Acad Ophthalmol New York: Raven, 1986, pp 478–488.

Krill AE: Hereditary Retinal and Choroidal Diseases, vol 2. Clinical Characteristics. Hagerstown, MD, Harper & Row. 1977, pp 359–369, 391–420, 1044–1108.

Lambert SR, Taylor D, Kriss A: The infant with nystagmus, normal appearing fundi, but an abnormal ERG. Surv Ophthalmol 34:173, 1989.

Margolis S, Scher BM, Carr RE: Macular colobomas in Leber's congenital amaurosis. Am J Ophthalmol 83:27, 1977.

Noble KG, Carr RE: Leber's congenital amaurosis. Arch Ophthalmol 96:818, 1978.

Roizenblatt J, Cunha LAP: Leber's congenital amaurosis with associated nephronophthisis. J Pediatr Ophthalmol Strabismus 17:154, 1980.

Sears ML, Peterson WS, Carr RE, Jampol LM: Leber's congenital amaurosis. Am J Ophthalmol 83:32, 1977.

Wagner RS, Caputo AR, Nelson LB, Zanoni D: High hyperopia in Leber's congenital amaurosis. Arch Ophthalmol 103:1507, 1985.

Nystagmus Associated With Strabismus

Dell'Osso LF, Daroff RB, Troost BT: Nystagmus and saccadic intrusions and oscillations. In Duane TD, Jaeger EA (eds): Clinical Ophthalmology. Philadelphia, Harper & Row, 1988.

Dell'Osso LF, Ellenberger C, Abel LA, Flynn JT: The nystagmus blockage syndrome. Invest Ophthalmol Vis Sci 24:1580, 1983a.

Dell'Osso LF, Schmidt D, Daroff RB: Latent, manifest latent and congenital nystagmus. Arch Ophthalmol 97:1877, 1979.

Dell'Osso LF, Traocis S, Abel LA: Strabismus: A necessary condition of latent and manifest latent nystagmus. Neuroophthalmology 3:247, 1983b.

Von Noorden GK, Wong SY: Surgical results in nystagmus blockage syndrome. Ophthalmology 93:1028, 1986.

Optic Nerve Hypoplasia

Acers TE: Optic nerve hypoplasia. Trans Am Ophthalmol Soc 79:425, 1981.

DeMorsier G: Études, sur les dysraphies cranioencéphaliques; agenesie du septum lucidum avec malformation du tractus optique. La dysplasia septo-optique. Schweiz Arch Neurol Psychiatr 77:267, 1956.

Edwards WC, Layden WE: Optic nerve hypoplasia. Am J Ophthalmol 70:950, 1970.

Frisen L, Holmegaard L: Spectrum of optic nerve hypoplasia. Br J Ophthalmol 62:7, 1978.

Hackenbruch Y, Meerhoff E, Besio R, Cardoso H: Familial bilateral optic nerve hypoplasia. Am J Ophthalmol 79:314, 1975.

Hotchkiss ML, Green WR: Optic nerve aplasia and hypoplasia. J Pediatr Ophthalmol Strabismus 16:225, 1979.

Hoty CS, Billson FA: Maternal anticonvulsants and optic nerve hypoplasia. Br J Ophthalmol 62:3, 1978.

Hoyt WF, Kaplan SL, Grumbach MM, Glaser JS: Septo-optic dysplasia and pituitary dwarfism. Lancet 2:893, 1970.

Lloyd L, Buncic JR: Hypoplasia of the optic nerve and disc. In Smith JL (ed): Neuroophthalmology Focus 1980. New York, Masson, 1980, pp 85–96.

Margalith D, Jan JE, McCormick AQ, et al: Clinical spectrum of congenital optic nerve hypoplasia: review of 51 patients. Dev Med Child Neurol 26:311, 1984.

McKinna AJ: Quinine-induced hypoplasia of the optic nerve. Can J Ophthalmol 1:261, 1966.

Peterson RA, Walton DS: Optic nerve hypoplasia with good visual acuity and visual field defects. Arch Ophthalmol 95:254, 1977.

Skarf B, Hoyt CS: Optic nerve hypoplasia in children. Arch Ophthalmol 102:62, 1984.

Stromland K: Ocular involvement in the fetal alcohol syndrome. Surv Ophthalmol 31:277, 1987.

Walton DS, Robb RM: Optic nerve hypoplasia, a report of twenty cases. Arch Ophthalmol 84:572, 1970.

Weiter JJ, McLean IW, Zimmerman LE: Aplasia of the optic nerve and disc. Am J Ophthalmol 83:569, 1977.

Pathological Nystagmus

Baloh RW, Honrubia V, Konrad HR: Periodic alternating nystagmus. Brain 99:11, 1976.

Burde RM, Henkind P: Downbeat nystagmus. Surv Ophthalmol 25:263, 1981.

Cogan DG: Neurology of the Ocular Muscles, ed 4. Springfield, IL: Thomas, 1969, pp 154, 191–193, 219–225.

Cogan DG: Downbeat nystagmus. Arch Ophthalmol 80:757, 1968.

Costlin JA, Smith JL, Emery S, et al: Alcoholic downbeat nystagmus. Ann Ophthalmol 12:1127, 1980.

Daroff RB: Upbeat nystagmus (letter to the editor). JAMA 225:312, 1973.

Daroff RB: See-saw nystagmus. Neurology 15:874, 1965.

Davis DG, Smith JL: Periodic alternating nystagmus. Am J Ophthalmol 72:757, 1971.

Donin JF: Acquired monocular nystagmus in children. Can J Ophthalmol 2:212, 1967.

Duke-Elder S, Scott GI: Neuroophthalmology. In Duke-Elder S (ed): System of Ophthalmology. St. Louis, Mosby, 1971, vol 12, pp 876–886.

Farmer J, Hoyt CS: Monocular nystagmus in infancy and early childhood. Am J Ophthalmol 98:504, 1984.

Fein JM, Williams RDB: See-saw nystagmus. J Neurol Neurosurg Psychiatry 32:202, 1969.

Fischer A, Gresty M, Chambers B, et al: Primary position upbeating nystagmus: A variety of central positional nystagmus. Brain 106:949, 1983.

Gilman N, Baloh RW, Tomiyasu U: Primary position upbeat nystagmus. Neurology 27:294, 1977.

Halmazzi GM, Rudge P, Giesty MA, et al: Downbeating nystagmus: A review of 62 cases. Arch Neurol 40:777, 1983.

Halmazzi GM, Rudge P, Giesty MA, et al: Treatment of periodic alternating nystagmus. Ann Neurol 6:609, 1980b.

Holmes GL, Hafford J, Zimmerman AW: Primary position upbeat nystagmus following meningitis. Ann Ophthalmol 13:935, 1981.

Huber A: Eye Symptoms in Brain Tumors, ed 2. St. Louis, Mosby, 1971, p 48.

Jan JE, Farrell K, Wong PK, McCormick AQ: Eye and head movements of visually impaired children. Dev Med Child Neurol 28:285, 1986.

Keane JR: Periodic alternating nystagmus with downward beating nystagmus. Arch Neurol 30:399, 1974.

Kischer A, Gresty M, Chambers B, et al: Primary position upbeating nystagmus: A variety of central positional nystagmus. Brain 106:949, 1983.

Leigh RJ, Robinson DA, Zee DS: A hypothetical explanation for periodic alternating nystagmus: Instability in the optokinetic-vestibular system. Ann NY Acad Sci 374:619, 1981.

Marquis DG: Effects of removal of visual cortex in mammals with observations on the retention of light discrimination in dogs. Proc Assoc Res Neur Ment Dis 13:558, 1934.

Pederson RA, Troost BT, Abel LA, et al: Intermittent downbeat nystagmus and oscillopsia reversed by suboccipital craniectomy. Neurology 30:1239, 1980.

Perenin MT, Ruel J, Hecaen H: Residual visual capacities in a case of cortical blindness. Cortex 16:605, 1980.

Shaw HE, Smith JL: Downbeat nystagmus: A clinical update. In Smith JL (ed): Neuroophthalmology Focus 1980. New York, Masson, 1980, p 433.

Smith JL, Zieper I, Gay AJ, Cogan DG: Nystagmus retractorius. Arch Ophthalmol 62: 864, 1959.

Walsh FB, Hoyt WF: Clinical Neuro-ophthalmology, ed 3. Baltimore, Williams & Wilkins, 1969, pp 270–289, 524.

Yanoff M, Rorke LB, Allman MI: Bilateral optic system aplasia with relatively normal eyes. Arch Ophthalmol 96:97, 1978.

Yee RD, Baloh RW, Honrubia V: Episodic vertical oscillopsia and downbeat nystagmus in a Chiari malformation. Arch Ophthalmol 102:723, 1984.

Yee RD, Jelks GW, Baloh RW, Honrubia V: Uniocular nystagmus in monocular visual loss. Ophthalmology 86:54, 1979.

Zee DS, Friendlich AR, Robinson DA: The mechanism of downbeat nystagmus. Arch Neurol 30:277, 1974.

Zee DS, Yee RD, Cogan DG, et al: Ocular motor abnormalities in hereditary cerebellar ataxia. Brain 99:207, 1976.

Physiological Nystagmus

Abel LA, Dell'Osso LR, Daroff RB: Analog model for gaze evoked nystagmus. IEEE Trans Biomed Eng 25:71, 1978a.

Abel LA, Parker L, Daroff RB, et al: End-point nystagmus. Invest Ophthalmol Vis Sci 17:539, 1978b.

Aschoff JC, Becker W, Rettelbach R: Voluntary nystagmus in five generations. J Neurol Neurosurg Psychiatry 39:300, 1976.

Nagle M, Bridgeman B, Stark L: Voluntary nystagmus, saccadic suppression and stabilization of the visual world. Vision Res 20:717, 1980.

Smith JL: Optokinetic Nystagmus. Springfield, IL, Thomas, 1963, pp 115–118.

Retinal Abnormalities

Balian JV, Falls HF: Congenital vascular veils in the vitreous. Arch Ophthalmol 63:92, 1960.

François J: Incontinentia Pigmenti and retinal changes. Br J Ophthalmol 68:19, 1984.

Manschot WA: Pathology of hereditary juvenile retinoschisis. Arch Ophthalmol 88:131, 1972.

Moore AT, Taylor DS, Harden A: Bilateral macular dysplasia ("colobomata") and congenital retinal dystrophy. Br J Ophthalmol 69:691, 1985.

Phillips CI, Stokoe NL, Newton M: Macular coloboma and retinal aplasia. Acta Ophthalmol 59:894, 1981.

Review Articles

Buckley EG: The clinical approach to the pediatric patient with nystagmus. Int Pediatr 5:225, 1990.

Calhoun JH: Cataracts and lens anomalies in children. In Nelson LB, Calhoun JH, Harley RD (eds): Pediatric Ophthalmology, 3rd ed. Philadelphia: Saunders 1991, pp 234–257.

Catalano RA: Nystagmus. In Nelson LB, Calhoun JH, Harley RD: Pediatric Ophthalmology, ed 3. Philadelphia, Saunders, 1991, pp 489–503.

Catalano RA, Calhoun JH: Ocular conditions associated with nystagmus. In Reinecke RD (ed): Ophthalmology Annual 1988. New York, Raven, 1988, pp 89–113.

DeLuise VP, Anderson DR: Primary infantile glaucoma (congenital glaucoma). Surv Ophthalmol 28:1, 1983.

Ellsworth RM: Retinoblastoma. In Duane TD, Jaeger EA (eds): Clinical Ophthalmology. Philadelphia, Harper & Row, 1988.

Flynn JT: An international classification of retinopathy of prematurity. Ophthalmology 97:987, 1985.

François J, Verchraegen-Spae MR, DeSutter E: The aniridia–Wilms' tumor syndrome and other associations of aniridia. Ophthalmol Peadiatr Genet 1:125, 1982.

Haddad R, Font RL, Reiser F: Persistent hyperplastic primary vitreous. Surv Ophthalmol 23:123, 1978.

McKusick VA: Mendelian Inheritance in Man, ed 2. Baltimore, Johns Hopkins, 1968.

Nelson LB, Spaeth GL, Nowinski TS, et al: Aniridia. A review. Surv Ophthalmol 28:621, 1984.

Pagon RA: Ocular coloboma. Surv Ophthalmol 25:223, 1981.

Perkins ES: Ocular toxoplasmosis. Br J Ophthalmol 57:1. 1973.

Schlaegel TR: Toxoplasmosis. In Duane TD, Jaeger EA (eds): Clinical Ophthalmology. Philadelphia, Harper & Row, 1988.

Stern JH, Catalano RA: Current status of diagnostic and therapeutic measures in infantile glaucoma. Sem Ophthalmol 5:166, 1990.

Tingley DH, Flynn JT: Perspectives on retinopathy of prematurity. Int Pediatr 5:232, 1990.

Townsend WM: Congenital corneal leukomas. Am J Ophthalmol 77:80, 1974.

Spasmus Nutans

Albright AL, Schlabassi RJ, Slamovitis TL, Bergman I: Spasmus nutans associated with optic gliomas in infants. J Pediatr 105:778, 1984.

Jayalakshmi P, Scott TF, Tucker SH, Schaffer DB: Infantile nystagmus: A prospective study of spasmus nutans, congenital nystagmus, and unclassified nystagmus of infancy. J Pediatr 77:177, 1970.

Lavery MA, O'Neill JF, Chu FC, Martyn L: Acquired nystagmus in early childhood: A presenting sign of intracranial tumor. Ophthalmology 91:425, 1984.

Sedwick LA, Burde RM, Hodges FJ: Leigh's subacute encephalomyelopathy manifesting as spasmus nutans. Arch Ophthalmol 102:1046, 1984.

Weissman BM, Dell'Osso LF, Abel LA, Leigh RJ: Spasmus nutans: Quantitative prospective study. In Keller EL, Zee DS (eds): Adaptive Process in Visual and Oculomotor Systems. New York, Pergamon, 1986. pp 479–483.

Vestibular Nystagmus

Baloh RW: Dizziness, Hearing Loss and Tinnitus: The Essentials of Neurology. Philadelphia, Davis, 1984.

Baloh RW, Honrubia V: Clinical Neurophysiology of the Vestibular System. Contemporary Neurology Series. Philadelphia, Davis, 1979.

Baloh RW, Sills AW, Honrubia V, et al: Caloric testing. Ann Otol Rhinol Laryngol 86(suppl 43):1, 1987.

Brandt T, Daroff RB: The multisensory physiological and pathological vertigo syndrome. Ann Neurol 7:195, 1980.

Paige GD: Caloric vestibular responses despite canal inactivation. Invest Ophthalmol Vis Sci 25:229, 1984.

Recker U: Peripheral–vestibular spontaneous nystagmus: Analysis of reproducibility and methodologies. Arch Otorhinolaryngol 336:225, 1980.

Zee DS, Preziosi TJ, Proctor LR: Bechterew's phenomenon in a human patient. Ann Neurol 12:495, 1982.

DISORDERS OF THE EYELIDS, LACRIMAL DRAINAGE SYSTEM, AND ORBIT

ESSENTIAL INFORMATION FOR PRIMARY CARE PRACTITIONERS

Eyelid Disorders

Capillary Hemangioma of the Eyelid

The most common vascular lesion of childhood is a capillary hemangioma. These benign tumors are composed of proliferating endothelial cells with anastomosing blood-filled channels. Occurring in 1 to 2 percent of newborns, they are usually first noted between birth and age 6 weeks. They grow rapidly during the first 6 months of life and may double in size in days to weeks. The surfaces of superficial lesions are elevated, red, and irregularly dimpled; hence the name **strawberry nevus** (Figs. 8–1 and 8–2). Unlike port wine stains, hemangiomas are spongy, blanch with pressure, and increase in size when the child cries. Deeper tumors can be bluish. One fourth of affected children have additional hemangiomas on the scalp, neck, face, or shoulders.

Resolution usually begins in the second year of life and is complete in 60 percent of cases by 4 years of age, and in 76 percent of cases by 7 years of age (Margileth & Museles, 1965). Small eyelid tumors can, however, induce astigmatism and anisometropic amblyopia. Large tumors can cause occlusion amblyopia and/or

strabismus. Amblyopia from an induced astigmatism requires glasses and patching therapy. Intralesional steroids may also be necessary. This involves injecting the tumor mass at several different sites with up to 40 mg of triamcinolone (prolonged acting) and 6 mg of an equal mixture of betamethasone sodium phosphate and betamethasone acetate (rapidly acting), using a 27-gauge needle. Because epinephrine can potentially enhance the action of the steroid, lidocaine hydrochloride 1 percent with 1:1,000,000 epinephrine is often

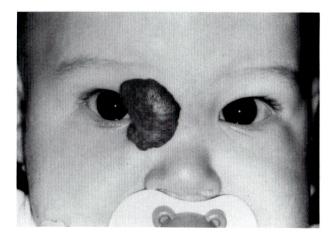

Figure 8–1. Capillary hemangioma involving only the skin.

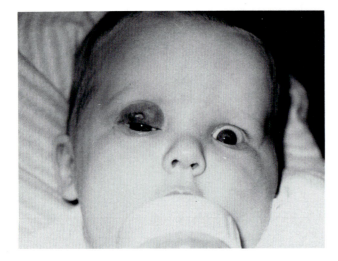

Figure 8–2. Capillary hemangioma involving the skin and subcutaneous tissue.

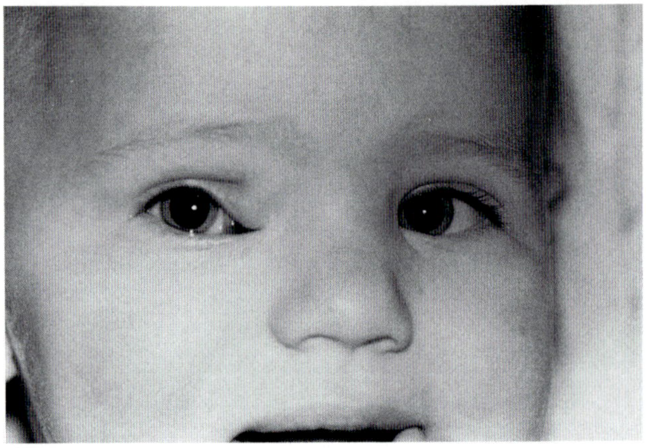

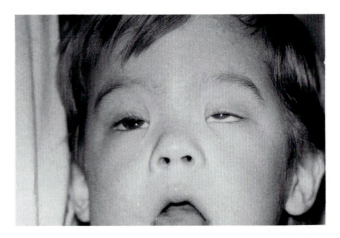

Figure 8–4. Redundant skin following spontaneous resolution of a capillary hemangioma involving the medial upper eyelid.

used as the dilutant for the steroid. If a response occurs, it will be noted within the first 2 weeks; regression can continue up to 5 weeks after injection. If a second injection is necessary, it can be performed 6 to 8 weeks after the first.

Complications of steroid injections into the eyelid include subcutaneous atrophy, eyelid necrosis, and skin depigmentation (Fig. 8–3). Complications of deep orbital injections include retrobulbar hemorrhage and central retinal artery occlusion from embolization of the steroid. Immunizations with live viruses should be withheld 1 week prior to or after a steroid injection.

Other treatment modalities include radiotherapy and systemic corticosteroids. Generally, these are reserved for tumors that are located far posterior in the orbit. Recently, hormone therapy directed at blocking estrogen receptors has been advocated in selected cases

(Carruthers et al, 1991). In addition to amblyopia and strabismus, another sequela is redundant skin. This is particularly likely if the medial upper eyelid and canthal angle are involved (Fig. 8–4); cosmetic plastic surgery may be required.

Epicanthus

Epicanthus is a common benign eyelid anomaly in infants and young children. It consists of a semilunar fold of skin that runs from the upper to the lower eyelid, covering the medial canthal angle. Epicanthus occurs most commonly as an isolated finding with an autosomal dominant transmission. Prominent epicanthal folds also are present in as many as 60 percent of children with Down syndrome. The epicanthal fold in Down syndrome, however, may differ from "true" epicanthus. In Down syndrome the epicanthal fold re-

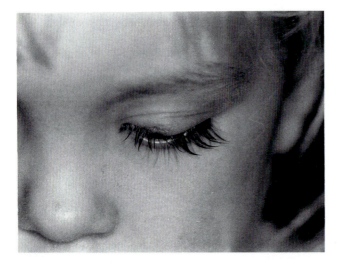

Figure 8–3. Subcutaneous atrophy following a steroid injection into a capillary hemangioma.

Figure 8–5. Epicanthus in Down syndrome. Note how it begins at the upper margin of the nasal tarsal fold, and ends below the inner canthus.

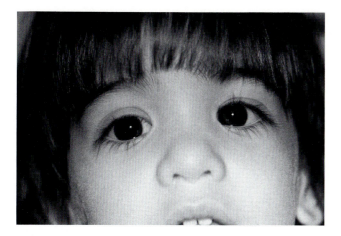

Figure 8–6. "True" epicanthus is more sharply curved and attaches to the lower eyelid.

sembles the fetal fold, extending from the nasal margin of the upper tarsal fold to the skin below the inner canthus (Fig. 8–5). True epicanthus is more sharply curved and attaches to the lower eyelid (Fig. 8–6).

The epicanthus of both Down syndrome and true epicanthus become less noticeable as the bridge of the nose grows forward. Surgery is, therefore, rarely necessary. The most striking appearance in many children is not the skin fold, but that of pseudostrabismus (the impression that the eyes are crossed). This results from less sclera being visible nasally than temporally; it too resolves as the child grows.

Congenital Ptosis

Congenital ptosis (an inability to elevate the upper eyelid) is the most common anomaly of the eyelid function. Most authorities reserve this term for developmental dystrophies of the levator muscle or its tendon. Ptosis resulting from an innervational, myogenic, or mechanical cause is usually considered "acquired" rather than congenital (Table 8–1). Two rare syndromes in which ptosis is a major component are

blepharophimosis and Marcus Gunn jaw-winking (described later in the chapter).

Congenital ptosis can be unilateral or bilateral. Most cases are not familial, although occasionally an autosomal dominant pedigree with a high penetrance is encountered. The severity of congenital ptosis varies widely. The deformity can be minimal and remain almost unnoticeable (Fig. 8–7), or the drooping upper eyelid can occlude the visual axis. In the latter cases, vision may be possible only by tilting the head backward (Fig. 8–8), or raising the eyelid with a finger (see Fig. 8–63). In marked cases, patients also wrinkle their forehead and contract their frontalis muscle in an effort to pull the eyelid upward.

Ptosis can be quantitated using several methods. The palpebral fissure can be measured with a millimeter ruler, and the level at which the eyelid crosses the cornea can be noted. In the normal resting state, the palpebral fissure is 9 to 10 mm wide, and the upper eyelid margin is 1 to 2 mm below the superior limbus. The distance between a reflected corneal light reflex and the upper eyelid margin can also be measured. This is normally about 4 mm. The excursion of the upper eyelid as the eye moves from downward to upward gaze gives an estimation of levator function. To accurately measure excursion the brow should be fixated by applying pressure just below the eyebrows. This prevents any contribution to eyelid elevation from frontalis contraction. The normal eyelid excursion is 15 mm; an excursion of 8 to 14 mm is considered good function; an excursion of 4 mm or less is considered poor levator function. Surgical correction via a levator approach is usually attempted when excursion is good; frontalis muscle suspension is indicated with poor function.

The function of the superior rectus muscle should also be evaluated. Some patients with ptosis have concomitant weakness of this muscle. Additionally, patients with a superior rectus muscle palsy can have a lower eye (hypotropia) and pseudoptosis. A strabis-

TABLE 8–1. CLASSIFICATION OF INFANTILE PTOSIS

Category	Abnormality	Entities
Congenital	Developmental dysgenesis of the levator muscle or tendon	Congenital ptosis
Myogenic	Localized or diffuse muscular disease; neuromuscular syndromes	Myasthenia gravis, progressive external ophthalmoplegia
Innervational	Congenital or acquired neurological disorder; aberrant neuronal connections	Third cranial nerve palsy, Horner's syndrome, Marcus Gunn jaw-winking
Aponeurotic	Disinsertion or stretching of the levator aponeurosis	Traumatic ptosis, chronic inflammation
Mechanical	Restricted movement of the upper eyelid	Large tumor (neurofibroma, capillary hemangioma)
Pseudoptosis	Reduced orbital volume due to a small eye or herniation of tissue outside the orbit; strabismus (hypotropia)	Microphthalmos, phthisis bulbi (blind, shrunken eye), orbital floor fracture, superior rectus muscle palsy

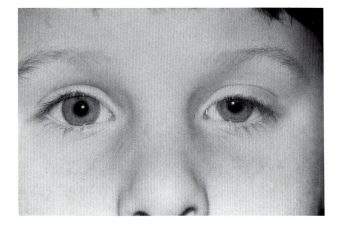

Figure 8–7. Minimal ptosis, left upper eyelid.

mus procedure is more appropriate in the latter instance than ptosis surgery. The surgical procedure chosen will also depend on whether the patient has an intact Bell's phenomenon (upward movement of the eye with eyelid closure) and a normal ability to produce tears. If either are deficient, the surgeon must be careful not to overcorrect the ptosis. A neuromuscular evaluation should also be performed. Corneal sensitivity should be documented by noting eyelid closure upon touching the cornea with a wisp of cotton. An infant with ptosis, orbicularis weakness, limited eye movements, poor feeding, and hypotonia should be evaluated for myasthenia gravis. If symptoms improve following an intramuscular or subcutaneous injection of 0.1 mg of edrophonium chloride (Tensilon test), the diagnosis is confirmed. Older children with juvenile myasthenia may also have prominent and life-threatening bulbar symptoms of dysphagia, shortness of breath, and nocturnal regurgitation of secretions. Finally, a finding of elevation of the ptotic eyelid with

yawning or mouth movement suggests Marcus Gunn jaw-winking (described later in the chapter).

Nonsurgical, temporizing measures include eyelid crutches attached to eyeglass frames and taping of the upper eyelids (Fig. 8–9). Although the surgical correction of ptosis is beyond the scope of this chapter, the surgeon should be aware that there is a five times greater incidence of congenital heart disease in infants with ptosis (Larned et al, 1986). Additionally, infants with ptosis have a higher risk of developing malignant hyperthermia under anesthesia. Parents should be told preoperatively that the goal of surgery is to improve the child's appearance while looking straight ahead. Lid lag on downward gaze (Fig. 8–10), or lagophthalmos (inability of the eyes to close entirely) (Fig. 8–11), can occur following surgery. Ocular lubricants may be needed during the immediate postoperative period, especially if the child does not close the eyes during sleep. This usually improves, however, with time. Parents should also be told that the eyelid may slowly come down again, and further surgery may be needed in the future.

Many authorities believe that surgery is best performed after 3 years of age, because by this age the eyelid tissue is sufficient to perform a levator resection if necessary. If there is potential for visual loss (for example, obstruction of the visual axis), or if the infant must maintain a chin elevation in order to see, surgery will be necessary at a young age.

Children with congenital ptosis should also be followed for the development of amblyopia. Amblyopia from occlusion of the visual axis by the droopy eyelid is rare. The ptotic eyelid can, however, induce an astigmatism, which if left uncorrected can result in anisometropic amblyopia. At each visit, the vision in an eye with a ptotic eyelid should be carefully evaluated, and the refraction of the eye should be followed regularly.

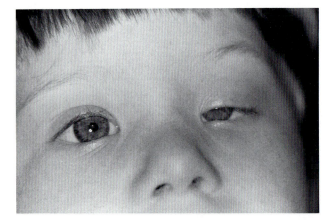

Figure 8–8. Marked ptosis, left upper eyelid. This child maintains a chin-up head position to see out of this eye.

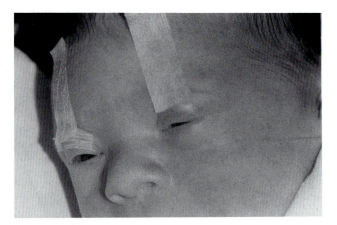

Figure 8–9. Taping the upper eyelid open, a temporizing measure for a child with marked bilateral ptosis.

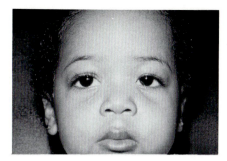

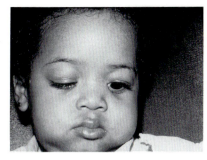

Figure 8–10. A. Excellent cosmetic appearance following ptosis surgery, left upper eyelid. **B.** Lid lag on downward gaze, same eye.

A   B

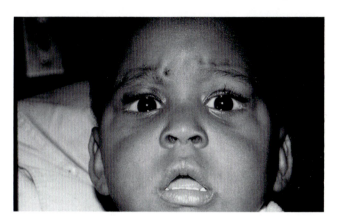

Figure 8–11. Lagophthalmos, or the inability to close the eyes, a temporary condition following ptosis surgery.

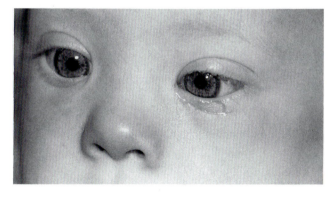

Figure 8–12. CNLDO due to an obstruction high in the lacrimal drainage system. Note the excessive tearing but absent discharge or conjunctival injection.

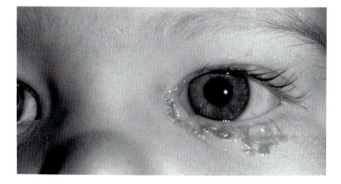

Figure 8–13. CNLDO due to an obstruction low in the lacrimal drainage system. Note the matted discharge on the eyelids.

Lacrimal Drainage System Disorders

Nasolacrimal Duct Obstruction

Congenital nasolacrimal duct obstruction (CNLDO), or dacryostenosis, is the most common disorder of the lacrimal system, occurring in up to 5 percent of newborn infants. (See also Chapter 14.)

The clinical presentation of CNLDO is somewhat variable. If the obstruction is at a higher level of the lacrimal drainage system (for example, in the punctum or canaliculi), the infant will tear, but is unlikely to have thick discharge or secondary infection (Fig. 8–12). If the obstruction is lower, mucoid material, produced by the goblet cells lining the lacrimal sac, can reflux from the sac onto the eye and accumulate on the eyelashes (Fig. 8–13).

The diagnosis of CNLDO can be confirmed with the fluorescein dye disappearance test. A drop of 2 percent fluorescein solution is instilled in the conjunctival fornix of each eye, and excess dye is wiped away from the skin of the eyelids. With blue-filtered light from an ophthalmoscope or a penlight, the child is observed from a distance of 3 to 4 feet in a semidarkened room. Normally, virtually all the dye is cleared from the tear lake within 5 minutes. When CNLDO is present, there is still obvious retention of dye after 10 minutes.

Controversy exists regarding the surgical management of CNLDO. Many studies have shown that spontaneous remittance occurs in 80 to 90 percent of affected infants by 9 to 12 months of life. For this reason, many ophthalmologists advocate temporizing measures during the first year of life. Antibiotics are used on an as needed basis, and compression over the lacrimal sac is instituted as often as four times a day. The latter is performed by placing a finger on the medial edge of the eyelid (over the common canaliculus) and firmly stroking down the side of the nose to increase hydrostatic pressure within the lacrimal sac. This maneuver has the potential to rupture a membranous obstruction within the nasolacrimal duct. Although the word "massage" is often used to describe this compression, it is misleading, because "massage" connotes a rubbing action.

Other ophthalmologists advocate early surgical probing of the lacrimal system (Figs. 8–14 to 8–16).

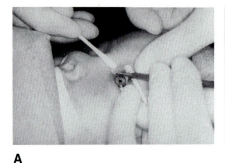

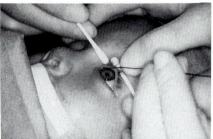

A

B

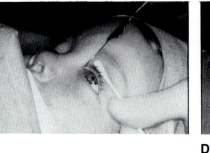

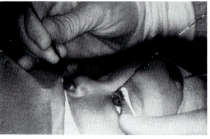

C

D

Figure 8–14. Technique of probing. **A.** The superior puncta is dilated with a punctal dilator. **B.** A Bowman probe is placed through the puncta into the superior canaliculus. **C.** The probe is then directed into the nasolacrimal duct. **D.** The position of the probe in the nose is checked with a second probe.

They note that because young infants require less restraint, probing at a young age can be performed in the office, avoiding the risks of general anesthesia. Proponents of late probing counter that the immobilization of the patient provided by general anesthesia is valuable in the performance of probing, which often relies on subtle tactile discrimination for success.

Proponents of early probing also cite evidence suggesting that the longer the surgery is delayed beyond 2 to 4 months of age, the poorer the prognosis for a successful initial probing in CNLDO. In a retrospective study of 427 patients with CNLDO involving 572 eyes, Nelson and associates (1985) reported success in 97 percent of cases when probing was performed before 13 months of age. Beyond 13 months, however, the success rate was found to decrease with age, to 76.4 percent between 13 and 18 months and 33.3 percent for pa-

tients probed after 24 months. Other studies have noted a cure rate of nearly 90 percent with first-time probing in children ranging in age from 1 to 7 years (El-Mansoury et al, 1986; Robb, 1986).

We believe that conservative management, which includes compression of the lacrimal sac, is appropriate for most infants less than 1 year of age with CNLDO. Antibiotic drops or ointment, up to several times a day, should be used when the discharge is more purulent. In resistant cases, ointment is preferred, as it is less easily washed out of the eye by tears. Early probing is suggested for infants with chronic, copious mucopurulent discharge, resistant to antibiotics. It is also recommended for any child who develops acute infection of the lacrimal sac (dacryocystitis), after treating this infection with systemic antibiotics. Additionally, early probing is recommended for children

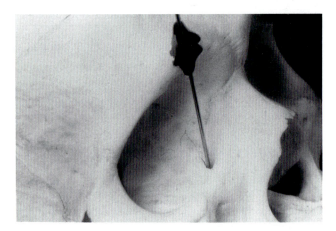

Figure 8–15. Probe passed through the bony nasolacrimal duct of a skull.

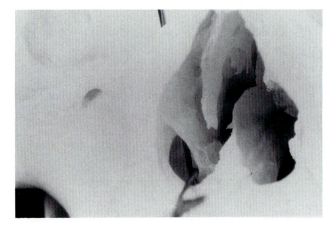

Figure 8–16. Same probe passing under the inferior turbinate into the nose.

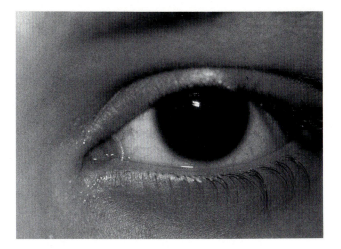

Figure 8–17. Silicone tube intubation, demonstrating the tube arcing between the superior and inferior puncta. The two ends of the tube are tied in the nose.

with lacrimal sac mucoceles, as these are associated with a high rate of infection.

Probings can be repeated one or two times. A subsequent failure should be managed by intubating the nasolacrimal system with a silicone tube (Fig. 8–17). This tube is left in place for 6 to 12 weeks to prevent closure of the nasolacrimal osteum during healing. Individuals with persistent symptoms, or with a bony obstruction not amenable to probing, require a more extensive surgical procedure to bypass the obstruction (dacryocystorhinostomy).

Developmental Anomalies of the Puncta and Canaliculi

Atresia or agenesis of the lacrimal puncta is an uncommon condition in which a thin membrane occludes the punctal opening and prevents entry of tears into a well-developed canalicular system. Either all four puncta or only the puncta of the lower eyelid may be involved. Affected individuals have epiphora, but because the puncta are blocked, they do not have regurgitation of mucopurulent material from the lacrimal sac. The atretic puncta can often be opened with a sharp pin. If the canaliculi are also atretic, a more involved surgical procedure to create an opening from the conjunctiva through the lacrimal sac into the nose (conjunctivodacryocystorhinostomy) will be necessary.

A rare developmental anomaly is the presence of supernumerary puncta and canaliculi. Also known as lacrimal anlage ducts or congenital lacrimal fistulae, these are usually asymptomatic, and do not require treatment.

Orbital Disorders

An orbital disorder should be suspected when a child presents with proptosis (a bulging eye), globe displacement, eyelid swelling, or restriction of ocular motility.

More common orbital disorders are reviewed here; rarer disorders are presented under "Comprehensive Information" later in the chapter.

Rhabdomyosarcoma

Rhabdomyosarcoma is the most common childhood primary malignant tumor of the orbit, and the third commonest tumor of children. It is composed of striated muscle cells in a pattern suggestive of neoplastic analogs of various stages of normal muscle embryogenesis. More than 90 percent of rhabdomyosarcomas present in children under the age of 16 years; the most common age of presentation is 7 to 8 years.

Between 15 and 25 percent of all rhabdomyosarcomas arise in the orbit; most commonly in the superior nasal quadrant. When it arises in this location, it presents with a rapid (days to weeks) downward and outward displacement of the globe (Fig. 8–18). A marked adnexal response with lid edema and discoloration is usually concomitant (Fig. 8–19). Sinus extension results in nasal stuffiness and nosebleeds. A history of antecedent trauma is not unusual, often causing a delay in diagnosis. Occasionally, rhabdomyosarcoma may present as a palpable subconjunctival or eyelid mass without proptosis.

If the mass is in the superior nasal quadrant, it may be palpable. CT scanning will demonstrate bone destruction in advanced cases (Fig. 8–20); ultrasonography findings include a relatively well-circumscribed mass with low to moderate internal reflections. To confirm the diagnosis, a biopsy should be performed. A transconjunctival or eyelid incision is recommended to prevent tumor seeding along the biopsy tract. The periosteum also presents a relative barrier and should not be violated. Spindle-shaped cells with prominent

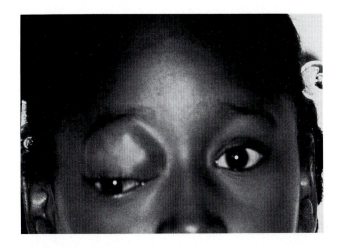

Figure 8–18. Rhabdomyosarcoma originating in the superior nasal quadrant, presenting as rapidly progressive exophthalmos with downward displacement of the globe. *(From Nelson LB, Brown GC, Arentsen JJ: Recognizing patterns of ocular childhood diseases. Thorofare, NJ, Slack, 1985, p 155, with permission.)*

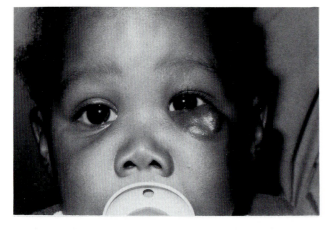

Figure 8–19. Rhabdomyosarcoma originating in the inferior orbit, presenting with upward displacement of the globe, eyelid edema, and discoloration.

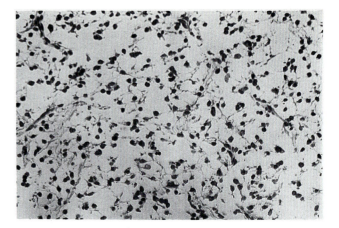

Figure 8–21. Rhabdomyoblasts, with an occasional spindle-shaped cell in poorly differentiated rhabdomyosarcoma. *(Courtesy of Albany Medical College slide collection.)*

cross-striations and "tadpole" cells with tapered cytoplasmic processes are hallmarks of the tumor in tissue biopsies (Fig. 8–21). Because these findings may be present only in more differentiated tumors, electron microscopy may be necessary. This requires glutaraldehyde fixation of fresh biopsy specimens.

Upon diagnosis, complete evaluation requires bone marrow biopsy, complete blood count, liver function tests, bone scanning, chest x-ray, and lumbar puncture to search for distant metastases. Therapy is based on guidelines established by the Intergroup Rhabdomyosarcoma Study. Local radiation of 45 to 60 Gy is given over 6 weeks, combined with systemic chemotherapy (vincristine, adriamycin, and cyclophosphamide). Extraorbital extension decreases 3-year survival from 90 to 30 percent.

Dermoid Cysts

A dermoid cyst is the most frequent, benign, childhood tumor of the orbit. It consists of histologically normal tissues that are not normally present at the involved site.

The typical dermoid cyst presents as a painless, smooth, oval, subcutaneous mass, mobile on palpation, and not attached to the overlying skin. It is most often located in the upper temporal quadrant (Figs. 8–22 and 8–23). Hemorrhage into the cyst or orbital inflammation in response to spontaneous or traumatic release of cyst contents can occasionally occur. Rarely, a fistulous tract between the cyst and the skin or conjunctival surface may produce drainage and signs of infection.

Dermoid cysts usually do not threaten vision, but

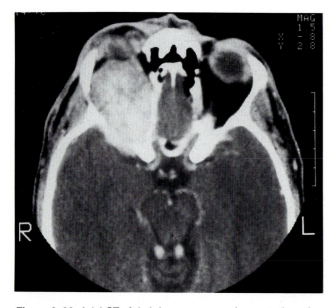

Figure 8–20. Axial CT of rhabdomyosarcoma, demonstrating a homogeneous mass in the superior orbit.

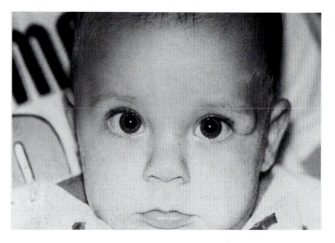

Figure 8–22. Dermoid cyst in the upper temporal quadrant of the left orbit. *(From Catalano RA: Ocular Emergencies. Philadelphia, Saunders, 1992, p 306, with permission.)*

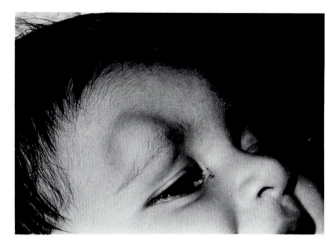

Figure 8–23. Side view of a dermoid cyst. *(Courtesy of Joseph H. Calhoun; from Nelson LB: Pediatric Ophthalmology. Philadelphia, Saunders, 1984, with permission.)*

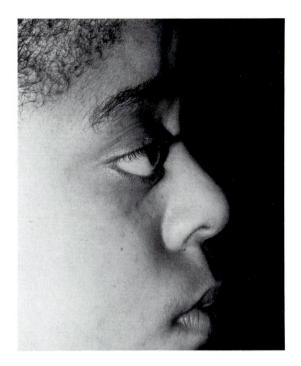

Figure 8–25. Lateral view of proptosis in another child with optic nerve glioma.

cosmetic consideration prompts parents to seek treatment. Because the tumors are relatively easy to dissect, the procedure of choice is surgical removal, usually through an anterior brow incision.

Optic Nerve Glioma

Optic nerve glioma (juvenile pilocytic astrocytoma) is a rare tumor occurring with an incidence of 1 in 176,000 individuals. The tumor usually becomes clinically apparent during the first decade of life; approximately 50 percent of cases are diagnosed prior to age 5 years. Females are slightly more affected than males.

The clinical presentation of glioma depends largely on the location of the tumor and the stage when diagnosed. The classic presentation is a gradual, painless proptosis with loss of vision and an afferent pupillary defect (Figs. 8–24 and 8–25). The visual loss is often slow, insidious, and asymptomatic, which may result

in the child presenting instead with nystagmus or strabismus.

Depending on the stage when diagnosed, disc edema (Fig. 8–26) or optic atrophy may be seen. Anteriorly located tumors can compromise the central retinal veins, manifested by their dilation and tortuosity; a hemorrhagic retinopathy can also occur. Proptosis initially occurs in an axial direction but eventually assumes a downward and outward direction conforming to the contour of the orbit. If the chiasm is involved (50 percent of cases), pituitary dysfunction and signs of increased intracranial pressure can be present. Intracran-

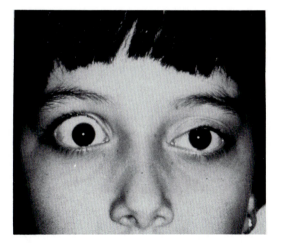

Figure 8–24. Proptosis in a child with a right optic nerve glioma. *(Courtesy of Joseph H. Calhoun.)*

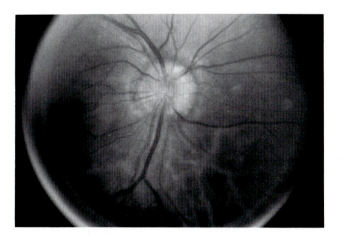

Figure 8–26. Optic disc edema in optic nerve glioma.

ial involvement is suggested by nystagmus, headache, vomiting, or seizures.

In children, optic nerve gliomas are almost always benign juvenile pilocytic (hairlike) astrocytomas, but some tumors progress. Plain-film x-rays and tomography will demonstrate enlargement of the optic foramen (Fig. 8–27); CT scan shows a fusiform enlargement of the nerve (Fig. 8–28) and optic chiasm involvement (Fig. 8–29). MRI scanning, however, best demonstrates the extent of intracranial involvement. Treatment of optic nerve gliomas is controversial. If the patient has good visual acuity and cosmetically acceptable proptosis, periodic clinical and radiological evaluation should be performed. If the tumor is growing, the affected eye is blind, and there is corneal exposure and disfigurement, or if a mass effect by the tumor causes increased intracranial pressure, surgical intervention is necessary. Radiation therapy can be used for nonresectable tumors involving the chiasm and optic radiations.

An important clinical relationship exists between optic nerve glioma and von Recklinghausen's neurofibromatosis. Among reports of glioma, the incidence of neurofibromatosis varies from 12 to 38 percent. Gliomas in patients with neurofibromatosis are occasionally bilateral and multicentric. These tumors also proliferate within the subarachnoid space. Tumors in patients without neurofibromatosis do not usually invade the dura.

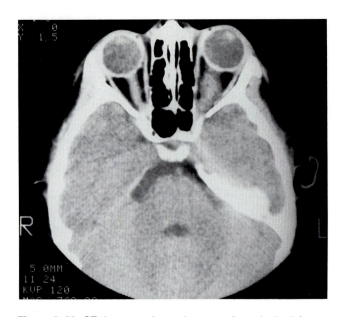

Figure 8–28. CT demonstrating optic nerve glioma in the left eye. *(From Catalano RA: Ocular Emergencies. Philadelphia, Saunders, 1992, p 54, with permission.)*

COMPREHENSIVE INFORMATION ON THE EYELIDS, LACRIMAL DRAINAGE SYSTEM, AND ORBIT

Uncommon Eyelid Disorders

Cryptophthalmos

Cryptophthalmos describes a condition in which a sheet of skin covers the eye. In complete cryptophthalmos, the sheet is continuous with the skin of the periorbital area, and there is no horizontal fissure or eyelashes (Fig. 8–30). This skin may be the most anterior surface of the underlying globe, with the skin substituting for or fusing with underlying corneal tissue. Partial cryptophthalmos also occurs (Fig. 8–31). The underlying globe is usually microphthalmic, with a de-

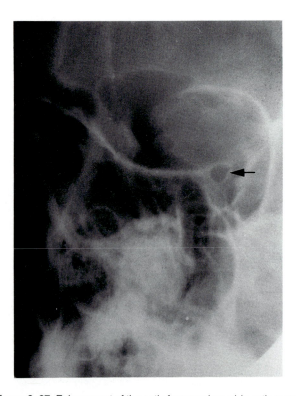

Figure 8–27. Enlargement of the optic foramen (*arrow*) in optic nerve glioma. *(From Catalano RA: Ocular Emergencies. Philadelphia, Saunders, 1992, p 53, with permission.)*

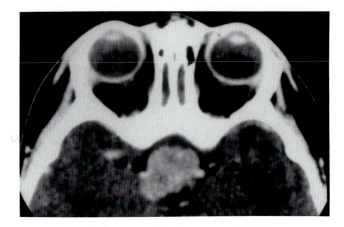

Figure 8–29. CT demonstrating optic chiasm involvement by glioma.

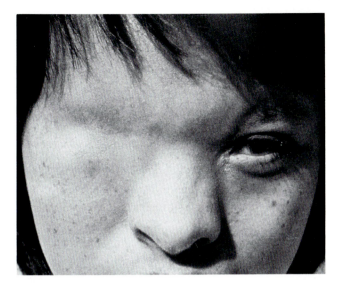

Figure 8–30. Unilateral cryptophthalmos. Note the continuous sheet of skin covering the right eye. *(Courtesy of Dario F. Savino; from Nelson LB, Folberg R: Ocular developmental anomalies. In Duane TD, Jaeger EA (eds): Biomedical Foundations of Ophthalmology. Philadelphia, Lippincott, 1984, with permission.)*

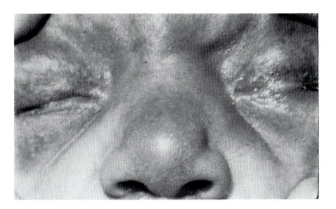

Figure 8–32. Ankyloblepharon (complete fusion of the eyelids in a newborn). *(Courtesy of Robinson D. Harley and Joseph C. Flanagan; from Harley RD (ed): Pediatric Ophthalmology. Philadelphia, Saunders, 1983, with permission.)*

fective or absent lens; the anterior chamber is usually shallow or nonexistent. The condition can occur as a part of a syndrome that is inherited in an autosomal recessive manner, which includes mental retardation, meningocele, cardiac anomalies, genitourinary anomalies, cleft lip and palate, ear and nose anomalies, and syndactyly.

The pathogenetic mechanisms responsible for cryptophthalmos are unknown. Among the possible explanations are (1) primary failure of mesodermal and ectodermal differentiation, resulting in the absence of

eyelid folds; (2) intrauterine inflammation, producing fusion of the eyelids to the globe (symblepharon); and (3) normal eyelid fold development with maldifferentiation of the conjunctiva, resulting in symblepharon.

Ankyloblepharon

Ankyloblepharon is characterized by fusion of the eyelid margins over a portion of their length, producing a shortening of the palpebral fissure (Fig. 8–32). Most commonly the eyelids are fused at the outer canthus (external ankyloblepharon); more rarely the inner canthus is involved (internal ankyloblepharon).

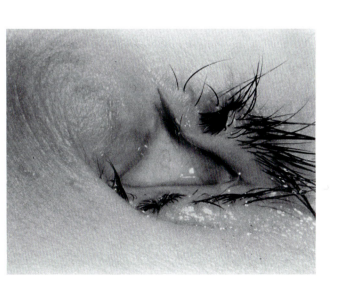

Figure 8–31. Partial cryptophthalmos. Note the coloboma in the upper eyelid separating the lateral eyelids from the medial cryptophthalmic area. *(From Waring GO, Shields JA: Partial cryptophthalmos with syndactyly, brachycephaly, and renal anomalies. Am J Ophthalmol 79:437, 1975, with permission.)*

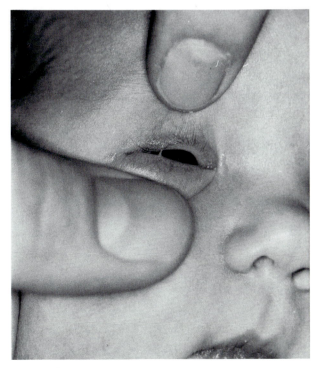

Figure 8–33. Ankyloblepharon filiforme adnatum (a band connecting the upper and lower eyelid margin).

A variant is ankyloblepharon filiforme adnatum (AFA), in which the lid margins are connected by fine strands of connective tissue (Fig. 8–33). The strands may be single or multiple, and unilateral or bilateral. The medial and lateral canthi, however, are spared. AFA is associated with cardiac anomalies, cleft lip and palate, syndactyly, and trisomy 18. All types of ankyloblepharon are treated by cutting the eyelid borders apart.

Eyelid Coloboma

An eyelid coloboma is a triangular defect of the eyelid, with the base of the triangle directed primarily at the lid margin. Colobomas are most common in the upper eyelid, where they usually occur nasally (Figs. 8–34 and 8–35). When the defect occurs in the lower eyelid, it is usually located laterally. If it is large, corneal exposure and ulceration may occur. Early surgical correction will be necessary to prevent corneal pathology from exposure.

Colobomas of the upper eyelid are a feature of Goldenhar's syndrome. When they occur concomitant with epibulbar dermoids, the eyelid notch often fits over the dermoid. A coloboma of the outer third of the lower eyelid is a feature of Treacher Collins syndrome. Isolated colobomas are usually unilateral. Associated findings in the ipsilateral eye are anterior polar cataract and lens dislocation.

Lid colobomas may result from the defective fusion of temporal and nasal waves of mesodermal tissue. Experiments also suggest that ischemia of the rapidly differentiating lid complex can cause infarction of the part of the eyelid that is farthest from the principal blood supply, resulting in a notch.

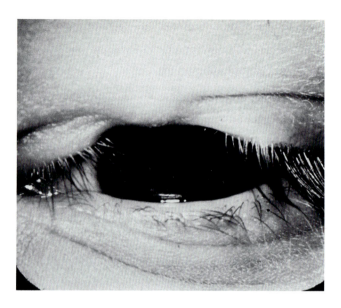

Figure 8–35. Coloboma involving the middle third of the upper eyelid. *(Courtesy of Robinson D. Harley; from Nelson LB, Brown GC, Arentsen JJ: Recognizing Patterns of Ocular Childhood Diseases. Thorofare, NJ, Slack, 1985, p 135, with permission.)*

Congenital Entropion

Congenital entropion is a rare disorder characterized by partial or complete inversion of the eyelid margin. It is caused by hypertrophy of the pretarsal fibers, specifically the fibers of the muscles of Riolan.

The extreme form of congenital entropion is the horizontal tarsal kink, which is characterized by a fixed, inward rotation of the distal tarsal margin (Fig. 8–36). This causes the eyelid margin to be turned in toward the globe, and the eyelashes to rub against the

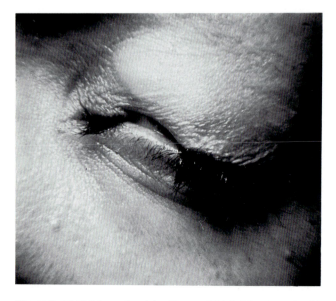

Figure 8–34. Coloboma involving the nasal third of the upper eyelid. *(From Harley RD: Disorders of the eyelid. In Nelson LB (ed): Pediatr Clin North Am 30:1145, 1983, with permission.)*

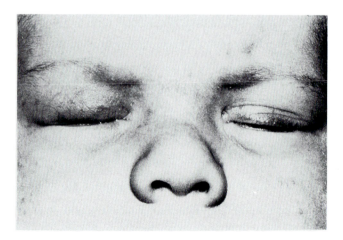

Figure 8–36. Congenital entropion, tarsal kink variant. Note the absence of the upper eyelid fold. *(From Biglan AW, Buerger GF: Congenital horizontal tarsal kink. Am J Ophthalmol 89:522, 1980, with permission.)*

cornea. This form of entropion needs to be corrected immediately to prevent corneal ulceration and scarring.

Congenital Ectropion

Congenital ectropion, or eversion of the edge of the eyelid at birth, is a rare disorder. The affected upper or lower eyelid(s) are thickened and edematous, and the palpebral conjunctiva is chemotic and hyperemic (Fig. 8–37). Congenital ectropion rarely occurs as a separate primary entity. Seven of the 20 reported cases, occurring in the absence of other major ocular abnormalities, have been in infants with Down syndrome (Catalano, 1990). Postulated pathogenic mechanisms include a constitutional weakness and flaccidity of the eyelid, and traumatic eversion during passage through the birth canal. Obstruction of venous outflow from prominent epicanthal folds, resulting in palpebral conjunctival edema and eversion of the eyelids, has also been surmised. Congenital eversion can also be associated with blepharophimosis if the skin is insufficient to allow the eyelids to close completely. Dermatologic conditions, such as hyperkeratosis and ichthyosis congenita, are rarely causative.

Mechanical inversion of the everted eyelid with repositioning of the conjunctiva, followed by a bland ointment and tight patching of the eyelids, should be the initial therapy. If the eyelids do not maintain their proper position after several days, or if they can not be inverted initially, surgical correction is indicated. It is notable that surgical intervention was needed for 5 of the 7 affected Down syndrome infants.

Epiblepharon

Epiblepharon is characterized by the presence of a redundant horizontal fold of skin across either the upper or the lower eyelid. Unlike congenital entropion, the

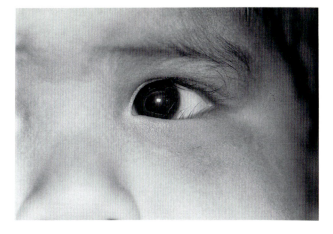

Figure 8–38. Epiblepharon. Note that the lashes are directed up toward the cornea.

lid margin in epiblepharon is correctly apposed to the eye and not inverted. The extra fold of skin can, however, turn the eyelashes against the cornea resulting in corneal irritation (Fig. 8–38). If this occurs, applying ointment to the eyelashes may redirect them away from the cornea. Surgical correction is rarely necessary, but when it is a simple excision of the extra skin fold with suturing of the superior border of the incision to deep tissues prior to closure is curative. In the majority of cases, the condition corrects itself as the face grows during the first 2 years of life.

Blepharophimosis

Blepharophimosis is characterized by a diminution of both the width and length of the palpebral fissure (Fig. 8–39). Comprising 3 to 6 percent of congenital ptosis cases, it consists of epicanthus inversus (large inverse epicanthal folds), ptosis, and telecanthus (widening of

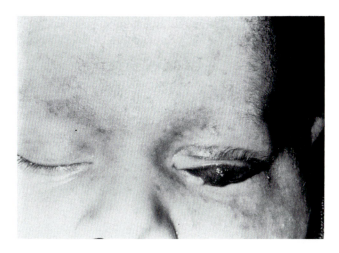

Figure 8–37. Congenital ectropion of the left upper eyelid. *(Courtesy of Joseph H. Calhoun; from Nelson LB: Pediatric Ophthalmology. Philadelphia, Saunders, 1984, with permission.)*

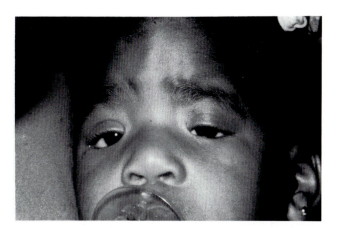

Figure 8–39. Blepharophimosis. Note the telecanthus (widely spaced orbits), ptosis, and large inverse epicanthal folds.

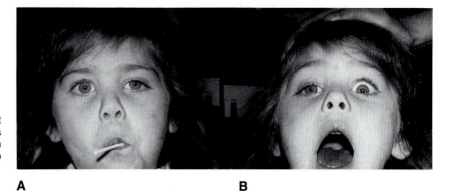

Figure 8–40. Marcus Gunn jaw-winking, left eye, in an older child. **A.** Ptosis when the jaw is moved toward the ipsilateral side. **B.** Elevation of the left upper eyelid when the jaw is moved to the opposite side.

A   **B**

the distance between the medial canthal tendons, with normally spaced orbits). Associated ocular findings include strabismus, nystagmus, microphthalmos, and lacrimal drainage system abnormalities.

Blepharophimosis is frequently transmitted in an autosomal dominant manner with essentially 100 percent penetrance. Transmission of the trait predominantly through the male parent may be due to primary amenorrhea. Although chromosomal studies are usually normal in these patients, duplication of 6p and 10q chromosomes has been reported. Surgical correction is usually deferred until the clinical features stabilize in the preschool years.

Marcus Gunn Jaw-winking Syndrome

From 4 to 6 percent of congenital ptosis cases are associated with the jaw-winking of Marcus Gunn's syndrome. This syndrome is characterized by elevation of the ptotic eyelid when the patient moves the jaw to the side opposite the involved eye (Figs. 8–40 and 8–41). Marcus Gunn jaw-winking ptosis is almost always unilateral and more frequently involves the left upper eyelid than the right. The ptosis varies from almost unnoticeable to cosmetically unacceptable. The syndrome may be associated with amblyopia, anisometropia, double elevator palsy, and superior rectus palsy. Some authorities believe that jaw-winking ptosis improves with age, while others are adamant that the anomaly persists but that the individual's adaptation to it im-

proves. Bilateral surgery to achieve a symmetrical postoperative appearance may be necessary.

The condition is usually sporadic, but occasionally, an autosomal dominant transmission is encountered. It results from congenitally misdirected fibers between the external pterygoid and levator muscles. Ordinarily the levator muscle is innervated by the third cranial nerve. In jaw-winking this is usurped or taken over by the fifth cranial nerve, which also innervates the muscles of mastication. As a result, stimulation to move the jaw is accompanied by an excess of impulses being sent to the ipsilateral levator muscle, which momentarily raises the eyelid.

Orbital Disorders in Children*

Pathological processes that involve the orbit present with proptosis (forward displacement of the eye) or as a mass, hemorrhage, or inflammation in or behind the eyelids. Orbital disorders in children should be evaluated with regard to the rate of progression (Table 8–2), presence of pain (Table 8–3), location of any mass (Table 8–4), and the presence of proptosis (Table 8–5). Figure 8–42 is a flowchart that can be used to narrow the differential diagnosis for the child who presents with signs and symptoms of orbital swelling or inflam-

---

*Modified from Catalano RA: Ocular Emergencies. Philadelphia, Saunders, 1992, pp 290–313, with permission.

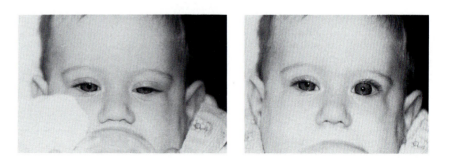

Figure 8–41. Marcus Gunn jaw-winking, left eye, elicited by an infant sucking on a bottle.

TABLE 8–2. DIFFERENTIAL DIAGNOSIS OF ORBITAL DISORDERS BY RATE OF PROGRESSION

Rate of Progression	Category	Entities
Days to weeks	Inflammation	Pseudotumor
	Infection	Cellulitis
	Hemorrhage	Lymphangioma
	Carcinoma	Rhabdomyosarcoma, neuroblastoma, granulocytic sarcoma, Burkitt's lymphoma
	Tumor	Capillary hemangioma (some)
Months to years	Tumors	Dermoid, neurofibroma, capillary hemangioma (most)
	Vascular	Orbital varix, lymphangioma

Modified from Catalano RA: Ocular Emergencies. Philadelphia, Saunders, 1992, pp 290–313, with permission.

TABLE 8–4. DIFFERENTIAL DIAGNOSIS OF ORBITAL MASSES BY LOCATION

Location	Entities	Features
Superior nasal	Encephalocele	Present in infancy, transilluminating, midline, pulsatile, fluctuant
	Plexiform neurofibroma	"Bag of worms" feel, "S"-shaped upper eyelid deformity, neurofibromatosis
	Dermoid	Smooth, firm, oval, mobile, nontender
	Capillary hemangioma	Compressible, violaceous, may have overlying skin hemangioma
Superior temporal	Dermoid	As above
	Pseudotumor	Proptosis, motility disturbance, injection, lid swelling, tender

TABLE 8–3. DIFFERENTIAL DIAGNOSIS OF ORBITAL PAIN

Category	Entities	Features
Headache	Tension	Bilateral, retrobulbar, worse in the evening, familial
Infection	Preseptal celulitis	Lid swelling and erythema
	Orbital cellulitis	Chemosis, proptosis, motility disturbance, and visual loss
	Sinusitis	Localized tenderness over sinus, upper respiratory infection
Inflammation	Optic neuritis	Aggravated by eye movement
	Foreign body	Chronic suppuration, tenderness
	Pseudotumor	Proptosis, motility disturbance, injection, lid swelling
	Posterior scleritis	Deep orbital pain radiating to the temple, mild proptosis, injection
Hemorrhage	Orbital varix, lymphangioma, blood dyscrasia	Sudden pain, proptosis, nausea, vomiting, ecchymosis, motility disturbance, visual loss
Ischemia	Sickle-cell disease	Subjective bruit, motility disturbance, episcleral injection, visual loss
Carcinoma	Neuroblastoma	Orbital hemorrhage with lid ecchymosis, under age 4 years
	Granulocytic sarcoma	Mean age 7 years, myelogenous leukemia
	Rhabdomyosarcoma	Rapid progression of proptosis, pain

mation. Additionally, several utrasonographic and pathognomonic features of certain orbital disorders are presented in Tables 8–6 and 8–7.

Alacrima

Reflex tearing normally begins shortly after birth, but may be delayed for several weeks. Psychogenic tearing appears later, typically between 2 and 4 months of age. Congenital absence or marked deficiency of tear production (alacrima) has been reported in association with aplasia of the lacrimal gland or brainstem nuclei that control lacrimation. It has also been reported with ectodermal dysplasia, and as an idiopathic occurrence in otherwise healthy individuals. Clinical manifestations of alacrima may include ocular irritation and photophobia, a viscous tear film, and punctate erosions of the corneal epithelium. In the case of aplasia of the main lacrimal gland, the ocular appearance is usually normal, as baseline tear production is unaffected.

Familial dysautonomia (Riley–Day syndrome) is a rare generalized disorder of the autonomic and sensory nervous systems. Systemic signs include dehydration due to cyclic vomiting and diarrhea, blotching of the skin, hyporeflexia, and insensitivity to pain. The disorder occurs almost exclusively in families of Ashkenazic Jewish descent, and is inherited in an autosomal recessive pattern. Ocular involvement is related to a variety of factors. Altered parasympathetic innervation of the lacrimal gland interferes with tear production. In addition, affected individuals usually have corneal hypesthesia or anesthesia, and often sleep with their eyes open. The combination of poor tearing, exposure, and altered sensation results in a keratitis that may be very difficult to control.

TABLE 8–5. DIFFERENTIAL DIAGNOSIS OF PROPTOSIS

Category	Entities	Category	Entities
Pseudoproptosis	Enlarged globe (high myopia, infantile glaucoma) Asymmetry of lid fissures Cranial nerve palsy Contralateral enophthalmos (post-traumatic) Contralateral Horner's syndrome Asymmetric palpebral fissures Asymmetric orbital size	Recurrent proptosis (*cont.*)	Pseudotumor Ruptured dermoid cyst with granulomatous reaction
		▪ *DISPLACEMENT OF GLOBE*	
		Axial	Optic nerve glioma or meningioma Carotid cavernous fistula Neurilemmoma Rhabdomyosarcoma (some)
Unilateral proptosis	Cellulitis Pseudotumor	Superior	Fibromatosis (firm, painless tumor)
Bilateral proptosis	Neuroblastoma Pseudotumor Leukemia	Inferior	Capillary hemangioma Fibrous dysplasia
		Inferior and medial	Dermoid
		Inferior and lateral	Rhabdomyosarcoma (some)
Recurrent proptosis	Orbital varix (with Valsalva maneuver) Lymphangioma (with upper respiratory infection)	Medial	Neuroblastoma with metastases to zygomatic bone

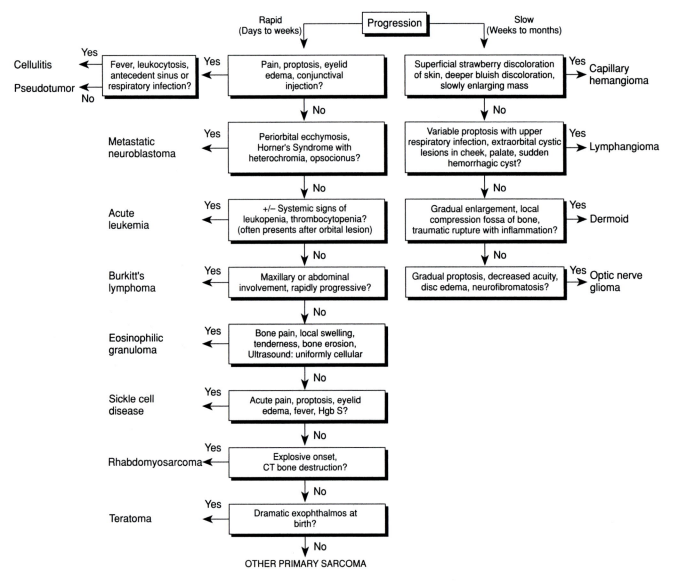

Figure 8–42. Flowchart for differentiating nontraumatic orbital disorders in children. (*From Catalano RA: Ocular Emergencies. Philadelphia, Saunders, 1992, p 296, with permission.*)

TABLE 8–6. DIFFERENTIAL FINDINGS OF ORBITAL DISORDERS ON ULTRASONOGRAPHY

Feature	Category	Entities
Good transmission	Cystic and angiomatous tumors	Dermoid Cavernous hemangioma Lymphangioma
Poor transmission	Solid and infiltrative tumors	Meningioma Glioma Neurofibroma Pseudotumor
Few internal echoes	Cystic lesions, tumors containing compact cells	Dermoid Burkitt's lymphoma
Strong internal echoes	Angiomatous tumors	Varix Lymphangioma
Rounded borders	Cystic and solid tumors	Dermoid Burkitt's lymphoma
Irregular borders	Infiltrative and angiomatous tumors	Rhabdomyosarcoma Invasive retinoblastoma
Thickened optic nerve	Optic nerve tumors	Glioma Meningioma

TABLE 8–7. PATHOGNOMONIC FEATURES OF CERTAIN ORBITAL DISORDERS

Feature	Entities	Feature	Entities
Corkscrew epibulbar vessels	Arteriovenous malformation Carotid–cavernous fistula Pseudotumor Orbital abscess	▪ *RADIOGRAPHIC SIGNS*	
		Ocular calcification	Retinoblastoma Phthisis bulbi Cicatricial retinopathy of prematurity
Strawberry birthmark	Capillary hemangioma	Orbital calcification	Hemangioma
Yellow, fleshy mass under conjunctiva	Dermolipoma		Varix Dermoid cyst
"S"-shaped lid, "bag of worms" texture	Plexiform neurofibroma	Absence of sphenoid wing	Neurofibromatosis
Bilateral ecchymoses	Neuroblastoma Granulocytic sarcoma	Local compression lacrimal gland fossa	Dermoid Lymphangioma
Immobility of the eye	Pseudotumor/myositis Orbital cellulitis Large orbital tumor	Enlargement of optic canal	Optic nerve glioma/meningioma Invasive retinoblastoma Optic nerve granuloma
▪ *ASSOCIATED OCULAR FINDINGS*		Optic nerve enlargement	Optic nerve glioma/meningioma Granulomatous disease Pseudoenlargement (contralateral optic atrophy)
Anterior uveitis	Scleritis Pseudotumor		
Optic nerve dysplasia	Encephalocele	Thickened extraocular muscles	Thyroid ophthalmopathy Myositis Arteriovenous fistulas
Optociliary shunt vessels at disk	Meningioma Chronic papilledema		
Choroidal folds	Papilledema Ocular hypotony Orbital tumor	Enlarged superior ophthalmic vein	Arteriovenous malformation or fistula
		Scleral enhancement	Scleritis Pseudotumor
Smooth indentation of globe	Orbital tumor		

Ischemic Orbital Disorder (Sickle-cell Disease)

Acute orbital pain, proptosis, eyelid edema, and fever can occur in sickle-cell disease with sickling crises. Orbital bones become infarcted with secondary inflammation. The disorder is differentiated from osteomyelitis with subperiosteal abscess by the decreased uptake of radionucleotides in sickle-cell infarction, but increased uptake in infection. Furthermore, subperiosteal abscesses are more likely to occur adjacent to an opacified sinus.

Orbital Inflammation

Pseudotumor. Children as young as age 3 can be afflicted with an idiopathic inflammation of the orbit called orbital pseudotumor. Patients with this disorder present with lid erythema and swelling, ptosis, and an S-shaped deformity of the upper eyelid (Fig. 8–43). Additionally, they can have restricted eye movements, orbital pain, proptosis, conjunctival chemosis and vascular congestion, and reduced corneal sensitivity. One third of children with pseudotumor present with bilateral involvement, and only rarely in children is there an associated systemic disorder.

Nearly half of the children with pseudotumor have headache, abdominal discomfort, fever, and lethargy. Eosinophilia, an elevated erythrocyte sedimentation rate, antinuclear antibodies, and mild spinal fluid pleocytosis are occasionally found. The absence of marked leukocytosis and a left shift helps differentiate this condition from bacterial orbital cellulitis. Children with pseudotumor may also have papillitis or iridocyclitis.

Clinical, CT, and ultrasound findings are often sufficiently characteristic to exclude the need for biopsy prior to treatment. CT may demonstrate infiltration within the retrobulbar fat and thickening of the extraocular muscles if a myositic component is present and/or contrast enhancement of the sclera (ring sign) if sclerotenonitis is present (Fig. 8–44). Neoplastic in-

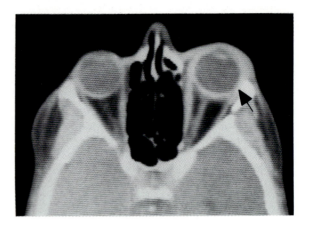

Figure 8–44. Scleral enhancement (*arrow*) in pseudotumor, also known as the "ring" sign. *(From Catalano RA: Ocular Emergencies. Philadelphia, Saunders, 1992, p 302, with permission.)*

volvement of an extraocular muscle usually produces more focal, globular enlargement. B-scan ultrasonography can demonstrate an acoustically hollow, edematous Tenon's capsule in sclerotenonitis and thickened extraocular muscles if myositis is present. Biopsy findings include patchy infiltrates of lymphocytes, plasma cells, and eosinophils (especially in children) and lymphoid hyperplasia embedded in a loose, fibrous stroma. Scarring (sclerosing pseudotumor) is a late finding.

Pseudotumor Variants. Pseudotumor variants include myositis (principally extraocular muscle involvement), sclerotenonitis (sclera and Tenon's capsule), dacryoadenitis (lacrimal gland), or papillitis (dural sheath of the optic nerve). Of these, myositis and dacryoadenitis are the most common forms encountered in children. The **Tolosa–Hunt** syndrome is another variant, in which inflammation primarily occurs around the superior orbital fissure and optic canal. Involvement of this area results in restriction of ocular movements and reduction of visual acuity.

ORBITAL HAMARTOMAS

A **hamartoma** is a tumor arising from tissue components normally present at the involved site. **Choristomas** contain tissue elements not normally found at the site.

Orbital Capillary Hemangiomas

Capillary hemangiomas can occur in the eyelid, orbit, or both locations (Figs. 8–45 to 8–47). Eyelid lesions are more common (described at the start of the chapter), and isolated orbital tumors may be difficult to diagnose with certainty. The most common site of orbital involvement is the superior nasal quadrant. Because of the propensity of encephaloceles and rhabdomyosarcomas to also involve the superior nasal quadrant, CT

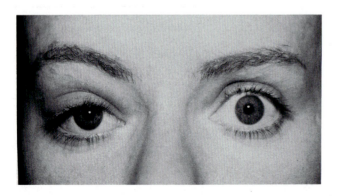

Figure 8–43. Orbital pseudotumor, right orbit. Note the S-shaped curve to the upper eyelid. *(From Catalano RA: Ocular Emergencies. Philadelphia, Saunders, 1992, p 300, with permission.)*

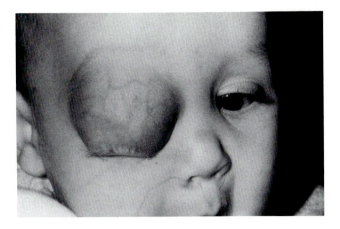

Figure 8–45. Capillary hemangioma of the right eyelid and orbit, causing marked distension of the eyelid.

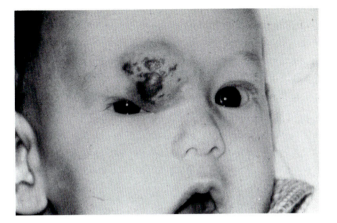

Figure 8–47. Capillary hemangioma of the right eyelid and superior nasal orbit. *(Courtesy of Joseph H. Calhoun.)*

scanning is advised prior to treating an orbital hemangioma in this area. A homogeneous mass, with possible orbital expansion but without bony clefts or destruction, is characteristic of an orbital hemangioma. Contrast enhancement is not useful because malignant tumors also enhance. A-scan ultrasonography of a hemangioma demonstrates high-amplitude spikes from vessel lumen/cellular interfaces, in contrast to the low-amplitude spikes seen in densely cellular rhabdomyosarcomas.

Orbital hemangiomas that cause proptosis or globe displacement may have to be treated. Deep orbital steroid injections carry increased risks of hemorrhage and retinal artery embolus of steroid. Concomitant visualization of the retinal artery is advised during injection, so that immediate measures can be instituted if embolization occurs. Other options include systemic prednisone (2 mg/kg per day or 4 mg/kg on alternate days; maximum 80 to 100 mg/day), orthovoltage radiotherapy (single treatment of 2 Gy), and surgical resection. Pediatric consultation is advised if systemic steroids

are used, as these may induce adrenal suppression, growth retardation, and cushinoid features.

Lymphangiomas

A lymphangioma is a benign, slowly progressive tumor. The lymphatic (or vascular) channels that comprise it are likely present at birth, but the tumor usually does not become apparent until several years of age. The child may have a history of variable proptosis, related to upper respiratory infections. Frequently, a multiloculated cystic mass of the bulbar conjunctiva develops, which may periodically fill with blood (Fig. 8–48). Spontaneous bleeding into the eyelid may produce ecchymosis in association with proptosis (Fig. 8–49). As orbital lymphangiomas slowly enlarge, the proptosis and conjunctival involvement worsen. Pressure on the globe from the mass can lead to secondary glaucoma, congestion of the optic nerve, and eventual visual loss.

Orbital roentgenograms usually shows a larger

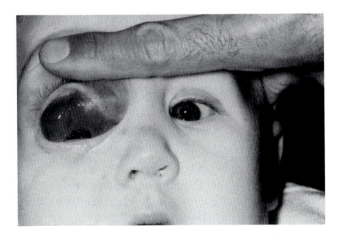

Figure 8–46. Same patient as in Figure 8–45, with the eyelid raised.

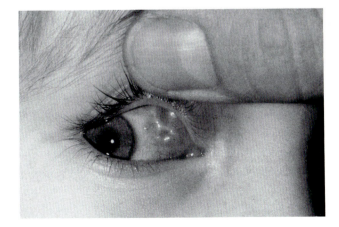

Figure 8–48. Lymphangioma appearing as multiloculated cysts in the bulbar conjunctiva.

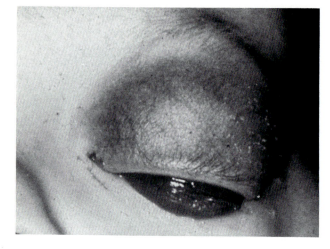

Figure 8–49. Spontaneous hemorrhage in a patient with a lymphangioma. *(Courtesy of the Wills Eye Hospital slide collection.)*

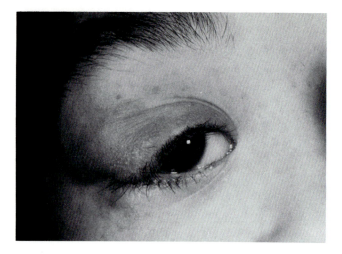

Figure 8–50. Plexiform neurofibroma in the right upper lid causing an S-shaped deformity to the eyelid. *(Courtesy of Dale R. Meyer; from Catalano RA: Ocular Emergencies. Philadelphia, Saunders, 1992, p 305, with permission.)*

orbit on the involved side, a finding consistent with a slow growing orbital tumor. B-scan ultrasonography demonstrates either a diffuse or a cystic pattern, both types of which have acoustic hollowness and good sound transmission. Orbital CT usually shows a multiloculated cystic mass within the orbital soft tissue.

Lymphangiomas usually stabilize in size by the third decade. Spontaneous regression can occur, but not as characteristically as with capillary hemangiomas. Unless massive proptosis and optic nerve compression occur, hemorrhagic cysts are treated conservatively. Uninvolved portions of a hemorrhagic lymphangioma should not be evacuated because of the risk of greater hemorrhage. Bovie electrocautery or carbon dioxide laser surgery may prevent this complication. Occasionally orbital decompression is necessary for cosmetic or functional treatment.

Neurofibromas

Neurofibromas are tumors composed of proliferating Schwann cells, axons, endoneural fibroblasts, and mucin. They are encountered in the von Recklinghausen form of neurofibromatosis (NF1). They may be discreet and nodular or diffuse and plexiform. Plexiform neurofibromas of the upper eyelid can cause an S-shaped deformity to the lid (Fig. 8–50). They have a texture similar to a bag of worms and are associated with a higher incidence of infantile glaucoma.

Plexiform orbital neurofibromas are enclosed within a perineural sheath. Similar to plexiform neurofibromas of the eyelid, they are more likely to be associated with neurofibromatosis and present during the first decade of life. Because the lesions are diffuse, enveloping the optic nerve, extraocular muscles, and lacrimal gland, their surgical removal is difficult. These

tumors frequently coexist with bony orbital defects, particularly of the sphenoid bone. When associated with neurofibromatosis, malignant transformation can occur in up to 10 percent of cases. **Neurilemmomas (schwannomas)** are composed only of Schwann cells. Like neurofibromas, they can be associated with neurofibromatosis (presenting at a younger age) or unassociated (presenting in middle age). Unlike neurofibromas, neurilemmomas rarely, if ever, undergo malignant transformation.

ORBITAL CHORISTOMAS

Dermoid and Epidermoid Cysts

Dermoid cysts arise from dermal elements and epidermoid cysts from epidermal elements that get pinched off at suture lines during embryonic development. Dermoid cysts are lined by keratinizing epithelium, and contain components of dermal appendages, such as hair, teeth, and sebaceous and sweat glands, in the cyst wall. Epidermoid cysts are lined by epidermis only. They are usually filled with keratin and do not contain dermal elements.

Dermoid and epidermoid cysts comprise as many as 10 percent of orbital masses. They usually appear during childhood; 25 percent are apparent at birth. Their natural course is slow expansion and, depending on their site, displacement of adjacent structures. There is no recognized heritable pattern.

Half of the cysts that present in childhood are located anterior to the orbital septum, in the lateral brow and upper eyelid, adjacent to the zygomaticofrontal suture (Fig. 8–51). Twenty-five percent of cysts occur at the nasofrontal suture. These need to be distinguished

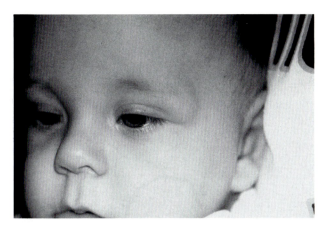

Figure 8–51. Orbital dermoid in the superior temporal quadrant of the left orbit.

from capillary hemangiomas and orbital encephaloceles. A bony defect and herniation of brain tissue on radiological studies are characteristic of the latter.

Dermoid and epidermoid cysts are smooth, oval, nontender, well-circumscribed masses of rubbery consistency. Superficial cysts present as 1 to 2 cm asymptomatic orbital masses in young infants. Their posterior surfaces are clinically palpable, and they can easily be removed by anterior orbitotomy. Because bony structures are under pressure from the cyst, well-corticated osseous depressions can occur. Usually no palpable bony defect is felt, but bony dehiscences can occur and can enlarge with time. This is particularly true of posteriorly located dermoids. Deep dermoids arise in older children, and have no palpable posterior limit. If the entire extent of the cyst cannot be palpated, radiological studies are indicated to rule out a dumbbell-shaped cyst with possible dural exposure at surgery, or an encephalocele.

Traumatic rupture of the cyst can lead to an acute inflammatory process, resembling orbital cellulitis or pseudotumor. Surgical excision through the upper eyelid crease is therefore generally suggested. Rarely, patients with orbital dermoids can present with spontaneous draining fistulas. Fistulas usually result after incomplete removal.

Lipodermoids

Lipodermoids are solid fat-containing tumors, usually located over the lateral surface of the globe beneath the conjunctiva (Fig. 8–52). They may extend deep toward the muscle cone, lacrimal gland, or levator muscle. Restrictive strabismus from fat–extraocular muscle adhesion can result from incomplete removal. Resection can also damage lacrimal gland ducts. Lipodermoids are therefore best left alone unless cosmetically disfiguring.

Teratomas

Teratomas are rare tumors that are evident at birth as grossly visible orbital masses (Figs. 8–53 and 8–54). They are almost always unilateral, with a female preponderance of 2:1. Histologically, they are composed of tissue elements from two or more germinal layers.

Teratomas are usually cystic and often contain intracranial contents. They displace the globe forward and upward, distend the eyelids and conjunctiva, and enlarge the bony orbit. Proptosis may increase progressively during the first few days or weeks of life. Prompt and continuous protection of the exposed proptotic eye should be maintained at all times.

An orbital teratoma should be differentiated from other lesions that may produce progressive proptosis at birth, such as a capillary hemangioma and, rarely, rhabdomyosarcoma. Ultrasonography of a teratoma reveals a semicystic mass, often in direct opposition to the posterior surface of the globe. CT shows an enlarged orbit with an irregular multiloculated soft tissue mass. Teratomas do not erode bone or extend intracranially, but they are not reducible. They are usually cystic and transilluminate, but occasionally are solid.

Malignant change, which occurs in about 20 percent of teratomas elsewhere in the body, has been reported only once in an orbital tumor. If left untreated, orbital teratomas can cause death by complications of intracranial erosion or compression of nasal or oral passages. Some teratomas can be removed without exenteration, preserving visual function (Fig. 8–55). Surgery should be performed as early as possible. In the interim, the exposed, proptotic eye should be continuously protected with ointments and a moisture chamber.

MALIGNANT ORBITAL NEOPLASMS

Rhabdomyosarcoma

See the "Rhabdomyosarcoma" section earlier in the chapter.

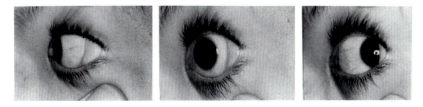

Figure 8–52. Lipodermoid, left eye. Note how the eye and bulbar conjunctiva slide under the tumor on ocular rotation.

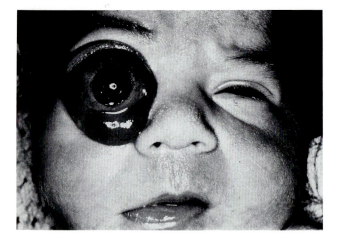

Figure 8–53. Frontal view of a 1-day-old infant with an orbital teratoma. *(From Chang DG, Dallow RL, Walton DS: Congenital orbital teratoma: Report of a case with visual preservation. J Pediatr Ophthalmol Strabismus 17:88, 1980, with permission.)*

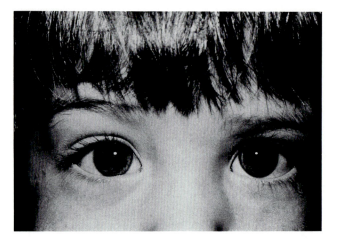

Figure 8–55. Same patient as Figures 8–53 and 8–54 at 18 months of age, following successful removal of the right orbital teratoma. *(From Chang DG, Dallow RL, Walton DS: Congenital orbital teratoma: Report of a case with visual preservation. J Pediatr Ophthalmol Strabismus 17:88, 1980, with permission.)*

Neuroblastoma

Neuroblastoma is the most common metastatic orbital tumor of childhood. It usually originates in the adrenal medulla or an adjacent retroperitoneal site but can arise in the neck or mediastinum. It generally presents between 18 and 36 months of age, but can present at birth or as late as the midteens.

Ophthalmologic findings occur in 20 percent of cases, and orbital findings can be the presenting feature. The classic orbital finding is periorbital ecchymo-sis. It occurs when the rapidly growing tumor outgrows its blood supply, causing hemorrhagic necrosis (Fig. 8–56). Proptosis can also occur (Fig. 8–57). Orbital presentations generally signify disseminated disease and herald a poor prognosis. Additional ocular findings include Horner's syndrome from involvement of the cervical sympathetic ganglia, and opsoclonus (chaotic, bilateral, back-to-back, rapid movements of the eyes in various directions). The latter is a paraneoplastic sign.

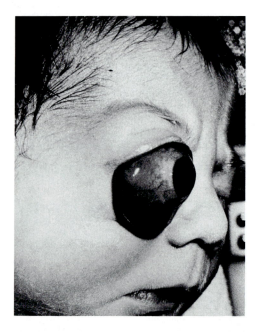

Figure 8–54. Lateral view of same patient with an orbital teratoma. *(From Chang DG, Dallow RL, Walton DS: Congenital orbital teratoma: Report of a case with visual preservation. J Pediatr Ophthalmol Strabismus 17:88, 1980, with permission.)*

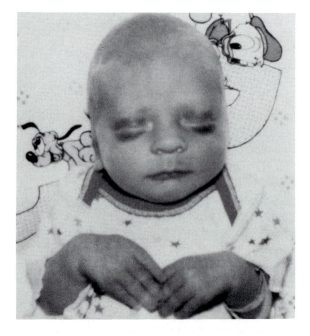

Figure 8–56. Infant with metastatic neuroblastoma, presenting with bilateral periorbital ecchymosis ("raccoon eyes"). *(From Catalano RA: Ocular Emergencies. Philadelphia, Saunders, 1992, p 309, with permission.)*

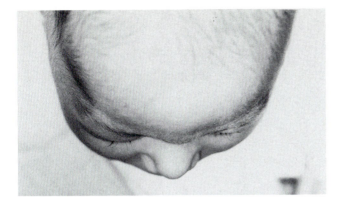

Figure 8–57. Proptosis in the right eye of an infant with neuroblastoma, demonstrated by gazing down at the orbits from the top of the head.

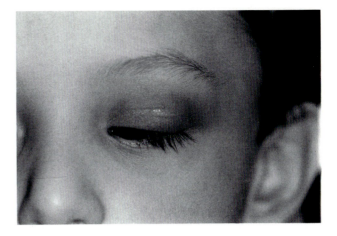

Figure 8–58. Chloroma, presenting with a swollen, discolored left upper eyelid and downward globe displacement.

Diagnostic studies include urinalysis for catecholamine metabolites, CT of the orbit to determine metastatic extent, and CT of the abdomen or thorax to demonstrate the primary tumor. Biopsy is required for definitive diagnosis, and specimens should be fixed in formalin for light microscopy and glutaraldehyde for electron microscopy. The latter may demonstrate neurosecretory granules containing catecholamines. Homer-Wright pseudorosettes are rarely found in orbital metastases. Management includes surgical excision, radiation and chemotherapy, and autogenous bone marrow transplantation.

Leukemia and Lymphoma

The most common malignancy in childhood is acute leukemia. Ocular and orbital involvement in childhood leukemia is usually secondary to disseminated lymphoblastic tumors. A rare form of granulocytic leukemia, however, disproportionately involves the orbit. These tumors, called **granulocytic sarcomas** or **chloromas,** can present months in advance of blood or bone marrow signs of leukemia. The initial signs can be swelling and discoloration of the eyelids, proptosis, and globe displacement (Fig. 8–58). Eyelid ecchymosis and bilateral involvement can follow. Computed tomography demonstrates a well-defined growth without bony erosion (Fig. 8–59). On biopsy, the tumors appear greenish owing to the pigment myeloperoxidase, hence the name "chloroma." Diagnosis is made with the Leder stain, which demonstrates cystoplasmic esterase activity in the cells. Electron microscopy may also reveal early granule formation. Formally, the prognosis was dismal; most patients died within 6 months. Chemotherapy and radiotherapy can prolong survival, but are most effective if they can be instituted prior to the development of the leukemic phase.

Burkitt's lymphoma is endemic in East Africa,

where it accounts for the majority of pediatric orbital tumors. It is rare but not unheard of in North America. It presents between ages 3 and 15 years (mean 7 years) with unilateral or bilateral proptosis or extranodal masses in the maxilla, mandible, or abdominal viscera. Its progression may be explosive, with a doubling time of only 24 hours. Histologically, the tumor demonstrates a "starry-sky" pattern due to the presence of large histiocytes interspersed among homogeneous neoplastic lymphocytes.

Eosinophilic granuloma (Langerhans cell granulo-

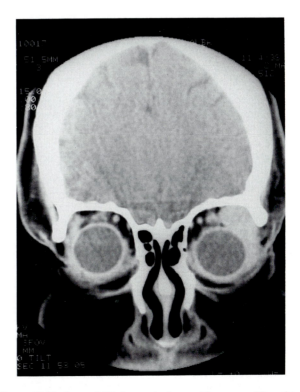

Figure 8–59. Coronal CT demonstrating a chloroma molding about the eye without bony erosion.

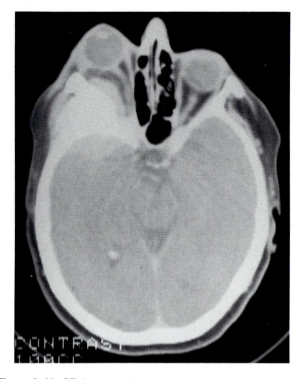

Figure 8–60. CT demonstrating sphenoid wing meningioma. *(From Catalano RA: Ocular Emergencies. Philadelphia, Saunders, 1992, p 328, with permission.)*

matosis) is a relatively benign and probably reactive lesion composed of histiocytes and mature eosinophils. It is the subset of histiocytosis X, which most commonly involves the orbit. It usually involves the superior temporal quadrant and occurs as a solitary lesion within bone rather than a systemic disorder. Symptoms include localized bone pain, tenderness, and swelling. Radiological studies demonstrate bone erosion similar to that which can occur with lacrimal tu-

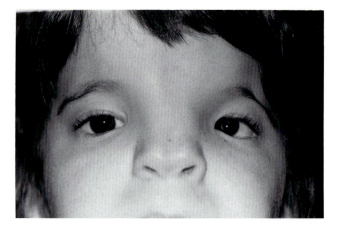

Figure 8–62. Congenital facial midline cleft.

mors. Ultrasonography, however, demonstrates its uniformly cellular nature, and electron microscopy reveals Langerhans or Birbeck granules in biopsy specimens. Treatment of an eosinophilic granuloma includes intralesion steroids, low-dose radiation, and surgical excision.

Other histiocytic tumors (Letterer–Siwe and Hand–Schüller–Christian disease) can also produce proptosis. In addition, they usually also cause lytic skull lesions, visceral abnormalities, and/or diabetes insipidus from encroachment of hypothalamus and pituitary gland. They should be excluded by bone scans, liver function tests, and a 24-hour urine collection after water deprivation.

Meningiomas

Orbital meningiomas occur more frequently in the second through fifth decades. Those that occur in childhood are more aggressive than those occurring in

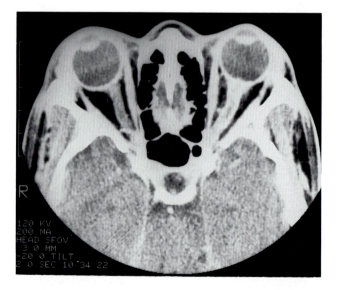

Figure 8–61. CT demonstrating meningioma of the left optic nerve sheath. *(From Catalano RA: Ocular Emergencies. Philadelphia, Saunders, 1992, p 327, with permission.)*

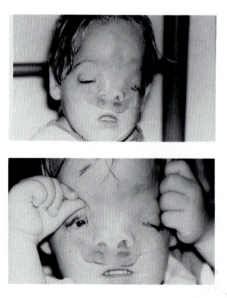

Figure 8–63. Another patient with a congenital facial midline cleft. Note how he raises his ptotic right eyelid in order to see.

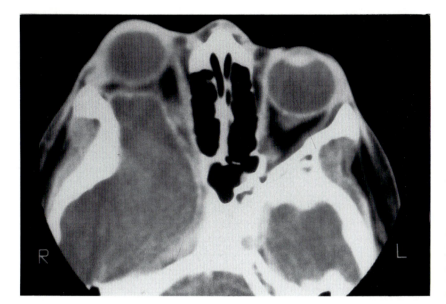

Figure 8–64. Axial CT demonstrating hypoplasia of the sphenoid wing, with herniation of the temporal lobe into the orbit, in a child with neurofibromatosis. *(From Catalano RA: Ocular Emergencies. Philadelphia, Saunders, 1992, p 313, with permission.)*

adulthood. Similar to optic nerve gliomas, there is a higher than expected incidence in patients with neurofibromatosis.

Meningiomas can arise within the cranium and invade the orbit secondarily; less commonly, they arise directly from the meninges of the optic nerve. They usually present with a progressive loss of vision or progressive exophthalmos. Visual field loss, optic atrophy, retinal striae, and/or optociliary shunt vessels are commonly found on examination. Meningiomas arising from the lateral portion of the sphenoid bone produce a temporal fossa mass and proptosis (Fig. 8–60). Orbital apex meningiomas can cause swelling of the lower eyelid.

Radiographic findings in sphenoid ridge meningiomas include hyperostosis (bone thickening), bone resorption and destruction, and blurring of the oblique (innominate) line. CT scanning demonstrates a lucid center in optic nerve sheath meningiomas (Fig. 8–61). In contrast, optic nerve gliomas have a denser center and a more fusiform shape (see Fig. 8–28). Surgical manipulation of optic nerve sheath meningiomas can result in blindness. Intervention is usually reserved for tumors that have already caused blindness, or threaten intracranial structures. Irradiation is not of value.

CONGENITAL FACIAL CLEFTS

Congenital facial clefts usually involve the orbit and/or maxilla (Figs. 8–62 and 8–63). Clefts involving orbital bones can result in the herniation of meninges (meningocele), brain tissue (encephalocele), or both (meningoencephalocele). Most commonly, these present as a subcutaneous mass near the medial canthus, over the bridge of the nose. Straining or crying may in-

crease the size of the mass, and the globe may be displaced. The differential includes an orbital capillary hemangioma.

Dysplasia of orbital bones can occur in neurofibromatosis. Hypoplasia of both the greater and lesser wing of the sphenoid, with elevation of the lesser wing, widening of the superior orbital fissure, and herniation of the temporal lobe into the orbit, can occur (Figs. 8–64 and 8–65). Transmission of the cerebrospi-

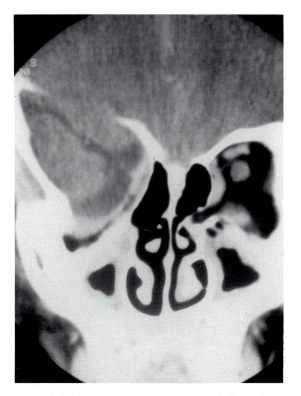

Figure 8–65. Coronal CT of same patient as in Figure 8–64.

nal fluid pulsation can result in a pulsatile exophthalmos, in concert with the radial pulse. Orbital neurofibromas are often associated with these bony defects.

REFERENCES

Ankyloblepharon

Duke-Elder S: Normal and abnormal development. In Duke-Elder (ed): System of Ophthalmology, vol 3. St. Louis, Mosby, 1963.

Ehlers N, Jensen IK: Ankyloblepharon filiforme congenitum associated with harelip and cleft palate. Acta Ophthalmologica 48:465, 1970.

Kazarian EL, Goldstein P: Ankyloblepharon, filiforme adnatum with hydrocephalus, meningomyelocele and imperforate anus. Am J Ophthalmol 84:355, 1977.

Long JC, Blanford SE: Ankyloblepharon filiforme adnatum with cleft lip and palate. Am J Ophthalmol 53:1265, 1962.

Blepharophimosis

Callahan A: Surgical correction of the blepharophimosis syndromes. Trans Am Ophthalmol Otolaryngol 77:687, 1973.

Jones CA, Collin JRO: Blepharophimosis and its association with female infertility. Br J Ophthalmol 68:533, 1984.

Kohn R: Additional lacrimal finding in the syndrome of blepharoptosis, blepharophimosis, epicanthus inversus and telecanthus. J Pediatr Ophthalmol Strabismus 20:98, 1983.

Kohn R, Romano PE: Blepharoptosis, blepharophimosis, epicanthus inversus, and telecanthus—a syndrome with no name. Am J Ophthalmol 72:625, 1971.

Townes PL, Meuchler EK: Blepharophimosis, ptosis, epicanthus inversus and primary amenorrhea: A dominant trait. Arch Ophthalmol 97:1664, 1979.

Capillary Hemangioma

Carruthers JDA, Shaw C, Cynader M, et al: Estrogen receptors in periocular hemangiomas of infancy. Paper presented at American Association for Pediatric Ophthalmology and Strabismus annual meeting, Hawaii 1991.

Haik BG, Jakobiec FA, Ellsworth RM, et al: Capillary hemangiomas of the lids and orbit: An analysis of the clinical features and therapeutics results in 101 cases. Ophthalmology 86:760, 1979.

Kushner BJ: Infantile orbital hemangiomas. Int Pediatr 5:249, 1990.

Kushner BJ: Treatment of periorbital infantile hemangioma with intralesional corticosteroid. Plast Reconstructive Surg 76:517, 1985.

Margileth A, Museles M: Cutaneous hemangiomas in children: Diagnosis and conservative management. JAMA 194:523, 1965.

Nelson LB, Melnick JE, Harley RD: Intralesional corticosteroid injections for infantile hemangioma of the eyelid. Pediatrics 74:241, 1984.

Robb RM: Refractive errors associated with hemangiomas of the eyelids and orbit in infancy. Am J Ophthalmol 83:52, 1977.

Stigmar G, Crawford JS, Ward CM, et al: Ophthalmic se-
quelae of infantile hemangiomas of the eyelids and orbit. Am J Ophthalmol 85:806, 1978.

Yee RD, Hepler RS: Congenital hemangiomas of the skin with orbital and subglottic hemangiomas. Am J Ophthalmol 75:876, 1973.

Colobomas of the Eyelids

Caset TA: Congenital colobomata of the eyelids. Trans Ophthalmol Soc UK 96:65, 1976.

Crawford JS: Congenital eyelid anomalies in children. J Pediatr Ophthalmol Strabismus 21:140, 1984.

Guibor P: Surgical repair of congenital colobomas. Trans Am Acad Ophthalmol Otolaryngol 9:671, 1975.

Kidwell EDR, Tenzel RR: Repair of congenital colobomas of the lids. Arch Ophthalmol 97:1931, 1979.

Patipa M, Wilkins RB, Guelzow KWL: Surgical management of congenital eye coloboma. Ophthalmic Surg 13:212, 1982.

Cryptophthalmos

Codere F, Brownstein S, Chen MF: Cryptophthalmos syndrome with bilateral and renal agenesis. Am J Ophthalmol 91:737, 1981.

Ehlers N: Cryptophthalmos with orbito-palpebral cyst and microphthalmos. Acta Ophthalmologica 44:84, 1966.

Varnek L: Cryptophthalmos, dyscephaly, syndactyly and renal aplasia: Report of a case. Acta Ophthalmologica 56:302, 1978.

Waring GO, Shields JA: Partial unilateral cryptophthalmos with syndactyly, brachycephaly and renal anomalies. Am J Ophthalmol 79:437, 1975.

Dermoid (Orbital)

Blei L, Chambers JT, Liotta LA, et al: Orbital dermoid diagnosed by computed tomographic scanning. Am J Ophthalmol 85:58, 1978.

Grove AS: Giant dermoid cysts of the orbit. Ophthalmology 86:1513, 1979.

Henderson JW: Orbital Tumors, ed 2. New York, Thieme-Stratton, 1980.

Nicholas DH, Green WR: Pediatric Ocular Tumors. New York, Masson, 1981.

Pollard ZF, Calhoun JH: Deep orbital dermoid with draining sinus. Am J Ophthalmol 70:310, 1975.

Pollard ZF, Harley RD, Calhoun JH: Dermoid cysts in children. Pediatrics 57:379, 1976.

Sherman P, Rootman J, LaPointe JS: Orbital dermoids: Clinical presentation and management. Br J Ophthalmol 68:642, 1984.

Shields JA: Diagnosis and Management of Orbital Tumors. Philadelphia, Saunders, 1989.

Ectropion (Congenital)

Catalano RA: Down syndrome. Surv Ophthalmol 34:385, 1990.

Gilbert HD, Smith RD, Barlow MH, et al: Congenital upper eyelid eversion and Down's Syndrome. Am J Ophthalmol 75:469, 1973.

Johnson CC, McGowan BL: Persistent congenital ectropion of

all four eyelids with megaloblepharon. Report of a case in a mongoloid child. Am J Ophthalmol 67:252, 1969.

Moaninie R, Kopelowitz N, Rosenfeld W, et al: Congenital eversion of the eyelids: A report of two cases treated with conservative management. J Pediatr Ophthalmol Strabismus 19:326, 1982.

Pico G: Congenital ectropion and distichiasis. Etiologic and hereditary factors. A report of cases and review of the literature. Am J Ophthalmol 47:363, 1959.

Stern EN, Campbell CH, Faulkner HW: Conservative management of congenital eversion of the eyelids. Am J Ophthalmol 75:319, 1973.

Entropion (Congenital)

Biglan AW, Buerger GJ Jr: Congenital horizontal tarsal kink. Am J Ophthalmol 90:522, 1980.

Crawford JS: Congenital eyelid anomalies in children. J Pediatr Ophthalmol Strabismus 21:140, 1984.

Fox SA: Primary congenital entropion. Arch Ophthalmol 56:839, 1956.

Hiles DA, Wilder LW: Congenital entropion of the upper lids. J Pediatr Ophthalmol 6:157, 1969.

Karlin DB: Congenital entropion, epiblepharon and antimongoloid obliquity of the palpebral fissure. Am J Ophthalmol 56:487, 1956.

Lacrimal Disorders

Calhoun JH: Disorders of the lacrimal apparatus in infancy and childhood. In Nelson LB, Calhoun JH, Harley RD (eds): Pediatric Ophthalmology, ed 3. Philadelphia, Saunders, 1991.

Christian CJ, Nelson LB: Lacrimal system disorders in infants and children. Ophthalmol Clin North Am 3:239, 1990.

El-Mansoury J, Calhoun JH, Nelson LB, Harley RD: Results of late probing for congenital nasolacrimal duct obstruction. Ophthalmology 93:1052, 1986.

Katowitz JA, Kropp TM: Congenital abnormalities of the lacrimal drainage system. In Hornblass A: Oculoplastic, Orbital, and Reconstructive Surgery. Baltimore, Williams & Wilkins, 1990, pp 1397–1416.

Katowitz JA, Welsh MG: Timing of initial probing and irrigation in congenital nasolacrimal duct obstruction. Ophthalmology 94:698, 1987.

Kushner B: Congenital lacrimal system obstruction. Arch Ophthalmol 100:597, 1982.

La Piana FG: Management of occult atretic lacrimal puncta. Am J Ophthalmol 74:332, 1972.

Liebman SD: Ocular manifestations of Riley–Day syndrome. Arch Ophthalmol 56:719, 1956.

Marshall D: Ectodermal dysplasia. Am J Ophthalmol 45:143, 1958.

Nelson LB, Calhoun JH, Menduke H: Medical management of congenital nasolacrimal duct obstruction. Ophthalmology 92:1187, 1985.

Paul TO: Medical management of congenital nasolacrimal duct obstruction. J Pediatr Ophthalmol Strabismus 22:68, 1985.

Petersen RA, Robb RM: The natural course of congenital obstruction of the nasolacrimal duct. J Pediatr Ophthalmol Strabismus 15:246, 1978.

Robb RM: Probing and irrigation for congenital nasolacrimal duct obstruction. Arch Ophthalmol 104:378, 1986.

Sjogren H: The lacrimal secretion in newborn, premature, and fully developed children. Acta Ophthalmol 33:557, 1955.

Sjogren H, Erikson A: Alacrima congenita. Br J Ophthalmol 34:691, 1950.

Lacrimal Sac Mucoceles

Bogan S, Simon JW, Nelson LB, et al: Astigmatism associated with adnexal masses in infancy. Arch Ophthalmol 105:1368, 1987.

Divine RD, Andersen RL, Brumsted RM: Bilateral congenital lacrimal sac mucoceles with nasal extension and drainage. Arch Ophthalmol 101:246, 1983.

Grin TR, Mertz JS, Stass-Isern M: Congenital nasolacrimal duct cysts in dacryocystocele. Ophthalmology 98:1238, 1991.

Hornblass A: Lacrimal evaluation. In Hornblass A: Oculoplastic, Orbital and Reconstructive Surgery. Baltimore, Williams & Wilkins, 1990, pp 1348–1355.

Levy NS: Conservative management of congenital amniotocele of the nasolacrimal sac. J Pediatr Ophthalmol Strabismus 16:254, 1979.

Mansour AM, Cheng KP, Mumma JV, et al: Congenital dacryocele. Ophthalmology 98:1744, 1991.

Scott, WE, Fabre JA, Ossoining KC: Congenital mucocele of the lacrimal sac. Arch Ophthalmol 97:1656, 1979.

Weinstein GS, Biglan AW, Patterson JH: Congenital lacrimal sac mucoceles. Am J Ophthalmol 94:106, 1982.

Leukemia and Lymphoma

Jordan DR, Noel LP, Carpenter BF: Chloroma. Arch Ophthalmol 109:734, 1991.

Rootman J, Robertson W, LaPointe JS, et al: Lymphoproliferative and leukemic lesions. In Rootman J (ed): Diseases of the Orbit. Philadelphia, Lippincott, 1988, p 227.

Rosenthal AR: Ocular manifestations of leukemia: A review. Ophthalmology 90:899, 1983.

Ziegler JL: Burkitt's lymphoma. Cancer 32:144, 1982.

Zimmerman LE, Font RL: Ophthalmologic manifestations of granulocytic sarcoma (myeloid sarcoma or chloroma). Am J Ophthalmol 80:975, 1975.

Lymphangiomas

Dryden RM, Wulc AE, Day D: Eyelid ecchymosis and proptosis in lymphangioma. Am J Ophthalmol 100:486, 1985.

Ileff WS, Green WR: Orbital lymphangiomas. Trans Am Acad Ophthalmol Otolaryngol 86:914, 1979.

Jones IS: Lymphangiomas of the ocular adnexa: An analysis of 62 cases. Trans Am Ophthalmol Soc 57:602, 1959.

Jordan DR, Nerad J, Hansen SO: Case report: Orbital lymphangioma. Ophthalmic Practice 8:242, 1990.

Rootman J, Hay E, Graeb D, et al: Orbital-adnexal lymphangiomas. A spectrum of hemodynamically isolated vascular hamartomas. Ophthalmology 93:1558, 1986.

Shields JA: Diagnosis and Management of Orbital Tumors. Philadelphia, Saunders, 1989.

Wilson ME, Parker PL, Chavis RM: Conservative management of childhood lymphangioma. Ophthalmology 96:484, 1989.

Marcus Gunn Jaw-winking Syndrome

Beard C: Ptosis, ed 4. St. Louis, Mosby, 1991.
Doucet TW, Crawford JS: The quantification, natural course and surgical results in 57 eyes with Marcus Gunn (jaw-winking) syndrome. Am J Ophthalmol 92:702, 1981.
Iliff CE: The optimum time for surgery in the Marcus Gunn phenomenon. Trans Am Acad Ophthalmol Otolaryngol 74:1005, 1970.
Pratt SG, Beyer CK, Johnson CC: The Marcus Gunn phenomenon: A review of 71 cases. Ophthalmol 90:27, 1984.
Sano K: Trigemino-oculomotor synkinesis. Neurologica 1:29, 1959.

Neuroblastoma

Bullock JD, Goldberg SH, Rakes SM, et al: Primary orbital neuroblastoma. Arch Ophthalmol 107:1031, 1989.
Musarella MA, Chan HSL, DeBoer G, et al: Ocular involvement in neuroblastoma: Prognostic implications. Ophthalmology 91:936, 1984.

Optic Nerve Glioma

Davis FA: Primary tumors of the optic nerve (a phenomenon of von Recklinghausen's disease): A clinical and pathologic study with a report of five cases and a review of the literature. Arch Ophthalmol 23:735, 1940.
Hoyt WF, Baghdassarian SA: Optic glioma of childhood. Natural history and rationale for conservative management. Br J Ophthalmol 53:793, 1969.
Lewis RA, Gerson PL, Axelson KA, et al: Von Recklinghausen's neurofibromatosis, II. Incidence of optic gliomata. Ophthalmology 91:929, 1984.
Shields JA: Diagnosis and Management of Orbital Tumors. Philadelphia, Saunders, 1989.
Stern J, Jakobiec FA, Housepian EM: The architecture of optic nerve gliomas with and without neurofibromatosis. Arch Ophthalmol 98:505, 1980.

Orbital Cellulitis

Catalano RA, Smoot CN: Subperiosteal orbital masses in children with orbital cellulitis: Time for a reevaluation? J Pediatr Ophthalmol Strabismus 27:141, 1990.
Char DH, Ablin A, Beckstead J: Histiocystic disorders of the orbit. Ann Ophthalmol 16:867, 1984.
Harris GJ: Subperiosteal abscess of the orbit. Arch Ophthalmol 101:751, 1983.
Hornblass A, Herschorn BJ, Stern K, et al: Orbital abscess. Surv Ophthalmol 29:169, 1984.
Israele V, Nelson JD: Periorbital and orbital cellulitis. Pediatr Infect Dis 6:404, 1987.
Lawless M, Martin F: Orbital cellulitis and preseptal cellulitis in children. Aust NZ J Ophthalmol 14:211, 1986.
Rubin SE, Rubin LG, Zito J, et al: Medical management of subperiosteal orbital abscess in children. J Pediatr Ophthalmol Strabismus 26:21, 1989.
Spires JR, Smith RJH: Bacterial infections of the orbital and periorbital soft tissues in children. Laryngoscope 96:763, 1986.
Steinkuller PG, Jones DB: Preseptal and orbital cellulitis and orbital abscess. In Linberg JV: Oculoplastic and Orbital Emergencies. Norwalk, CT, Appleton & Lange, 1990, pp 51–66.

Orbital Disorders (General)

Krohel GB, Stewart WB, Chavis RM: Orbital Disease: A Practical Approach. New York, Grune & Stratton, 1981.
Krohel GB, Wright JE: Orbital hemorrhage. Am J Ophthalmol 88:254, 1979.
Shields JA, Bakewell B, Augsburger JJ, et al: Space-occupying orbital masses in children. Ophthalmology 93:379, 1986.
Shorr N, Lessner AM, Goldberg RA: Proptosis: A systematic approach to its diagnosis and management. Ophthalmic Pract 8:95, 1990.
Stefanyszyn MA, Harley RD, Penne RB: Disorders of the orbit. In Nelson LB, Calhoun JH, Harley RD: Pediatric Ophthalmology, ed 3. Philadelphia, Saunders, 1991, pp 355–381.

Pseudotumor

Abdul-Rahim AS, Savino PJ: Orbital apex syndrome. In Linberg JV (ed): Oculoplastic and Orbital Emergencies. Norwalk, CT, Appleton & Lange, 1990, pp 125–143.
Barthold HJ, Harvey A, Markoe AM, et al: Treatment of orbital pseudotumors and lymphoma. Am J Clin Oncol 9:527, 1986.
Curtin HD: Pseudotumor. In: Imaging in Ophthalmology, part I. Radiol Clin North Am. 25:583, 1987.
Kennerdell JS, Dresner SC: The nonspecific orbital inflammatory syndromes. Surv Ophthalmol 29:93, 1984.
Kline LB: The Tolosa–Hunt syndrome. Surv Ophthalmol 27:79, 1982.
Kwan ESK, Wolpert SM, Hedges TR, et al: The Tolosa–Hunt syndrome revisited: Not necessarily a diagnosis of exclusion. Am J Radiol 150:413, 1988.
Leone CR Jr, Lloyd WC III: Treatment protocol for orbital inflammatory disease. Ophthalmology 92:1325, 1985.
Mauriello JA, Flanagan JC: Management of orbital inflammatory disease. Surv Ophthalmol 29:104, 1984.
Mottow LS, Jakobiec FA, Smith M: Idiopathic inflammatory orbital pseudotumor in childhood, II. Results of diagnostic tests and biopsies. Ophthalmology 88:565, 1981.
Weber AL, Mikulis DK: Inflammatory disorders of the paraorbital sinuses and their complications. Radiol Clin North Am 25:615, 1987.

Ptosis (Congenital)

Anderson RL, Baumgartner SA: Amblyopia and ptosis. Arch Ophthalmol 98:1068, 1980.
Beard C: Ptosis, ed 4. St. Louis, Mosby, 1991.
Hoyt C, Lambert S: Lids. In Taylor D (ed): Pediatric Ophthalmology. London, Blackwell Scientific, 1990.
Larned DC, Flanagan JC, Nelson LB, et al: The association of congenital ptosis and congenital heart disease. Ophthalmology 93:492, 1986.
Merrian WW, Ellis RD, Helveston EM: Congenital blepharoptosis, anisometropia and amblyopia. Am J Ophthalmol 89:401, 1980.

Rhabdomyosarcoma

Abramson DH, Ellsworth RM, Tretter P, et al: The treatment of orbital rhabdomyosarcoma with irradiation and chemotherapy. Ophthalmology 86:1330, 1979.

Char DH, Norman D: Orbital tumor diagnosis: Imaging techniques. Ophthalmic Forum 3:16, 1985.

Maurer HM, Donaldson M, Gehan EA, et al: The intergroup rhabdomyosarcoma study: Update—November 1978. J Natl Cancer Inst Monograph 56:61, 1981.

Sagerman RH, Tretter P, Ellsworth RM: Orbital rhabdomyosarcoma in children. Trans Am Acad Ophthalmol Otolaryngol 78:602, 1974.

Shields JA: Diagnosis and Management of Orbital Tumors. Philadelphia, Saunders, 1989.

Shields JA: Rhabdomyosarcoma of the orbit. In Hornblass A (ed): Ophthalmic Plastic and Reconstructive Surgery. Baltimore, Williams & Wilkins, 1987.

Weichselbaum RR, Cassady JR, Albert DM, et al: Multimodality management of orbital rhabdomyosarcoma. Int Ophthalmol Clin 20:247, 1980.

Wharam M, Beltangady M, Haye D, et al: Localized orbital rhabdomyosarcoma. An interim report of the intergroup rhabdomyosarcoma study committee. Ophthalmology 94:251, 1987.

Teratoma (Orbital)

Barber JC, Barber LF, Guerry D, et al: Congenital orbital teratoma. Arch Ophthalmol 91:45, 1974.

Chang DF, Dallow RL, Walton DS: Congenital orbital teratoma: Report of a case with visual preservation. J Pediatr Ophthalmol Strabismus 17:88, 1980.

Garden JW, NcManis JC: Congenital orbital–intracranial teratoma with subsequent malignancy: Case report. Br J Ophthalmol 70:111, 1986.

Iele CH, Daves WE, Black SPW: Orbital teratoma. Arch Ophthalmol 96:2093, 1978.

Itanik K, Traboulsi ET, Karim FWA, et al: Conservative surgery in orbital teratoma. Orbit 5:61, 1986.

Levin ML, Leone CR Jr, Kincaid MC: Congenital orbital teratomas. Am J Ophthalmol 102:476, 1986.

DISORDERS OF THE CORNEA

ESSENTIAL INFORMATION FOR PRIMARY CARE PRACTITIONERS

Corneal abnormalities are usually conspicuous. Most adults will readily notice that something is amiss when a child's corneas are cloudy or of abnormal size. Although urgent ophthalmologic evaluation should never be delayed, not all corneal abnormalities are treatable, and not all portend a poor visual prognosis. In this section a few differential findings will be reviewed, to help the nonophthalmologist identify treatable corneal disorders.

Cloudy Cornea(s) in Infancy

The most common corneal abnormality in childhood is a cloudy cornea(s). There are three reasons why the cornea can appear "cloudy." The first two categories encompass losses of clarity due to edema (Fig. 9–1) or ulceration (Fig. 9–2). The third category includes corneas that never developed translucency, those with a congenital opaqueness or opacity.

It is most important to distinguish an edematous or ulcerated cornea from a developmental corneal opacity. Although corneal edema can result from trauma due to forceps injury, a metabolic disease, or a biochemical abnormality of the cornea, it most commonly is a manifestation of glaucoma. Glaucoma is a disorder

caused by, or related to, elevated pressure within the eye. By the time corneal edema arises in infantile glaucoma, the condition is already advanced. Urgent ophthalmologic referral is needed. Chapter 10 is entirely devoted to this subject. It is worth reiterating, however, that glaucoma should be suspected if the infant with a hazy cornea has one or more of the following signs or symptoms: tearing (Fig. 9–3), light sensitivity, eyelid

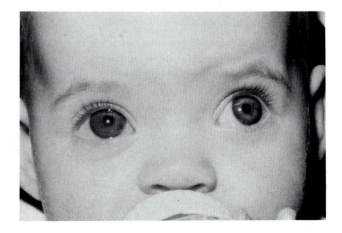

Figure 9–1. Edematous "cloudy" cornea in the right eye secondary to infantile glaucoma.

177

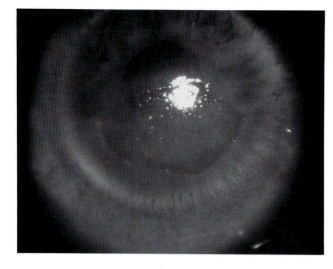

Figure 9–2. Ulcerated "cloudy" cornea due to chronic herpes infection.

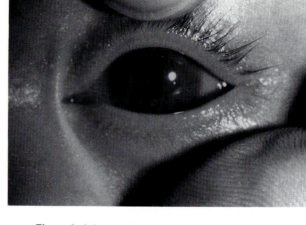

Figure 9–4. Large cloudy cornea in infantile glaucoma.

squeezing, eye rubbing, large eyes or corneas (Fig. 9–4), or red eyes. The diagnosis is confirmed by the presence of elevated ocular pressure, enlarged corneal diameters, and/or optic disc cupping.

Corneal ulcers can be secondary to exposure and desiccation, or to infection (most commonly in infancy due to herpes simplex). These are also treatable conditions, again implying the need for urgent ophthalmologic referral. Although severe cases of corneal edema will result in punctate (point-like) erosions of the surface layer of the cornea, a corneal ulcer should be suspected when there is a large disruption of the corneal surface and minimal or no deeper corneal haze. Large ulcers can be detected by instilling fluorescein dye into the eye and illuminating it with cobalt blue light. A Wood's lamp may be used for illumination (see Chap-

ter 2). Unfortunately, smaller ulcers may be difficult to see without the magnification afforded by a slit lamp. Corneal erosions secondary to desiccation usually occur in association with readily apparent eyelid malformations, which prevent complete closure of the eyelids or a normal blink. These are treated with ocular lubricants and surgery.

Corneal opacities due to developmental dysgenesis are usually nonprogressive. Ophthalmologic referral is required, but not as urgently as with corneal edema or ulceration. These can often be distinguished because there is usually at least some part of the cornea that is clear (Fig. 9–5). There may also be other readily identified developmental anomalies of the eye or other body parts, such as facial clefts (Fig. 9–6) and iris, ear, or skeletal abnormalities.

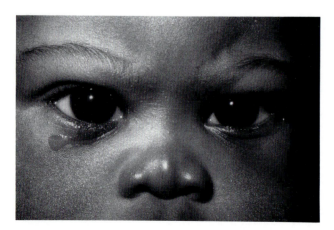

Figure 9–3. Tearing in infantile glaucoma in a child with Down syndrome.

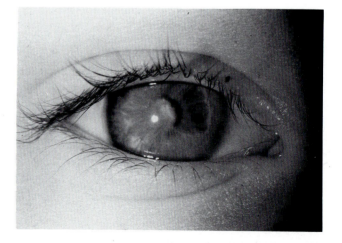

Figure 9–5. Posterior corneal opacity in Peter's anomaly. Note the iris strands extending to the edge of the opacity, and the area of clear cornea.

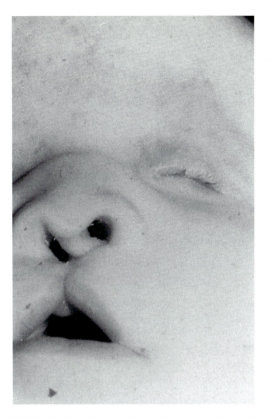

Figure 9–6. Midfacial cleft in a patient with small, maldeveloped eyes (microphthalmos).

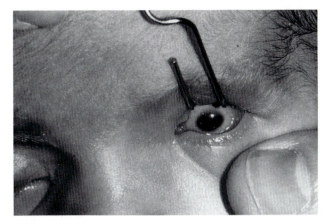

Figure 9–8. Microphthalmos. The entire eye is small.

Abnormally Sized Corneas

The average horizontal diameter of the newborn cornea is 10 mm. By 2 years of age it has grown to 11.75 mm, approaching the average adult diameter. In a newborn, a corneal diameter less than 10 mm is called microcornea; a diameter greater than 12 mm is called megalocornea.

Microcornea can occur as an isolated abnormality (Fig. 9–7) or in association with other ocular malforma-

tions. The term "microphthalmos" (Fig. 9–8) is used when the entire globe, not just the cornea, is small. Ultrasonography can differentiate the two. Either may be associated with a variety of other ocular abnormalities (Fig. 9–9). Autosomal dominant, recessive, and sporadic cases of microcornea and microphthalmos have been described.

Megalocornea can also present as an isolated abnormality (Fig. 9–10) or can be associated with other ocular dysgenesis (Fig. 9–11). When all of the structures of the anterior eye are enlarged, the term "anterior megalophthalmos" is used.

Corneal Dystrophies and Degenerations

Corneal dystrophies are rare heritable diseases. They are caused by localized, probably biochemical, abnormalities of the cornea, and have no associated systemic

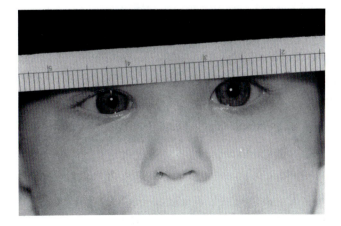

Figure 9–7. Microcornea. A small cornea, but otherwise normal eye.

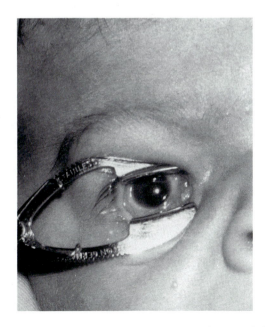

Figure 9–9. Microphthalmic eye with a coloboma (a congenital cleft in the inferior eye due to incomplete closure of the fetal fissure).

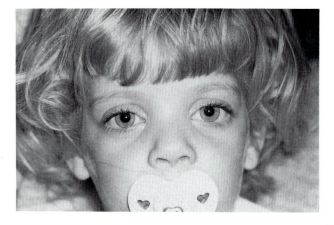

Figure 9–10. Megalocorneas. Large corneas, but otherwise normal eyes.

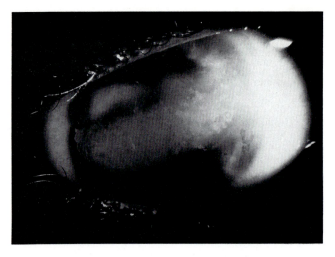

Figure 9–12. Band keratopathy in a child with juvenile rheumatoid arthritis, characterized by calcium deposit extending in a band across the anterior cornea.

findings. Usually bilateral, they are characterized by a slow but progressive loss of corneal transparency, beginning several years after birth. Examples include granular, macular, lattice, and Reis–Bucklers' dystrophy. Keratoconus and keratoglobus are usually classified as ectatic corneal dystrophies. Visual loss can result in the latter stages of most dystrophies, necessitating corneal transplantation.

Corneal degenerations result secondary to other ocular or systemic disorders. Most present in adulthood, but a few can arise in childhood or adolescence. They are not heritable and are often unilateral or asymmetric. Examples of corneal degenerations in children include band keratopathy (Fig. 9–12) and the corneal changes in primary and secondary infantile glaucoma.

COMPREHENSIVE INFORMATION ON CORNEAL DISORDERS

Cloudy Cornea(s) in Infancy

The differential diagnosis of a cloudy cornea in infancy is presented in Table 9–1. In developing this differential it is important to recognize that different corneal abnormalities can all be perceived as "cloudiness" to the untrained eye. These include corneal edema, corneal ulcers (disruption of the epithelial covering of the cornea), and developmental anomalies in which part or most of the cornea is opaque rather than translucent. If one can differentiate between edematous, ulcerated, and opaque cornea the differential diagnosis can be greatly reduced. The "cloudiness" in the first five disorders in Table 9–1 is primarily due to corneal edema. The "cloudiness" in the next three is due to ulcerated cornea, and the final six due to opaque cornea or corneal opacities. These will be discussed in order.

Corneal Cloudiness Due to Edema

Prompt referral is required when corneal edema is detected, because this almost always means glaucoma, which is treatable. The presence of elevated ocular pressure and/or optic nerve damage (Figs. 9–13 and 10–6) distinguishes glaucoma from the other causes of cloudy corneas in infancy. The glaucoma may be either primary (due to an isolated anomaly of the drainage system of the eye) or secondary (due to an associated ocular or systemic abnormality). In the early stages of **primary infantile (congenital) glaucoma,** especially in older infants, the cornea may not be cloudy. The presence of corneal edema suggests more advanced disease, requiring prompt treatment. A triad of findings of tearing, light sensitivity, and eyelid squeezing in-

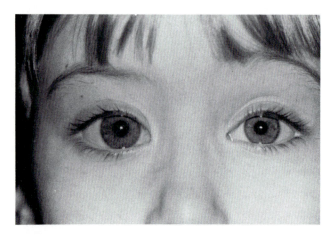

Figure 9–11. Pseudo-megalocornea (right eye). A secondarily enlarged cornea due to arrested infantile glaucoma.

TABLE 9–1. DIFFERENTIAL DIAGNOSIS OF A CLOUDY CORNEA IN INFANCY

Diagnosis	Laterality	Ocular Pressure	Other Findings
▪ **CORNEAL EDEMA**			
Infantile glaucoma	Bilateral > Unilateral (2:1)	Elevated	Tearing, light sensitivity, enlarged cornea
Forceps injury	Unilateral	Normal	Forceps markings on skin, possible intraocular hemorrhage
Congenital hereditary endothelial dystrophy	Bilateral	Normal	Autosomal recessive, stromal edema, cornea thickened
Congenital rubella	Bilateral	Normal or elevated	Eye may be small, with cataract and/or retinal pigment mottling
Congenital syphilis	Bilateral	Normal	Intraocular inflammation within first 30 days of life, late corneal vascularization
▪ **CORNEAL ULCER**			
Exposure	Unilateral or bilateral	Normal	Eyelid abnormalities, central corneal ulcer
Dysautonomia (Riley–Day syndrome)	Bilateral	Normal	Corneal hypesthesia, decreased tear formation, failure to thrive, insensitivity to pain, Jewish predilection, autosomal recessive
Herpes simplex infection	Unilateral	Normal	Epithelial (surface) defect which stains with fluorescein dye
▪ **CORNEAL OPACITY**			
Peter's anomaly	Unilateral or bilateral	Normal or elevated	Central opacity, iris strands may extend to the margins of the opacity
Sclerocornea	Unilateral or bilateral	Normal or elevated	Cornea blends with the sclera, clearest centrally, cornea appears flat
Dermoid	Unilateral or bilateral	Normal	White mass, more often located temporally, may contain hair
Congenital hereditary stromal dystrophy	Bilateral	Normal	Autosomal dominant, flaky, feathery opacities in the corneal stroma, normal corneal thickness, not progressive
Mucopolysaccharidosis, mucolipidosis	Bilateral	Normal	Rarely present at birth, progressive, majority are autosomal dominant
Cystinosis	Bilateral	Normal	Cystine crystals in the cornea and conjunctiva, failure to thrive, rickets, progressive renal failure, autosomal recessive

creases the suspicion of this disorder, but only about one third of affected infants develop this classic symptom complex. **Secondary glaucomas** are associated with certain congenital anomalies (such as Peter's anomaly or sclerocornea), phakomatoses, metabolic diseases, inflammatory disease (for example, congenital rubella), mitotic diseases (such as retinoblastoma), and chromosomal abnormalities (such as Down syndrome) (see Fig. 9–3). These disorders are more fully discussed in Chapter 10.

Forceps injury to the cornea can also give rise to corneal edema. Distinguishing features include unilaterality, presence at birth, absence of elevated ocular pressure, localization of the edema to the area of corneal damage, vertical orientation of a white ridge (where the tear in Descemet's membrane of the inner

cornea occurred), and the presence of periorbital skin injuries that align with the corneal tear (see Fig. 10–16). This injury may induce a large astigmatism in an infant, which if untreated with spectacles or contact lenses can result in a permanent reduction of central visual acuity.

Congenital hereditary dystrophy (CHED) is a disorder in which the cornea, including the corneal epithelium, is diffusely edematous and thick. This may be noticed at birth or soon thereafter. It is differentiated from congenital glaucoma by the absence of elevated ocular pressure and absence of an increased corneal diameter. Corneal transplantation is the definitive treatment.

Congenital **syphilis** and **rubella** can also account for corneal edema in infancy. In addition to transient

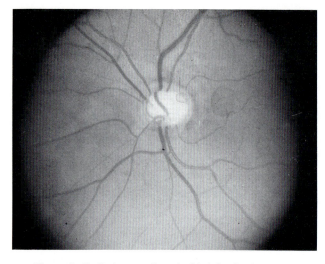

Figure 9–13. Optic nerve "cupping" in infantile glaucoma.

corneal edema, both are characterized by intraocular inflammation (uveitis) within the first 30 days of life. Additional signs of congenital syphilis will develop as the child grows. These include a saddle nose, bossing of the frontal bones, poor development of the maxilla (Fig. 9–14), anterior bowing of the tibias, and "Hutchinson's teeth." The latter maldevelopment of the permanent dentition consists of widely spaced, centrally notched upper incisors, tapered like screwdrivers. Additional findings in congenital rubella syndrome are described below. The treatment for syphilis is systemic steroids; for rubella topical cycloplegics (drugs that temporarily put the ciliary muscle at rest, dilating the pupil and paralyzing accommodation) and corticosteroids are used.

Corneal Cloudiness Due to Ulcerated Cornea

The corneas can become desiccated and subsequently ulcerate if **congenital anomalies of the eyelids** (see Chapter 7) prevent reflex closure of the cornea. A congenital sensory neuropathy of the cornea can cause similar findings in the absence of lid anomalies. Most notable is the **Riley–Day syndrome** (dysautonomia). These infants, of predominantly Jewish descent, have both corneal hypesthesia and decreased tear function, resulting in frequent corneal epithelial breakdown. Failure to thrive, insensitivity to pain, and the absence of fungiform papillae on the tongue are additional findings. "Exposed" corneas are treated with artificial tears and lubricants, soft contact lenses, collagen shields, or surgery to correct an eyelid malformation.

Herpes simplex keratitis is the most common cause of corneal ulceration seen in developed countries. The virus can be transmitted perinatally, by passage through an infected birth canal. Infected neonates can develop vesicular skin lesions (Fig. 9–15), perioral ulcers, and infection of the cornea and conjunctiva. In two thirds of cases, dissemination to the liver, adrenal glands, lungs, and central nervous system occurs; mortality in disseminated cases may be as high as 80%. Corneal ulcers (dendritic, Fig. 9–16; geographic, Fig. 9–17; or punctate) may occur; massive yellow-white retinal exudation may develop, and a cataract may form.

In the absence of a perinatal infection, it is very unusual for a herpes infection to present during the first 3 months of life. This is due to the protection afforded by maternal antibodies against the virus. After this period infection likely occurs readily following close contact with someone with an active herpetic lesion. The primary infection is inapparent in most children. Although the majority do not develop obvious herpetic lesions, by 5 years of age over 90 percent of children have developed antibodies to herpes simplex, confirming that exposure and infection did occur. When manifest, primary ocular herpetic disease presents with a herpetic lid lesion, with or without conjunctival and corneal involvement.

Recurrent herpes simplex ocular infection often presents as a "red eye." Precipitating influences include stress, upper respiratory infection, fever, sunburn, and minor trauma. A primary care physician

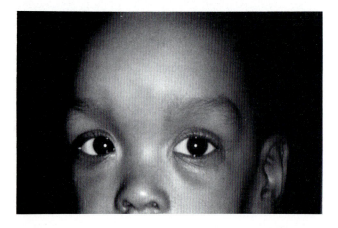

Figure 9–14. Facies of congenital syphilis characterized by frontal bossing, saddle nose, and maxillary hypoplasia. *(From Calalano RA: Ocular Emergencies. Philadelphia, Saunders, 1992, p 251, with permission.)*

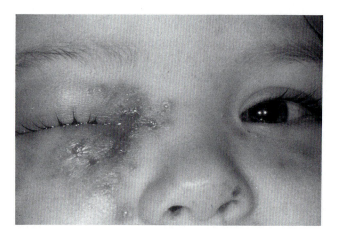

Figure 9–15. Herpetic skin lesions. Note the clear vesicles and crusting.

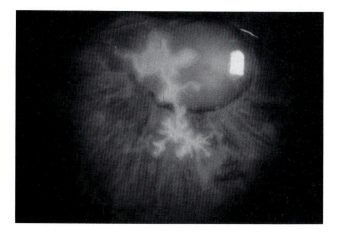

Figure 9–16. Dendritic ulcer secondary to herpes simplex infection. *(From Catalano RA: Ocular Emergencies. Philadelphia, Saunders, 1992, p 480, with permission.)*

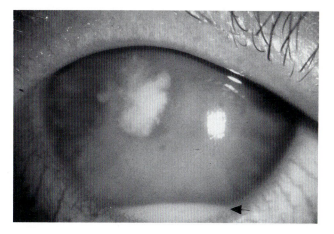

Figure 9–18. Staphylococcal corneal ulcer characterized by corneal infiltrate, cloudy cornea, and hypopyon (layering of inflammatory cells in the anterior chamber of the eye—*arrow*). *(From Catalano RA: Ocular Emergencies. Philadelphia, Saunders, 1992, p 477, with permission.)*

should instill fluorescein dye into the conjunctival sac and examine the eye with either a Wood's lamp (see Chapter 2) or blue-filtered penlight. Corneal ulceration will appear bright green; its shape can be dendritic, geographic, or punctate. Unfortunately, it is often difficult to detect small ulcers without the use of a slit lamp. Treatment with an antibiotic is ineffective; treatment with a corticosteroid can markedly exacerbate the herpes infection. Ophthalmologic referral should be requested for slit-lamp examination in any child with a red eye unresponsive to medication. Corticosteroids should never be used unless a herpetic infection has been ruled out. The mainstay of treatment is debridement of a corneal dendrite, and topical application of an antiviral agent (for example, Vira A ointment five times per day).

Bacterial infections (Figs. 9–18 and 9–19) are less

common causes of corneal ulceration in infants. Another infrequent cause is severe burns secondary to the instillation of an excessive concentration of **silver nitrate** or the inappropriate use of a caustic silver nitrate stick, for ocular prophylaxis against *Neisseria gonorrhoeae.* This cause should rank high on the differential of corneal ulcers appearing within the first 24 hours of life. Conjunctival edema (chemosis) is an associated finding.

Corneal Cloudiness Due to Opaque Corneal or Corneal Opacities

A host of developmental abnormalities of the anterior eye have been described. Reese and Ellsworth (1966) first used the term **anterior chamber cleavage syndrome** to describe them, and Waring and associates (1975) categorized them in a stepladder fashion, clari-

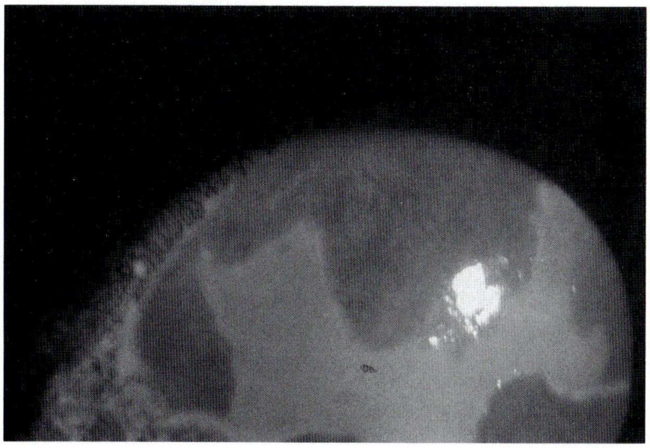

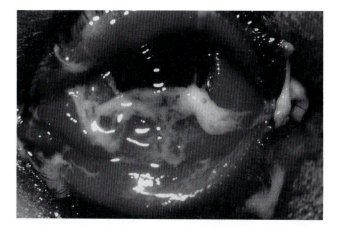

Figure 9–17. Geographic ulcer secondary to herpes simplex infection.

Figure 9–19. *Neisseria gonorrhoeae* infection characterized by marked purulent conjunctival exudation. Untreated this infection can lead to corneal perforation and blindness. *(From Catalano RA: Ocular Emergencies. Philadelphia, Saunders, 1992, p 465, with permission.)*

fying that these disorders represent a continuum of increasing dysgenesis. Because many of these disorders may have developmental glaucoma they are reviewed in Chapter 10. Central anterior chamber cleavage abnormalities deserve mention here, however, as they are more likely to be associated with corneal opacity.

The latter group of abnormalities share a basic abnormality of the posterior surface of the cornea. In each, the central corneal endothelium and Descemet's membrane are either attenuated or absent, and a corneal opacity overlies this defect. **Peter's anomaly** is the most common dysgenesis in this group (see Figs. 9–5 and 9–20). The simplest form of Peter's anomaly is characterized solely by a defect in the posterior cornea inducing an overlying opacity. Greater dysgenesis is characterized by an adherence of iris strands to the edge of the posterior defect, adhesion of the lens to the posterior corneal defect, and central cataract formation. Over 80 percent of the time Peter's anomaly is bilateral; glaucoma is associated in approximately half the cases. Although most cases are the result of developmental dysgenesis, it has been postulated that some may be secondary to intrauterine inflammation. The latter is suggested by congenital vascularization of the opacity.

Sclerocornea is the term used to describe a developmental dysgenesis of the cornea (Fig. 9–21). In place of translucent cornea, "scleral-like" tissue develops. Instead of clearly demarcated cornea, white, feathery, often ill-defined and vascularized tissue develops in the peripheral cornea, appearing to blend with and extend from the sclera. The central cornea is usually clearer, but rare cases of total replacement of the cornea with sclera have been reported. The entire corneal periphery, or only a small arc, may be involved. The clear cornea that does exist is usually flatter than normal. Potentially coexisting abnormalities include a shallow anterior chamber, iris abnormalities, and microphthalmos. Associated skeletal, chromosomal, and cen-

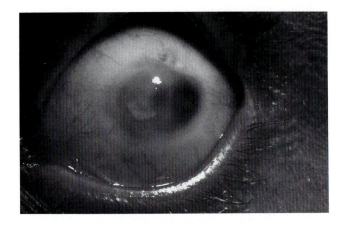

Figure 9–21. Sclerocornea.

tral nervous system abnormalities have been described, but there are no invariable systemic findings.

Dermoids are benign tumors composed of tissues normally not found in the involved area. Corneal dermoids appear as solid, pink-white, round masses. They are usually solitary and small (<5 mm in diameter), and are commonly located at the junction of the cornea and sclera (the limbus) (Fig. 9–22). Occasionally they are multiple, large, and/or located entirely within the cornea. Histologically, they are composed of fibrofatty tissue covered by keratinized epithelium; they can contain hair follicles, sebaceous glands, and sweat glands.

If the dermoid is small and located over the limbus, it usually does not affect visual acuity. Visual impairment occurs when the dermoid encroaches on the visual axis or induces an astigmatism. In these instances surgical excision should be considered.

One third of infants with corneal dermoids will be

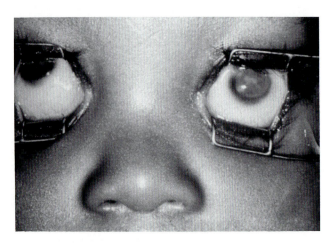

Figure 9–20. Bilateral Peter's anomaly.

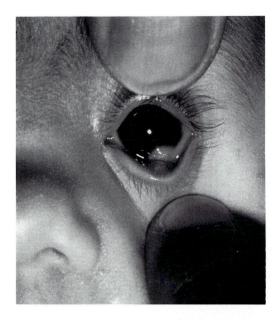

Figure 9–22. Corneal dermoid in the inferior cornea.

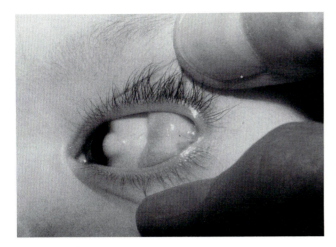

Figure 9–23. Corneal dermoid and subconjunctival lipodermoid in the same eye of a patient with Goldenhar's syndrome.

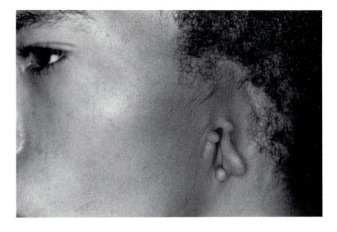

Figure 9–25. Maldeveloped, posteriorly placed ear in a patient with Goldenhar's syndrome.

found to have additional developmental abnormalities. The most common association is **Goldenhar's syndrome,** characterized by ocular dermoids, preauricular appendages, and vertebral abnormalities. The ocular dermoids in this syndrome include the corneal dermoids described above, which are usually located in the inferotemporal quadrant, and subconjunctival lipodermoids, which are usually located in the superotemporal quadrant (Fig. 9–23). The latter are white, soft, fleshy masses composed of fatty tissue. They can be covered with keratinized epithelium, and can contain hair follicles. Additional ocular findings in this syndrome include Duane's syndrome (see Chapter 6), lacrimal duct stenosis, and colobomas of the upper eyelid at the junction of the inner and middle third.

Auricular anomalies in Goldenhar's syndrome include preauricular appendages (Fig. 9–24), small and/or posteriorly placed ears (Fig. 9–25), and stenosis of the external auditory meatus. Vertebral anomalies include fused cervical vertebrae and spina bifida. Dental anomalies and facial malformations can also occur.

Congenital hereditary stromal dystrophy (CHSD) is a disorder in which flaky, feathery opacities develop in the corneal stroma (Fig. 9–26). These can be manifest at birth. Unlike CHED and congenital glaucoma, corneal and epithelial edema are not present, and the cornea is not thickened. Because this disorder is heritable (often autosomal dominant), family members should be examined.

Readily detectable corneal opacities develop in most of the **mucopolysaccharidoses** (disorders of carbohydrate metabolism; MPS) and **mucolipidoses** (disorders of glycoprotein catabolism). The cornea is usually clear at birth, but progressively becomes diffusely cloudy, starting peripherally. In only a few of the disorders are the opacities apparent early in life. These are MPS I-H (Hurler syndrome), MPS I-S (Scheie's syndrome), gangliosidosis I, and mucolipidoses type IV. In

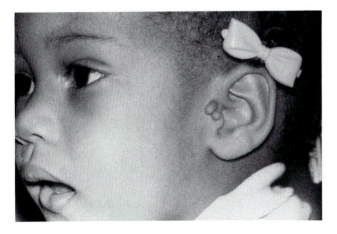

Figure 9–24. Periauricular appendages in a patient with Goldenhar's syndrome.

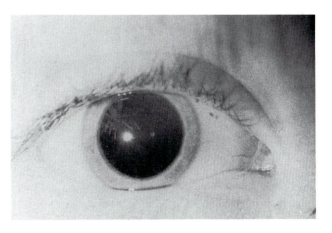

Figure 9–26. Congenital hereditary stromal dystrophy.

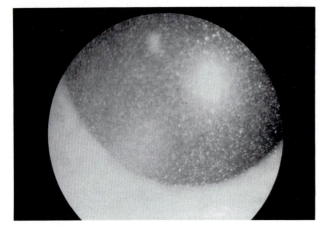

Figure 9–27. Cornea in cystinosis. *(Courtesy of John W. Simon.)*

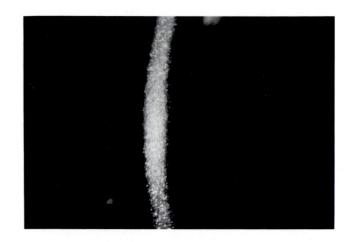

Figure 9–28. Slit-lamp view of the cornea in cystinosis (same eye as in Figure 9–27) demonstrating thin needle-like crystals throughout the entire thickness of the cornea. *(Courtesy of John W. Simon.)*

the other metabolic diseases, systemic findings are present by the time corneal opacification appears. In contrast to the corneal edema seen in infantile glaucoma, the corneal epithelium is smooth and unedematous in metabolic disease. Associated systemic findings include psychomotor retardation and musculoskeletal and visceral abnormalities. The diagnosis is made by urinalysis, or by electronmicroscopic examination of a conjunctival biopsy.

Cystinosis is a rare metabolic disorder in which the amino acid cystine cannot be transported across lysosomal membranes and accumulates in tissues as crystals. Three forms exist, the most common of which is the infantile or nephropathic form. Within the first year of life affected infants show signs of failure to thrive, rickets, and progressive renal failure (Fanconi's syndrome). Affected infants usually have blond hair and a fair complexion. By 6 to 15 months of age, needle-like, iridescent crystals begin to appear throughout the entire thickness of the cornea (Figs. 9–27 and 9–28). Their presence results in photophobia and reduced visual acuity. Cystine crystals also deposit in various other tissues of the body, including the conjunctiva. A peripheral pigmentary retinopathy also develops within the first year of life (Fig. 9–29). The two other subtypes of this disorder have a later onset and milder symptoms. In each, conjunctival biopsy may be diagnostic.

Abnormally Sized Corneas

Small Corneas

Microcornea can be isolated or associated with other deformities of the anterior eye including Peter's anomaly and aniridia (see Chapter 10). It may also accompany congenital cataracts, particularly in eyes with persistent hyperplastic primary vitreous (see Chapter 11).

Microphthalmos can be a part of numerous systemic syndromes of genetic, environmental, or un-

known cause. Autosomal dominant, recessive, and X-linked disorders, as well as chromosomal disorders have been described in which microphthalmos is one component. The same can be said for presumed viral embryopathies due to cytomegalovirus, rubella, herpes virus, and Epstein–Barr virus, and fetal irradiation. Two systemic syndromes of unknown etiology are also characterized by microphthalmos. The first is Hallermann–Streiff syndrome, which is further characterized by a bird-like facies, dental anomalies, and congenital cataracts. The second is the CHARGE association, an acronym for *C*olobomatous microphthalmos, *H*eart defects, choanal *A*tresia, *R*etarded growth, *G*enital anomalies, and *E*ar anomalies or deafness.

As in the latter syndrome, microphthalmos is often associated with ocular coloboma (a congenital cleft in the eye due to failure of the fetal fissure to completely close; Fig. 9–30). A multitude of other ocular abnormalities are also associated with microphthalmos. An ex-

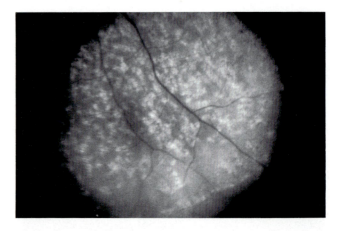

Figure 9–29. Peripheral pigmentary retinopathy in cystinosis. Cystine crystals accumulate predominantly in the retinal pigment epithelium. (Courtesy of John W. Simon.)

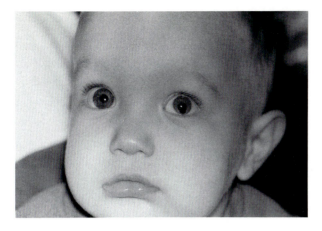

Figure 9–30. Unilateral microphthalmos and coloboma, left eye.

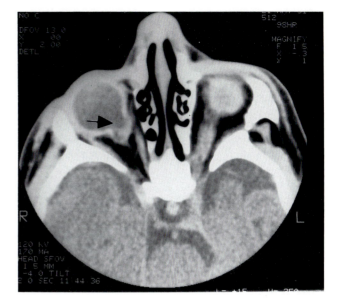

Figure 9–32. Computed tomogram demonstrating microphthalmos with cyst in the right eye (*arrow*). The plane is not true axial; the inferior globe and inferior rectus is seen in the left orbit. *(From Catalano RA: Ocular Emergencies. Philadelphia, Saunders, 1992, p 70, with permission.)*

ample is congenital rubella syndrome. In addition to microphthalmos, these eyes may have chronic inflammation of the iris and ciliary body, congenital cataracts, glaucoma, iris hypoplasia, corneal opacification, and a salt-and-pepper type retinopathy (Fig. 9–31).

Microphthalmos with cyst occurs due to a fault in the embryonic development of the eye. The cyst is apparent as a bluish, fluctuant mass under the lower eyelid attached to a variably sized globe above (Fig. 9–32).

Nanophthalmos denotes that the entire eye is smaller than normal, but without substantial structural abnormality. High hyperopia (farsightedness) is usually present due to the reduced anteroposterior diameter of the eye. Later in life these eyes are susceptible to developing angle-closure glaucoma, uveal effusion syndrome, and exudative retinal detachment.

Large Corneas

Isolated (simple) megalocornea is a bilateral, heritable, and nonprogressive condition. There is no corneal edema, and it does not result in visual loss. **Anterior**

megalophthalmos is a disorder in which abnormalities in the iris, anterior chamber angle, and ciliary body are associated with congenital, nonprogressive, symmetrically enlarged corneas. Most cases are inherited as an X-linked recessive disorder; occasionally megalophthalmos is a feature of Marfan syndrome (see Chapter 11).

A common complication of megalophthalmos is subluxation of the ocular lens (Fig. 9–33). This occurs because the normal sized lens can not be held in place by the enlarged ciliary body. The anterior stroma of the iris may be hypoplastic; it may also transilluminate. Vision in adults is threatened by a high incidence of glau-

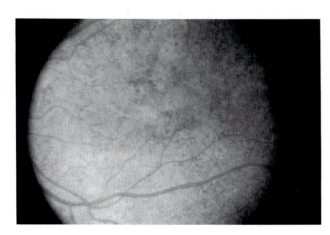

Figure 9–31. "Salt-and-pepper" retinopathy of congenital rubella.

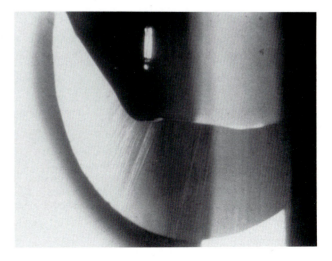

Figure 9–33. Lens subluxation in anterior megalophthalmos.

TABLE 9–2. DIFFERENTIATION OF CORNEAL DISORDERS IN INFANTS AND CHILDREN

Congenital Anomaly	Corneal Degeneration	Corneal Dystrophy
Developmental malformation	Secondary to other ocular or systemic disease or disorder	Localized biochemical abnormality without systemic associations
Evident at birth	Can be congenital, but most become apparent after infancy	Most become apparent several years after birth
Most are bilateral, can be asymmetric	Often unilateral or very asymmetric	Bilateral and symmetric
Variable heritable patterns	Variable heritable patterns	Autosomal dominant (most)
Most nonprogressive	Slowly progressive (most)	Very slowly progressive
Can involve the entire eye	Peripheral cornea primarily involved	Central cornea primarily involved
Avascular	Vascular (many)	Avascular

coma, the lens subluxation, and the early development of cataracts. These complications rarely present in childhood.

Megalocornea and anterior megalophthalmos are more likely than infantile glaucoma to be present at birth, bilateral, symmetric, and nonprogressive. They are also asymptomatic.

Corneal Degenerations and Dystrophies

Although it is useful to categorize corneal disorders by signs such as cloudiness or abnormal size (as above), learned reviews usually categorize corneal abnormalities into congenital anomalies, corneal degenerations, or corneal dystrophies (Table 9–2). The differentiation of the three categories relates to the age at which they present, etiology, bilaterality, heritability, propensity to progress, and association with other ocular or systemic findings. Table 9–3 lists common corneal disorders in children by classification. The congenital anomalies were discussed earlier in the chapter; corneal degenerations and dystrophies will now be reviewed.

Corneal Degenerations

The term corneal degeneration is used to denote a change or abnormality in the cornea brought about by an extrinsic ocular or systemic disorder. An example is **infantile glaucoma,** in which the corneal changes (edema, increased size, breaks in Descemet's membrane) occur as a result of elevated ocular pressure. Other degenerations result from abnormal deposits or accumulations within the cornea due to inborn errors in metabolism. A few degenerations are secondary to infectious diseases, environmental exposure, or trauma. Although a great many corneal degenerations have been described, this review will be limited to only those commonly found in infants or children. Infantile glaucoma is reviewed earlier in this chapter and in Chapter 10.

Band keratopathy denotes calcium deposition in the region of the cornea between the eyelid fissures. The peripheral cornea, at the 3:00 and 9:00 positions, is most involved; but the deposit may extend in an arc across the central cornea (see Fig. 9–12). Tiny translucent areas devoid of calcium are usually visible, corresponding to sites where nerves penetrate the cornea. This gives the band a Swiss-cheese-like appearance. In children, band keratopathy is most commonly secondary to chronic inflammation and iritis due to juvenile rheumatoid arthritis. Less common causes include hyperparathyroidism, vitamin D intoxication, renal

TABLE 9–3. COMMON CORNEAL DISORDERS IN CHILDREN BY CLASSIFICATION

Congenital Anomalies	Corneal Degenerations	Corneal Dystrophies
Microcornea	Primary and secondary infantile glaucoma	Cogan's
Microphthalmos	Keratectasia	Meesmann's
Nanophthalmos	Band keratopathy	Reis–Bucklers'
Megalocornea	Wilson's Disease	Granular
Anterior megalophthalmos	Arcus juvenilis	Macular
Anterior chamber	Fabry's disease	Lattice
cleavage syndrome	Mucolipidoses	Schnyder's
Sclerocornea	Mucopolysaccharidoses	Congenital hereditary stromal
Dermoids		Congenital hereditary endothelial
		Posterior polymorphous
		Keratoconus
		Keratoglobus

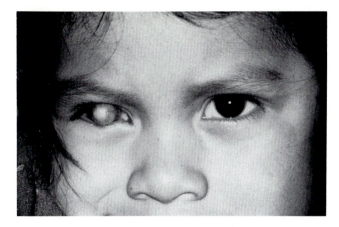

Figure 9–34. Keratectasia of the right eye secondary to intrauterine infection.

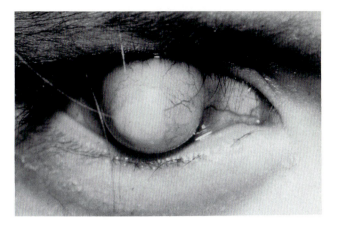

Figure 9–35. Close-up of the right eye in Figure 9–34. Note the opaque, metaplastic cornea.

failure, sarcoidosis, and sequelae to a severe alkali burn. Chelating agents are used to strip the deposits from the cornea, but they may recur if the underlying disorder is not controlled.

Keratectasia describes a bulging, thin, opaque, metaplastic cornea that presents at birth. The cornea is usually greatly enlarged and protrudes through the palpebral fissures (Figs. 9–34 and 9–35). Most cases are believed to result secondary to an intrauterine corneal infection, but some may be secondary to a developmental dysgenesis. Corneal tissue becomes metaplastic, resembling skin. Only the cornea is involved, and most cases are unilateral.

Wilson's disease (hepatolenticular degeneration) results from a deficiency in cerruloplasmin, the copper binding serum protein. Copper accumulates throughout the body, but particularly in the cornea, basal ganglia, liver, and kidneys. Symptoms include ataxia and progressive neurological impairment. Signs include hepatosplenomegaly and a Kayser–Fleischer ring in the peripheral cornea. This ring is 1 to 3 mm wide and begins right at the limbus (the junction of the cornea and sclera; Fig. 9–36). Unlike most peripheral corneal deposits there is no interval of clear cornea before the deposition begins. The ring may be brown, red, blue, green, or any mixture of these colors. In most affected individuals it appears around 10 years of age; it disappears upon treatment with chelating agents and dietary restriction. An associated ocular finding is anterior subcapsular cataracts. These have been called "sunflower cataracts" because of their characteristic color and petaloid shape.

Arcus juvenilis results secondary to elevated blood cholesterol levels. Similar to the disorder seen in older adults, cholesterol deposits in the peripheral cornea. It is distinctive in arising during the early teen years. Even with regulation of the blood cholesterol level the corneal deposits remain, but being peripheral they do not affect vision.

Fabry's disease is a lipid storage disease that often presents in childhood with the appearance of characteristic corneal changes. Lipid deposits in a whorl pattern radiating from the central to the peripheral cornea. Fabry's disease is an X-linked recessive disorder. Vision is unaffected and there is no known treatment. Cardiovascular, renal, gastrointestinal, and central nervous system complications (hemiplegia, cerebellar disorders, and strokes) occur in middle adult years.

The **mucolipidoses** and **mucopolysaccharidoses** are heritable metabolic disorders resulting from deficiencies in lysosomal enzymes. They are characterized by excessive accumulations of sphingolipids, glycolipids, and mucopolysaccharides in the eye, brain, viscera, and skin, and by musculoskeletal syndromes. Ocular manifestations vary by syndrome, but include corneal deposits (Fig. 9–37), a "cherry red spot" in the retina (Fig. 9–38), spoke-like cataracts, glaucoma, optic atrophy, and retinal degeneration. Systemic manifesta-

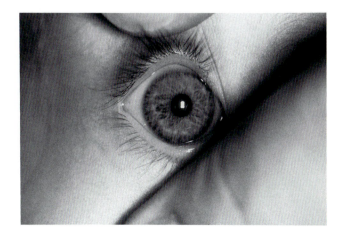

Figure 9–36. Wilson's disease. Note the peripheral corneal ring of copper, which begins at the limbus.

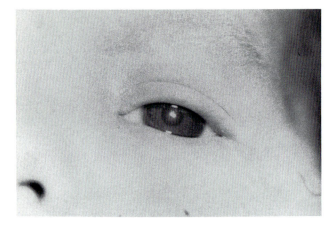

Figure 9–37. Cloudy cornea in a young infant with Hurler syndrome (mucopolysaccharidosis I-H).

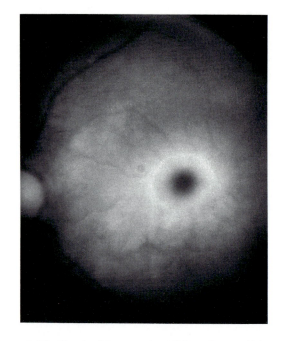

Figure 9–38. Macular "cherry red spot" in a 5-year-old boy with generalized gangliosidoses (G_{M1}). This appearance is due to lipid deposition in the retina surrounding the fovea.

tions also vary by syndrome, but include psychomotor retardation, hepatomegaly, gargoyle-like facies, small stature, scoliosis, short neck, thickened tongue, hypertrophic gums, and thickened skin. Most are inherited as autosomal recessive traits. With the exception of the four disorders mentioned under the earlier discussion of cloudy corneas in infancy, the systemic aspects of these disorders are evident by the time corneal opacities develop.

Corneal Dystrophies

Corneal dystrophies are localized disorders without systemic associations. Each arises secondary to a probable unique biochemical abnormality. They are bilateral and symmetric, with a predilection for the central cornea. Most dystrophies are heritable as autosomal dominant traits and are very slowly progressive. Although they occasionally present in childhood, most are not detected until adolescence or adulthood.

Most reviewers classify the dystrophies according to the level of the cornea involved: anterior cornea, stroma, or posterior cornea (Table 9–4). Keratoconus and keratoglobus are classified as ectactic dystrophies.

This categorization is useful in relating symptoms and signs in the different dystrophies. Anterior dystrophies are associated with recurrent corneal erosions and ocular irritation, stromal dystrophies with more markedly reduced vision, and posterior dystrophies with corneal edema and thickening. A multitude of corneal dystrophies have been described. Some are very rare, and found in only one family line. The more common disorders, particularly those likely to present in childhood, are reviewed below.

Anterior Dystrophies. Cogan's microcytic (map-dot-fingerprint) dystrophy is the most common corneal dystrophy, but only rarely presents in childhood. It is characterized by the presence of microcysts and fine, geographic appearing "map" and "fingerprint"

TABLE 9–4. CORNEAL DYSTROPHIES BY ANATOMIC LOCATION

Classification	Anatomic Level	Symptoms/Signs	Examples
Anterior	Epithelium, basement membrane, Bowman's membrane	Pain and foreign body sensation secondary to recurrent erosions, blurred vision	Cogan's, Meesmann's, and Reis–Bucklers' dystrophies
Stromal	Stroma	Reduced vision, recurrent erosions (lattice dystrophy)	Granular, macular, lattice, Schnyder's, and congenital hereditary stromal dystrophies
Posterior	Descemet's membrane, endothelium	Corneal edema, corneal thickening	Congenital hereditary endothelial and posterior polymorphous dystrophies
Ectactic	Bowman's membrane, stroma, Descemet's membrane	Blurred vision, corneal thinning	Keratoconus and keratoglobus dystrophies

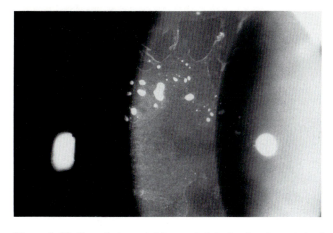

Figure 9–39. Cogan's (map-dot-fingerprint) dystrophy, characterized by dots; the small, sharply defined opacities; and maps, which are larger, lighter, and more diffuse. *(From Catalano RA: Ocular Emergencies. Philadelphia, Saunders, 1992, p 245, with permission.)*

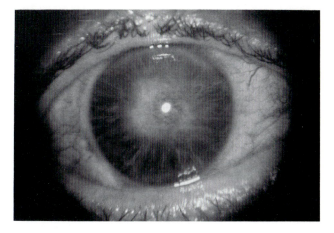

Figure 9–41. Reis–Bucklers' dystrophy, characterized by gray white opacification in the central cornea.

lines in the epithelial layer (Fig. 9–39). It results from an abnormality in epithelial maturation and turnover, associated with an abnormal production of basement membrane. The abnormal epithelial layer is prone to recurrent erosions, resulting in ocular discomfort and transient blurring of vision. These erosions are more likely to begin in the middle years, but can start in childhood or adolescence. Treatments include lubricating drops and ointments, 5 percent sodium chloride ointment at night, patching, bandage contact lenses, epithelial scraping, and anterior stromal puncture.

Meesmann's dystrophy is a rare disorder, which becomes manifest by 3 to 4 years of age. Tiny bubble-like vesicles, containing a PAS-positive material of unknown composition, occur throughout the epithelial layer (Fig. 9–40). Symptoms are mild, and include slight irritation and blurring of vision. Most cases require no treatment.

Reis–Bucklers' dystrophy is a progressive disorder that presents within the first years of life. It is characterized by the presence of a gray-white, reticular opacification at the level of Bowman's membrane (Figs. 9–41 and 9–42). By midlife the disorder has usually progressed to the point where painful epithelial erosions are recurring regularly, and visual acuity is reduced. Secondary inflammation and vascularization result. Partial or full thickness corneal transplantation is usually required at this stage, but the disorder commonly recurs in the grafted tissue.

Stromal Dystrophies. There are three classic stromal dystrophies: granular, macular, and lattice. They are clinically differentiated by the signs noted in Table 9–5.

Granular dystrophy presents early in life but progresses very slowly. Visual acuity is rarely reduced below 20/200. Focal, discrete, white "granules" con-

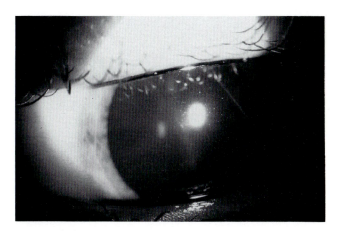

Figure 9–40. Meesmann's dystrophy, characterized by tiny vesicles on the anterior corneal surface.

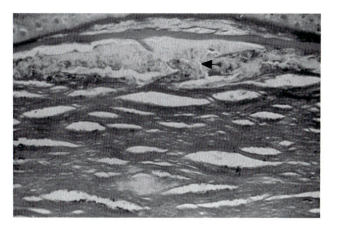

Figure 9–42. Histopathology of Reis–Bucklers' dystrophy. Note the thick, avascular fibrous tissue, and fragmentation of Bowman's membrane (*arrow*), under the epithelial layer of the cornea. *(Courtesy of the Albany Medical College slide collection.)*

TABLE 9–5. CLINICAL DIFFERENTIATION OF THE STROMAL DYSTROPHIES

Granular	Macular	Lattice
▪ OPACITIES		
Discrete, white, granular, surrounded by clear cornea	Gray-white amid a diffuse haze, no clear cornea	Refractile lines, ground-glass appearance
▪ LOCATION		
Does not extend to limbus	Extends to limbus	More prominent centrally
▪ HEREDITY		
Autosomal dominant	Autosomal recessive	Autosomal dominant
▪ NOTABLE FEATURES		
Onset is early, but progresses slowly Acuity reduced late	Involves full thickness of the stroma Extends peripherally Acuity reduced early	Recurrent erosions Onset is early, but vision good until age 30–40 years
▪ RECURRENCE IN GRAFT		
After many years	After several years	More likely than in other dystrophies
▪ COMPOSITION		
Hyaline	Mucopolysaccharide	Amyloid
▪ STAINING		
Masson trichrome	Alcian blue	Congo red, PAS

taining hyaline accumulate in the central cornea. These granules are separated by clear cornea, and do not extend to the peripheral cornea (Figs. 9–43 to 9–45). Corneal transplant may be necessary in later life; recurrence of the dystrophy in the graft is less than with the other stromal dystrophies.

Macular dystrophy differs from the other stromal dystrophies in being transmitted as an autosomal recessive trait. It is also the most visually debilitating dystrophy as the entire thickness of the stroma may be involved with a diffuse haze, punctuated by gray-white opacities (Fig. 9–46). Acuity is reduced early, often necessitating corneal transplantation in childhood. Recurrence of the dystrophy is expected within several years. The abnormal material is a mucopolysaccharide, glycosaminoglycan; the underlying etiology is believed to be an inability of the cornea to adequately metabolize keratin sulfate.

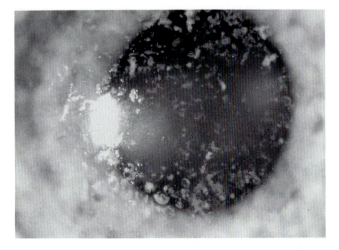

Figure 9–43. Granular dystrophy. Note the intervening clear area of cornea. *(Courtesy of James McCulley.)*

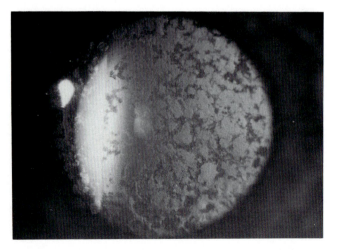

Figure 9–44. Retroillumination of granular dystrophy, same eye as in Figure 9–43. *(Courtesy of James McCulley.)*

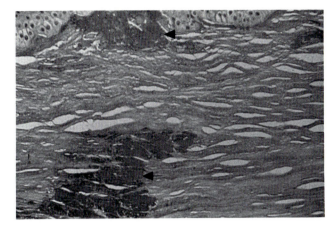

Figure 9–45. H&E staining of "granules" in granular dystrophy (*arrows*). *(Courtesy of the Albany Medical College slide collection.)*

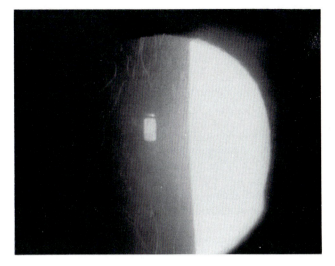

Figure 9–47. Lattice dystrophy. Note the fine, translucent, refractile lines.

Lattice dystrophy results from an accumulation of amyloid in the superficial corneal stroma. Affected corneas have a ground glass appearance with superimposed refractile lines and white dots (Fig. 9–47). The central cornea is predominantly involved. The disorder is slowly progressive, and vision is usually good until the third or fourth decade of life. This dystrophy is distinguished from the other stromal dystrophies in being associated with recurrent epithelial erosions. It is also more likely than the others to recur following corneal transplantation.

Schnyder's (central crystalline) dystrophy is a rare autosomal dominant dystrophy characterized by the accumulation of minute yellow-white crystals in the anterior corneal stroma. Additionally, the stroma may be diffusely hazy. It begins within the first year of life, but is every slowly progressive, and is usually not detected for many years. The accumulations are of choles-

terol and neutral fats, suggesting a localized lipid abnormality. There is, however, no associated systemic hyperlipidemia or hypercholesterolemia. Corneal erosions are not associated, and vision is rarely reduced to a level that would justify corneal transplantation.

Congenital hereditary stromal dystrophy was described earlier in the chapter.

Posterior Dystrophies. **Congenital hereditary endothelial dystrophy** was described earlier in the chapter.

Posterior polymorphous dystrophy is an autosomal dominant dystrophy that presents early in life but is very slowly progressive. It is characterized by variable findings of grouped vesicles on the posterior surface of the cornea, broad endothelial bands, and stromal edema (Fig. 9–48). In addition, the pupil may be misshapen (Fig. 9–49), and there may be areas of iris-

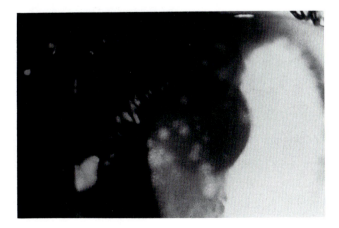

Figure 9–46. Macular dystrophy. Note the diffuse haze punctuated by gray-white opacities.

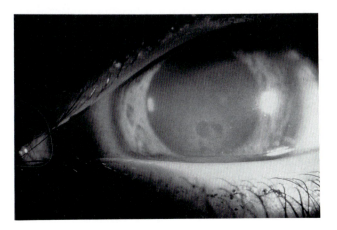

Figure 9–48. Posterior polymorphous dystrophy.

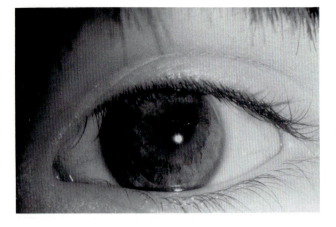

Figure 9–49. Misshapen pupil in posterior polymorphous dystrophy.

corneal adhesion. Histopathologically, the endothelial cells are abnormal and resemble epithelial cells or fibroblasts. Visual reduction is either inapparent or very mild.

Ectactic Dystrophies. **Keratoconus** is a disease of unclear pathogenesis characterized by progressive thinning and bulging of the central cornea, which becomes cone shaped (Fig. 9–50). Although familial cases are known, most cases are sporadic. Eye rubbing and contact lens wear have been implicated as pathogenic, but the evidence to support this is equivocal. An increased incidence occurs in individuals with atopy, Down syndrome, Marfan syndrome, and retinitis pigmentosa. There is also a slight female predominance.

Most cases are bilateral, but the eyes may be very asymmetrically involved. The disorder usually presents and progresses rapidly during adolescence; pro-

gression slows and stabilizes when the individual reaches full growth. Signs of keratoconus include Munson's sign (bulging of the lower eyelid upon looking downward) and the presence of a Fleischer's ring (a deposit of iron in the epithelium at the base of the cone). Corneal transplantation is indicated if satisfactory visual acuity can not be attained with the use of hard contact lenses. The prognosis following transplantation is excellent.

Acute hydrops is a complication of keratoconus. It occurs suddenly when a break in Descemet's membrane develops, and results in marked corneal edema (Fig. 9–51). The break heals spontaneously in 6 to 10 weeks, and the corneal edema slowly resorbs. Visual acuity, already reduced by the irregularly distended cornea, may be further reduced if the cornea has been scarred from the hydrops. Individuals with Down syndrome are particularly prone to develop acute hydrops as a complication of keratoconus; the reason for this is unknown. Hydrops is not an indication for surgery; most cases resolve with a conservative regimen of hypertonic agents, patching, and soft contact lens wear.

Keratoglobus is a very rare, autosomal recessive disorder, in which the cornea has a normal diameter but is quite thin and bulging, arcing high over the iris. It is most commonly seen as part of Ehlers–Danlos syndrome, which is further characterized by hyperextensible joints, neurosensory hearing loss, and blue sclera. The thin cornea and sclera may rupture with even minor trauma (Fig. 9–52); affected children should refrain from contact sports and wear protective polycarbonate spectacles with side eyeguards. Spectacle correction is also needed to correct the high axial myopia present in these elongated eyes.

Keratoglobus is differentiated from keratoconus by the location of maximal thinning. In keratoglobus the thinning is greatest in the midperiphery; in kerato-

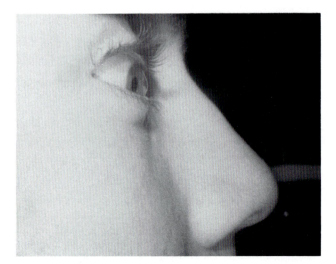

Figure 9–50. Keratoconus.

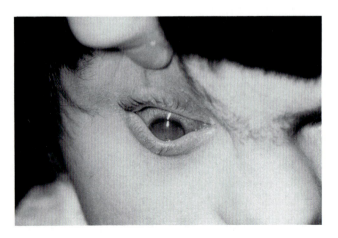

Figure 9–51. Acute hydrops in an adolescent with Down syndrome and keratoconus.

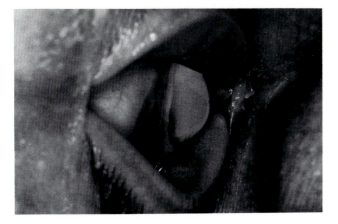

Figure 9–52. Acute hydrops in a patient with keratoglobus.

conus it is at the apex of the cornea. Keratoconus creates a conical bulging; keratoglobus a more globular protrusion. Due to this difference, the prognosis for successful corneal transplantation is much poorer in keratoglobus than in keratoconus.

REFERENCES

Akiya S, Brown S: Granular dystrophy of the cornea. Arch Ophthalmol 84:179, 1970.

Baum JL, Feingold M: Ocular aspects of Goldenhar's syndrome. Am J Ophthalmol 75:250, 1973.

Biglan AW, Brown SI, Johnson BL: Keratoglobus and blue sclera. Am J Ophthalmol 83:225, 1977.

Bron AJ, Williams HP, Carruthers ME: Hereditary crystalline stromal dystrophy of Schnyder. Br J Ophthalmol 56:383, 1972.

Burns RP: Meesmann's corneal dystrophy. Trans Am Ophthalmol Soc 66:530, 1968.

Caldwell DR: Postoperative recurrence of Reis–Bucklers' corneal dystrophy. Am J Ophthalmol 85:577, 1978.

Cibis GW, Tripathi RC: The differential diagnosis of Descemet's tears (Haab's striae) and posterior polymorphous dystrophy bands. Ophthalmology 89:614, 1982.

Cross HE, Yoder F: Familial nanophthalmos. Am J Ophthalmol 81:300, 1976.

Dorfman A, Matalon R: The mucopolysaccharidoses. In Stanbury JB, Wyngaarden JB, Fredrickson DS (eds): The Metabolic Basis of Inherited Disease, ed 3. New York, McGraw-Hill, 1972.

Dubord PJ, Krachmer JH: Diagnosis of early lattice corneal dystrophy. Arch Ophthalmol 100:788, 1982.

Friedlander MH, Smolin G: Corneal degenerations. Ann Ophthalmol 11:1485, 1974.

Goldstein JE, Cogan DG: Sclerocornea and associated congenital anomalies. Arch Ophthalmol 67:761, 1962.

Grayson M: Diseases of the Cornea, ed 2. St. Louis, Mosby, 1983, pp 238–278.

Grayson M, Pieroni D: Severe silver nitrate injury to the eye. Am J Ophthalmol 70:227, 1970.

Hall P: Reis–Bucklers' dystrophy. Arch Ophthalmol 91:170, 1974.

Hofmann RF, Paul TO, Pentelei-Molnar J: The management of corneal birth trauma. J Pediatr Ophthalmol Strabismus 18:45, 1981.

Howard RO, Abrahams IW: Sclerocornea. Am J Ophthalmol 71:1254, 1971.

Judisch GF, Maumenee IH: Clinical differentiation of recessive congenital hereditary endothelial dystrophy and dominant congenital hereditary endothelial dystrophy. Am J Ophthalmol 85:606, 1978.

Kenyon KR, Maumenee AE: Further studies of congenital hereditary endothelial dystrophy of the cornea. Am J Ophthalmol 76:419, 1973.

Kivlin JD, Fineman RM, Crandall AS, Olson RJ: Peters' anomaly as a consequence of genetic and nongenetic syndromes. Arch Ophthalmol 104:61, 1986.

Klintworth GK: Lattice corneal dystrophy. Am J Pathol 50:371, 1967.

Klintworth GK, Ferry AP, Sugar A, Reed J: Recurrence of lattice corneal dystrophy type 1 in the corneal grafts of 2 siblings. Am J Ophthalmol 94:540, 1982.

Klintworth GK, Reed J, Stainer GA, Binder PS: Recurrence of macular corneal dystrophy within grafts. Am J Ophthalmol 95:60, 1983.

Klintworth GK, Smith CF: Macular corneal dystrophy. Am J Pathol 89:167, 1977.

Krachmer JH, Feder RS, Belin MW: Keratoconus and related noninflammatory corneal thinning disorders. Surv Ophthalmol 28:293, 1984.

Kuwabara Y, Ciccarelli EC: Meesmann's corneal dystrophy. Arch Ophthalmol 71:676, 1964.

Laibson PR, Waring GO: Diseases of the cornea. In Nelson LB, Calhoun JH, Harley RD: Pediatric Ophthalmology, ed 3. Philadelphia, Saunders, 1991, pp 191–233.

Lanier JD, Fine M, Tongi B: Lattice corneal dystrophy. Arch Ophthalmol 94:921, 1976.

Malbran ES: Corneal dystrophies: A clinical, pathological, and surgical approach. Am J Ophthalmol 74:771, 1972.

Malbran E, Dodds R: Megalocornea and its relation to congenital glaucoma. Am J Ophthalmol 49:908, 1960.

Mondino BJ, Raj CVS, Skinner M, Cohen AS: Protein AA and lattice corneal dystrophy. Am J Ophthalmol 89:377, 1980.

Morgan G: Macular dystrophy of the cornea. Br J Ophthalmol 50:57, 1966.

O'Connor GR: Calcific band keratopathy. Trans Am Ophthalmol Soc 70:58, 1972.

Read J, Goldberg MF, Fishman G, Rosenthal I: Nephropathic cystinosis. Am J Ophthalmol 76:791, 1973.

Reese AB, Ellsworth RM: The anterior chamber cleavage syndrome. Arch Ophthalmol 75:307, 1966.

Richler M, Milot J, Quigley M, O'Regan S: Ocular manifestations of nephropathic cystinosis. Arch Ophthalmol 109:359, 1991.

Riedel KG, Zwaan J, Kenyon KR, et al: Ocular abnormalities in mucolipidosis IV. Am J Ophthalmol 99:125, 1985.

Sanderson PO, Kuwabara T, Stark WJ, et al: Cystinosis: A clinical, histopathologic and ultrastructural study. Arch Ophthalmol 91:270, 1974.

Schneider JA, Wong V, Seegmiller JE: The early diagnosis of cystinosis. J Pediatr 74:114, 1969.

Sher NA, Letson RD, Desnick RJ: The ocular manifestations of Fabry's disease. Arch Ophthalmol 97:671, 1979.

Spaeth GL, Frost P: Fabry's disease. Arch Ophthalmol 74:760, 1965.

Sturrock GD: Lattice corneal dystrophy. Br J Ophthalmol 67:629, 1983.

Sugar J: Corneal manifestations of the systemic mucopolysaccharidoses. Ann Ophthalmol 11:531, 1979.

Townsend WM, Font RL, Zimmerman LE: Congenital corneal leukomas, I. Central defect in Descemet's membrane. Am J Ophthalmol 77:80, 1974.

Tremblay M, Dube I: Meesmann's corneal dystrophy. Am J Ophthalmol 17:24, 1982.

Tripathi RC, Garner A: Corneal granular dystrophy. Br J Ophthalmol 54:361, 1970.

Waring GO: Congenital and neonatal corneal abnormalities. In Leibowitz HM: Corneal Disorders. Philadelphia, Saunders, 1984, pp 29–56.

Waring GO, Rodrigues MM, Laibson PR: Corneal dystrophies, I. Dystrophies of the epithelium, Bowman's layer and stroma. Surv Ophthalmol 23:71, 1978.

Waring GO, Rodrigues MM, Laibson PR: Corneal dystrophies, II. Endothelial dystrophies. Surv Ophthalmol 23:147, 1978.

Waring GO, Rodrigues MM, Laibson PR: Anterior chamber cleavage syndrome. A stepladder classification. Surv Ophthalmol 20:3, 1975.

Witschel H, Fine BS, Grutzner P, et al: Congenital hereditary stromal dystrophy of the cornea. Arch Ophthalmol 96:1043, 1978.

Wood WJ, Green WR, Marr WG: Megalocornea: A clinicopathologic clinical case report. Md State Med J 23:57, 1974.

Yanoff M, Fine BS, Colosi NJ, Katowitz JA: Lattice corneal dystrophy. Arch Ophthalmol 95:651, 1977.

Infantile and Juvenile Glaucoma

ESSENTIAL INFORMATION FOR PRIMARY CARE PRACTITIONERS

Glaucoma is a general term used to indicate damage to the optic nerve caused by, or related to, elevated pressure within the eye. It is classified according to the affected individual's age at presentation and the association of other ocular or systemic conditions. Glaucoma that begins within the first 3 years of life is called infantile (congenital); that which begins between the ages of 3 and 30 years is called juvenile. Adult glaucoma arises beyond this age.

Primary glaucoma indicates that the etiology is an isolated anomaly of the drainage apparatus of the eye (the trabecular meshwork). More than 50 percent of infantile glaucoma is primary. **Secondary glaucoma** indicates that other ocular or systemic abnormalities are associated, even if a similar developmental defect of the trabecular meshwork is also present. "Secondary" is also used when the trabecular meshwork develops normally, but mechanical obstruction to aqueous outflow occurs from an associated ocular abnormality.

Primary (open-angle) juvenile glaucoma is a very rare disorder. It is similar to the open-angle glaucoma of adults, but arises at a younger age. Primary and secondary infantile glaucoma are more common, but still rare.

Unless greatly advanced, the diagnosis of infantile glaucoma can be difficult to make. Severe signs are not present in every case, and mild findings and symptoms overlap with more benign ocular disorders. The importance of an accurate and timely diagnosis is evident by the availability of therapy, which can be vision-saving only if applied within a relatively early time-frame. Without treatment, an affected child will face a lifetime of severe visual handicap.

Epidemiological Characteristics of Primary Infantile Glaucoma

Primary infantile glaucoma (trabeculodysgenesis) occurs with an incidence of only 0.02%. The general ophthalmologist may see only one case every 5 years, and the pediatrician only one case every 10 years. The epidemiological characteristics of the disorder are enumerated in Table 10–1.

Secondary Infantile and Juvenile Glaucoma

Secondary infantile or juvenile glaucoma can arise from dysgenesis of the eye, metabolic or inflammatory disease, ocular tumors, or trauma. "Secondary" glaucoma can also be one of a spectrum of ocular findings in the phakomatoses and certain chromosomal and developmental disorders. These associations are reviewed later in the chapter.

TABLE 10–1. EPIDEMIOLOGICAL CHARACTERISTICS OF PRIMARY INFANTILE GLAUCOMA

Incidence	1:10,000–12,500 births
Presentation	80% by 1 year of age; may be present at birth
Male versus female	Under 3 months of age: male = female
	Over 3 months of age: 2 males:1 female
Bilaterality	Under 3 months of age: bilateral in 90%
	Over 3 months of age: bilateral in 60%
Inheritance	Sporadic/multifactorial
	10% familial (autosomal recessive)
	More common in twin siblings
Ethnicity	Increased incidence in caucasian males
	Increased incidence in Japanese females (?)
	Increased incidence in consanguineous populations
Genetic risks	Affected next sibling in sporadic case: 5%
	Affected next sibling in familial case: 25%
	Sporadically affected parent having an affected child: 5%
Other	No relationship to open-angle glaucoma of adults
	No relationship to steroid-induced glaucoma

Modified from Stern JH, Catalano RA: Current status of diagnostic and therapeutic measures in infantile glaucoma. Semin Ophthalmol 5:169, 1990, with permission.

Symptoms and Signs of Infantile Glaucoma

The symptoms of infantile glaucoma are presented in Table 10–2. The classic triad of symptoms includes epiphora (tearing; Fig. 10–1), photophobia (sensitivity to light), and blepharospasm (eyelid squeezing; Fig. 10–2). Each of these can be attributed to corneal irritation. Only about one third of affected infants, however, demonstrate the classic symptom complex. Parents are just as likely to notice signs. These include corneal edema, corneal and ocular enlargement, ocular injection (red eye), and visual impairment (Table 10–3).

Under 3 months of age the cornea is very sensitive to elevated intraocular pressure. Corneal signs, including edema and breaks in the endothelial basement membrane (Descemet's membrane), are present in more than 90 percent of affected infants. Haziness of the cornea confirms edema (Fig. 10–3), and a sudden increase in haziness suggests that breaks in Descemet's membrane (**Haab's striae**) have occurred. The latter are visible as horizontal, edematous lines that cross or curve around the central cornea (Fig. 10–4). They rarely occur beyond 3 years of age, or in corneas less than 12.0

TABLE 10–2. SYMPTOMS OF PRIMARY INFANTILE GLAUCOMA

Epiphora (tearing)
Photophobia (sensitivity to light)
Blepharospasm (eyelid squeezing)
Eye rubbing

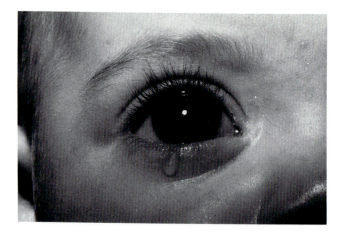

Figure 10–1. Epiphora (tearing) in infantile glaucoma.

mm in diameter. Older infants, with a gradual and moderate rise in intraocular pressure, may have only mild corneal edema.

Until approximately 3 years of age, the cornea and sclera of the eye can be distended by elevated intraocular pressure. Glaucoma is suggested by a corneal diameter of greater than 12.0 mm in an infant. With long-standing glaucoma, enlargement of the entire globe or **buphthalmos** (Greek: ox eye) can occur (Fig. 10–5).

Other signs, cupping of the optic nerve head in particular, are detected by ocular examination. The infant's optic nerve is easily distended by excessive pressure. Deep, central cupping (Fig. 10–6) readily occurs and may regress with normalization of pressure. Progressive myopia (nearsightedness) also suggests glaucoma, but this is often counteracted by corneal flattening.

Visual Prognosis in Infantile Glaucoma

The visual prognosis for children with congenital glaucoma is correlated to their age at presentation and the successful treatment of associated amblyopia. Corneal

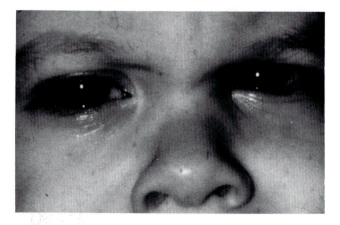

Figure 10–2. Blepharospasm (eyelid closure) secondary to photophobia (light sensitivity) in infantile glaucoma.

TABLE 10–3. SIGNS OF PRIMARY INFANTILE GLAUCOMA

Buphthalmos (large eyes)
Injection (red eye)
Visual impairment
Hazy large corneas
Breaks in Descemet's membrane of the cornea (Haab's striae)
Elevated intraocular pressure
Increased cup to disc ratio (> 0.3)
Myopic (nearsighted) refraction

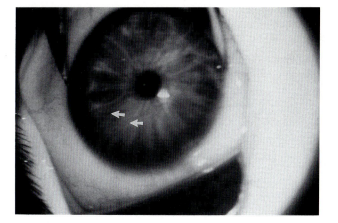

Figure 10–4. Haab's striae (breaks in Descemet's membrane of the cornea) in infantile glaucoma (*arrows*).

edema within the first 3 months of life results in a visual acuity of less than 20/200 in 50 percent of affected infants. This number is reduced to 20 percent in infants who present after 3 months of age. The visual prognosis is also poor if the corneal diameter is 14.0 mm or greater at the time of diagnosis. Profound amblyopia, from corneal clouding or a refractive error, is the most common cause of poor vision. Other causes include optic nerve damage, corneal opacity, and corneal irregularity.

COMPREHENSIVE INFORMATION ON INFANTILE AND JUVENILE GLAUCOMA

Differential Diagnosis of Primary Infantile Glaucoma

The principal disorder in the differential diagnosis of infantile glaucoma is congenital nasolacrimal duct obstruction. This presents with epiphora, but not with photophobia or blepharospasm. In infantile glaucoma, the nasolacrimal duct is patent and the ipsilateral nostril is often wet (Fig. 10–7). With nasolacrimal duct obstruction, the nostril is dry. Additional findings that suggest nasolacrimal duct obstruction include the expression of mucus through the inferior punctum from

pressure on the tear sac, crusting about the eyelids, and secondary infection (Fig. 10–8).

The differential diagnosis of corneal haziness includes cystinosis, metabolic diseases, corneal dystrophies, trauma, and keratitis. In all of these conditions, the cornea may be hazy, but not enlarged. The infantile form of **cystinosis** (Fanconi's syndrome) is an autosomal recessive disorder characterized by polyuria, growth retardation, rickets, and progressive renal failure. Cystine crystals deposit in the cornea and conjunctiva by 6 to 15 months of age and cause photophobia and blepharospasm. They are homogeneously distributed, and give the cornea an iridescent, and the conjunctiva a ground-glass, appearance (Fig. 10–9). In early life vision is not impaired, and the cornea does not enlarge. By 7 years of age, however, corneal sensitivity is usually markedly reduced. An additional finding of cystinosis is a peripheral retinopathy, which is characterized by generalized or patchy depigmentation (Fig. 10–10). The diagnosis of cystinosis can be made by assaying for cystine in biopsied conjunctiva.

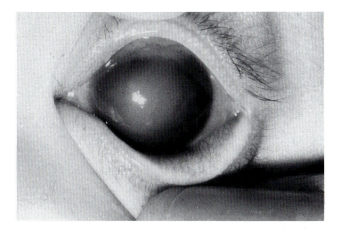

Figure 10–3. Hazy large cornea in infantile glaucoma.

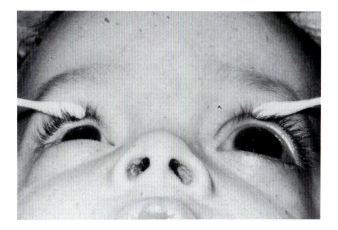

Figure 10–5. Buphthalmic (ox-like) left eye in infantile glaucoma.

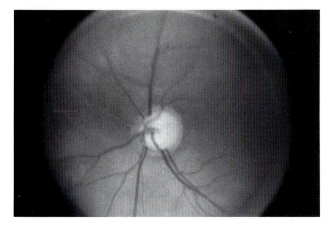

Figure 10–6. Deep central cupping of the optic nerve in infantile glaucoma.

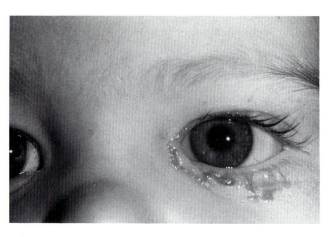

Figure 10–8. Obstructed nasolacrimal duct. Note discharge and crusting about the eyelashes.

The mucopolysaccharidoses and mucolipidoses are rare lysosomal storage diseases, in which enzyme deficiencies cause abnormal accumulations within keratocytes. Most are inherited as autosomal recessive traits, and are associated with dwarfism and extreme lumbar kyphosis (hunchback). Corneal opacification gradually occurs within the first years of life, and is diffuse and symmetrical. Four disorders which present with corneal haziness very early in life can be confused with infantile glaucoma. These are Hurler (MPS I-H), Scheie (MPS I-S), GM$_1$ gangliosidosis I, and mucolipidosis IV. Distinguishing characteristics from infantile glaucoma are the absence of epithelial involvement and the normal size of the cornea. Corneal clouding is characterized by a diffuse gray stromal haze due to the progressive accumulation of fine punctate opacities in the posterior stroma (Fig. 10–11). The peripheral cornea is preferentially involved and the visual acuity may be better than expected.

Rarer disorders in the differential diagnosis of infantile glaucoma include the corneal dystrophies of Meesmann's, Reis–Buckler's, and congenital hereditary epithelial dystrophies. Meesmann's juvenile dystrophy is a bilateral, symmetric, autosomal dominant disorder that presents during the first year of life with tiny epithelial vesicles (Fig. 10–12). In infants the vesicles rarely break through the epithelial surface, causing mild ocular irritation and photophobia. Affected children are typically asymptomatic, but the tiny blebs on the surface of the cornea can be mistaken for corneal edema. Reis–Buckler's dystrophy is also bilaterally symmetric and inherited as an autosomal dominant trait. It appears during the first years of life, and is characterized by subepithelial, linear opacifications in a ring or fishnet pattern in the central cornea (Fig. 10–13). Painful epithelial erosions are common, distinguishing this from Meesman's dystrophy and infantile glaucoma. Congenital hereditary epithelial dystrophy

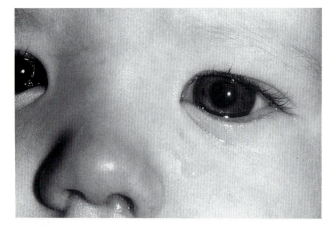

Figure 10–7. Wet nostril ipsilateral to a tearing eye. This finding is consistent with infantile glaucoma, and inconsistent with obstructed nasolacrimal duct.

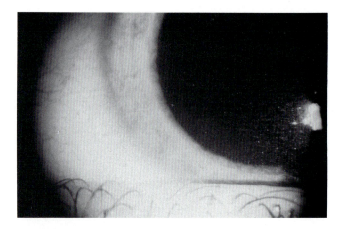

Figure 10–9. Corneal crystals in cystinosis. *(Courtesy of John W. Simon.)*

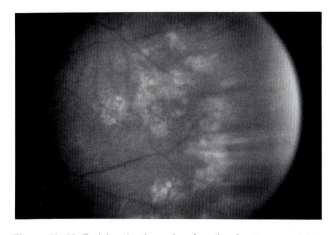

Figure 10–10. Peripheral retinopathy of cystinosis. *(Courtesy of John W. Simon.)*

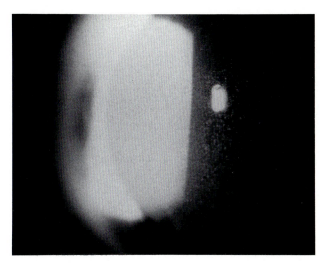

Figure 10–12. Juvenile Meesmann's dystrophy.

can be inherited as an autosomal recessive or dominant trait. The recessive form presents at birth with a ground-glass corneal opacification (Fig. 10–14). The cornea is also thickened two to three times the normal size, and may be mildly edematous. Affected infants usually develop a searching nystagmus by 3 to 4 months of age. The autosomal dominant form of this disorder does not present until the first or second year of life. It is slowly progressive and, unlike the recessive form, can present with photophobia and tearing. Nystagmus, however, is infrequent. Neither is associated with glaucoma, iris involvement, or other ocular abnormality.

The cornea can be enlarged but without edema or Haab's striae in **congenital megalocornea.** This is a rare, benign, X-linked condition in which the corneal diameter is usually greater than 14.0 mm (Fig. 10–15). Corneal striae, edema, and irritation are not present.

The most common disorder in the differential diagnosis of a congenital break in Descemet's membrane is **forceps injury.** Breaks due to forceps injuries are usually vertical or oblique (Fig. 10–16) as opposed to horizontal or curvilinear in glaucoma. Periorbital skin injuries are also usually seen with birth trauma.

Included in the differential diagnosis of optic disc cupping are congenital malformations of the nerve head such as an optic nerve head coloboma (Fig. 10–17), pit (see Fig. 13–18), staphyloma (see Fig. 5–14), and physiological cupping. These occur in the absence of increased intraocular pressure. Heredofamilial temporal optic atrophy appears in older children, and degeneration from infiltrative tumors and hydrocephalus, can usually be ascertained by associated neurological findings.

Table 10–4 provides a summary of the differential diagnosis of signs and symptoms in infantile glaucoma.

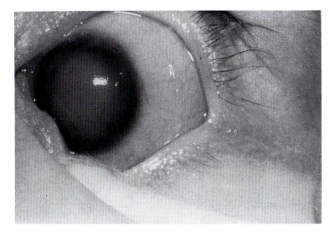

Figure 10–11. Mucopolysaccharidoses. Note the normal size of the cornea (compare with Fig. 10–3).

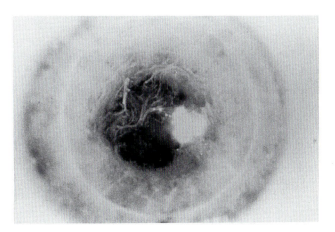

Figure 10–13. Reis–Buckler's dystrophy.

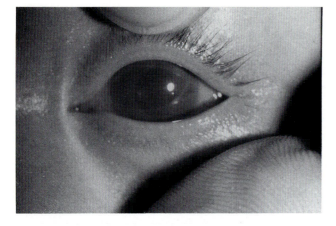

Figure 10–14. Congenital hereditary epithelial dystrophy.

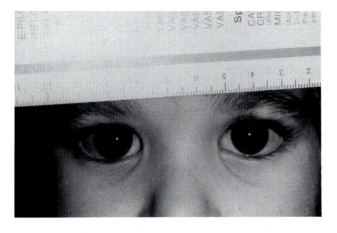

Figure 10–15. Congenital megalocornea.

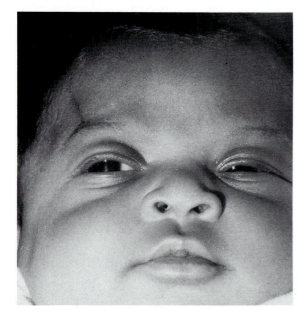

Figure 10–16. Forceps injury to the cornea. Note the oblique vertical orientation of the break in Descemet's membrane and the extension onto the forehead.

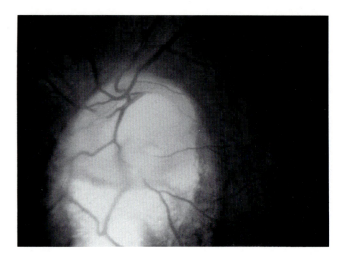

Figure 10–17. Optic nerve head coloboma. Note extension to the retina inferiorly.

TABLE 10–4. DIFFERENTIAL DIAGNOSIS OF SIGNS AND SYMPTOMS OF INFANTILE GLAUCOMA

Tearing
  Nasolacrimal duct obstruction
Corneal irritation
  Abrasion or foreign body
  Keratoconjunctivitis
  Keratitis
  Iritis
Corneal haziness
  Cystinosis
  Mucopolysaccharidoses
  Mucolipidoses
  Meesmann's dystrophy
  Reis–Buckler's dystrophy
  Congenital hereditary endothelial dystrophy
  Interstitial keratitis (rubella or syphilis)
Corneal enlargement
  Congenital megalocornea
Corneal stria
  Forceps injury
Scleral distension
  Progressive pathological axial myopia
Optic nerve head cupping
  Physiological cupping
  Heredofamilial optic atrophy
  Optic pits or coloboma
  Hydrocephalus
  Compressive or infiltrative neuropathy due to tumor

Modified from Stern JH, Catalano RA: Current status of diagnostic and therapeutic measures in infantile glaucoma. Semin Ophthalmol 5:170, 1990, with permission.

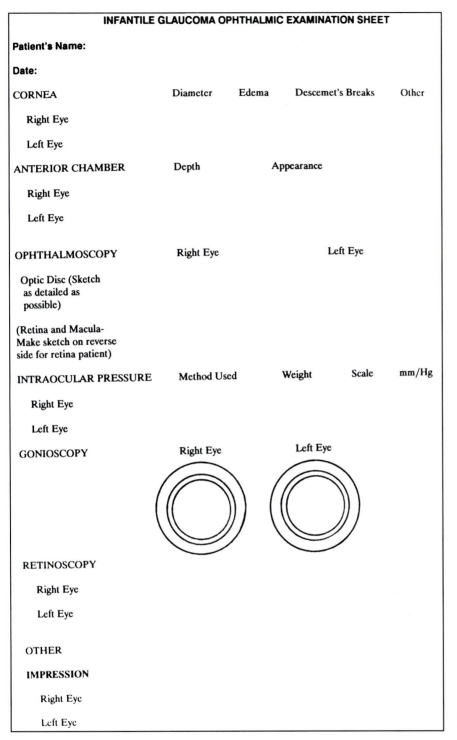

INFANTILE GLAUCOMA OPHTHALMIC EXAMINATION SHEET

Patient's Name:

Date:

CORNEA   Diameter   Edema   Descemet's Breaks   Other

   Right Eye

   Left Eye

ANTERIOR CHAMBER   Depth   Appearance

   Right Eye

   Left Eye

OPHTHALMOSCOPY   Right Eye   Left Eye

Optic Disc (Sketch
as detailed as
possible)

(Retina and Macula-
Make sketch on reverse
side for retina patient)

INTRAOCULAR PRESSURE   Method Used   Weight   Scale   mm/Hg

   Right Eye

   Left Eye

GONIOSCOPY   Right Eye   Left Eye

RETINOSCOPY

   Right Eye

   Left Eye

OTHER

IMPRESSION

   Right Eye

   Left Eye

Figure 10–18. Infantile glaucoma ophthalmic examination record.

Examination of the Eye When Infantile Glaucoma Is Suspected

The ocular examination of an infant suspected of having glaucoma includes measurement of visual function, intraocular pressure, corneal diameter and clarity, optic nerve cupping, and refractive error. Figure 10–18 is a worksheet useful for recording the findings in infants with suspected glaucoma. Table 10–5 lists the average findings in normal and glaucomatous infant eyes.

The intraocular pressure in infants can be measured with either a Schiotz (Fig. 10–19) or hand-held applanation tonometer (Fig. 10–20). Schiotz tonometry is easier to perform, but may be inaccurate if the cornea is markedly edematous or irregular. With cooperative older children, applanation tonometer at the slit lamp can be attempted (Fig. 10–21).

TABLE 10–5. AVERAGE FINDINGS IN NORMAL AND GLAUCOMATOUS INFANT EYES

	Normal Eyes	Glaucoma
Corneal size		
< 3 months of age	10.0–10.5 mm	12.0 +/– 2.0 mm
12 months	11.5 mm	≥ 11.5 mm
24 months	12.0 mm	≥ 12.0 mm
Central corneal thickness	0.99 mm	0.6 mm
Corneal radius of curvature	7.8 mm	11.8 mm
Anterior chamber depth	2.6 mm	2.6–6.3 mm
Intraocular pressure	18.5 +/– 2.3 mm	≥ 20–45 mm
Axial length		
< 3 months of age	17.5–20.0 mm	17.5–32.0 mm
12 months	22.0 mm	22.0–32.0 mm
Optic nerve cup to disc ratio	< 0.3	0.1 to 1.0
Refraction in 67% of affected infants	+1 to +4D (hyperopia)	≥ –3D (myopia)

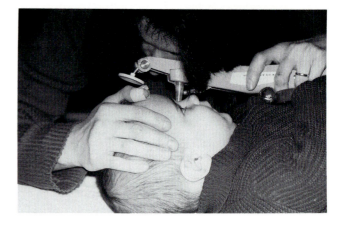

Figure 10–20. Intraocular pressure measurement by hand-held Perkins applanation tonometry.

Sedation or general anesthesia may be necessary to perform an adequate examination. Commonly used agents, however, can greatly alter intraocular pressure measurements. Barbituates and opiates usually lower the pressure, whereas ketamine usually raises it. General anesthetics (such as halothane and enflurane) usu-

ally lower intraocular pressure, but in the absence of intubation and succinylcholine, halothane–nitrous oxide induction may not substantially reduce the pressure for at least 10 minutes. Given these effects, an elevated pressure obtained under anesthesia is considered highly suggestive of glaucoma, and a normal or reduced pressure under anesthesia should not be the sole criteria used to rule out glaucoma.

Corneal findings are of great importance in the diagnosis of infantile glaucoma. The size of the cornea can be measured with calipers (see Fig. 10–4) or by photographing the child with a millimeter ruler held above the eyes (see Fig. 10–15). The horizontal meridian should be measured because the margins of the vertical meridian of the cornea are less distinct due to encroachment of the sclera superiorly. Corneal edema can be detected by observing the reflex of a penlight from the corneal surface. With corneal edema, the reflex lacks its usual luster and varies irregularly as the light moves across the corneal surface (Fig. 10–22). Cor-

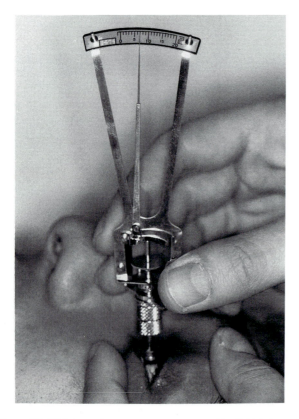

Figure 10–19. Intraocular pressure measurement by Schiotz tonometry.

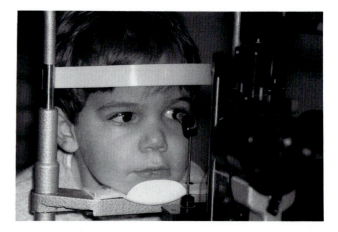

Figure 10–21. Intraocular pressure measurement by Goldmann applanation tonometry in an older child.

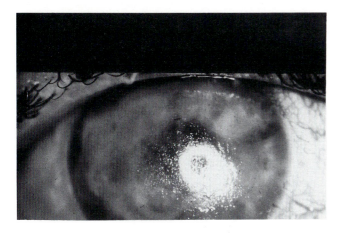

Figure 10–22. Corneal edema diffuses the usually crisp light reflex.

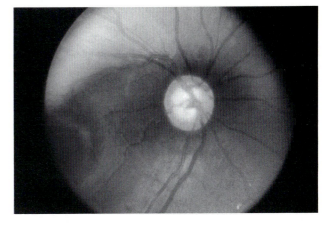

Figure 10–24. Optic nerve cupping in infantile glaucoma prior to treatment. *(Courtesy of John W. Simon.)*

neal striae can be observed with the direct ophthalmoscope by reflecting light off the retina and retro-illuminating the cornea. Descemet's breaks appear as lines traversing an otherwise homogeneous red reflex. These breaks are horizontal and linear when they occur in the central cornea, and parallel and curvilinear in the peripheral cornea. In the absence of edema, the cornea thins and its radius of curvature increases. These are difficult, however, to measure in infants.

Developmental anomalies in the anterior chamber angle have been described in both primary and secondary infantile glaucoma (discussed later in the chapter). Gonioscopy describes the technique used to examine this area of the eye. A special lens (several different types are available) is necessary because the opaque sclera and corneal limbus prevent direct visualization. Hypertonic ointment may be used to dehydrate an edematous cornea. A gonioscopic view of the angle is shown in Figure 10–23.

Optic nerve damage defines glaucoma, and appears as cupping of the nerve head. As opposed to

adult glaucoma, the neuroretinal rim initially remains intact in infants, without notching or a marked nasal shift of vessels (Fig. 10–24). Less than 2 percent of normal infants have a cup to disc ratio greater than 0.3; less than 10 percent have asymmetry in the cup to disc ratio between the eyes. Optic nerve cupping correlates with corneal diameter. When the corneal diameter is greater than 12.5 mm, the cup to disc ratio usually exceeds 0.3; cupping increases by about 20 percent for every 0.5 mm increase in corneal size.

The distensibility of the sclera should be considered when interpreting the cup to disc ratio. Increased intraocular pressure can stretch the scleral optic nerve canal as well as damage the optic nerve. The observation that cupping is somewhat reversible with normalization of pressure is consistent with this hypothesis (Figs. 10–24 and 10–25). Reversal of cupping is usually noted in children less than 1 year of age; recovery of up to 50 percent of the initial cup loss has been reported. Experimental studies have also suggested that elevated intraocular pressure may be less damaging to the in-

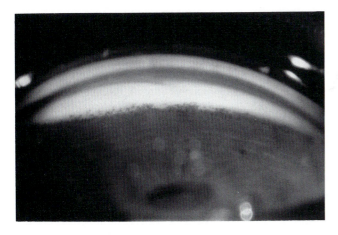

Figure 10–23. Gonioscopy in infantile glaucoma demonstrating concave iris insertion (see also Fig. 10–30).

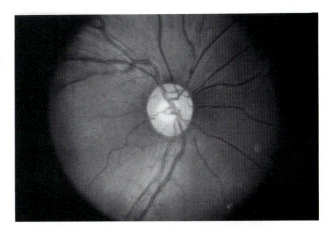

Figure 10–25. Reversal of optic nerve cupping subsequent to normalization of intraocular pressure. *(Courtesy of John W. Simon.)*

fant than the adult optic nerve. The possibility that mechanisms other than elevated intraocular pressure may cause optic nerve damage has not been excluded.

The axial length of the eye usually increases in infantile glaucoma, resulting in axial myopia (nearsightedness). It may, however, lie within the normal range, and an enlarged corneal diameter is a more reliable diagnostic finding.

Complications of Infantile Glaucoma

Profound visual loss occurs in infantile glaucoma due to damage of the optic nerve, cornea, or amblyopia. Severe visual loss should be suspected when the patient presents with an inward (esotropic) or outward (exotropic) deviating eye (Fig. 10–26). Amblyopia can result from corneal edema or a high refractive error. Myopia can result from scleral stretching, and astigmatism invariably occurs when Haab's striae are present. A rarer complication is a dislocated ocular lens (ectopia lentis; Fig. 10–27). This results when the zonules are disrupted due to equatorial expansion of the ciliary body. Iatrogenic medical complications secondary to systemic absorption of topically applied drugs, and surgical complications (such as cataract or hyphema), are not uncommon.

Pathogenesis and Anatomical Classification of Infantile Glaucoma

Although the mechanism underlying primary infantile glaucoma remains uncertain, developmental defects of the anterior chamber angle are commonly found (trabeculodysgenesis). During normal development, neural crest tissue forms a primitive iris root that inserts anterior to the trabecular meshwork. The iris migrates during the third trimester of gestation to a more posterior position, behind the scleral spur (Fig. 10–28). Failure of iris migration is believed to result in anterior

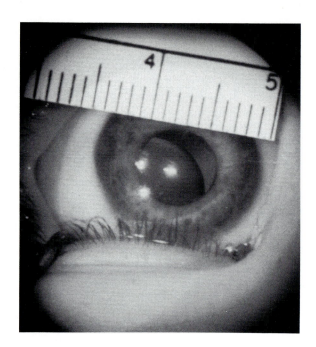

Figure 10–27. Dislocated ocular lens in infantile glaucoma.

insertion of the iris on the ciliary body. This has been observed histopathologically in the eyes of several infants with primary glaucoma. Anderson (1981) hypothesized that abnormally thickened collagen lattice elements in the trabecular meshwork inhibit this migration in infantile glaucoma. These thickened trabecular beams are also thought to result in the membranous appearance of the trabecular meshwork that is often observed on gonioscopy. An alternative hypothesis is that high fibrin and fibrinogen levels in the aqueous lead to clot formations, which thicken trabecular beams and obstruct outflow through the meshwork (Lam et al, 1983).

Hoskins and associates (1984) have suggested a classification scheme for the developmental glaucomas. The importance of classification is that it facilitates communication and provides standardized terminology. The most common maldevelopment of the trabecular meshwork (trabeculodysgenesis) is characterized by a flat, abrupt insertion of the iris into a thickened trabecular meshwork (Fig. 10–29). The iris can insert either anterior or posterior to the scleral spur; in either case, small iris processes often extend onto the trabecular surface. Less commonly, the plane of the iris is concave but its anterior portion sweeps upward, over the trabecular meshwork, and inserts just posterior to Schwalbe's line (Fig. 10–30). Dense sheets of tissue, or an arborizing network, cover the meshwork. Dense sheets of tissue, however, may be a normal finding of the anterior chamber angle during the first years of life.

It remains uncertain how often anterior iris insertion occurs in the absence of glaucoma, but it is be-

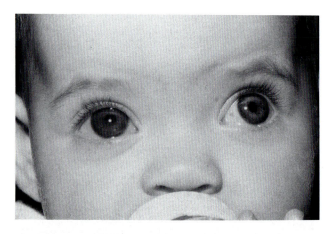

Figure 10–26. Profound visual loss in glaucomatous right eye, heralded by outward turning (exotropia) of the eye. The child is looking to the left (fixating with her left eye).

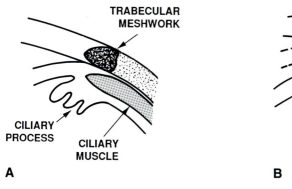
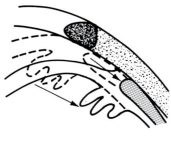

Figure 10–28. Normal development of the anterior chamber angle. **A.** Early developmental state. **B.** Posterior migration of the iris during the third trimester of gestation. *(Modified from Anderson DR: The development of the trabecular meshwork and its abnormality in primary infantile glaucoma. Trans Am Ophthalmol Soc 79:458, 1981, with permission.)*

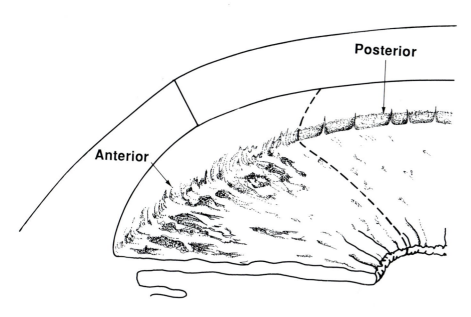

Figure 10–29. Trabeculodysgenesis: Flat iris insertion into a thickened trabecular meshwork, either anterior or posterior to the scleral spur. *(Modified from Hoskins, HD Jr, Shaffer RN, Hetherington J: Anatomical classification of the developmental glaucomas. Arch Ophthalmol 102:1331, 1984, with permission.)*

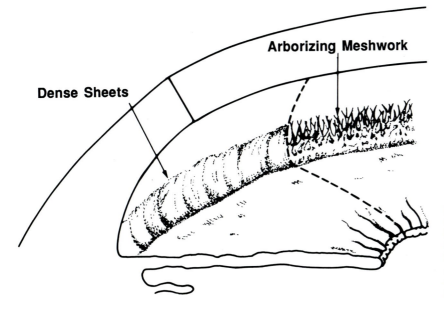

Figure 10–30. Trabeculodysgenesis: Concave iris insertion posterior to Schwalbe's line, with either dense sheets of tissue or an arborizing network of tissue covering the trabecular meshwork. *(Modified from Hoskins, HD Jr, Shaffer RN, Hetherington J: Anatomical classification of the developmental glaucomas. Arch Ophthalmol 102:1331, 1984, with permission.)*

lieved that the iris inserts flatly into the ciliary body, posterior to the scleral spur in the normal infant eye. The principal difference between glaucomatous and normal infant eyes is that the angle recess and ciliary body is not visible in the former. The presence of a membrane that covers the trabecular meshwork (Barkan's membrane) remains controversial. Most investigators have not been able to confirm its presence histologically.

Secondary Infantile Glaucoma

It is estimated that approximately 50 percent of infantile glaucoma is not isolated to a developmental anomaly of the anterior chamber angle. When older children are included, more than 75 percent of childhood glaucoma is secondary. The wide variety of secondary glaucomas is usually categorized according to the presence of a congenital neural crest dysgenesis, phakomatoses, hamartoma, tumor, or inflammatory, metabolic, or other congenital abnormality.

The anterior iris insertion of primary glaucoma has been described in several of the secondary glaucomas, including Rieger's syndrome, aniridia, maternal rubella syndrome, posterior polymorphous dystrophy, neurofibromatosis, Sturge–Weber syndrome, and oculo-dento-osseous dysplasia. It must be emphasized,

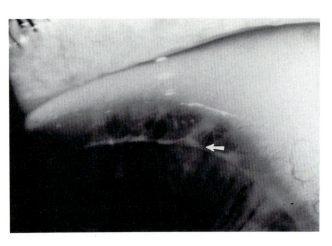

Figure 10–31. Anterior Schwalbe's line (posterior embryotoxin) in Rieger's syndrome (*arrow*).

however, this is not an invariable finding in these disorders, and anterior iris insertion may be found in nonglaucomatous infants. A different pathogenesis is suggested when a secondary glaucoma responds poorly to a treatment that is efficacious for primary glaucoma.

Table 10–6 lists disorders secondarily associated with infantile glaucoma. Many of these anomalies are reviewed in Chapter 4. The discussion that follows emphasizes the glaucomatous aspects of these disorders.

Anterior Chamber Cleavage Syndromes
The common neural crest origin of the trabecular meshwork and other structures of the anterior eye may explain the occurrence of glaucoma in the anterior chamber cleavage syndromes.

Rieger's syndrome is a bilateral, autosomal dominant condition characterized by an anteriorly located Schwalbe's line (Fig. 10–31) to which fine iris strands insert (Fig. 10–32). These strands bridge the anterior chamber angle and also insert on the trabecular meshwork. Additional findings include iris hypoplasia, correctopia (misshapen pupil), and ectropion uvea (outward turning of the inside margin of the pupil)

TABLE 10–6. SECONDARY INFANTILE GLAUCOMA

A. Associated with mesodermal neural crest dysgenesis
  1. Iridocorneotrabeculodysgenesis
    a. Rieger's syndrome (AD)   }   Anterior chamber
    b. Peter's anomaly (AR > AD) }   cleavage syndrome
    c. Marfan syndrome (AD)
    d. Weill–Marchesani syndrome (AD)
  2. Iridotrabeculodysgenesis
    a. Aniridia (AD, S)
B. Associated with phakomatoses and hamartomas
  1. Neurofibromatosis (Von Recklinghausen) (AD)
  2. Encephalofacial angiomatosis (Sturge–Weber) (AD, S)
  3. Angiomatosis of the retina (von Hippel) (AD, S)
  4. Oculodermal melanocytosis (AD, S)
C. Associated with metabolic disease
  1. Oculocerebrorenal syndrome (Lowe's) (XL)
  2. Homocystinuria (AR)
D. Associated with inflammatory disease
  1. Congenital rubella syndrome
  2. Herpes simplex iridocyclitis
E. Associated with mitotic disease
  1. Juvenile xanthogranuloma
  2. Retinoblastoma (AR, S)
F. Associated with other congenital disease
  1. Trisomy 21 (Down syndrome)
  2. Trisomy 13–15 (Patau syndrome)
  3. Rubinstein–Taybi syndrome
  4. Persistent hyperplastic primary vitreous

AD = autosomal dominant; AR = autosomal recessive; XL = X-linked; S = sporadic
Modified from DeLuise VP, Anderson DR: Primary infantile glaucoma (congenital glaucoma). Surv Ophthalmol 28:2, 1983, with permission.

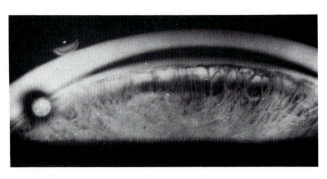

Figure 10–32. Anterior insertion of iris strands to Schwalbe's line in Rieger's syndrome.

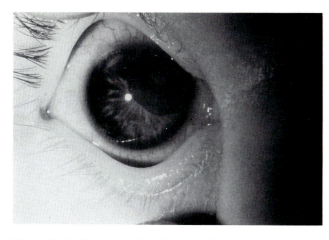

Figure 10–33. Correctopia (misshapen pupil), and ectropion uvea in Rieger's syndrome.

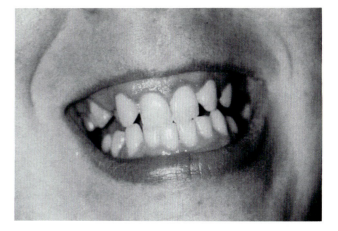

Figure 10–35. Missing and malformed teeth are common findings in oculosystemic syndromes such as Rieger's syndrome and incontinentia pigmenti (this patient). *(From Catalano RA: Incontinentia pigmenti. Am J Ophthalmol 110:696, 1990, with permission. Copyright the Ophthalmic Publishing Company.)*

(Figs. 10–33 and 10–34). The iris may be markedly distorted and misshapen, and changes may continue to progress after birth. Associated findings include reduction in the crown size and number of teeth (Fig. 10–35). The maxillary bone may be hypoplastic, causing the midface to be flat and the upper lip to recede.

More than half of affected individuals develop glaucoma, which usually appears in childhood or young adulthood. Glaucoma is believed to arise secondary to a developmental arrest of the anterior eye. Endothelial cells overlying the trabecular meshwork and iris do not resorb. Their eventual contraction leads to maldevelopment of the anterior eye and glaucoma.

In adults, Rieger's syndrome is occasionally confused with the **iridocorneal endothelial (ICE) syndrome.** The latter is unilateral, has an onset in young adulthood, and predominantly affects females. A positive family history is common in Rieger's syndrome, but is unusual in ICE. The latter syndrome is believed to result when abnormal corneal endothelium grows over the trabecular meshwork and iris, blocking aqueous outflow.

Peter's Anomaly

Peter's anomaly is characterized by a central opacity of the posterior cornea, local absence of Descemet's membrane, and adhesions of the central iris to the periphery of the corneal opacity (Fig. 10–36). Glaucoma occurs in 50 to 70 percent of cases, and anterior polar cataracts are common. The mechanism of obstruction of aqueous humor outflow in Peter's anomaly has not been fully elucidated. It may be due to dysgenesis of the anterior chamber angle or mechanical blockage of the trabecular meshwork. In contrast to primary infantile glaucoma, the cornea is not enlarged and there is often a distinct discontinuity between clear and opaque cor-

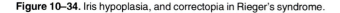

Figure 10–34. Iris hypoplasia, and correctopia in Rieger's syndrome.

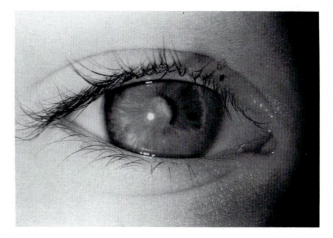

Figure 10–36. Peter's anomaly.

nea in Peter's anomaly. In addition, the anterior chamber is generally shallow, and the corneal opacity does not resolve when the intraocular pressure is normalized.

Aniridia

Aniridia is a rare, bilateral, condition occurring in 1 in 64,000 to 96,000 live births. Three genetic types exist. The first (AN1) is an isolated defect of the eye. The second (AN2) is associated with Wilms' tumor, genitourinary anomalies, and mental retardation. The third (AN3) is associated with cerebellar ataxia, congenital cataracts, and mental retardation. Both AN1 and AN2 are inherited as autosomal dominant conditions. AN1 is associated with a deletion on the short arm of chromosome 2, and AN2 with a deletion on the short arm of chromosome 11. AN3 is an autosomal recessive disorder. One third of all cases occur sporadically; twenty five percent of these will develop Wilms' tumor.

The term "aniridia" is a misnomer, as at least a small rudimentary iris invariably exists (Fig. 10–37). The cornea may be small and occasionally a cellular infiltrate (pannus) develops in the superficial layers of the peripheral cornea. Clinically this appears as a gray opacification (Fig. 10–38). Cataracts occur in a characteristic fashion for each subtype in 50 to 85 percent of individuals. In AN1, optically insignificant cortical opacities occur at birth, and progress to require extraction by the second or third decade of life. In AN2, dense nuclear cataracts can occur in the neonatal period.

In addition to cataract formation, the ocular lens can also dislocate. Macular hypoplasia occurs in both AN1 and AN2, and is believed to be responsible for the associated findings of visual reduction, nystagmus, and optic nerve hypoplasia (Fig. 10–39). Glaucoma occurs in as many as 75 percent of individuals with aniridia. It is unusual in the neonatal period, and for this

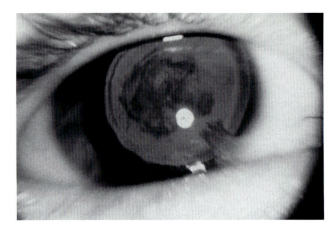

Figure 10–38. Aniridia with pannus (inferiorly) and cataract.

reason buphthalmos and Haab's striae rarely occur. Glaucoma in AN2 is thought to arise secondary to an underdeveloped filtration apparatus and anterior iris insertion. In AN1, progressive closure of the trabecular meshwork by the rudimentary iris, during the first decades of life, can result in angle-closure glaucoma. The latter has also been reported following cataract or glaucoma surgery in every type of aniridia.

Infants with aniridia are photophobic, and have reduced vision to 20/100 or worse. Pendular nystagmus is typical, regardless of acuity. Wilms' tumor usually presents before the third birthday. Most reported cases of aniridia and Wilms' tumor have had near total absence of the iris. Infants at risk should be screened using abdominal ultrasonography.

Lowe's Syndrome

Lowe's syndrome is an X-linked recessive condition consisting of renal tubular acidosis; dense, white, nuclear or posterior cataracts; glaucoma; mental and motor retardation; muscular hypotonia; and failure to

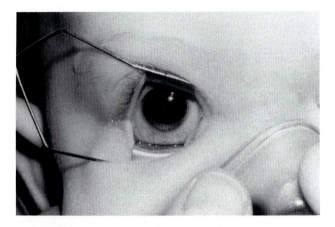

Figure 10–37. Aniridia demonstrating rudimentary iris. *(Courtesy of John W. Simon; from Catalano RA: Ocular Emergencies. Philadelphia, Saunders, 1992, p 253, with permission.)*

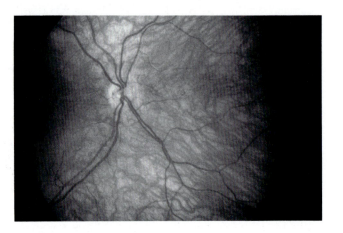

Figure 10–39. Macular and optic nerve hypoplasia in aniridia.

thrive (Fig. 10–40). The cataracts are bilateral and present at birth, and the anterior chamber angle is anatomically similar to that seen in primary infantile glaucoma. A searching nystagmus develops within months.

The typical child has a chubby habitus, pale skin, and prominent frontal bossing. He or she exhibits blindisms (such as pressing on the eye; Fig. 10–41), inattentiveness, hyperexcitability, and repetitive movements of the extremities. The child may emit high-pitched screams and assume bizarre positions due to the hypermobility of the joints and poor muscle tone.

The Phakomatoses

Sturge–Weber syndrome (encephalofacial angiomatosis) is the only phakomatosis commonly associated with glaucoma. This syndrome is characterized by nevus flammeus (port wine stain) and intracranial calcified hemangiomas. Glaucoma occurs in 30 percent of affected individuals according to a bimodal distribution. Sixty percent present within the first 2 years of life and remainder present in later childhood. The glaucoma is usually unilateral, on the same side as the nevus flammeus, and is more common if the upper eyelid, including the tarsus and conjunctiva, is involved (Fig. 10–42). If choroidal hemangioma is also present, the risk of glaucoma rises to 90%.

The pathogenesis of the glaucoma may involve two mechanisms. Infants with early-onset, but not late-onset, glaucoma have been observed to have anterior iris insertion. Infants with either early- or late-onset glaucoma have also been noted to have elevated episcleral venous pressure. This is believed to mediate glaucoma by elevating the pressure within Schlemm's canal and slowing aqueous outflow. It is possible that both mechanisms may occur in early-onset disease, but only the hemodynamic component is present in late-onset glaucoma.

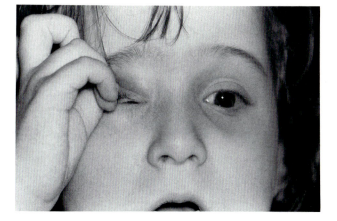

Figure 10–41. Young boy with Lowe's syndrome pressing on blind right eye. This action is called a "blindism."

Glaucoma can rarely occur in **neurofibromatosis,** usually secondary to direct tumor involvement of angle structures. It is almost always unilateral, and may be heralded by a plexiform neurofibroma of the upper eyelid. Occasionally, anterior iris insertion has been described in neurofibromatosis.

Juvenile Xanthogranuloma

Juvenile xanthogranuloma (nevoxanthoendothelioma) is a rare disorder that invariably occurs in infants less than 2 years of age. It is characterized by a benign proliferation of cells that resemble reactive histiocytes. The most frequent area of involvement is the dermis, producing single or multiple, yellow to reddish-brown, papular lesions that vary in size from a few millimeters to several centimeters (Fig. 10–43). Most commonly they are distributed over the head, neck, and trunk.

Similar accumulations can occur in the eye, but usually only one eye is affected. The tumor involves the iris either locally or diffusely (Fig. 10–44). Sponta-

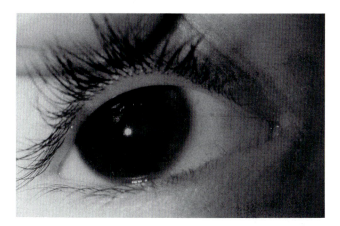

Figure 10–40. Congenital cataract with glaucoma in Lowe's syndrome.

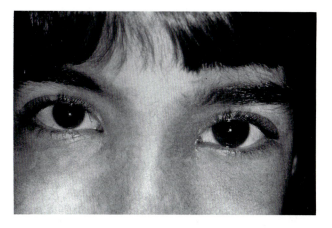

Figure 10–42. Glaucoma associated with Sturge–Weber syndrome. Note the nevus flammeus involving the left upper eyelid and buphthalmic left eye.

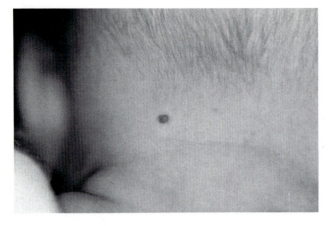

Figure 10–43. Skin lesion in juvenile xanthogranuloma.

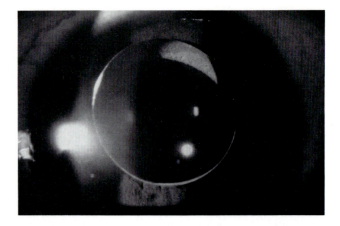

Figure 10–45. Anteriorly dislocated lens in Marfan syndrome.

neous hyphema, unilateral glaucoma, heterochromia of the iris, and a red eye with signs of uveitis can all occur. Glaucoma may progress to cause corneal edema, breaks in Descemet's membrane, and buphthalmos. Without treatment (corticosteroids or radiotherapy), repeated hemorrhage and progressive glaucoma lead to loss of vision. The skin lesions undergo spontaneous remission by 5 years of age.

Marfan Syndrome, Homocystinuria, and Weill–Marchesani Syndrome

Dislocated ocular lenses (ectopia lentis) and secondary glaucoma occur in a heredofamilial group of systemic syndromes, which also share skeletal dysplasia as a common feature. **Marfan syndrome** is a dominantly inherited disorder in which greater than 50 percent of affected individuals develop bilateral lens subluxation or dislocation (Fig. 10–45). Other associated abnormalities include joint hyperextensibility, arachnodactyly (long, slender fingers and limbs), pectus excavatus,

and scoliosis. Aortic arch dilatation and cardiac valve abnormalities are the most serious abnormalities, and can lead to premature death. **Homocystinuria** is a recessively inherited disorder in which the amino acid homocysteine cannot be metabolized into methionine and/or cysteine. Affected persons have a tall, thin habitus similar to individuals with Marfan syndrome. Lens dislocations occur in over 90 percent of these persons; associated findings include osteoporosis and cognitive disorders. Death usually occurs secondary to a thromboembolic event.

Weill–Marchesani syndrome is characterized by brachymorphia (short stocky build and short digits), limited joint mobility, and microspherophakia. Microspherophakia describes a lens that is increased in the anterior to posterior dimension, and decreased in the horizontal dimension, resulting in a more spherical shape. The small lens size contributes to the frequency of lens dislocations in the anterior chamber of the eye and secondary glaucoma (Fig. 10–46).

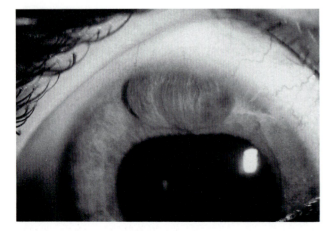

Figure 10–44. Iris nodule in juvenile xanthogranuloma. *(Courtesy of James McCulley.)*

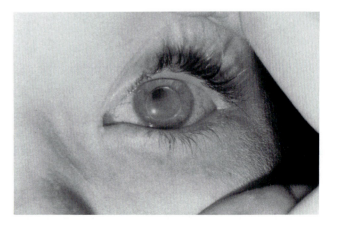

Figure 10–46. Secondary pupillary block glaucoma from an anteriorly dislocated lens in Weill–Marchesani syndrome.

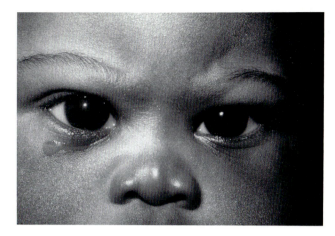

Figure 10–47. Infantile glaucoma in Down syndrome.

Other Congenital Disease

Infantile glaucoma has rarely been reported in **Down syndrome** (Fig. 10–47), and may be a chance concordance. The combination of infantile glaucoma, severe myopia, and cataracts in Down syndrome infants, however, portends a poor visual outcome. **Patau syndrome** (trisomy 13) is characterized by cleft lip and/or palate, sloping forehead, bulbous nose, severe retardation, congenital cataract, secondary infantile glaucoma, microphthalmia, persistent hyperplastic primary vitreous, intraocular cartilage, and retinal dysplasia. Over 90 percent of affected infants do not survive to their first birthday.

Rubenstein–Taybi syndrome is a syndrome of unknown heritable pattern distinguished by broad, elongated toes and thumbs (Fig. 10–48), short stature, mental retardation, and low-set ears. Cardiac, renal, and vertebral anomalies can also occur. The eye can be involved with coloboma, glaucoma, cataract, strabismus, and/or optic atrophy.

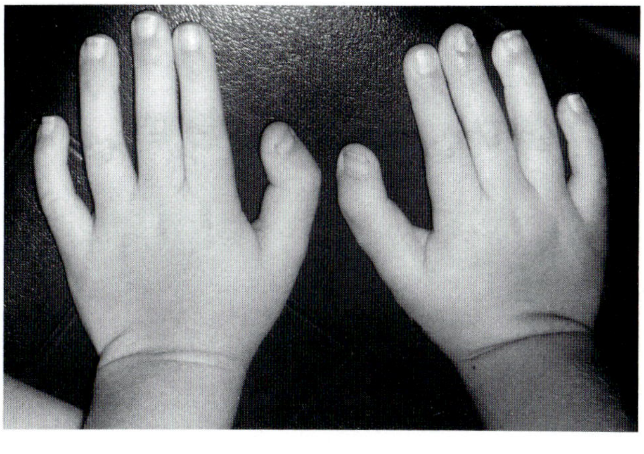

Figure 10–48. Broad, elongated thumbs in Rubenstein–Taybi syndrome.

Primary Juvenile Glaucoma

Primary juvenile (open-angle) glaucoma is a very rare condition. It is similar to its adult counterpart, but arises at a younger age. There is often evidence of familial inheritance. Unlike infantile glaucoma, there are no associated abnormalities of the anterior chamber angle, no enlargement of the cornea, and no breaks in Descemet's membrane. Juvenile glaucoma is always bilateral, but may be asymmetric.

Children with this disorder may be asymptomatic, presenting only with an insidious loss of peripheral vision. Photophobia does not occur, and complaints of browache, headache, or the appearance of colored halos around lights are rare. Most reported cases have occurred in school-age children. Large diurnal variation in pressure, between 30 and 50 mm Hg, are common.

The management of these children can be difficult. Compliance with the long-term use of medications is often poor in young individuals. Furthermore, a child's eye may respond to a surgical procedure with great inflammation.

REFERENCES

Abbassi V, Lowe CU, Calcagno PL: Oculo-cerebro-renal syndrome. Am J Dis Child 115:145, 1968.

Anderson DR: The development of the trabecular meshwork and its abnormality in primary infantile glaucoma. Trans Am Ophthalmol Soc 79:458, 1981.

Arias S, Rolo M, Gonzalez N: Terminal deletion of the short arm of chromosome 2, informative for acid phosphotase (ACP1), malate dehydrogenase (MDH1), and coloboma of iris loci. Cytogen Cell Genet 37:401, 1984.

Barsoum-Homsy M, Chevrette L: Incidence and prognosis of childhood glaucoma: A study of 63 cases. Ophthalmology 93:1323, 1986.

Chew E, Morin JD: Glaucoma in children. In Nelson LB (ed): Symposium on pediatric ophthalmology. Ped Clin North Am 30:1043, 1983.

Cibis GW, Tripathi RC, Tripathi BJ: Glaucoma in Sturge–Weber syndrome. Ophthalmology 91:1061, 1984.

DeLuise VP, Anderson DR: Primary infantile glaucoma (congenital glaucoma). Surv Ophthalmol 28:1, 1983.

Dowling JL, Albert DM, Nelson LB, Walton DS: Primary glaucoma associated with iridotrabecular dysgenesis and ectropion uvea. Ophthalmology 92:912, 1985.

Francke U, Holmes LB, Atkins L, Riccardi VM: Aniridia–Wilms' tumor association: Evidence for specific deletion of 11p13. Cytogen Cell Genet 24:185, 1979.

François J: Congenital glaucoma and its inheritance. Ophthalmologica 181:61, 1980.

Ginsberg J, Bove KE, Fogelson MH: Pathologic features of the eye in oculocerebrorenal (Lowe) syndrome. J Pediatr Ophthalmol Strabismus 18:16, 1981.

Gregor Z, Hitchings RA: Rieger's anomaly: A 42 year follow-up. Br J Ophthalmol 64:56, 1980.

Hoskins HD Jr, Shaffer RN: Evaluation techniques for congenital glaucoma. J Pediatr Ophthalmol Strabismus 8:81, 1971.

Hoskins HD Jr, Shaffer RN, Hetherington J: Anatomical classification of the developmental glaucomas. Arch Ophthalmol 102:1331, 1984.

Jay MR, Rice NSC: Genetic implications of congenital glaucoma. Metabol Ophthalmol 2:257, 1978.

Kenyon KR: Mesenchymal dysgenesis in Peter's anomaly, sclerocornea and congenital endothelial dystrophy. Exp Eye Res 21:125, 1975.

Khodadoust AA, Zini M, Biggs SL: Optic disc in normal newborns. Am J Ophthalmol 66:502, 1965.

Kupfer C, Kaiser-Kupfer MI: Observations on the development of the anterior chamber angle with reference to the pathogenesis of congenital glaucoma. J Pediatr Ophthalmol Strabismus 22:149, 1985.

Lam KW, Mansour Am, Fox RR, et al: Fibrinogen concentration in the aqueous humor of buphthalmic rabbits. Curr Eye Res 2:153, 1983.

Layman PR, Anderson DR, Flynn JT: Frequent occurrence of hypoplastic optic disks in patients with aniridia. Am J Ophthalmol 77:513, 1974.

Levy NS: Juvenile glaucoma in the Rubenstein–Taybi syndrome. J Pediatr Ophthalmol 13:141, 1976.

Luntz MH: Congenital, infantile and juvenile glaucoma. Ophthalmology 86:793, 1979.

Mackman G, Brightbill FS, Opitz JM: Corneal changes in aniridia. Am J Ophthalmol 87:497, 1979.

Margo CE: Congenital aniridia: a histopathologic study of the anterior segment in children. J Pediatr Ophthalmol Strabismus 20:192, 1983.

Morin JD: Primary congenital glaucoma—diagnosis and therapy. In Cairns JE (ed): Glaucoma. London, Grune & Stratton, 1986, vol 2, pp 731–786.

Morin JD: Primary infantile glaucoma: Influence of age of onset. Can J Ophthalmol 18:233, 1983.

Morin JD, Bryars J: Causes of loss of vision in congenital glaucoma. Arch Ophthalmol 98:1575, 1980.

Morin JD, Coughlin WA: Corneal changes in primary congenital glaucoma. Trans Am Ophthalmol Soc 78:123, 1980.

Nelson LB, Spaeth GL, Nowinsky TS, et al: Aniridia. A review. Surv Ophthalmol 28:621, 1984.

Parks MM: Management of infantile glaucoma. Trans New Orleans Acad Ophthalmol. New York, Raven, 1986, pp 193–200.

Quigley HA: The pathogenesis of reversible cupping in congenital glaucoma. Am J Ophthalmol 84:358, 1977.

Richardson HT: Optic cup symmetry in normal newborn infants. Invest Ophthalmol Vis Sci 7:137, 1968.

Robin AL, Quigley HA, Pollack IP, Maumenee AE, Maumenee IH: An analysis of visual acuity, visual fields, and disc cupping in childhood glaucoma. Am J Ophthalmol 88:847, 1979.

Schottenstein EM: Peter's anomaly. In Ritch R, Shields MB, Krupin T: The Glaucomas. St. Louis, Mosby, 1989, vol 2, pp 897–903.

Seidman DJ, Nelson LB, Calhoun JH, et al: Signs and symptoms in the presentation of primary infantile glaucoma. Pediatrics 77:399, 1986.

Shaffer RN, Cohen JS: Visual reduction in aniridia. J Pediatr Ophthalmol 12:220, 1975.

Shields MB: Axenfeld–Rieger syndrome: A theory of mechanism and distinctions from the iridocorneal endothelial syndrome. Trans Am Ophthalmol Soc 81:736, 1983.

Shields MB: Axenfeld-Rieger syndrome. In Ritch R, Shields MB, Krupin T: The Glaucomas. St. Louis, Mosby, 1989, vol 2, pp 885–895.

Soong HK, Raizman MB: Corneal changes in familial iris coloboma. Ophthalmology 93:335, 1986.

Stern JH, Catalano RA: Current status of diagnostic and therapeutic measures in infantile glaucoma. Semin Ophthalmol 5:166, 1990.

Traboulsi EI, Jaafar MS, Wilson ME, Parks MM: Hypoplasia of the iris: The aniridia spectrum. Int Pediatr 5:275, 1990.

Traboulsi EI, Levine E, Mets M, et al: Infantile glaucoma in Down's syndrome. Am J Ophthalmol 105:389, 1988.

Tripathi RC, Cibis GW, Tripathi BJ: Lowe's syndrome. Trans Ophthalmol Soc UK 100:132, 1980.

Walton DS: Juvenile open-angle glaucoma. In Epstein DL (ed): Chandler and Grant's Glaucoma, ed 3. Philadelphia, Lea & Febiger, 1986, pp 528–529.

Waring GO, Bourne WM, Edelhauser HF, Kenyon KR: The corneal endothelium, normal and pathologic structure and function. Ophthalmology 89:531, 1982.

Waring GO, Rodrigues MM, Laibson PR: Anterior chamber cleavage syndrome: A stepladder classification. Surv Ophthalmol 20:3, 1975.

Zimmerman LE: Ocular lesions of juvenile xanthogranuloma: Nevoxanthoendothelioma. Trans Am Acad Ophthalmol Otolaryngol 69:412, 1965.

CATARACTS AND LENS DISLOCATION IN CHILDREN

ESSENTIAL INFORMATION FOR PRIMARY CARE PRACTITIONERS

Cataracts in Infants and Young Children

Congenital and early developmental cataracts are common ocular abnormalities; one of every 250 newborns (0.4 percent) has some form of congenital cataract. Although some are located outside the visual axis and do not affect vision, most childhood cataracts are deleterious to visual development. The importance of detecting infantile cataracts is underscored by the fact that the visual loss they cause is usually remediable.

The Greeks used the word "cataract" to describe a downpouring of water (a waterfall). Physicians in the late middle ages adopted the term to describe cloudiness in the normally crystalline ocular lens. The handicap of a cataract can be likened to looking through a dirty car windshield. Affected adults readily perceive this as a hindrance, and seek ophthalmic care early. Infants and young children, however, have not developed a perception of what the world should look like. Coupled with their inability to communicate, the frequently encountered delay in diagnosis of infantile cataracts is easily understood. The even greater delay in diagnosing unilateral cataracts is attributable to the fact that children with unilateral cataracts usually have good visual function and performance.

The Diagnosis of Infantile Cataracts

When the cataract involves the anterior portion of the lens, it may be visible as a white reflex in the child's pupil (leukokoria; Fig. 11–1). Other times cataracts are revealed upon examination of a child who is visually inattentive, or has nystagmus, reduced vision, or a deviated eye (Table 11–1).

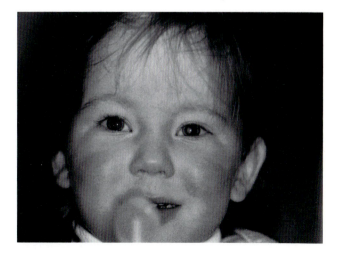

Figure 11–1. Leukokoria, the appearance of a white pupil due to the presence of a cataract in the left eye.

TABLE 11–1. PRESENTING SIGNS AND SYMPTOMS OF INFANTILE CATARACTS

Leukokoria (white pupil)
Visual inattentiveness
Poor visual fixation reflexes
Progressive visual deficits
Nystagmus (searching/wandering conjugate eye movements)
Strabismus (deviated eye)
Microphthalmos (small eye)
Photophobia (sensitivity to light)
Absent or irregular red reflex
Inability to observe retinal details with the ophthalmoscope
Behavioral or emotional change when the normally seeing eye is covered (monocular cataract)
Family history of childhood cataracts

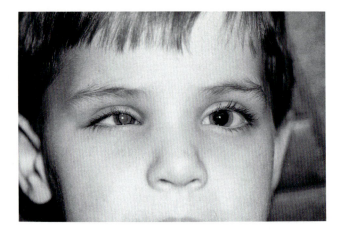

Figure 11–3. Esotropia, the inward deviation of an eye, in this case secondary to poor vision in the right eye due to a cataract.

Infants who are born with significant bilateral lens opacities develop profound visual impairment and nystagmus if a clear, focused retinal image cannot be achieved within the first 3 months of life (Fig. 11–2). The nystagmus is of the searching or wandering type (see Chapter 7). When measured by preferential looking techniques, visual acuity in these children is 20/200 or less. The infant 3 months of age or older who has apparent bilateral cataracts but no nystagmus is usually found by preferential looking to have an acuity of approximately 20/100 to 20/200. Cataracts that are discovered in the absence of nystagmus or parental concern are usually less incapacitating. Parents may not appreciate the reduced visual performance caused by lens opacities that blur the vision from approximately 20/50 to 20/100 until the child is about 3 or 4 years of age.

Monocular cataracts may go undetected for longer periods, as affected children do not develop nystagmus and do not appear to be visually handicapped. The loss or impedance of binocularity, however, creates a severe obstacle to proper ocular alignment. Because of this sensory obstacle to fusion, the visually impaired eye may change its position relative to the fixating eye and turn in (become esotropic; Fig. 11–3) or out (exotropic). Microphthalmos (a small eye) is an additional frequent finding in unilateral cataracts (Fig. 11–4).

Occasionally, a lens opacity creates so much scattering of light or glare that light sensitivity (photophobia) is a presenting symptom. Typically, the cataracts that cause photophobia are of the lamellar or zonular type (discussed later in the chapter).

Because parents often do not notice cataracts, it is important for nonophthalmic medical and paramedical personnel to be familiar with the red reflex test, which is an excellent screen for many ocular abnormalities. This test is performed by looking at an infant or small child in a darkened room through the "0" lens of

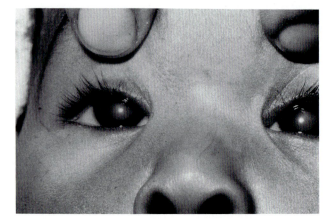

Figure 11–2. Dense, bilateral congenital cataracts. This child had nystagmus.

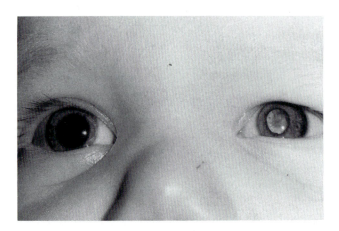

Figure 11–4. Microphthalmos, a small eye, in a patient with persistent hyperplastic primary vitreous and cataract in the left eye.

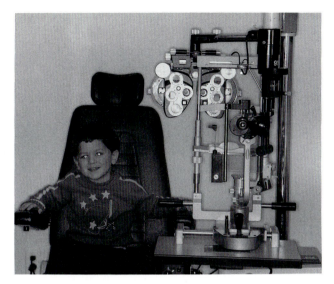

Figure 11–5. A normal red reflex in each eye.

an ophthalmoscope from a distance of 1 to 3 feet (30 to 90 cm). The infant should be supine in the bassinet; the toddler should be sitting comfortably. The examiner looks for an orange-red reflex in the pupil (Fig. 11–5). Its presence rules out gross corneal lesions, cataracts or other opacities in the ocular media, and complete detachment of the retina. Cataracts will appear as black forms against the red background (Fig. 11–6). The red reflex test should be part of all infant evaluations in the newborn nursery and during the first year of life. In the newborn nursery it may be necessary to dilate the pupils to obtain an adequate view. This can usually be accomplished by instilling one drop each of 0.5 percent cyclopentolate and 2.5 percent phenylephrine into the

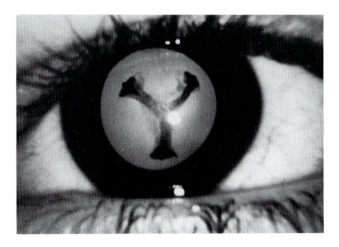

Figure 11–6. An abnormal red reflex. The black opacity in the otherwise homogeneous bright band is a "sutural" cataract. *(Courtesy of Stephen B. Lichtenstein; from Nelson LB: Pediatric ophthalmology. Philadelphia, Saunders, 1984, with permission.)*

eyes. All children with an abnormal red reflex should be immediately referred to an ophthalmologist for a more definitive diagnosis.

Lens Dislocation

A dislocated lens refers to any lens that is not in its normal anatomic position in the eye. The term "subluxation" is used when the lens is partially dislocated. A subluxated lens remains in the pupillary area, whereas a dislocated lens may migrate anteriorly to the front of the eye (anterior chamber) or posteriorly (vitreous cavity).

Children with ectopia lentis usually present because of a concern over poor vision. Their parents may have noticed visual difficulties, or the child may have failed a vision screening test. Blurred vision occurs because the optics of the eye are misaligned. With subluxated lenses, light rays strike the edge of the lens and bend abnormally, resulting in a blurred (astigmatic) image on the retina. An additional distortion with dislocated lens is an induced nearsightedness. This results because the unattached lens is more spherical than normal.

Occasionally, children with dislocated lenses will present with acute glaucoma. A free-floating lens can block the normal flow of aqueous humor. If aqueous cannot egress the eye, the ocular pressure will increase and the child will experience sudden pain and blurred vision. Glaucoma is more likely to occur if the lens dislocates anteriorly. Rarely, parents may notice a fine quivering movement of their child's iris(es) with ocular movement (iridodonesis).

The Diagnosis of Dislocated Lens

The appearance of a clear, round disc is easily recognized when a total dislocation into the anterior eye occurs. This should still be evident even if the cornea is somewhat edematous and cloudy due to an induced glaucoma (see Fig. 11–45). In the absence of total anterior dislocation, iridodenesis can often be noticed by closely observing the child's eye when she moves her head or eye, or by gently moving the eye, using light finger pressure to the upper eyelid. Dilation of the pupil makes visible the fine, shimmering lens movement (phacodonesis). With marked subluxation or dislocation, the edge of the lens may be seen. Usually this is rounded (Fig. 11–7), but if there is a localized zonular defect (the fine tissue strands that attach the lens to the ciliary body of the eye), the visible edge of the lens may appear flat (Fig. 11–8). The best diagnostic tool to detect mildly dislocated lenses is the retinoscope. Either an irregular astigmatism, or the edge of the lens within the red reflex, may be seen. Older children can sit at the slit lamp, allowing greater visibility of phacodenesis, lens edges, and in more substantial dislocations, zonular fibers (Fig. 11–9). Table 11–2 summarizes the presenting signs and symptoms of lens dislocation.

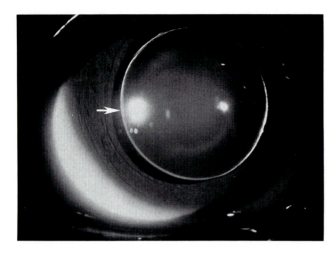

Figure 11–7. A dislocated small (microspherophakic) ocular lens. Note the round edge of the lens seen within the pupillary aperture (*arrow*). *(Courtesy of the Scheie Eye Institute library; from Nelson LB, Maumenee IH: Ectopia lentis. Surv Ophthalmol 27:143, 1982, with permission.)*

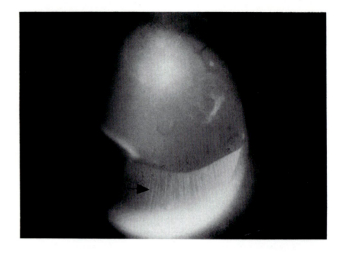

Figure 11–9. Slit-lamp view of a dislocated lens demonstrating zonular fibers (*arrow*). *(From Catalano RA: Ocular Emergencies. Philadelphia, Saunders, 1992, p 252, with permission.)*

COMPREHENSIVE INFORMATION ON CATARACTS AND OTHER LENS ANOMALIES IN CHILDREN

Infantile Cataracts

Etiology and Workup of Infants and Children With Cataracts

A search for an etiology should always be made when a child is born with a cataract. In some children the cause is obvious, as with familial congenital cataracts. In others, a detailed physical examination and elaborate laboratory tests are necessary (Tables 11–3 and 11–4). The basic approach is to determine whether the cataract is an isolated finding in an otherwise healthy child or whether the cataract is part of a systemic disorder. Although the list of causes and associations of congenital cataracts is quite long, many disorders can be readily ruled out by the lack of associated findings (Table 11–5).

As Table 11–5 indicates, cataracts can be heritable or acquired secondary to injuries, insults, infections, tumors, or other anomalies of the eye. They can also be isolated, or a component of a systemic syndrome. Systematic associations are usually obvious, and the pediatrician caring for the child likely will have initiated appropriate investigations in children with multiple congenital anomalies. Delay in diagnosis is more likely in infants with developmental delay or failure to thrive.

When evaluating a child with cataracts who is otherwise normal, one should remember that approximately one third of cases are idiopathic, and approximately 50 percent of all hereditary cataracts are new mutations (Fraser & Freedman, 1967). Parents, siblings, and even cousins should be examined to determine if the cataracts are familial. Table 11–3 summarizes the laboratory test available when heritable cataracts cannot be confirmed. The use of these tests should be

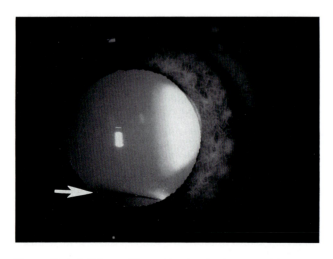

Figure 11–8. A dislocated lens with a localized zonular defect causing the edge of the lens to be flat (*arrow*).

TABLE 11–2. PRESENTING SIGNS AND SYMPTOMS OF LENS DISLOCATION

Decreased vision
Iridodonesis (quivering-like movement of the iris)
Phacodonesis (quivering movement of the lens)
Glaucoma secondary to pupillary block
Lens in the anterior chamber
Family history of Marfan syndrome
Other ocular or systemic disorder (e.g., aniridia, homocystinuria)

TABLE 11–3. LABORATORY EVALUATION OF PATIENTS WITH INFANTILE AND CHILDHOOD CATARACTS

Category of Test	Substance	Potential Disorder
Urine studies	Reducing substances	Galactosemia
	Glucose	Diabetes mellitus
	Amino acids	Lowe syndrome, homocystinuria
	Blood/protein	Alport's syndrome
	Lipid bodies	Fabry's disease
	Sediment	Alport's syndrome (maltese cross under polarized light)
	Ketones	Homocystinuria
Blood studies	Glucose	Hypoglycemia, diabetes mellitus
	Calcium/phosphorus	Hypoparathyroidism, Lowe syndrome
	Amino acids	Lowe syndrome, homocystinuria
	Serological	TORCH titers, syphilis
	Platelet count	Rubella (thrombocytopenia)
	Rubella titer	Rubella
Red blood cells	Galactose enzymes	Galactosemia
	G-6-PD activity	G-6-PD deficiency
White blood cells	Mannosidase activity	Mannosidosis
Plasma	Phytanic acid	Refsum's disease

Modified from Nelson LB: Diagnosis and management of congenital and developmental cataracts. Semin Ophthalmol 5:157, 1990; data from DelMonte MA: Diagnosis and management of congenital and developmental cataracts. Pediatr Clin North Am 37:205, 1990, with permission.

patient directed. Table 11–4 lists tests that should be considered in the presence of specific associated findings.

Galactokinase deficiency should be ruled out in all children with congenital cataracts who are otherwise healthy. Two enzymatic disorders of galactose metabolism are known to occur. The first results from a deficiency of galactose-1-phosphate uridyl transferase. Infants with this disorder develop hepatomegaly, jaundice, vomiting, diarrhea, and failure to thrive within 1 to 2 weeks of receiving galactose-containing formulas. Lens opacification characteristically starts as an "oil-

drop" cataract and progresses through a lamellar cataract to maturity. The second enzymatic defect is a deficiency of the enzyme galactose kinase. Although galactosuria occurs, the only significant manifestation is the development of bilateral, lamellar cataracts. The simplest screening test for either cause of galactosuria is a urine test for reducing substances. Galactosuria causes a positive Clinitest reaction, but a negative reaction to a glucose oxidase dipstick (Clinistix). Definitive diagnosis is established by assaying red blood cells for the deficient enzyme. Because both forms of galactosuria are treatable if detected at an early age, it is recom-

TABLE 11–4. PATIENT-DIRECTED LABORATORY EVALUATION IN INFANTS WITH CATARACTS

Finding	Test
No familial history/healthy child	Urinalysis for reducing substances (Clinitest), proteinuria, hematuria
Small-for-date infant	Fasting blood glucose
Seizures	Fasting blood glucose, serum calcium, chromosomal analysis
Neonatal jaundice	TORCH titers, RBC assays for galactose transferase or glucose-6-phosphate dehydrogenase deficiency
Failure to thrive	TORCH titers, RBC assay for galactose transferase deficiency, urinalysis for proteinuria and hematuria, chromosomal analysis
Hearing loss	Plasma assay for phytanic acid, urinalysis for proteinuria and hematuria, child and maternal rubella IgG and IgM
Skeletal anomalies	X-rays of epiphyseal plates
Somatic anomalies	Chromosomal analysis, genetic evaluation
Uveitis	Antinuclear antibody for JRA, serological tests for syphilis, ELISA for Toxocara, indirect fluorescent antibody and hemagglutination test for toxoplasmosis
Aniridia	Chromosomal analysis (11p–)

TABLE 11–5. INFANTILE CATARACTS: ETIOLOGIC CLASSIFICATION

Category	Entity	Findings
Mendelian Inheritance	Autosomal dominant	Most common; often lamellar or "milky way" appearance, may be associated with microphthalmos, variable expressivity and penetrance is typical
	Autosomal recessive	Sutural opacities, may be associated with microphthalmos
	X-linked	Rare, all reported cases have been dominant, carrier females may have sutural cataracts
Intrauterine infection	Rubella	Regurgitative jaundice during the first days of life, thrombocytopenic purpura, failure to thrive, microcephaly, deafness, congenital heart defects, microphthalmos, uveitis, glaucoma, corneal opacity, retinopathy
	Mumps	Painful swelling of the parotid gland, conjunctivitis, uveitis
	Herpes simplex	Vesicular skin eruption, perioral ulcers, dissemination to the liver, adrenals, lungs, and central nervous system
	Syphilis	Frontal bossing, saddle nose, maxillary hypoplasia, uveitis within the first 30 days of life
	Toxoplasmosis	Congenital infection results in jaundice, hepatomegaly, hyperpyrexia, and purpura; cataract follows uveitis
	Cytomegalovirus	Jaundice within the first 24 hours, hepatosplenomegaly, petechiae, erythroblastoma
Prematurity		Associated with hypoxia; may be transient
Metabolic disorders	Galactose transferase deficiency	Jaundice by the first or second week of life, hepatomegaly, feeding difficulties, failure to thrive, vomiting, diarrhea, autosomal recessive (chromosome 9)
	Galactose kinase deficiency	Cataracts are the only major manifestation, galactosuria, autosomal recessive (chromosome 17)
	Alport's syndrome	Glomerulonephritis, hematuria, proteinuria, neurosensory hearing loss, autosomal dominant
	Lowe syndrome	Glaucoma, cloudy corneas, hypotonia, areflexia, aminoaciduria, glycosuria, renal tubular acidosis, mental retardation, bone rarefraction, X-linked recessive
	Hypoglycemia	Episodes of flushing, pallor, or cyanosis, irritability, tremors, convulsions, apnea, poor feeding, unstable temperature, high pitched cry, hypotonia, rolling eye movements; diabetic mother, hemolytic (RF) factor disease, or perinatal stress
	Hypocalcemia	Tremor, irritability, apnea, seizures, feeding difficulty, failure to thrive, hypoparathyroidism
	Glucose-6-phosphate-dehydrogenase deficiency	Hemolytic reactions, anemia, hyperbilirubinemia, X-linked
	Mannosidosis	Hepatosplenomegaly, mental retardation, kyphosis, coarse facies, anterior capsular cataracts, corneal opacities (chromosome 19)
	Refsum disease	Elevated phytanic acid, hearing loss, ataxia, ichthyosis, pigmentary retinopathy
	Wilson's disease	Defect in copper metabolism, jaundice, cerebellar dysfunction, sunflower cataract of the anterior capsule
Chromosomal disorders	Trisomy 21	Down syndrome: mental retardation, simian crease, congenital heart defects, upward-slanting palpebral fissures, epicanthal folds, speckled irises
	Trisomy 18	Edwards' syndrome: mental retardation, failure to thrive, high-pitched cry, microphthalmos, prominent occiput, rocker bottom feet, congenital heart defects
	Trisomy 13	Patau's syndrome: mental retardation, motor seizures, microcephaly, holoprosencephaly, microphthalmos, cleft lip/palate, polydactyly, congenital heart defects
	5q–	Cri du chat syndrome: mental retardation, microcephaly, oblique palpebral fissures, micrognathia, epicanthal folds, cat-like cry
	11p–	Aniridia: near-total absence of iris, foveal hypoplasia, glaucoma, Wilms' tumor
Craniofacial dysostosis	Crouzon syndrome	Oxycephaly, beak shaped nose, protruding mandible, hypoplastic maxilla, exophthalmos, exotropia, optic atrophy, deafness, autosomal dominant
	Apert syndrome	Flattened occiput, prominent forehead, hypertelorism, syndactyly, exophthalmos, sporadic
Systemic syndromes	Cockayne	Premature aging, deafness, mental retardation, dwarfism, microcephaly, photodermatitis
	Conradi	Epiphyseal calcifications, dysplastic skeletal changes, short limbs, joint contractures
	Hallermann–Streiff	Parrot-beak-like nose, sparse hair, hypoplasia of teeth, micrognathia, small stature
	Kutner	Green (fluorescent) cataracts, mental retardation, dwarfism, dry skin, pancreatic insufficiency

(continued)

TABLE 11–5. INFANTILE CATARACTS: ETIOLOGIC CLASSIFICATION (continued)

Category	Entity	Findings
	Marinesco–Sjögren	Mental retardation, hypotonia, dwarfism, ataxia
	Meckel	Encephalocele, polycystic kidneys, polydactyly, congenital heart defects
	Neurofibromatosis II	Bilateral acoustic neuromas, posterior subcapsular and central posterior cortical cataracts, epiretinal membranes, RPE hamartoma
	Rubenstein–Taybi	Mental retardation, broad thumbs and great toes, short stature, vertebral, cardiac, renal anomalies, strabismus
	Schafer	Mental retardation, dwarfism, hyperkeratosis, nail abnormalities
	Smith–Lemli–Opitz	Mental retardation, microcephaly, syndactyly of toes, cryptorchism, broad nasal tip with anteverted nares, low-set ears, micrognathia, ptosis
	Stickler	Arthritis, kyphosis, deafness, micrognathia, cleft palate
	Sotos	Prominent forehead, high arched palate, gigantism, large hands and feet, mental retardation
	Myotonic dystrophy	Progressive muscle wasting, hypotonia, hypogonadism, progressive mental deterioration, ptosis, fixed facial expression. Cataracts: rarely evident before age 10 years, multicolored (crystalline)
Dermatologic disorders	Dyskeratosis congenita	Leukoplakia and hyperpigmentation of skin, pancytopenia, visceral cancers, X-linked recessive
	Incontinentia pigmenti	Vesicular skin eruptions evolving to verrucous skin lesions, retinal detachment, X-linked dominant
	Atopic dermatitis	Associated with asthma, chronic conjunctivitis, chemosis
	Rothmund–Thomson syndrome	Dermal atrophy, telangiectasias, short stature, sparse hair, hypogonadism
Ocular associations	Aniridia	Near-total absence of iris, foveal hypoplasia, glaucoma, Wilms' tumor
	Coloboma	Keyhole-shaped pupil with defect inferiorly, can involve retina, optic nerve, autosomal dominant
	Peter's anomaly	Central corneal opacity, with or without iris strands to the edge of opacity
	Norrie's disease	Mental retardation, deafness, retinal dysplasia, corneal opacification, blindness, X-linked recessive
	Persistent hyperplastic primary vitreous	Unilateral (90%), small eye (80%), fibroglial and vascular proliferation in the retrolental space, glaucoma, sporadic
	Persistent pupillary membranes	Iris strands crossing over and attached to the lens, sporadic
	Microphthalmos	Associated with multiple ocular anomalies (see Chapter 9)
	Uveitis	Etiologies: juvenile rheumatoid arthritis, sarcoidosis, toxocariasis
	Retinoblastoma	Retinal tumor, presents with leukokoria, strabismus, or visual inattentiveness

Modified from Nelson LB: Diagnosis and management of congenital and infantile cataracts. Semin Ophthalmol 5:156, 1990, with permission.

mended that the Clinitest test be performed for all infants with cataracts.

It is also important to know that some infantile cataracts may be transient. These include cataracts associated with prematurity (presumably secondary to hypoxia), galactosemia, hyperglycemia, and steroids.

Cataract Subtypes

The ocular lens is composed of three separate structures: the lens capsule, lens epithelium, and lens substance. The lens capsule completely surrounds the lens and acts as a semipermeable membrane, allowing the free transport of water, nutrients, and oxygen into and out of the lens substance. This "capsule" is actually the basement membrane of the lens epithelium (anteriorly), and nuclear lens cells (posteriorly). Inside the anterior capsule lies a single row of cuboidal cells, the lens epithelium. Between this and the posterior lens capsule lies the lens substance. The latter consists of

newly formed soft lens fibers, the cortex, surrounding a zone of older, compressed lens fibers, the nucleus.

The lens nucleus is not homogeneous. Instead, it consists of several distinct layers created by the laying down of fibers of different optical densities during different stages of development. These layers are separated by bright bands called zones of discontinuity. These zones, which are apparent by biomicroscopy, are as follows:

1. The **embryonic nucleus**—an optically clear central zone formed in embryonic life (months 1 to 3) from primary lens fibers.
2. The **fetal nucleus**—formed from secondary lens fibers in months 3 to 8 of fetal life.
3. The **infantile nucleus**—formed in the last weeks of fetal life through puberty.
4. The **adult nucleus**—formed after puberty and throughout adult life.

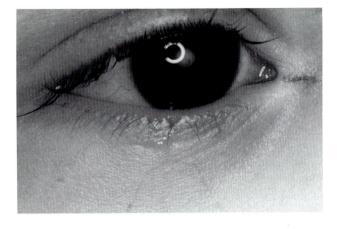

Figure 11–10. Anterior polar cataract. Most are even smaller than this.

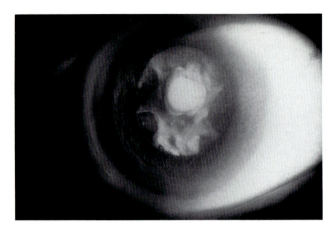

Figure 11–12. Progression of an anterior polar cataract to total cataract, a rare occurrence.

Normal lens transparency depends on the special spatial arrangement of the lens fibers and their protein constituents. Denaturation of the lens protein and loss of transparency result in opacification (cataract), which may interfere with vision.

Infantile cataracts are commonly classified according to their location and morphology. Three main types are described: (1) **polar cataracts,** opacities of the anterior or posterior pole of the lens involving the capsule and underlying lens; (2) **zonular cataracts,** opacities involving an entire layer or zone of the lens, leaving other parts of the lens transparent; and (3) **total cataracts,** opacities involving the entire lens.

Anterior Polar Cataracts.

Anterior polar cataracts can assume a number of morphological forms. Visual impairment varies, depending on the size of the opacity. Most anterior polar cataracts are very small, not exceeding 1 to 2 mm in diameter (Fig. 11–10). They are often bilateral and symmetric, and occasionally project forward into the anterior chamber, forming a pyrami-

dal cataract (Fig. 11–11). They usually remain stationary and traditionally have been considered to have little or no effect on vision. Rarely, however, an anterior polar cataract will progress to become a significant opacity requiring surgery (Fig. 11–12). Occasionally, eyes with anterior polar cataracts have a corneal astigmatism of greater than 1.5 diopters. Spectacle or contact lens correction may be required in these cases. This type of cataract may be inherited as an autosomal dominant condition or occur sporadically.

Anterior lenticonus is a rare condition in which the anterior surface of the lens bulges centrally (Fig. 11–13). A developmental weakness of the anterior lens capsule is assumed causative. It is bilateral in 75 percent of cases, and all bilateral cases reported after 1966 have been in patients with Alport's syndrome.

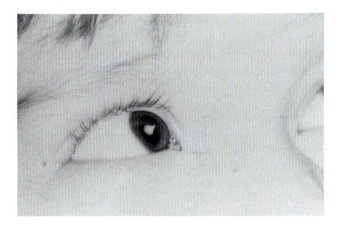

Figure 11–11. "Pyramidal" anterior polar cataract.

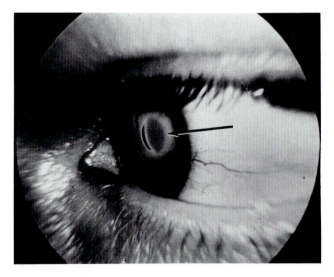

Figure 11–13. Anterior lenticonus with bulging of the anterior surface of the lens centrally (*arrow*). (*From Sand BJ, Abraham SV: Anterior lenticonus: An operated case and review of the literature. Am J Ophthalmol 53:636, 1962, with permission.*)

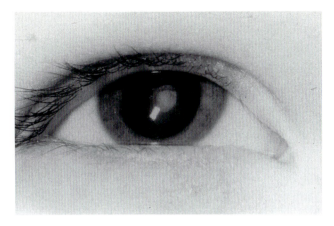

Figure 11–14. Small, posterior polar cataract.

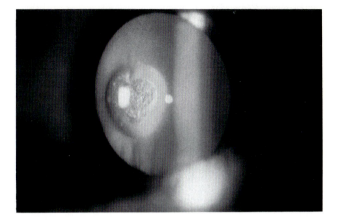

Figure 11–16. Posterior lenticonus, early stage. Note the circumscribed, oval, "oil-droplet" appearance.

Posterior Polar Cataracts. Posterior polar cataracts are usually larger than anterior ones, ranging in diameter from 1 to 4 mm (Figs. 11–14 and 11–15). Because of their larger diameter and closeness to the optical nodal point of the eye, posterior polar cataracts may significantly affect visual acuity. Although these lens opacities are usually stationary, progressive cases have been documented.

Posterior polar cataracts may be familial or may occur sporadically. The familial type is usually an autosomal dominant disorder, although autosomal recessive inheritance has been reported. Posterior polar cataracts may also occur in familial syndromes such as Alport's syndrome.

Posterior Lenticonus (Lentiglobus). Posterior lenticonus is a circumscribed round or oval bulge of the posterior lens capsule into the vitreous. In the early

stages, by the red reflex test, this may look like an oil droplet (Fig. 11–16). With the slit lamp the central portion of the posterior lens capsule can be seen to protrude posteriorly. Usually the lens material within and surrounding the capsular bulge eventually becomes opacified (Fig. 11–17). This disorder of the posterior lens capsule is most often unilateral. It is usually sporadic, although several familial cases (usually bilateral involvement) consistent with autosomal dominant inheritance have been reported. Because there is usually a period of normal visual development before posterior lenticonus appears or progresses, the visual prognosis following surgery for this cataract is usually favorable.

Nuclear Cataracts. Nuclear cataracts may involve the embryonic nucleus alone or both the embryonic and the fetal nucleus. These lens opacities are usually

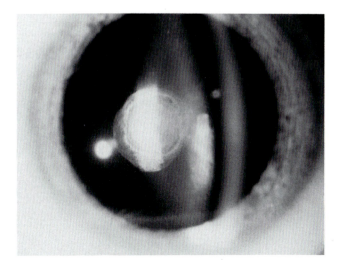

Figure 11–15. Larger, posterior polar cataract. *(Courtesy of Stephen B. Lichtenstein; from Nelson LB: Pediatric Ophthalmology. Philadelphia, Saunders, 1984, with permission.)*

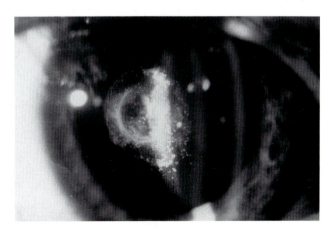

Figure 11–17. Posterior lenticonus, more advanced stage.

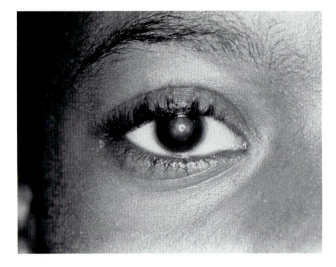

Figure 11–18. Lamellar cataract. Note the surrounding rim of clear lens.

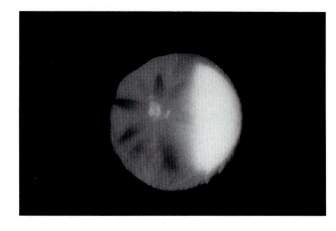

Figure 11–20. Stellate cataract.

bilateral and range in diameter from 2 to 4 mm. They typically cause significant visual impairment. Nuclear cataracts are inherited in an autosomal dominant, recessive, or X-linked manner.

Lamellar (Zonular) Cataracts. Lamellar cataracts are the most common type of congenital lens opacity. They can occur prenatally or during postnatal development. The typical lamellar cataract presents as a circular zone of opacity within the lens substance, surrounded by clear lens (Fig. 11–18). A distinctive feature is the presence of associated opacities called "riders." These are recognized as arcuate linear opacities bending around the equator; their tapered ends are directed axially (Fig. 11–19).

Lamellar cataracts are frequently hereditary, with autosomal dominant transmission. They may also be associated with systemic disorders, particularly neonatal hypoglycemia and galactosemia. A child's visual acuity with lamellar cataract depends on the density of the opacity. If the cataract is translucent, visual acuity may be quite good, but when it is dense, visual acuity may be as low as 20/400.

Other Cataract Types. Many other rarer opacities within the lens have been described. These include sutural (see Fig. 11–6), stellate (Fig. 11–20), cerulean (Fig. 11–21), crystalline (Fig. 11–22), and pulverulent (Fig. 11–23), to name a few.

Persistent Hyperplastic Primary Vitreous

Persistent hyperplastic primary vitreous (PHPV) results when the embryonic hyaloid artery in the posterior eye does not atrophy at the appropriate stage of

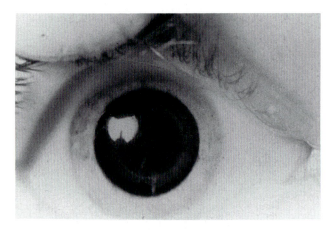

Figure 11–19. Lamellar cataract with a prominent "rider" at 6:00 (*arrow*).

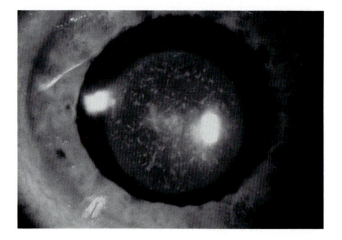

Figure 11–21. Cerulean cataract, characterized by minute, nonprogressive, opaque dots and strands. (*Courtesy of Malcolm N. Luxenberg.*)

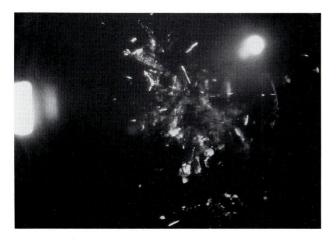

Figure 11–22. Crystalline (coralliform) cataract. The consistency of the opacity resembles coral. Branches radiate out into the lens cortex in a radial pattern. *(Courtesy of Malcolm N. Luxenberg.)*

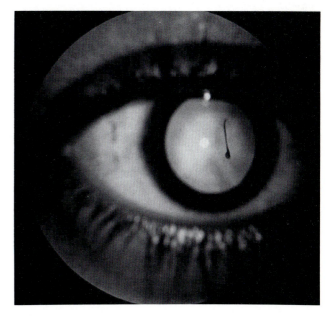

Figure 11–24. Persistent hyaloid artery, floating in the vitreous. *(From Degenhart W, Brown GC, Augsburger JJ, et al: Congenital vascular anomalies of the optic nerve head. Trans PA Acad Ophthalmol Otolaryngol 34:152, 1981, with permission.)*

ocular development. Various degrees of abnormality can be present, ranging from a collapsed arterial strand floating in the vitreous (Fig. 11–24) to a Mittendorf dot on the posterior lens capsule (see Fig. 13–11), to a patent hyaloid artery and a fibrovascular membrane attaching to the posterior surface of the lens (Fig. 11–25). A cataract may already be present at birth, or the lens may gradually opacify starting posteriorly. Spontaneous intraocular hemorrhage or retinal detachment can occur with progressive traction of the retrolental membrane on the ciliary processes (Fig. 11–26). The majority of cases are unilateral. Eventually the affected eye will be smaller than its pair, but this may not be apparent at birth. In questionable cases, ultrasonography is helpful in demonstrating a stalk running from the posterior

surface of the lens to the optic disc. It is best to treat these eyes, because left untreated most eyes with PHPV develop secondary glaucoma. The poor visual outcome in these eyes is also related to an often associated foveal hypoplasia.

Surgical Indications
Any cataract in an infant or child substantial enough to interfere with normal visual development should be removed. For the infant who presents at several

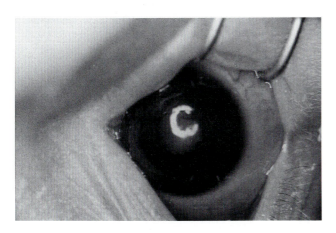

Figure 11–23. Pulverulent cataract. A semitranslucent cataract of the fetal nucleus, typically spherical or ovoid in shape.

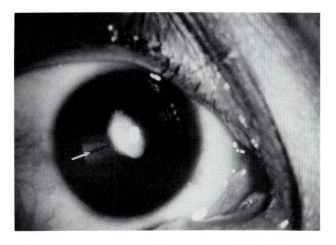

Figure 11–25. Persistent hyperplastic primary vitreous with central lens opacity and retrolental fibrovascular stalk (*arrow*). *(Courtesy of William Tasman; from Nelson LB, Brown GC, Arentsen JJ: Recognizing Patterns of Ocular Childhood Diseases. Thorofare, NJ, Slack, 1985, p 73, with permission.)*

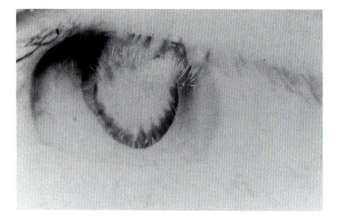

Figure 11–26. Persistent hyperplastic primary vitreous with retrolental membrane causing traction on the ciliary processes. *(Courtesy of William Tasman; from Nelson LB, Brown GC, Arentsen JJ: Recognizing patterns of ocular childhood diseases. Thorofare, NJ, Slack, 1985, p 73, with permission.)*

months of age with dense bilateral cataracts and nystagmus, the decision to operate is easy. These children have significant visual impairment; surgical treatment is absolutely indicated if there is to be any hope for visual development.

The decision is more difficult for the child with cataracts who does not have nystagmus and cannot cooperate for an objective measurement of visual acuity using eye charts. The absence of nystagmus indicates either that the vision is better than 20/200 or the lens opacities became denser after 2 or 3 months of age. A careful history of the child's overall performance is useful for these children. Parents should be asked how well the child explores the environment, and whether he or she can find small objects while crawling along the floor. How well the child functions in new environments may also be a useful indicator of vision. Frequently, a child with a moderately severe visual impairment will function reasonably well in a familiar environment, such as the home. The child will be reluctant, however, to explore a strange area without parental assistance.

An objective indicator of the severity of a cataract is its density centrally. A dense cataract larger than 3 mm in the center of the lens is almost always amblyogenic. Ophthalmoscopic examination should, therefore, include an estimate of the size, location, and density of the cataract. This can be accomplished using the hand-held slit lamp, retinoscope, or ophthalmoscope. If a retinoscopic reflex cannot be obtained sufficient to secure an adequate refraction, or if the retina cannot be visualized with a direct ophthalmoscope, the cataract is likely significant enough to require surgical intervention.

In young infants, vision is assessed by evaluating visual fixation reflexes. The ability to fixate and follow small objects on cover testing, and to develop op-

tokinetic nystagmus (see Chapter 2), are sought. Preferential looking techniques and pattern reversal visual evoked responses can also be incorporated in the testing. Differences between the two eyes using these techniques provides particularly useful information. When cataracts are very dense, an electroretinogram may be useful in assessing retinal function. When a child reaches 3 years of age, vision can usually be measured directly using picture or illiterate "E" charts.

Although there are no steadfast rules, some ophthalmologists believe that with minimally obstructive cataracts there remains some benefit in having the natural lens in the eye, even if the acuity is not perfectly clear. This is because the natural lens can accommodate to focus objects at different distances. Most ophthalmologists believe that this advantage is negated when the cataract prevents a best acuity of 20/50 to 20/60. Similarly, the age and functional needs of the child have to be considered. A 3-year-old child with 20/70 vision would probably appear quite content, but a school-age child with the same visual acuity would be more disabled, due to greater visual demands.

Monocular cataracts present an even greater clinical challenge. A poor visual prognosis exists due to the potential for irreversible deprivation amblyopia. Associated ocular defects, such as microphthalmos, which occur in 30 to 70% of eyes with monocular cataracts, further complicate the management and prognosis of unilateral congenital cataracts.

Even in older children with monocular cataracts, the lack of assurance in achieving good visual results should not be an absolute deterrence to surgery. Occasionally, it may be difficult to distinguish between a cataract present at birth and an early-onset developmental cataract; children with the latter may have an excellent visual result. Good results are common in children with posterior lenticonus or traumatic cataracts, if they had normal vision before developing the lens opacity. In other children, even if visual acuity does not improve following cataract removal, the peripheral field of vision will be enlarged, possibly enhancing peripheral fusion, and reducing the tendency toward strabismus. The cosmetic and psychological benefits of a clear black pupil, to both parents and child, must also be considered. Finally, unilateral cataracts associated with persistent hyperplastic primary vitreous should be removed to reduce the risks of late complications even though the final visual result in these eyes is often poor.

Management of Infantile Cataracts

The definitive treatment of the vast majority of significant congenital cataracts is surgical lens removal. Occasionally, however, this treatment modality can be delayed. For example, if a child with a zonular or lamellar cataract has reasonably good vision, and complains primarily of photophobia, the use of either sunglasses

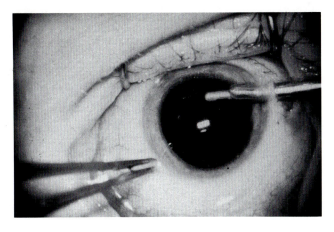

Figure 11–27. Procedure to remove infantile cataract using an automated vitrectomy instrument.

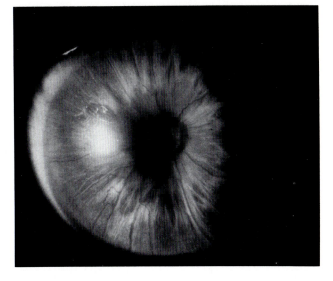

Figure 11–29. Pupillary-block glaucoma following infantile cataract surgery. *(From Catalano RA: Ocular Emergencies. Philadelphia, Saunders, 1992, p 272, with permission.)*

or a broad-rimmed hat may be all that is necessary. When only a small central opacity exists, a trial of a long-acting mydriatic agent may be attempted. The latter technique, however, is rarely tolerated over a long period of time in pediatric patients. The large pupil may aggravate photophobia, and the cycloplegic effect of these drugs paralyzes accommodation, necessitating reading glasses for near work.

The discussion of surgical techniques used to remove infantile cataracts is beyond the scope of this book. Suffice it to mention that the development of automated vitrectomy instruments with cutting and aspirating capabilities have substantially improved the surgical outcome, and reduced the incidence of postoperative complications (Fig. 11–27).

Postoperative Complications

Late complications following congenital cataract surgery include the development of secondary opacities (Fig. 11–28), glaucoma (Fig. 11–29), and retinal detachment (Fig. 11–30).

Secondary opacities result when membranes grow or cloudiness develops on the posterior lens capsule. To prevent visually significant opacities from developing, most ophthalmologists advocate removing the central 3 mm of the posterior capsule at the time of surgery. Membranes result when capsular epithelial cells proliferate and undergo pseudometaplastic change. These membranes may occlude or seclude the pupil; their removal requires a second operation.

Glaucoma may develop as an early or late compli-

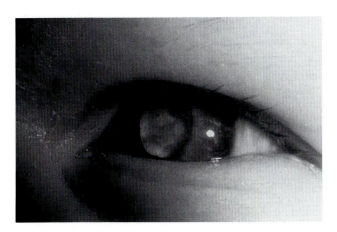

Figure 11–28. Membrane growing across a retained posterior lens capsule, resulting in a secondary opacity.

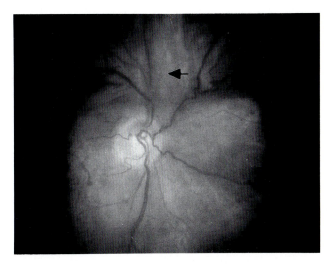

Figure 11–30. Retinal detachment (*arrow*) following infantile cataract surgery.

cation of infantile cataract surgery. Pupillary-block glaucoma can result following the development of a secondary membrane and seclusion of the pupil. It can also result when the vitreous face occludes the pupil and/or iridotomy opening. To prevent the latter, some surgeons advocate performing an anterior vitrectomy at the time of cataract surgery. Glaucoma can also develop insidiously, many years after infantile cataract surgery. The etiology of this glaucoma remains elusive; it may be due to a concordant developmental defect or surgically induced trauma to the anterior chamber angle. Typically, the glaucoma is open angle and asymptomatic; it may develop in as many as 24 percent of eyes by 60 months after surgery (Simon et al, 1991). Because of this possibility, individuals who undergo cataract surgery as children should be followed as glaucoma suspects for the rest of their lives.

The incidence of retinal detachment following infantile cataract surgery has been greatly reduced with the use of vitrectomy instrumentation to remove the cataract. Two recent studies of children who underwent newer surgical techniques showed the incidence of postoperative retinal detachment to be between 1.5 (Chrousos et al, 1984) and 19 percent (Keech et al, 1989). These studies, however, had much shorter follow-up periods than earlier studies; it may be many years before the true incidence of retinal detachment using current techniques is known.

Optical Rehabilitation

The removal of the cataractous lens is the most rudimentary step in treating these children. Once the lens has been removed the eye remains with poor vision, due to its inability to focus, and a commonly associated amblyopia. Postoperative treatment includes correction for the aphakia (absence of the ocular lens) and treatment of a superimposed amblyopia.

The correction of aphakia can include spectacles

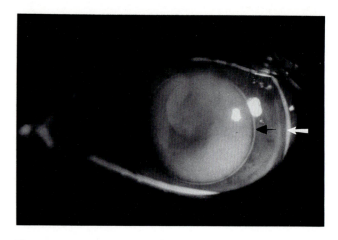

Figure 11–32. Silicone contact lens after the instillation of fluorescein solution. Note the steeper central area of the lens (*black arrow*) and the lens edge (*white arrow*).

(Fig. 11–31), contact lenses (Fig. 11–32), intraocular lenses, or epikeratophakia (Fig. 11–33). In general, children under 3 years of age are corrected such that their sharpest vision is for objects 50 cm away. By the time the child reaches school age, either bifocals (if spectacles are worn) or reading glasses are used to provide focused distant and near images.

Spectacles are an imperfect solution because they result in alterations in the peripheral field of vision, distortion, and prismatic effects. In addition, obtaining stable centration with the heavy thick lenses is difficult, and the optical center of the lens does not move with the eye. Spectacles are never used to correct monocular aphakia because the image through the aphakic spectacle is approximately 25 percent larger than the image that occurs in the normal eye. This retinal image disparity makes spectacle correction impractical for monocular aphakia.

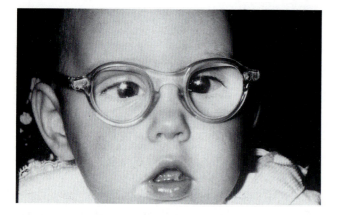

Figure 11–31. Spectacle correction of bilateral infantile aphakia. *(Courtesy of Joseph H. Calhoun from Nelson LH, Calhoun JC, Harley RD: Pediatric Ophthalmology, 3rd ed. Philadelphia, Saunders, 1992, p 246, with permission.)*

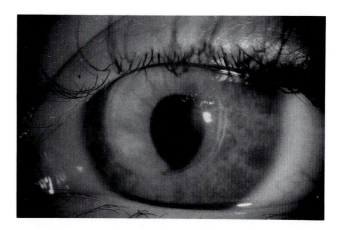

Figure 11–33. Epikeratophakia for the correction of pediatric aphakia.

Most ophthalmologists use extended-wear contact lenses to correct pediatric aphakia (Fig. 11–32). A preferred lens is the Silsoft extended-wear contact lens. This lens is composed of 100 percent silicone polymer, making it extremely gas permeable; it is also an excellent thermal conductor. Its small size and rigidity allows for easy insertion, and keratotomy readings are not necessary for fitting. Because the lens is hydrophobic, medications can be given with the lens in the eye, without a buildup of preservatives producing symptoms of irritation.

Problems with contact lens include intolerance, downward displacement of the lens with induced vertical diplopia, and residual image disparity (image size is 6 percent larger than normal). These problems have prompted some ophthalmologists to advocate intraocular lens implants for pediatric aphakia. The need to change the refractive power of the lens several times during the first year of life, as the axial length of the eye increases, contraindicates the use of intraocular lenses in children under 1 year of age. Frequent postimplantation complications, including iris erosion, dislocation of the lens, corneal edema, and glaucoma, are additional reasons to advocate a conservative approach to intraocular lenses. Finally, the long-term effects of intraocular lens implantation are unknown.

A recently developed corneal surgery technique, epikeratophakia, has also been advocated for optical correction following pediatric cataract surgery. This technique uses a lathed lamellar corneal disk, which is sutured to the front surface of the recipient's cornea (Fig. 11–33). Epikeratophakia corrects the optical error by changing the anterior curvature of the cornea. The technique is advantageous in being entirely extraocular and reversible. It does not damage the central cornea, and may be performed at the time of cataract operation or as a secondary procedure. Disadvantages include graft failure caused by persistent epithelial defects, infection, or mechanical trauma. Interface opacities may develop, and the need for suture removal after 3 weeks necessitates a second anesthesia in young children. Finally, amblyopia therapy is generally delayed for 4 to 6 weeks following epikeratophakia.

For monocular or asymmetric cataracts, optical correction is generally of little use without concomitant occlusion therapy to treat the coexisting deprivation amblyopia. The authors begin with approximately 4 hours of occlusion for infants less than 3 months of age, increasing to 80 to 90 percent of awake hours by 6 months of age. Preferential looking techniques may be useful in helping to titrate patching regimens (Fig. 11–34). Patching is maintained until maximum visual improvement has been documented and visual acuity in the aphakic eye is stable.

Visual Prognosis for Infants and Children With Cataracts

The prognosis for vision varies with the age at which the cataract developed, the presence of other ocular anomalies, and the success of aphakic correction and amblyopia treatment. The prognosis is better if the cataract developed beyond infancy, and vision was unimpaired for a period of time. In one study, only 6 percent of eyes with nystagmus and/or microphthalmos had a postoperative visual acuity of 20/50 or better, as compared to 81 percent of eyes without associated abnormalities (Scheie et al, 1967).

The presence of associated ocular anomalies, such as microphthalmos (Fig. 11–35), foveal hypoplasia (Fig. 11–36), or strabismus, adversely affects the visual prognosis. A relative afferent pupillary defect (see Chapter 2) is another poor prognostic sign, usually indicating significant asymmetrical optic nerve or retinal dysfunction. Retinal detachments, vitreous opacities, in-

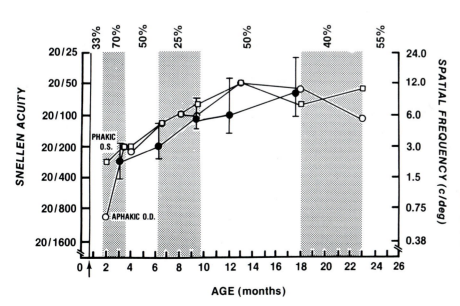

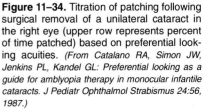

Figure 11–34. Titration of patching following surgical removal of a unilateral cataract in the right eye (upper row represents percent of time patched) based on preferential looking acuities. *(From Catalano RA, Simon JW, Jenkins PL, Kandel GL: Preferential looking as a guide for amblyopia therapy in monocular infantile cataracts. J Pediatr Ophthalmol Strabismus 24:56, 1987.)*

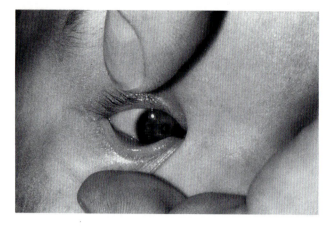

Figure 11–35. Congenital cataract in a microphthalmic eye.

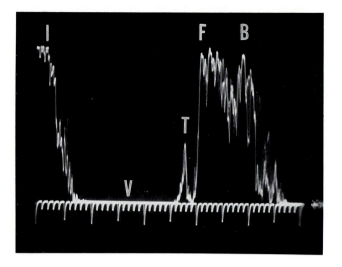

Figure 11–37. A-scan ultrasound demonstrating an intraocular tumor (I = initial spike, V = vitreous, T = tumor, F = fundus, B = orbital bone spike). *(From Catalano RA: Ocular Emergencies. Philadelphia, Saunders, 1992, p 46, with permission.)*

traocular foreign bodies, and posterior segment tumors also reduce the prognosis. These can be detected preoperatively with ultrasonography (Fig. 11–37) or neuroimaging (Fig. 11–38), when direct visualization of the posterior eye is inadequate.

Until recently, visual rehabilitation for monocular congenital cataracts was virtually unknown. During the past decade success has been reported with early surgery (within the first weeks of life) followed by immediate optical correction and occlusion therapy. Early surgery also improves the prognosis with bilateral cataracts. In one series, 60 percent of eyes operated on before 8 weeks of age achieved an acuity of 20/60 or better, whereas only 1 of 7 patients operated on after the

age of 8 weeks achieved a visual acuity better than 20/200 (Gelbart et al, 1982).

Lens Dislocation (Ectopia Lentis)

The lens is suspended in the eye by the zonule. This structure is composed of fine fibrils of modified collagenous tissue, which attach the lens capsule to the ciliary body (see Fig. 1–4). Contraction of the ciliary body releases tension on the zonule. The elastic lens capsule

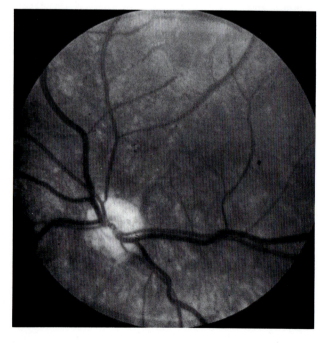

Figure 11–36. Foveal hypoplasia. Note the absence of the macular reflex.

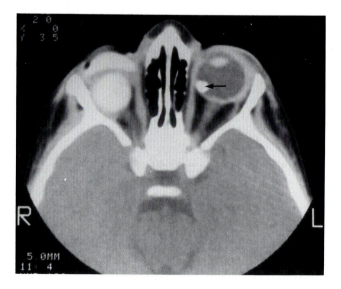

Figure 11–38. Computerized tomography demonstrating calcification in the left eye due to retinoblastoma (*arrow*). The right eye has undergone enucleation; a prosthesis is present in the right socket. *(From Catalano RA: Ocular Emergencies. Philadelphia, Saunders, 1992, p 68, with permission.)*

TABLE 11–6. LENS DISLOCATION: ETIOLOGIC CLASSIFICATION

Category	Entity	Associated Findings
Hereditary	Marfan syndrome	Arachnodactyly, cardiovascular defects, pectus excavatum, hyperextensible joints
	Homocystinuria	Mental retardation, fine/fair hair, osteoporosis, thromboses, malar flush
	Weill–Marchesani syndrome	Short stature, short fingers and toes, malformed teeth, stiff joints
	Ehlers–Danlos syndrome	Short stature, hyperextensible skin, kyphoscoliosis, blue sclera, retinal detachment, easily ruptured sclera, keratoconus, angioid streaks
	Hyperlysinemia	Mental retardation, seizures, hypertonia
	Sulfite oxidase deficiency	Mental retardation, severe neurological impairment, infantile death
	Refsum's disease	Ataxia, deafness, polyneuropathy, muscular weakness, icthyosis, defect in phytanic acid metabolism
Ocular syndrome	Simple ectopia lentis	Dislocated lenses are the only finding, autosomal dominant
	Ectopia lentis et pupillae	Pupils displaced in one direction, lens in opposite direction, autosomal recessive
	Aniridia	Near total absence of iris, foveal hypoplasia, glaucoma, Wilms' tumor, 11p–
	Infantile glaucoma (advanced)	Corneal edema, corneal enlargement, optic nerve cupping, tearing, photophobia, blepharospasm
	Anterior megalophthalmos	Congenital, nonprogressive, symmetrically enlarged corneas, X-linked recessive
	Coloboma	Keyhole-shaped pupil with defect inferiorly, can involve retina, optic nerve, autosomal dominant
	Medulloepithelioma	Cyst or mass in iris, anterior chamber, or ciliary body, glaucoma, exophthalmos, orbital mass, uveitis, strabismus, hyphema
Trauma	Blunt trauma	Iris sphincter tears, angle recession, choroidal rupture, commotio retinae, retinodialysis
	Child abuse	Ocular hemorrhages, retinal detachment, long bone fractures, dislocated joints, subdural hematoma, burns

then relaxes, allowing the lens to become more spherical. This in turn increases its power. Known as accommodation, this process occurs physiologically to focus near objects upon the retina.

When the zonular fibers become lax, torn, or broken, the lens can no longer be held in its proper anatomic location. It may partially (subluxation) or totally dislocate. This condition, known as ectopia lentis, is caused by a variety of factors, and is associated with a number of syndromes (Table 11–6).

Etiologic Classification of Ectopia Lentis

Ectopia lentis continues to be a diagnostic and therapeutic challenge for most ophthalmologists. A thorough systemic and ocular evaluation is necessary to establish the etiology and to initiate the appropriate therapeutic and prophylactic measures (Table 11–7).

Although trauma remains the most common cause of isolated ectopia lentis, two other ocular syndromes have been described in which no other significant ocular or systemic abnormalities exist. Simple ectopia lentis, either congenital or of delayed onset, is characterized solely by dislocated ocular lenses. In this autosomal dominant disorder the dislocation may be relatively stationary or progressive. Ectopia lentis et pupillae is an unrelated recessive disorder in which the lens and pupil are dislocated in opposite directions (Figs. 11–39 and 11–40). The lens usually moves na-

sally; the pupil temporally. The degree of pupillary displacement varies from slight to marked. The opposite displacements of the lens and pupil may render the patient functionally aphakic.

Another ocular condition in which the lens frequently dislocates is aniridia. This condition is characterized by near total absence of iris, foveal hypoplasia, and glaucoma. Lens dislocation in aniridia is usually minimal (Fig. 11–41). Lens dislocation can also occur as a secondary event in advanced infantile glaucoma and in anterior megalophthalmos. Dislocation in these disorders occurs when enlargement and stretching of the ciliary body causes compensatory stretching of the zo-

TABLE 11–7. LABORATORY EVALUATION OF PATIENTS WITH LENS DISLOCATION

Finding	Test
Family history of Marfan syndrome	None
No family history of Marfan syndrome	Urine amino acid assay (homocystinuria)
	Methionine loading (homocystinuria)
	Urine sodium nitroprusside test (homocystinuria)
	Urine sulfite assay (sulfite oxidase deficiency)
	Serum lysine (hyperlysinuria)

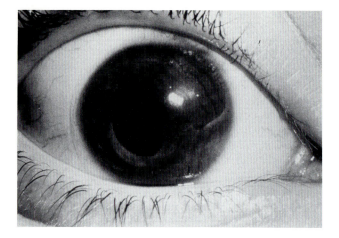

Figure 11–39. Ectopia lentis et pupillae. Temporal dislocation of the pupil. *(Courtesy of Joseph H. Calhoun.)*

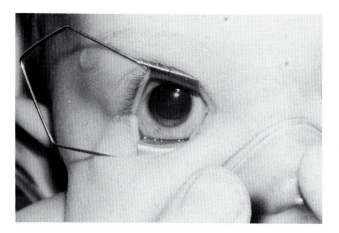

Figure 11–41. Minimal lens dislocation in aniridia. *(Courtesy of John W. Simon; from Catalano RA: Ocular Emergencies. Philadelphia, Saunders, 1992, p 253, with permission.)*

nule. As with aniridia, the lens rarely dislocates out of the pupillary area in either of these disorders.

Ectopia lentis is also an important diagnostic clue to the presence of several systemic disorders, including Marfan and Weill–Marchesani syndromes, and homocystinuria.

Marfan syndrome is a dominantly inherited disorder caused by a point mutation in the fibrillin gene. Fibrillin is a major component of microfibrils, which are ubiquitous in connective tissue. They make up the suspensory ligament of the lens (the zonule) as well as the scaffolding of elastic fibers surrounding the lens. More than 50 percent of affected individuals develop bilateral ectopia lentis. The direction of dislocation is most commonly superotemporal. Other associated abnormalities include joint hyperextensibility, arachnodactyly (slender, long fingers and limbs; Fig. 11–42),

pectus excavatum, and scoliosis. The major cardiovascular complications of aortic arch dilation, dissecting aortic aneurysm and cardiac valve abnormalities, often lead to premature death.

Homocystinuria refers to a group of recessively inherited inborn errors of amino acid metabolism in which homocysteine and methionine cannot be converted into cysteine, or homocysteine into methionine. These enzyme deficiencies lead to an accumulation of methionine and/or homocysteine in both urine and blood. Patients appear tall and thin, similar to the Marfan habitus. In addition, however, there is generalized osteoporosis. Mental retardation occurs in approximately 50 percent of patients and may be progressive. Death usually occurs secondary to thromboembolic events. Ectopia lentis occurs in approximately 90 percent of patients with homocystinuria. The dislocation is bilateral and symmetrical. In contrast to Marfan syndrome, the lenses usually migrate either inferiorly or inferonasally (Figs. 11–43 and 11–44). An additional distinction is that the zonular fibers are usually broken in homocystinuria, but intact in Marfan syndrome. Because clinical improvement occasionally follows vitamin supplements (pyridoxine, folate, or cobalamin), urine screening for homocystinuria should be performed in all cases of nontraumatic lens dislocation.

Weill–Marchesani syndrome is comprised of brachymorphia (short, stocky build and short digits), limited joint mobility, and microspherophakia. Microspherophakia is commonly present prior to dislocation of the lens and is responsible for the significant myopia that develops in these patients. Abnormal zonules, which frequently appear abnormally elongated and lax, may contribute to the development of spherophakia and ectopia lentis. The elongated zonules also permit the lens to move forward, increasing its area of contact with the iris. A resultant progressive shallow-

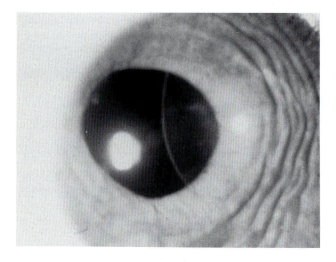

Figure 11–40. Ectopia lentis et pupillae. Nasal dislocation of the lens. *(Courtesy of Joseph H. Calhoun.)*

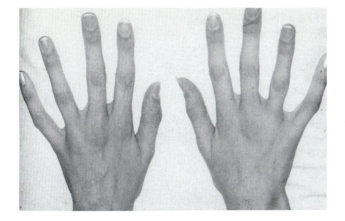

A

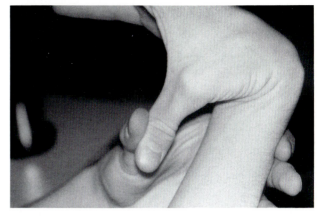

B

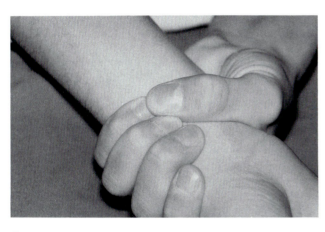

C

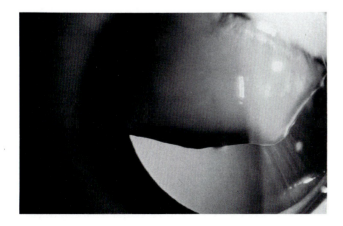

D

Figure 11–42. Hand signs in Marfan syndrome. **A.** Arachnodactyly (long, slender fingers). **B.** Hyperextensibility. **C.** Wrist sign (thumb overlaps fingers wrapped around the wrist). **D.** Thumb sign (thumb extends beyond clenched fingers).

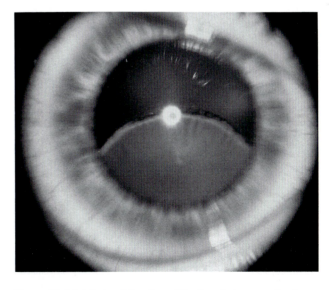

Figure 11–43. Superotemporal dislocation of the lens in a Marfan patient. Note the parallel arrangement of the zonular fibers. *(From Nelson LB, Maumenee IH: Ectopia lentis. Surv Ophthalmol 27:143, 1982, with permission.)*

Figure 11–44. Inferior dislocation of the lens in homocystinuric patient. Note the absence of zonular fibers. *(From Nelson LB, Maumenee IH: Ectopia lentis. Surv Ophthalmol 27:143, 1982, with permission.)*

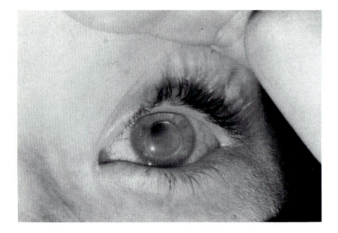

Figure 11–45. Pupillary-block glaucoma secondary to anterior lens dislocation in a patient with Weill–Marchesani syndrome. *(From Catalano RA: Ocular Emergencies. Philadelphia, Saunders, 1992, p 273, with permission.)*

ing of the anterior chamber can result in pupillary-block glaucoma (Fig. 11–45).

Although much rarer, lens dislocations have also been reported in Ehlers–Danlos syndrome, hyperlysinemia, sulfite oxidase deficiency, and Refsum disease.

Management of Ectopia Lentis

The presenting ophthalmic problem in children with dislocated lenses is usually blurred vision. Retinoscopy may reveal a significant refractive error, usually myopia and astigmatism. Occasionally an accurate refraction may be extremely difficult because of tilting or dislocation of the lens. In these cases an aphakic refraction should be attempted through an aphakic portion of the pupil. Lysing zonular fibers with the neodymium:YAG laser may further dislocate a subluxed lens to achieve a clear aphakic axis. It is notable that the amplitude of accommodation is rarely significantly reduced in an eye with a subluxated lens. Typically, a bifocal lens is needed only when an aphakic correction is used.

Occasionally, the lens may dislocate into the anterior chamber, inducing pupillary-block glaucoma. This is more likely to occur in homocystinuria. The first line of management should be to try to draw the lens back into the posterior chamber. The child should lie supine to effect gravitational pull. Pupillary dilation with phenylephrine may be helpful, but anticholinergic agents, which paralyze the pupillary sphincter, should not be used. When the lens has returned to the posterior chamber, a miotic agent should be instilled to reverse the dilation and keep the lens posterior. If successful, these patients should be kept on long-term miotics indefinitely. If the lens can not be repositioned into the posterior chamber it must be removed surgically. Repeated anterior dislocation is another indication for surgical removal.

REFERENCES

Abbassi V, Lowe CU, Calcagno PL: Oculo-cerebro-renal syndrome. Am J Dis Child 115:145, 1968.

Amos CF, Lambert SR, Buncic JR, Musarella MA: Rigid gas permeable contact lens correction of aphakia following congenital cataract removal during infancy. J Pediatr Ophthalmol Strabismus 29:243, 1992.

BenEzra D, Paez JH: Congenital cataract and intraocular lenses. Am J Ophthalmol 96:311, 1983.

Beutler E, Matsumoto F, Kuhl W, et al: Galactokinase deficiency as a cause of cataracts. N Engl J Med 288:1203, 1973.

Birch EE, Stager DR: Prevalence of good visual acuity following surgery for congenital unilateral cataract. Arch Ophthalmol 106:40, 1988.

Bouzas AG: Anterior polar cataract and corneal astigmatism. J Pediatr Ophthalmol Strabismus 29:210, 1992.

Calhoun JH: Cataracts and lens anomalies in children. In Nelson LB, Calhoun JH, Harley RD (eds): Pediatric Ophthalmology, Philadelphia, Saunders, 1991, pp 234–257.

Catalano RA, Simon JW, Jenkins PL, Kandel GL: Preferential looking as a guide for amblyopia therapy in monocular infantile cataracts. J Pediatr Ophthalmol Strabismus 24:56, 1987.

Chrousos GA, Parks MM, O'Neill JF: Incidence of chronic glaucoma, retinal detachment and secondary membrane surgery in pediatric aphakic patients. Ophthalmology 91:1238, 1984.

Cibis GW, Waeltermann JM, Whitcraft CT, et al: Lenticular opacities in carriers of Lowe's syndrome. Ophthalmology 93:1041, 1986.

Cordes FC: Galactosemia cataract: A review. Am J Ophthalmol 50:1151, 1960.

Crouch ER Jr, Parks MM: Management of posterior lenticonus complicated by unilateral cataract. Am J Ophthalmol 85:503, 1978.

DelMonte MA: Diagnosis and management of congenital and developmental cataracts. Pediatr Clin North Am 37:205, 1990.

Drummond GT, Scott WE, Keech RV: Management of monocular congenital cataracts. Arch Ophthalmol 107:45, 1989.

Federman JL, Shields JA, Altman B, et al: The surgical and nonsurgical management of persistent hyperplastic primary vitreous. Ophthalmology 90:452, 1982.

France TD, Frank JW: The association of strabismus and aphakia in children. J Pediatr Ophthalmol Strabismus 19:12, 1981.

François J: Glaucoma and uveitis after congenital cataract surgery. Ann Ophthalmol 3:131, 1971.

François J: Congenital Cataracts. Springfield, IL, Thomas, 1963.

Fraser GR, Freedman AL: The Causes of Blindness in Childhood: A Study of 776 Children with Several Visual Handicaps. Baltimore, Johns Hopkins, 1967.

Gelbart SS, Hoyt CS, Jastrebski G, et al: Long-term visual results in bilateral congenital cataracts. Am J Ophthalmol 93:615, 1982.

Ginsberg J, Bove KE, Fogelson MH: Pathological features of the eye in the oculocerebrorenal (Lowe) syndrome. J Pediatr Ophthalmol Strabismus 18:16, 1981.

Haddad R, Font RL, Reeser F: Persistent hyperplastic primary vitreous. A clinicopathologic study of 62 cases and review of the literature. Surv Ophthalmol 23:123, 1978.

Hiles DA: Intraocular lens implantation in children with monocular cataracts, 1974–1983. Ophthalmology 91:1231, 1984.

Hiles DA: Infantile cataracts. Pediatr Ann 12:556, 1983.

Hiles DA: The need for intraocular lens implantation in children. Ophthalm Surg 8:162, 1977.

Jaafa MS, Robb RM: Congenital anterior polar cataract: A review of 63 cases. Ophthalmology 91:249, 1984.

Jain IS, Pillai P, Gangwar DN, et al: Congenital cataract: Management and results. J Pediatr Ophthalmol Strabismus 20:243, 1983.

Jaureguy BM, Hall JG: Isolated congenital ectopia lentis with autosomal dominant inheritance. Clin Genet 15:97, 1979.

Kanski JJ, Elkington AR, Daniel R: Retinal detachment after congenital cataract surgery. Br J Ophthalmol 58:92, 1974.

Karr DJ, Scott WE: Visual acuity results following treatment of persistent hyperplastic primary vitreous. Arch Ophthalmol 104:662, 1986.

Keech RV, Tongue AC, Scott WE: Complications after surgery for congenital and infantile cataracts. Am J Ophthalmol 108:136, 1989.

Kelley CG, Keates RH, Lembach RG: Epikeratophakia for pediatric aphakia. Arch Ophthalmol 104:680, 1986.

Kohn BA: The differential diagnosis of cataracts in infancy and childhood. Am J Dis Child 130:184, 1976.

Krill AE, Woodbury G, Bowman JE: X-chromosomal-linked sutural cataracts. Am J Ophthalmol 68:867, 1969.

Kushner BJ: Visual results after surgery for monocular juvenile cataracts of undetermined onset. Am J Ophthalmol 102:468, 1986.

Levin AV, Edmonds SA, Nelson LB, et al: Extended-wear contact lenses for the treatment of pediatric aphakia. Ophthalmology 95:1107, 1988.

Levy NS, Krill AE, Beutler E: Galactokinase deficiency and cataracts. Am J Ophthalmol 74:41, 1972.

Maumenee IH: The eye in the Marfan syndrome. Trans Am Ophthalmol Soc 69:685, 1981.

Merin S: Congenital cataracts. In Renie WA (ed): Goldberg's Genetic and Metabolic Eye Disease. Boston, Little, Brown, 1986, p 369.

Merin S, Crawford JS: The etiology of congenital cataracts. Can J Ophthalmol 6:178, 1971.

Merin S, Lapithis AG, Horovitz D, et al: Childhood blindness in Cyprus. Am J Ophthalmol 74:538, 1972.

Metz H: Keeping glasses on an infant. J Pediatr Ophthalmol 9:250, 1972.

Morgan KS, Arffa RC, Marvelli TL, Verity SM: Five year follow-up of epikeratophakia in children. Ophthalmology 93:423, 1986.

Morgan KS, Ellis GS Jr, Marvelli TL, Arffa RC: Epikerato-

phakia in children with traumatic cataracts. J Pediatr Ophthalmol Strabismus 23:108, 1986.

Mostafa MS, Temtamy S, El-Gamma MY, et al: Genetic studies of congenital cataracts. Metab Pediatr Ophthalmol 5:233, 1981.

Nankis SJ, Scott WE: Persistent hyperplastic primary vitreous. Arch Ophthalmol 95:240, 1977.

Nelson LB: Diagnosis and management of congenital and developmental cataracts. Semin Ophthalmol 5:154, 1990.

Nelson LB, Calhoun JH, Simon JW, Harley RD: Progression of anterior polar cataracts in childhood. Arch Ophthalmol 103:1842, 1985.

Nelson LB, Cutler SI, Calhoun JH, et al: Silsoft extended wear contact lenses in pediatric aphakia. Ophthalmology 92:1529, 1985.

Nelson, LB, Maumenee IGH: Ectopia lentis. Surv Ophthalmol 27:143, 1982.

Nielson CE: Lenticonus anterior and Alport's syndrome. Acta Ophthalmol 56:518, 1978.

O'Neill JF: Cataracts in infants and children. Pediatr Ann 9:419, 1980.

Potter WS, Nelson LB: Congenital cataracts: Current diagnosis and management. Ophthalm Pract 8:154, 1990.

Pyeritz RE, McKusick VA: The Marfan syndrome: Diagnosis and management. N Engl J Med 300:772, 1979.

Robb RM, Mayer DL, Moore BD: Results of early treatment of unilateral congenital cataracts. J Pediatr Ophthalmol Strabismus 24:178, 1987.

Scheie HG, Rubenstein RA, Kent RB: Aspiration of congenital or soft cataracts: Further experience. Am J Ophthalmol 63:3, 1967.

Shih VE, Abrams IF, Johnson JL, et al: Sulfite oxidase deficiency: Biochemical and clinical investigations of a hereditary metabolic disorder in sulfur metabolism. N Engl J Med 297:1022, 1977.

Simon JW, Mehta N, Simmons ST, et al: Glaucoma after pediatric lensectomy/vitrectomy. Ophthalmology 98:670, 1991.

Stambolian D: Galactose and cataract. Surv Ophthalmol 32:333, 1988.

Tchah H, Larson RS, Nichols BD, Lindstrom RL: Neodymium:YAG laser zonulysis for treatment of lens subluxation. Ophthalmology 96:230, 1989.

Townes PL: Ectopia lentis et pupillae. Arch Ophthalmol 94:1126, 1976.

Tripathi RC, Cibis GW, Tripathi BJ: Lowe's syndrome. Trans Ophthalmol Soc UK 100:132, 1980.

Wilson WA, Richards W, Donnell GN: Oculo-cerebral-renal syndrome of Lowe. Arch Ophthalmol 70:5, 1963.

Winder AF: Laboratory screening in the assessment of human cataract. Trans Ophthalmol Soc UK 101:127, 1981.

Young ID, Fielder AR, Casey TA: Weill–Marchesani syndrome in mother and son. Clin Genet 30:475, 1986.

DISORDERS OF THE RETINA
AND VITREOUS

ESSENTIAL INFORMATION FOR PRIMARY CARE PRACTITIONERS

Retinopathy of Prematurity

Retinopathy of prematurity (ROP) is a disorder of the developing retinal vasculature. It occurs most frequently in the smallest, sickest, premature infants, and accounts for severe visual impairment in 300 to 500 children each year in the United States alone. Multiple risk factors are involved (Table 12–1). At highest risk are infants born at 23 to 28 weeks of gestation, who weigh less than 1000 g (2 lbs 3 oz) at birth. Associated medical disorders in these children are listed in Table 12–2.

Infants are not born with ROP; they are born with immaturity of the retina and develop ROP. Not all premature infants, even those at greatest risk, develop the disorder, and ROP resolves without treatment in 90 percent or more of infants who do develop it (Flynn, 1991). A recently completed multicenter trial demonstrated that when ROP does not resolve, but rather progresses to certain stages, cryotherapy can significantly reduce the final incidence of blindness (Cryotherapy for ROP Cooperative Group, 1990a, 1990b). Cryotherapy is the application of a cold probe to the surface of the eye to freeze the underlying part of the retina where blood vessels did not grow. Because this ther-

apy is effective in many cases, it is important to screen those infants who are at the greatest risk for nonregression. The American Academy of Pediatrics (AAP) has published guidelines for the selection of "at risk" infants, and for the timing of initial and follow-up examinations.

Screening Guidelines for ROP

The AAP guidelines suggest that all infants born at less than 30 weeks of gestation or weighing less than 1300 g at birth should have a screening eye examination regardless of oxygen exposure (AAP, 1988). In addition, all neonates less than 35 weeks of gestation or less than 1500 g at birth, who required supplemental oxygen, should be examined. Because the cryotherapy for ROP study included only babies who weighed less than 1251 g at birth, uncertainty remains regarding the appropriateness of these upper limits on birthweight and gestational age. Local standards vary, but it is not uncommon for many communities to follow arbitrary screening criteria, such as a birthweight of less than 1750 or 2000 g, a gestational age of less than 37 weeks, and oxygen use of more than 17 hours (Schaffer, 1990).

According to the Guidelines for Perinatal Care (AAP, 1990), the examination should be performed prior to hospital discharge or at 5 to 7 weeks of age if the infant is still hospitalized. There have been reports, however, of very young (gestational age less than 26

TABLE 12–1. RISK FACTORS AND PROTECTIVE FACTORS FOR THE DEVELOPMENT OF RETINOPATHY OF PREMATURITY

Factors	Comment
▪ RISK FACTORS	
Birthweight	Neonates < 1000 g have the highest incidence of ROP. The severity of ROP is also inversely related to the birthweight (Valentine et al, 1989). Very few vision-threatening cases of ROP occur in infants weighing more than 1700 g at birth.
Gestational age	Greatest risk is for those infants born at 23 to 28 weeks gestational age; significant risk remains through 32 weeks of gestation; risk is small after 37 weeks gestation.
Oxygen	Despite a long tradition of being implicated as the leading cause of ROP, it is neither necessary nor sufficient, in itself, to cause the disorder. A critical blood level of oxygen that induces ROP, or a regimen of care that prevents it, have not been established.
Carbon dioxide	Enhances the effect of oxygen damage in animal models. Postulated to cause vasodilation, resulting in greater exposure to, and damage from oxygen (Flowers et al, 1982); not substantiated by Biglan et al (1984).
Aspirin/indomethacin	Similar effects and postulates as carbon dioxide (Flowers et al, 1982).
Blood products	Fetal hemoglobin binds oxygen more strongly than adult hemoglobin. Transfusion with adult blood may result in more oxygen being set free in the vicinity of immature capillaries, potentiating the risk of ROP; most studies, however, have not confirmed this.
Steroids	The use of steroids for lung disease may be associated with the need for cryotherapy (Batton et al, 1992); see below, however.
Other	Other implicated factors that remain unconfirmed include sepsis, intraventricular hemorrhage, apnea spells, chronic in-utero hypoxia, acidosis (discussed by Flynn, 1991); bright nursery lights (Fielder et al, 1992); and seizures (Biglan et al, 1984). Unconfirmed associated risk factors include being white and being one of a multiple birth (Schaffer et al, 1990).
▪ PROTECTIVE FACTORS	
Vitamin E	Early reports that it protected against ROP have not been substantiated. Its effect may be small, and it may affect only the severity, not the incidence, of disease. Serum levels between 1.2 and 3.0 µg/dL appear most prudent to avoid complications of necrotizing enterocolitis, sepsis, altered immune response, and intraventricular and retinal hemorrhages.
D-penicillamine	One report that its use protects against ROP (Lakatos et al, 1986) remains unconfirmed.
Steroids	Prolonged (>24 days) treatment with steroids may reduce the likelihood that ROP will reach threshold criteria for cryotherapy (Sobel & Philip, 1992); see "Steroids" under RISK FACTORS, above, however.
Surfactant	The use of calf–lung surfactant extract (Infasurf) at the time of birth in infants with birthweights less than 1000 g was associated with a reduction in the incidence of ROP in all racial and gender groups (Repka et al, 1991); unconfirmed.

weeks) and small (birthweight less than 1000 g) infants needing cryotherapy during their fourth or fifth weeks of life. Therefore, an experienced examiner has suggested that infants with birthweights of less than 1500 g have their first examination at 4 to 6 weeks of age, and that infants over 1500 g have their first examination at 6 to 8 weeks of age (Schaffer, 1990).

The zone of immaturity or stage and zone of the ROP governs the timing for repeat examination. Be-

TABLE 12–2. MEDICAL DISORDERS IN HIGH-RISK PREMATURE INFANTS

Retinopathy of prematurity
Intraventricular hemorrhage
Bronchopulmonary dysplasia
Respiratory distress syndrome
Right-to-left shunting of blood with hypoxia
Necrotizing enterocolitis with sepsis
Electrolyte imbalance

cause severe ROP can rapidly progress, eyes found to have greater degrees of involvement, particularly prethreshold disease, need close follow-up (described in the "Comprehensive Information" section later in the chapter).

Examination for ROP

Examination requires manipulation of the premature infant's eyelids and eyes, and dilation of the pupils. These activities can affect the respiratory, cardiac, and gastrointestinal systems of these small infants. Complications can include ileus, cardiac arrhythmias, and increased blood pressure. In most cases these effects are short lived, and do not deter further examination. One study found that respiratory and cardiac rates, blood pressure, and oxygen saturation were not affected by the use of a topical anesthetic during the examination (Saunders & Miller, 1991). The protocol for pupil dilation is given in Table 12–3. The examiner should be aware that poor dilation is a sign of severe ROP. When

TABLE 12–3. PROTOCOL FOR PUPIL DILATION IN PREMATURE INFANTS

	Light Irides	Dark Irides
Drops	Cyclopentolate hydrochloride 0.2% and phenylephrine 1.0%	Tropicamide 1.0% and phenylephrine 2.5%
Administer	Give twice at 5-minute intervals	Give three times at 15-minute intervals
Examine	30 minutes after the last drop	15 minutes after the last drop

this occurs, dilation drops should be repeated; the child's exam should not be deferred to the next visit of the ophthalmologist.

Retinoblastoma

Retinoblastoma, a malignant tumor of the photoreceptor layer of the retina, is the most common intraocular malignancy of childhood. It occurs in approximately 1 in 18,000 infants; 250 to 300 new cases are diagnosed in the United States annually. Hereditary and nonhereditary patterns of transmission occur; there is no sex or race predilection. The tumor occurs bilaterally in 25 to 35 percent of cases. The average age at diagnosis for bilateral tumors is 12 months; unilateral cases are diagnosed, on average, at 21 months. Occasionally, the tumor is discovered at birth, during adolescence, or even in adulthood.

The prognosis for patients with retinoblastoma is directly related to the size and extension of the tumor.

Most tumors that are confined to the eye can be cured; the prognosis is poor when orbital or optic nerve extension has occurred. The suspicion of retinoblastoma, therefore, warrants prompt referral to an ophthalmologist.

Clinical Manifestations of Retinoblastoma

The clinical manifestations of retinoblastoma vary depending on the stage at which the tumor is detected. The initial sign in the majority of patients is a white pupillary reflex (leukocoria). This is usually first noticed by the child's parents or the pediatrician. Leukocoria results because of the reflection of light off the white tumor. With small tumors, it is noticed only when the eye is turned in a particular direction. This phenomenon is illustrated in Figures 12–1 and 12–2, and accounts for the occasionally given history of "sometimes seeing something white in the pupil." At times, leukocoria is captured in photographs of the child (Fig. 12–3).

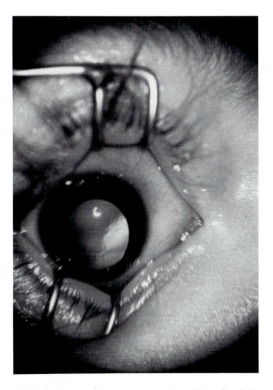

Figure 12–1. Leukocoria, the presence of a white reflex in the pupil due to retinoblastoma. Notice how only part of the pupil appears white.

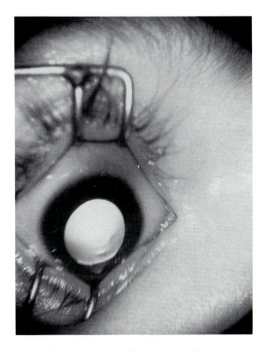

Figure 12–2. Same eye as in Figure 12–1. The eye has moved slightly; now the entire pupil appears white.

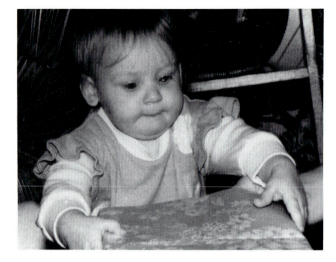

Figure 12–3. The leukocoria present in this photograph led to the discovery of a retinoblastoma in the peripheral retina. The parents never noticed a white reflex at any other time.

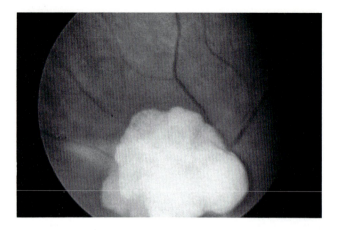

Figure 12–4. Indirect ophthalmoscopic view of a retinoblastoma.

The second most frequent initial sign of retinoblastoma is strabismus (misaligned eyes). Less frequent presenting signs include pseudohypopyon (tumor cells layered inferiorly in front of the iris), caused by tumor seeding in the anterior chamber of the eye; hyphema (blood layered in front of the iris), secondary to iris neovascularization; vitreous hemorrhage; or signs of orbital cellulitis. Tumors that grow anteriorly from the retina, seeding the vitreous (endophytic growth), may simulate endophthalmitis (intraocular infection). Tumors that grow into the subretinal space (exophytic growth) may resemble Coats' disease (described later in this chapter).

Diagnosis of Retinoblastoma

Retinoblastoma is diagnosed by ophthalmic examination, with the occasional assistance of computed tomography, ultrasonography, and other ancillary tests. A dilated fundus examination will reveal most retinoblastomas (Fig. 12–4). If a tumor is not detected on ophthalmoscopy, but the entire retina cannot be visualized with the child awake, an examination under anesthesia is necessary.

Computerized tomography is useful in delineating orbital extension and concurrent pinealoblastomas (described later in this chapter). Areas of calcification within the tumor may also be detected (Figs. 12–5 and 11–38). A-scan ultrasound of a retinoblastoma demonstrates markedly high internal reflectivity with prominent echo spikes corresponding to foci of calcification (Fig. 12–6). B-scan ultrasound demonstrates internal solidity and orbital shadowing. Fluorescein angiography and an anterior chamber tap, to analyze the aqueous for lactose dehydrogenase and cells, is sometimes needed when retinoblastoma can not be differentiated from other causes of leukocoria (see Table 12–8).

Retinitis Pigmentosa (RP)

Retinitis pigmentosa (RP) refers to a group of related disorders characterized by progressive pigmentary degeneration of the retina. Hereditary causes occur with an incidence of 1 in 3700. Every mode of inheritance has been described, each with a similar phenotypic expression but a differing onset and severity of illness. The most common heritable pattern is autosomal recessive, followed by autosomal dominant and X-linked recessive.

Although symptoms can appear at any age, most

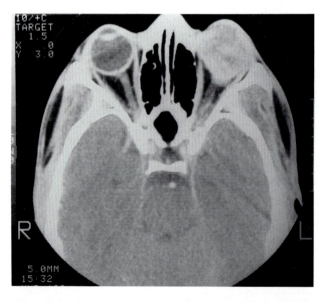

Figure 12–5. Computerized tomography demonstrating retinoblastoma filling the left eye. Areas of brighter intensity represent calcification.

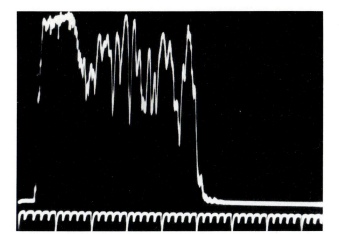

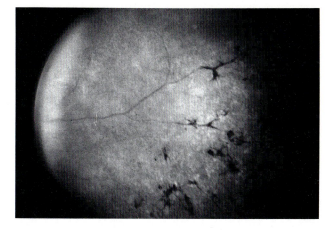

Figure 12–6. A-scan ultrasound of an eye with retinoblastoma. The multiple prominent echo spikes represent foci of calcification within the tumor. *(From Nelson LB, Brown GC, Arentsen JJ: Recognizing Patterns of Ocular Childhood Diseases. Thorofare, NJ, Slack, 1985, p 117, with permission.)*

Figure 12–7. Retinitis pigmentosa demonstrating the bone-corpuscle, peripheral, perivascular pigmentation.

affected individuals begin to notice difficulty with night blindness during youth or young adulthood. Later they notice a reduction in peripheral vision. Certain patients have symptoms primarily related to the cone system, such as poor central vision and difficulty with bright lights. The symptoms of RP are usually slowly progressive, and may vary from day to day. When more than one family member is affected, the rate of progression is usually similar within the family.

RP is characterized by progressive photoreceptor and retinal pigment epithelium (RPE) degeneration. Early features of the disorder include fine stippling of the RPE, and secondary striae of the internal limiting membrane. These subtle anatomic changes can usually be observed only with the greater magnification of the direct ophthalmoscope. With more advanced disease, clumps and strands of black pigment ("bone-corpuscle") become evident in the midperipheral retina. This is distributed in a perivascular pattern due to the predominance of pigment within vessel walls (Fig. 12–7). Clinical features of advanced disease include attenuated retinal arterioles and waxy pallor of the optic disc, as well as advanced pigmentary changes (Fig. 12–8). Advanced findings can be appreciated with the indirect ophthalmoscope.

Many systemic abnormalities have been noted to have a pigmentary retinopathy similar to RP (Table 12–4). These include syndromes associated with deafness, and central nervous system, metabolic, and chromosomal disorders (Fig. 12–9). Retinitis pigmentosa-like findings (nongenetic) can also be observed with congenital rubella (Fig. 12–10), congenital syphilis (Fig. 12–11), and following trauma (Fig. 12–12).

No treatment is available to arrest the progression

of retinitis pigmentosa, but many children and adults are benefited by low-vision aids. These include NOIR glasses, telescopes, night vision aids, large-print typewriters, closed-circuit TV, reading machines, and talking computers. There is no scientific evidence that normal light worsens the symptoms of RP, but affected individuals should be encouraged to protect their eyes from long exposure to bright light. Organizations that can provide support and assistance for patients and their families include the National Retinitis Pigmentosa Foundation, 8331 Mindale Circle, Baltimore, MD 21207, (800) 638–5682; and RP International, P.O. Box 900, Woodland Hills, CA 91365, (800) FIGHT-RP.

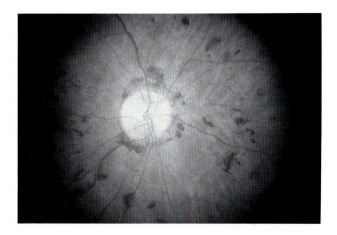

Figure 12–8. Retinitis pigmentosa, advanced stage, demonstrating waxy pallor of the optic disc and narrowed retinal arterioles.

TABLE 12–4. SYSTEMIC DISORDERS WITH RETINAL CHANGES SIMILAR TO RETINITIS PIGMENTOSA

Category	Disorder	Features
Central nervous system	Bassen–Kornzweig	Abetalipoproteinemia, cerebellar signs, acanthocytosis, vitamin A deficiency, malabsorption, celiac syndrome, anemia
	Batten disease	Mental deterioration, seizures, prominent macular involvement, ceroid lipofuscinosis, "amaurotic familial idiocy"
	Infantile form	Onset 1 year of age, ataxia, hypotonia, myoclonic jerks
	Juvenile form	Onset 6–7 years of age, visual loss, seizures
	Charot–Marie–Tooth syndrome	Atrophy of small muscles of hands and feet progressing to proximal muscles, optic atrophy
	Friedreich's ataxia	Ataxia, posterior column disease, nystagmus
	Hallervorden–Spatz syndrome	Parkinsonism, dementia, early death
	Kearns–Sayre syndrome	Ptosis, progressive external ophthalmoplegia, heart block
	Pelizaeus–Merzbacher disease	Ataxia, spasticity, mental deterioration, X-linked
Associated with deafness	Alström syndrome	Diabetes mellitus, obesity, nystagmus
	Bardet–Biedl syndrome	Mild mental retardation, obesity, polydactyly, hypogenitalism, diabetes mellitus, renal disease, predominantly males
	Cockayne's syndrome	Precocious aging, dwarfism, mental retardation, optic atrophy, cachexia, ocular albinism, cataracts
	Flynn–Aird syndrome	Ataxia, dementia, seizures, cataracts
	Laurence–Moon syndrome	Mild mental retardation, spastic paraplegia, hypogenitalism, predominantly males
	Refsum disease	Increased plasma phytanic acid, polyneuropathy, ataxia, muscular weakness, baldness, icthyosis
	Usher syndrome	Congenital deafness with or without vestibulocerebellar ataxia, psychosis, or mental retardation
	van der Hoeve's syndrome	See Osteogenesis imperfecta, below
	Wolfram syndrome	Diabetes mellitus, diabetes insipidus, optic atrophy
Associated with renal disease	Bardet–Biedl syndrome	See above
	Cystinosis	Corneal crystals, aminoaciduria, renal tubular acidosis (Fanconi's syndrome), small stature
Associated with bone disease	Marfan syndrome	Ectopia lentis, arachnodactyly, cardiac abnormalities, pectus excavatus, scoliosis
	Osteogenesis imperfecta	(van der Hoeve syndrome), bone fractures, dental defects, hyperflexible joints, scoliosis, deafness
	Osteopetrosis	(Albers–Schönberg disease), thick, dense, fragile, "marble" bone, pancytopenia, hypocalcemia
	Paget's disease	Decalcification and hyperostosis of skull, pelvis and long bones, optic atrophy, pancytopenia
Mucopoly-saccharidoses	Type I (Hurler)	Early corneal clouding, mental retardation, gargoyle facies, dwarfism, hepatosplenomegaly
	Type IS (Scheie)	Early corneal clouding, coarse facies, normal intellect, aortic regurgitation
	Type II (Hunter)	Mental retardation, facial and skeletal abnormalities, hepatosplenomegaly, X-linked
	Type III (Sanfilippo)	Severe mental retardation, optic atrophy
	Type IV (Morquio)	Cloudy corneas, facial and skeletal abnormalities
Chromosomal disorder	Klinefelter's syndrome	Karyotype XXY, XXXY, or XXXXY, mental deficiency, hypotonia, hypogenitalism
	Turner's syndrome	Karyotype XO, short stature, thick neck, infertility, shield chest, low hairline
Other syndromes	Gaucher's disease	Hepatosplenomegaly, ocular motor apraxia, abnormal bruising, fractures, with or without failure to thrive and spasticity
	Kartagener's syndrome	Dextrocardia, bronchiectasis, sinusitis
	Myotonic dystrophy	Mask-like facies, cataracts, mental deficiency, cardiac changes, hypogonadism, ptosis, temporalis wasting
Pseudoretinitis pigmentosa	Congenital syphilis	Saddle nose, maxillary hypoplasia, Hutchinson's teeth
	Drug-induced	Phenothiazines, indomethacin, quinine, chloroquine
	Rubella	Deafness, congenital cataracts, glaucoma, cardiac anomalies, growth retardation, bone defects
	Trauma	Blunt, penetrating, and obstetrical trauma, and radiotherapy

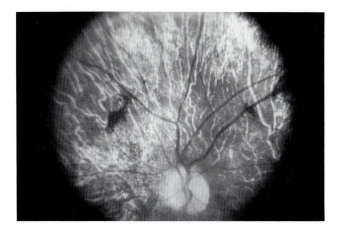

Figure 12–9. Refsum disease. Note the narrowed retinal arterioles and optic pallor, but absence of bone–corpuscle pigmentation.

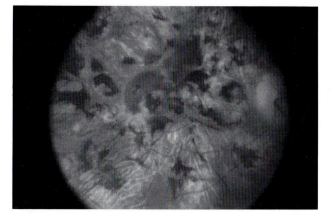

Figure 12–12. Pigmentary retinopathy following trauma. Note that the pigmentary changes are not perivascular, or predominantly peripheral.

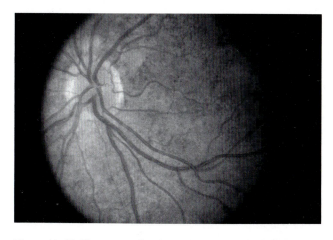

Figure 12–10. Pigmentary disturbance in congenital rubella, demonstrating diffuse stippling, without bone–corpuscle distribution.

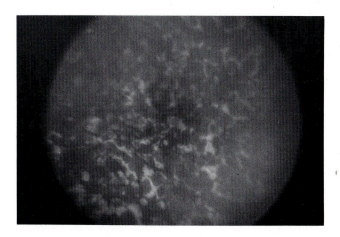

Figure 12–11. Pigmentary disturbance in congenital syphilis. Note the marked hyperpigmentation with lacunae of hypopigmentation.

COMPREHENSIVE INFORMATION ON DISORDERS OF THE RETINA AND VITREOUS

Retinopathy of Prematurity (ROP)

Classification of ROP

Retinopathy of prematurity (ROP) begins with an arrest in retinal vascular maturation. This is followed by an ophthalmoscopically visible response to injury. In 90 percent or more of cases, spontaneous regression, with minimal scarring and visual loss, occurs. In the remainder, abnormal vascularization and cicitrization occurs, leading to retinal dragging or detachment. Accurate descriptions of pathological findings require that the location (zone), extent, and severity (stage) of the disease be specified. In 1984, an international group of ophthalmologists systematized the classification of these characteristics.

The **location** of the disease is divided into three zones based on the natural progression of retinal vascularization (Fig. 12–13). The center of each zone is the optic nerve head. This was chosen because retinal vascularization proceeds outward from the optic nerve head toward the peripheral retina in an orderly fashion. Zone I extends from the optic nerve to twice the disc-to-macula distance, or 30 degrees in all directions. Zone II extends from the outer border of zone I to the ora serrata (the peripheral edge of the retina) nasally, and to approximately the equator of the eye temporally. Zone III extends from the outer edge of zone II in a crescentic fashion to the temporal ora serrata. The **extent** of involvement is specified by the number of clock hours involved.

The **stage** or degree of retinal vascular abnormality is divided into five categories (Table 12–5). **Stage 1** is characterized by the presence of a demarcation line that separates posterior vascularized retina from ante-

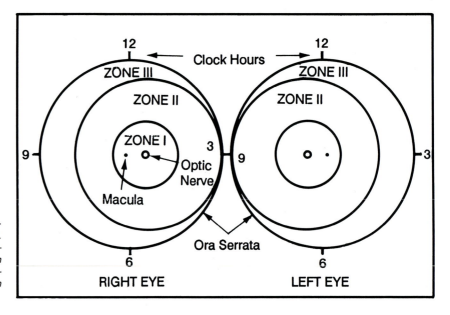

Figure 12–13. Diagram of zones of retinal involvement, used in the classification of ROP. *(Modified from Committee for the Classification of Retinopathy of Prematurity: An international classification of retinopathy of prematurity. Redrawn from Arch Ophthalmol 102:1130, Fig. 1, copyright 1984, American Medical Association, with permission.)*

rior avascular retina (Fig. 12–14). The line is thin, white, circumferentially located, and flat (within the plane of the retina). When the line lies within zone I or posterior zone II, the term **rush disease** is sometimes used, to indicate that successive stages can occur rapidly.

Stage 2 results when the demarcation line of stage 1 acquires volume and increases in height and width, to become a ridge (Figs. 12–15 and 12–16). It remains, however, intraretinal. The ridge may change from white to pink, and vessels may leave the plane of the retina to enter the ridge, but the retina remains attached.

Stage 3 is characterized by the presence of extraretinal fibrovascular proliferation added to the ridge of stage 2. Abnormal blood vessels and fibrous tissue extend through the internal limiting membrane of the retina, over the surface of the vascularized retina, and into the vitreous (Figs. 12–17 and 12–18). In later stages, this tissue may proliferate over the surface of the avascular retina, ciliary body, and lens. Neovascular fronds usually arise as small tufts along the posterior edge of the

ridge. Hemorrhages on or near the ridge, from these vessels, are common. The vessels that do enter the ridge are dilated and tortuous.

Stage 4 is defined by the presence of a retinal detachment with (4a) or without (4b) macular involvement (Figs. 12–19 and 12–20). Detachment occurs secondary to exudation and traction exerted by proliferating tissue in the vitreous or on the retinal surface. The

TABLE 12–5. STAGES OF RETINOPATHY OF PREMATURITY

Stage	Characteristic
1	Demarcation line
2	Ridge
3	Ridge with extraretinal fibrovascular proliferation
4	Subtotal retinal detachment[a]
5	Total retinal detachment

Plus disease denotes the accompanying presence of dilated veins and tortuous arterioles in the posterior retina, and is designated by a + sign (e.g., stage 3+)

[a]Stage 4a denotes that the macula is not involved.
Stage 4b denotes macular involvement.

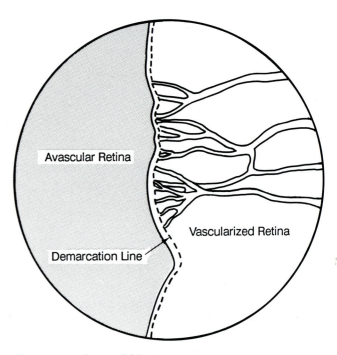

Figure 12–14. Stage 1 ROP. *(Modified from Committee for the Classification of Retinopathy of Prematurity: An international classification of retinopathy of prematurity. Redrawn from Arch Ophthalmol 102:1130, Fig. 2, copyright 1984, American Medical Association, with permission.)*

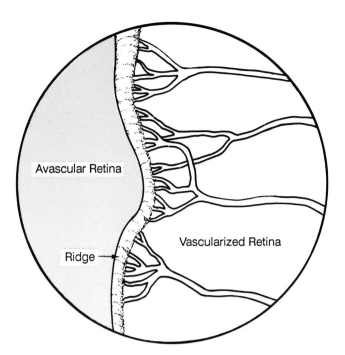

Figure 12–15. Stage 2 ROP. *(Modified from Committee for the Classification of Retinopathy of Prematurity: An international classification of retinopathy of prematurity. Redrawn from Arch Ophthalmol 102:1130, Fig. 3, copyright 1984, American Medical Association, with permission.)*

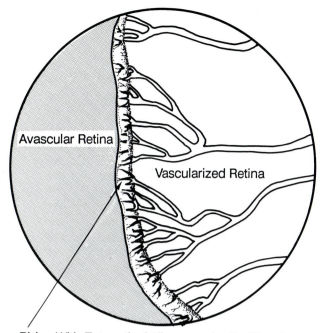

Ridge With Extraretinal Fibrovascular Proliferation

Figure 12–17. Stage 3 ROP. *(Modified from Committee for the Classification of Retinopathy of Prematurity: An international classification of retinopathy of prematurity. Redrawn from Arch Ophthalmol 102:1130, Fig. 4, copyright 1984, American Medical Association, with permission.)*

detachment usually starts in the periphery and envelops the retina posterior to the ridge. When the macula becomes involved, typically presenting as a traction fold within it, the prognosis for vision is poor.

Stage 5 is characterized by total, funnel-shaped retinal detachment with very poor visual prognosis (Fig.

12–21). The funnel is divided into an anterior and posterior part and commonly assumes either an open or closed form.

Plus disease represents a more florid stage of ROP, characterized by enlarged veins and tortuous arterioles in the posterior retina (Fig. 12–22). Plus disease usually

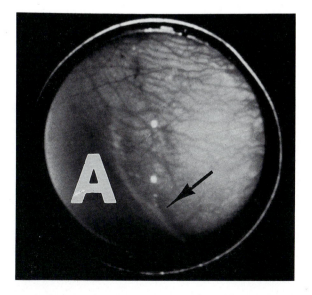

Figure 12–16. Stage 2 ROP. A ridge *(arrow)* is seen separating avascular (**A**) and vascular retina. *(From Nelson LB, Brown GC, Arentsen JJ: Recognizing Patterns of Ocular Childhood Diseases. Thorofare, NJ, Slack, 1985, p 119, with permission.)*

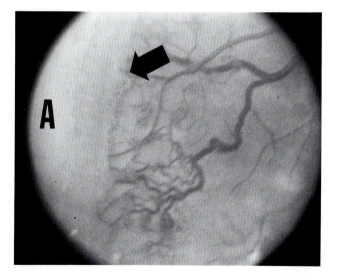

Figure 12–18. Stage 3 ROP. Extraretinal fibrovascular proliferation *(arrow)* is present separating avascular (**A**) and vascular retina. *(From Nelson LB, Brown GC, Arentsen JJ: Recognizing Patterns of Ocular Childhood Diseases. Thorofare, NJ, Slack, 1985, p 119, with permission.)*

Subtotal
Retinal Detachment

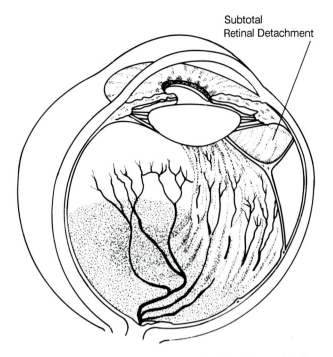

Figure 12–19. Stage 4a ROP, subtotal retinal detachment that does not involve the retina. *(Modified from Tingley DH, Flynn JT: Perspectives on retinopathy of prematurity. Int Pediatr 5:232, 1990, Fig. 4, with permission.)*

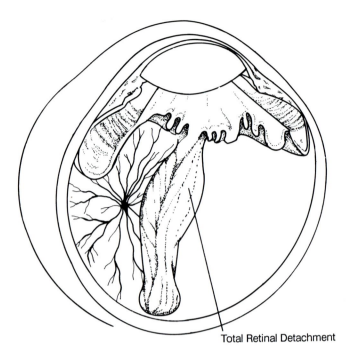

Total Retinal Detachment

Figure 12–21. Stage 5 ROP, total retinal detachment in a funnel configuration. *(Modified from Tingley DH, Flynn JT: Perspectives on retinopathy of prematurity. Int Pediatr 5:232, 1990, Fig. 4, with permission.)*

occurs only if the severity of ROP is stage 3 or greater, and its presence is a risk factor for rapid progression of the retinopathy. Iris vascular engorgement, pupillary rigidity, and vitreous haze can accompany plus disease.

Treatment of ROP

Once discovered, eyes with ROP should be followed until spontaneous resolution occurs, or until a need for treatment arises. Treatment considerations are based on the findings of the Cryotherapy for ROP Cooperative Group, which were published in 1990. This study

of very-low-birthweight (<1251 g) infants with advanced ROP found that cryoablation of the residual avascular retina significantly reduced the final incidence of blindness. Eligible infants had stage 3 ROP, involving 5 or more contiguous clock hours of retina (or 8 separate clock hour sectors) in zone I or zone II, and plus disease (Table 12–6). Transscleral cryotherapy (average of 50 applications per eye) was applied to the avascular retina in one eye; the other eye was observed as a control.

Cryotherapy was found to reduce the frequency of posterior retinal detachment, retinal folds (usually in-

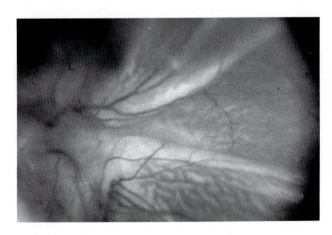

Figure 12–20. Stage 4 ROP, subtotal retinal detachment.

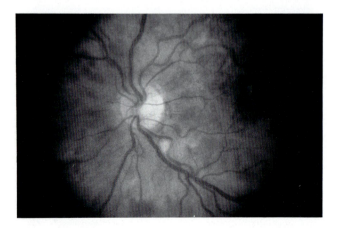

Figure 12–22. Plus disease in ROP. Note the venous dilation and prominent arterioles.

TABLE 12–6. CRITERIA FOR PRETHRESHOLD AND THRESHOLD RETINOPATHY OF PREMATURITY

Prethreshold Disease	Threshold Disease
ROP in Zone I—any stage, but less than threshold ROP in Zone II—stage 2+ ROP in Zone II—stage 3 or 3+, but less than 5 clock hours	At least 5 contiguous or 8 cumulative 30-degree clock hours of stage 3 ROP in the presence of plus disease (stage 3+)

TABLE 12–7. SEQUELAE OF REGRESSED RETINOPATHY OF PREMATURITY

- *REFRACTIVE*

  1. Myopia (6 or more diopters)
  2. Astigmatism

- *RETINAL*

  1. Failure of the peripheral retina to vascularize
  2. Retinal pigmentation
  3. Dragging of the retina
  4. Retinal folds
  5. Elevated retinal vessels
  6. Lattice-like degeneration
  7. Traction/rhegmatogenous retinal detachments

- *OTHER*

  1. Strabismus
  2. Pseudostrabismus
  3. Amblyopia
  4. Cataract
  5. Glaucoma
  6. Developmental structural abnormalities of the anterior segment including angle abnormalities, posterior synechiae, and visible iris or angle vessels

volving the macula), and retrolental tissue from 51.4 percent of control eyes to 31.1 percent of treated eyes, 3 months following treatment. Consistent results were found at 12 months following treatment. Furthermore, the percentage of infants who had a favorable acuity outcome (as assessed with the Teller acuity card procedure at the 12-month follow-up exam) was significantly greater in treated (66.1 percent) than in untreated (45.5 percent) eyes (Dobson, 1990). Cryotherapy, however, has been associated with the late occurrence of retinal detachment, and the long-term prognosis for vision in these eyes is unknown.

In the study all eyes with prethreshold disease were reexamined at a minimal interval of 1 week. If threshold disease was found, cryotherapy was performed within 72 hours. All eyes with zone I ROP or zone II ROP with either stage 2+ or stage 3 ROP were considered prethreshold (Table 12–6).

The natural course of ROP is for most zone II disease to go on to regression. The follow-up standard for zone II disease that is not prethreshold is, therefore, 2 weeks. Eyes with vascularization into zone III can be followed up in 6 to 10 weeks. The AAP guidelines suggest that all affected infants have at least one final follow-up examination during their first 6 months of life, and an annual follow-up exam is recommended for infants who had significant active disease. These infants are at a high risk to develop large refractive errors, strabismus, and amblyopia.

In addition to cryotherapy, infants may also be treated with laser therapy. Laser treatments are delivered through a modified indirect ophthalmoscope, the same type of instrument used to examine the infant's retina. This treatment is similar to cryotherapy in destroying avascular retinal tissue and reducing the growth of abnormal blood vessels. It is advantageous, however, in being less likely to be associated with intraocular hemorrhage. It is also less painful than cryotherapy. Reduced pain results in a reduced incidence of bradycardia, arrythmia, cardiac or respiratory arrest, cyanosis, and hypoxemia. Cryotherapy may require general anesthesia; this is less likely to be needed with laser treatment. Finally, laser treatment results in less swelling after treatment, and because it is more focused, less associated injury to the eye than cryother-

apy. The efficacy of laser therapy, however, has not been studied as extensively as cryotherapy.

Residual Changes in ROP

The acute, active phase of ROP may last for 3 to 4 months. Whereas regression is the most common outcome, residual changes can be detected in many eyes with regressed ROP (Table 12–7).

A common sequela of ROP is myopia, occurring in as many as 80 percent of affected children. It may be noted within the first 3 months of life, and usually progresses during early childhood to 6 diopters or greater. The myopia appears to be related to forward displace-

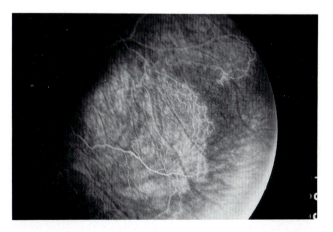

Figure 12–23. Fluorescein angiography demonstrating avascular peripheral retina in regressed retinopathy of prematurity.

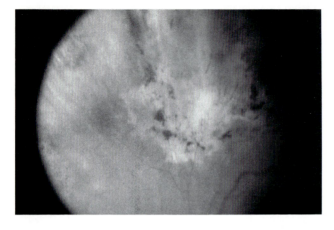

Figure 12–24. Peripheral pigment clumping in regressed retinopathy of prematurity.

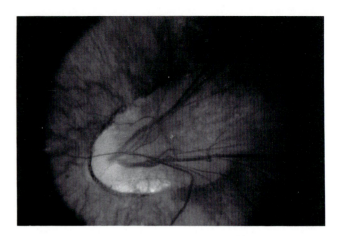

Figure 12–27. Temporal dragging of the retina due to retinopathy of prematurity. Note the prominent temporal straightening of the retinal vessels.

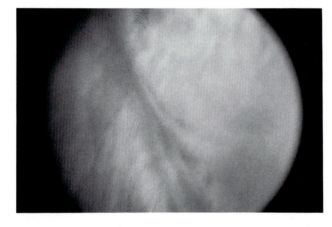

Figure 12–25. Peripheral retinal fold in regressed retinopathy of prematurity.

ment of the lens iris diaphragm, rather than increased axial length (Tasman, 1984).

Other common findings of regressed ROP include astigmatism, strabismus, pseudostrabismus, and glaucoma. The latter may occur secondary to developmental structural abnormalities of the anterior segment (Hartnett et al, 1990). Sequelae found near the site of the active phase of ROP include lack of vascularization (Fig. 12–23), pigment clumping (Fig. 12–24), retinal folds (Fig. 12–25), lattice-like degeneration, retinal breaks, and elevated retinal vessels (which can hemorrhage; Fig. 12–26). Dragging of the retina is another common finding in regressed ROP (Fig. 12–27). Usually this occurs to the temporal side and includes the macula, resulting in pseudoexotropia (Fig. 12–28). In

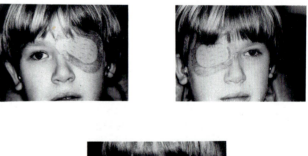

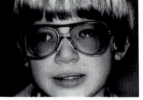

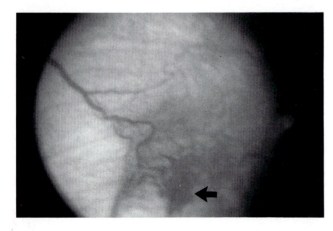

Figure 12–26. Elevated peripheral retinal vessels with hemorrhage (*arrow*) in regressed retinopathy of prematurity.

Figure 12–28. Pseudostrabismus and high myopia in a child with regressed retinopathy of prematurity (same patient as in Fig. 12–27). In the center photograph the child appears to have divergent eyes (exotropia). Patching of either eye, however, demonstrates that the child fixates with his eyes turned outward, because his maculas have been dragged temporally.

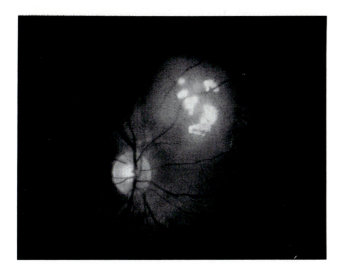

Figure 12–29. Small retinoblastoma appearing as a translucent, white, slightly elevated retinal mass.

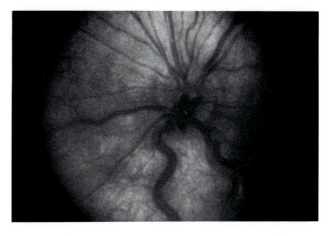

Figure 12–31. A peripheral retinoblastoma was suspected in this infant because of the presence of the dilated blood vessels noted in the posterior retina.

more severe cases, a falciform retinal fold, running through the macula, can occur. This reduces vision, and if it occurs bilaterally, nystagmus secondary to poor vision can result.

Retinal detachment can occur in the chronic as well as active phase of ROP. Detachments can result from traction, or secondary to multiple retinal breaks (rhegmatogenous). Tractional detachments occur mostly in newborns. Rhegmatogenous detachments can occur in young children, but more commonly arise during adolescence. Children whose birthweight was less than 1000 g are at the greatest risk.

Intraocular Tumors

Retinoblastoma

Ophthalmoscopic Appearance of Retinoblastoma.
In its earliest clinical stage, a small retinoblas-

toma will appear ophthalmoscopically as a translucent, white, slightly elevated lesion in the sensory retina (Fig. 12–29). With an increase in size, dilated retinal blood vessels that feed and drain the tumor can be appreciated (Fig. 12–30). With small peripheral tumors this may be the only sign of tumor visible in the posterior pole (Fig. 12–31). Larger tumors may show foci of chalk-like calcifications, and resemble cottage cheese in their appearance (Fig. 12–32).

As the tumor continues to enlarge, it assumes either an endophytic (inward; Fig. 12–33) or exophytic (outward) growth pattern. Histopathologically, poorly differentiated tumors consist of round cells with large basophilic nuclei and scanty cytoplasm. Well-differentiated tumors are characterized by the presence of fleurettes and Flexner–Wintersteiner rosettes, both of which represent attempts at photoreceptor differentiation (Fig. 12–34). Tumors with these features have a more favorable prognosis.

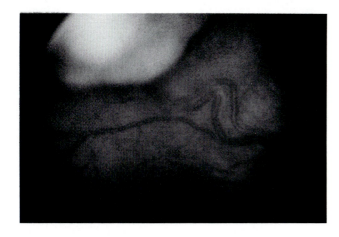

Figure 12–30. Dilated blood vessels feeding and draining a medium-sized retinoblastoma.

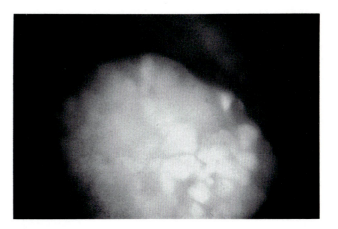

Figure 12–32. Foci of calcification (*brighter areas*) noted within a retinoblastoma.

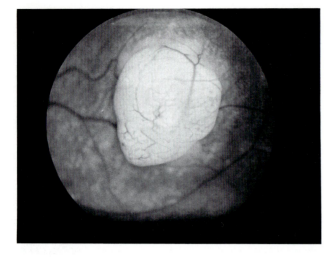

Figure 12–33. Endophytic growth pattern of a retinoblastoma. *(From Nelson LB, Brown GC, Arentsen JJ: Recognizing Patterns of Ocular Childhood Diseases. Thorofare, NJ, Slack, 1985, p 117, with permission.)*

TABLE 12–8. DIFFERENTIAL DIAGNOSIS OF LEUKOCORIA IN A CHILD

A. Corneal abnormality
   1. Peter's anomaly
   2. Congenital corneal opacity
B. Congenital cataract
C. Persistent hyperplastic primary vitreous
D. Ocular tumor
   1. Retinoblastoma
   2. Medulloepithelioma
   3. Retinal astrocytoma
   4. Combined hamartoma of the retina and RPE
E. Congenital developmental defect
   1. Coloboma of the choroid and retina
   2. Medullated nerve fibers
   3. High myopia with retinal degeneration
   4. Retinal dysplasia
   5. Juvenile retinoschisis
   6. Falciform fold of retina/congenital retinal detachment
   7. Morning glory disc anomaly
F. Progressive retinal disorder
   1. Cicatricial retinopathy of prematurity
   2. Coats' disease
   3. Organized vitreous hemorrhage
   4. Incontinentia pigmenti
   5. Norrie's disease
   6. Familial exudative vitreoretinopathy
   7. Retinal astrocytoma (tuberous sclerosis or neurofibromatosis)
G. Infectious
   1. Nematode endophthalmitis (toxocariasis)
   2. Congenital toxoplasmosis
   3. Congenital cytomegalovirus retinitis
   4. Herpes simplex retinitis
   5. Metastatic endophthalmitis

Differential Diagnosis of Retinoblastoma. The differential diagnosis of retinoblastoma is that of leukocoria (Table 12–8). The three entities that are most frequently misdiagnosed as retinoblastoma are Coats' disease (Fig. 12–35), presumed ocular toxocariasis (see Fig. 12–86), and retinal astrocytoma (Fig. 12–36). Other causes of leukocoria are more easily differentiated. Corneal opacities can be readily recognized, as can congenital cataracts, either directly or with a hand-held slit lamp. A small eye suggests persistent hyperplastic primary vitreous (Fig. 12–37) or incontinentia pigmenti. Vitreous haze in an older child suggests toxocariasis (infection with the larval stage of an intestinal parasite of dogs). Cells in the anterior chamber of the eye (pseudohypopyon), and/or the presence of abnormal vessels on the iris, suggest retinoblastoma.

Management of Retinoblastoma. Enucleation is recommended when tumors are so advanced that there is no hope for vision. With smaller tumors, episcleral plaque therapy, external beam irradiation, photocoagulation, or cryotherapy are employed with the hope of

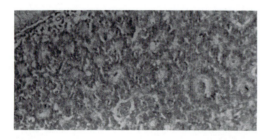

Figure 12–34. Histopathology of retinoblastoma demonstrating Flexner–Wintersteiner rosettes. *(Courtesy of the Albany Medical College slide collection.)*

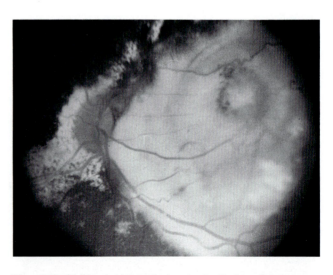

Figure 12–35. Massive intraretinal and subretinal exudate in an eye with Coats' disease. *(From Nelson LB, Brown GC, Arentsen JJ: Recognizing Patterns of Ocular Childhood Diseases. Thorofare, NJ, Slack, 1985, p 97, with permission.)*

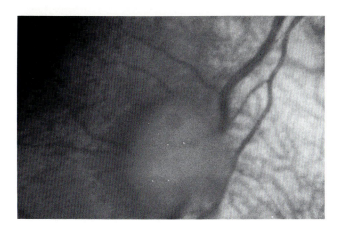

Figure 12–36. Retinal astrocytoma in a patient with tuberous sclerosis.

preserving some vision. Follow-up is dictated by the clinical findings noted 3 to 4 weeks after treatment.

Metastatic disease to the bone marrow, spinal cord, viscera, and lymph nodes develops in less than 10 percent of affected patients. At the time of diagnosis, demonstrable cerebral spinal fluid or bone marrow involvement is infrequent. In the absence of signs, symptoms, or histological evidence of dissemination, bone marrow aspiration and lumbar puncture may not need to be performed (Pratt et al, 1989). Three factors appear to be independently associated with the development of metastases: optic nerve invasion, choroidal invasion, and older age at diagnosis. The role of chemotherapy in the absence of overt metastases is controversial; it may enhance the development of second cancers in children with heritable retinoblastoma. With overt metastases, or extraocular orbital involvement, however, systemic chemotherapy with vincristine, cyclophosphamide, and adriamycin is used.

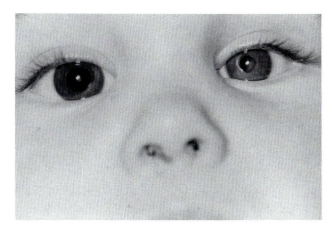

Figure 12–37. Persistent hyperplastic vitreous, left eye. Note the small eye and leukocoria.

The opposite eye of patients with unilateral sporadic retinoblastoma should be examined every 3 to 6 months under general anesthesia, unless DNA sequencing demonstrates that the individual is not at greater risk. This should continue until the child reaches 4 to 5 years of age, followed by yearly examinations in the office. The cure rate is greater than 90 percent; many children with the hereditary form of tumor, however, will develop other cancers (described in the next section).

Associated Tumors in Individuals With Hereditary Retinoblastoma. A high percentage of children with the hereditary form of retinoblastoma develop pinealoblastomas during their first 3 years of life. Pinealoblastomas are embryologically, pathologically, and immunologically identical to retinoblastomas. They are almost always primary rather than metastatic from a retinoblastoma. The term "trilateral" retinoblastoma is used when patients present with a pineal (or other intracranial neuroblastic tumor) and bilateral retinoblastoma.

These patients may also develop orbital sarcomas, regardless of whether radiation therapy was given, and are more likely to die from a second nonocular tumor than metastatic retinoblastoma. Osteogenic sarcoma of the femur is the most common nonocular tumor; others include leukemia, glioma, neuroblastoma, malignant melanoma, rhabdomyosarcoma, sebaceous and squamous cell carcinomas, and chondrosarcoma. Therapeutic modalities such as chemotherapy and radiation therapy may enhance the risk of second nonocular tumors.

Genetics of Retinoblastoma. Retinoblastoma was the first tumor proven to be caused by the absence of a normally occurring tumor suppressor gene. This antioncogene is located on band q14 of chromosome 13. Individuals homozygous for the absence of this gene—whether due to loss, deletion, mutation, or inactivation—develop the tumor. Individuals who retain one copy of the gene (heterozygous) will develop the tumor if this copy becomes inactivated. It is postulated that viral or environmental oncogenic factors are responsible for loss of the second gene (Knudson's two-hit hypothesis).

Approximately 40 percent of retinoblastomas are hereditary (familial), meaning that the mutation is present in germ cells. In the past many children with retinoblastoma did not procreate. Therefore, the majority (75 percent) of hereditary retinoblastomas are caused by new germ-cell mutations. The remaining 60 percent of retinoblastomas are not hereditary. In these individuals, mutations are present only in somatic cells, and the affected individual has no capacity to pass the gene to offspring. The predominance of nonhereditary tumors, and the limited offspring of individuals with hereditary tumors, accounts for the fact that the family history is positive in only 6 to 10 percent of newly diagnosed retinoblastoma cases.

Because both copies of the antioncogene must be lost as a prerequisite for tumor formation, retinoblastoma is, in actuality, a recessive disorder. Transmission of the hereditary form of retinoblastoma, however, follows an autosomal dominant mode of inheritance, with a penetrance of about 90 percent. This is because the rate of spontaneous mutation is so high that on average several heterozygous retinal cells will become homozygous for loss of the suppressor gene during normal development. Of the hereditary cases, 60 to 75 percent have bilateral tumor involvement.

It is now possible to perform DNA testing from tumor or blood samples of patients with retinoblastoma and their relatives. Sequencing is helpful in identifying individuals with unilateral retinoblastoma that are at high risk of developing a tumor in their other eye. It can also identify relatives at high risk. This testing is available via the Retinoblastoma Diagnostic Service at the Massachusetts Eye and Ear Infirmary, at a cost of approximately $1200 for a family of up to four members. It can be cost effective if it identifies children who are at no increased risk, eliminating the need for periodic eye examinations under anesthesia. The testing, however, does not identify the mutation in all cases. Useful information is more frequently provided for families with two or more affected individuals, or when a solitary member has bilateral disease. Sequencing is less likely to provide useful information when only one member of a family is affected with unilateral disease, and no tumor fragment is available.

Combined Hamartoma of the Retina and Retinal Pigment Epithelium

Combined hamartoma of the retina and retinal pigment epithelium (RPE) is a rare, benign lesion characterized by a greenish-gray sheen and traction of the internal limiting membrane of the retina. The latter distorts the blood vessels that run through the lesion (Figs. 12–38 and 12–39). Combined hamartomas usually arise near the optic nerve, and can evolve to produce progressive local effects. Pathologically they are comprised of excess vascular and glial tissue and cords of hyperpigmented, proliferated RPE cells in the sensory retina. Recent reports have suggested an association with neurofibromatosis type II and tuberous sclerosis (Ellis et al, 1991). Surgical intervention (epiretinal membrane stripping) has been successful in a few cases (Sappenfield & Gitter, 1990). Because the hamartoma is a part of the retina, however, it cannot be removed.

Congenital RPE Hypertrophy

Congenital RPE hypertrophy is characterized by solitary (Fig. 12–40) or grouped (Fig. 12–41) hyperpigmentation of the retina. Multifocal or grouped pigmen-

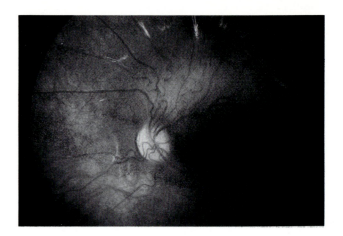

Figure 12–38. Combined hamartoma of the retina and RPE. Note the irregular sheen and traction on the internal limiting membrane that distorts the traversing blood vessels.

tations have been called "bear tracks" because of their resemblance to a bear paw walking across the retina. Individual areas are usually flat and well delineated; the anomaly is benign and nonprogressive. Histologically, affected RPE cells contain closely packed, large, spherical melanin granules in their cytoplasm. Unlike congenital hyperplasia, the reactive hyperplasia that follows trauma or inflammation is more likely to be elevated and have irregular margins.

Medulloepithelioma

Two forms of medulloepithelioma (diktyoma) have been described. The first consists of a pure proliferation of embryonic nonpigmented ciliary epithelium, containing a mucopolysaccharide identical to vitreous. The second also contains heteroplastic elements such as cartilage. Both types can be either benign or malignant.

Medulloepitheliomas are usually located in the cili-

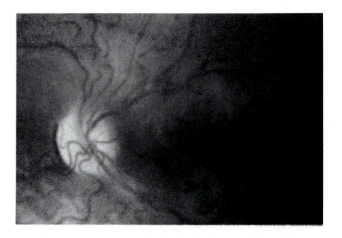

Figure 12–39. Higher magnification of combined hamartoma shown in Figure 12–38.

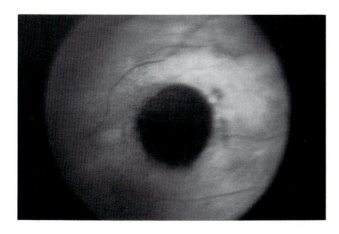

Figure 12–40. Solitary congenital RPE hypertrophy.

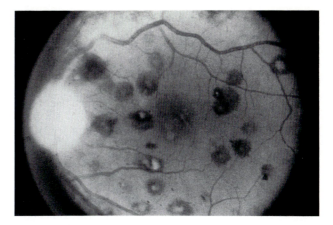

Figure 12–42. White-centered retinal hemorrhages in leukemia.

ary body region. Clinically, they can produce a "lens coloboma" in the quadrant of the mass due to a localized zonular defect (see Fig. 11–8). With progression, a fleshy, cystic-appearing mass may grow into the anterior chamber of the eye. Complications include subluxation of the lens, cataract, and neovascular glaucoma. Unless extraocular extension occurs, the prognosis is good. Enucleation may be necessary if complications ensue, but metastases are rare.

Leukemia

Metastatic leukemia in children can produce retinal hemorrhages (often with a white center) (Fig. 12–42), and neoplastic infiltration of the retina, optic nerve, choroid, and iris (Fig. 12–43). Optic nerve infiltration is associated with permanent and profound visual loss in most cases. Most children with optic nerve and central nervous system involvement survive less than 2 years despite treatment. Ocular disease is treated with irradiation and systemic chemotherapy.

Pigmentary Disorders

Retinitis Pigmentosa

There are several forms of retinitis pigmentosa (RP), each with a presumably different or separate cause. Although pedigrees generally demonstrate similar findings, many pedigrees have been described in which typical and atypical findings overlap. This suggests some variability in the expression of the disorder.

The X-linked form is the most severe. In this variant, the visual acuity is routinely reduced to 20/200, or worse, by age 30. X-linked as well as recessive RP often progresses to total blindness (Fig. 12–44). Rarely, vision is preserved into the sixth and seventh decade. The dominant form has the latest onset, and is the least severe. In dominant RP, the central visual acuity usually remains 20/30 to 20/100 until the sixth decade. In one family with autosomal dominant transmission, an abnormality in the gene coding for rhodopsin on chromosome 3 has been identified (Dryja et al, 1990).

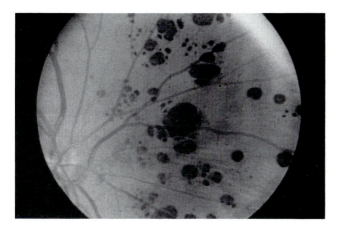

Figure 12–41. Grouped congenital RPE hypertrophy ("bear tracks"). *(Courtesy of the Wills Eye Hospital slide collection.)*

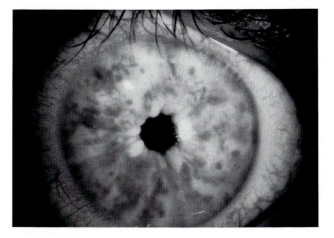

Figure 12–43. Leukemic infiltration of the iris. *(Courtesy of Robert Kalina.)*

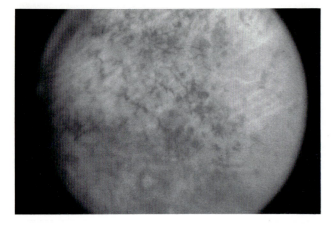

Figure 12–44. Peripheral, "bone-corpuscle" pigmentation in retinitis pigmentosa.

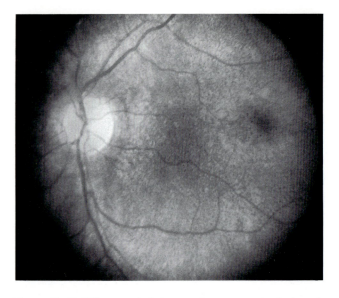

Figure 12–46. Diffuse mottled pigmentation, narrowed retinal arterioles, and optic pallor in Leber's congenital amaurosis. *(From Brown GC: Congenital fundus abnormalities. In Duane TD (ed): Clinical Ophthalmology. Hagerstown, MD, Harper & Row, 1982, vol 3, pp 15–18, with permission.)*

The dark adaptation curve in RP initially shows an increased rod threshold with a normal cone response. As the disease progresses, both rod and cone dysfunction become evident, and the curve becomes monophasic. The electroretinogram (ERG) becomes abnormal or absent prior to subjective visual deterioration or ophthalmoscopically visible changes. A decreased scotopic b-wave is seen early. Widespread rod involvement may precede cone involvement, or rod and cone dysfunction may deteriorate concurrently. Progression results in a nonrecordable state.

The initial visual field defect is an inferotemporal scotoma that enlarges to form a ring (annular) scotoma. With further progression the scotomatous area breaks out to the periphery and infringes on the central field. In advanced disease only a small area of vision re-

mains, sometimes associated with a temporal island. Other significant ocular findings in RP include posterior subcapsular cataract (Fig. 12–45), anterior vitreous cells, cystoid macular edema, progressive macular atrophy, glaucoma, myopia, and keratoconus.

Leber's Congenital Amaurosis

Leber's congenital amaurosis (LCA), also known as congenital retinitis pigmentosa, is a congenital retinal dystrophy originally described in 1869. The disease is characterized by profound visual loss (≤ 20/200) at or

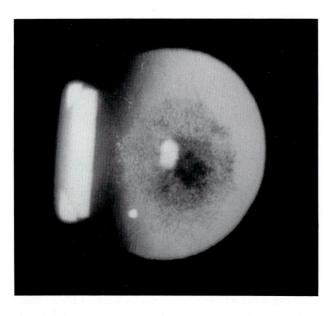

Figure 12–45. Posterior subcapsular cataract in retinitis pigmentosa.

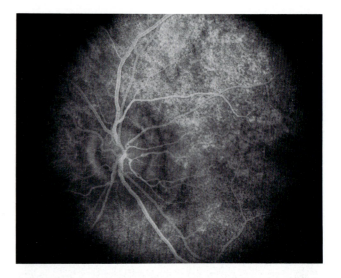

Figure 12–47. Fluorescein angiogram corresponding to Figure 12–46 demonstrating a pattern of mottled hyperfluorescence due to pigment changes. *(From Brown GC: Congenital fundus abnormalities. In Duane TD (ed): Clinical Ophthalmology. Hagerstown, MD, Harper & Row, 1982, vol 3, pp 15–18, with permission.)*

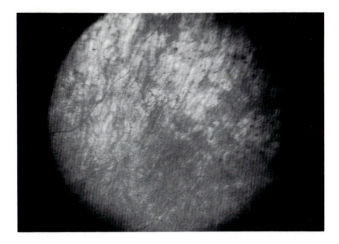

Figure 12–48. "Marbleized" pigment epithelial loss and clumping in Leber's congenital amaurosis. *(From Brown GC: Congenital fundus abnormalities. In Duane TD (ed): Clinical Ophthalmology. Hagerstown, MD, Harper & Row, 1982, vol 3, pp 15–18, with permission.)*

shortly after birth, searching nystagmus, and minimally reactive pupils. It occurs with an incidence of 2 to 3 per 100,000 births, and in most cases is transmitted as an autosomal recessive trait.

Although the fundus may be normal initially, irregular pigmentation, attenuated arterioles, and pale optic nerves usually become apparent by the end of the first decade (Figs. 12–46 to 12–48). Cataracts and keratoconus frequently develop in older children, and rarely patients will develop macular colobomas or optic disc edema. The diagnosis is established in infants by the presence of a nonrecordable or barely present ERG performed under photopic and scotopic conditions (Fig. 12–49).

LCA has been reported with various systemic conditions including structural abnormalities of the central nervous system, neurological disorders (mental retardation, seizures, hydrocephalus), skeletal anomalies, and renal disease. The incidences of these abnormalities in LCA are difficult to determine because of differences in patient selection and referral patterns in various institutions. Several investigators have attempted to differentiate a form of LCA that was associated with marked hyperopia, but had no systemic abnormalities. Other authors, however, have found a similar magnitude of hyperopia in all patients with LCA, whether complicated or uncomplicated.

Cone Disorders

Cone Dystrophies

Cone dystrophies are characterized by decreased central vision, photophobia, and color blindness. Night blindness and loss of peripheral vision, common complaints in retinitis pigmentosa, are unusual even in advanced cases of cone dystrophy. Both eyes are symmetrically involved. The mode of inheritance is usually autosomal recessive, but most familial cases are autosomal dominant.

Ocular symptoms usually develop during the first or second decade of life. Visual loss and photophobia typically precede definite macular changes on ophthalmoscopic examination. Because of this, and because of the age of onset, these children are often initially misdiagnosed as having Stargardt's disease or juvenile macular degeneration. Eventually, one of three types of macular lesions will become evident.

The most common macular abnormality is the "bull's-eye" lesion. This consists of a homogeneous dark red area of varying size, surrounded by a sharply defined, doughnut-like zone of atrophic pigment epithelium (Fig. 12–50). In some patients, a third peripheral zone of noninvolvement may appear to stand out, probably due to contrast (Fig. 12–51). These patients

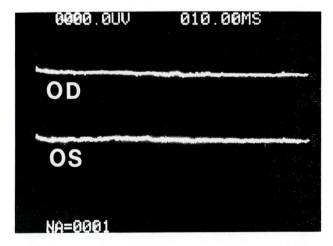

Figure 12–49. Flat electroretinogram in each eye; the pathognomonic test in Leber's congenital amaurosis. *(From Brown GC: Congenital fundus abnormalities. In Duane TD (ed): Clinical Ophthalmology. Hagerstown, MD, Harper & Row, 1982, vol 3, pp 15–18, with permission.)*

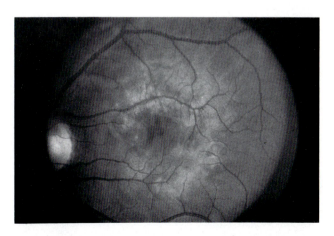

Figure 12–50. "Bull's-eye" lesion of cone dystrophy. A central area of more darkly pigmented retina is surrounded by a zone of atrophic pigment epithelium.

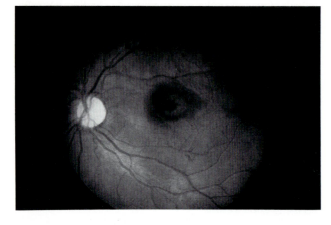

Figure 12–51. Smaller "bull's-eye" lesion of a different patient with cone dystrophy, demonstrating the variability of appearance of this finding. This patient also demonstrates a third peripheral zone of noninvolvement.

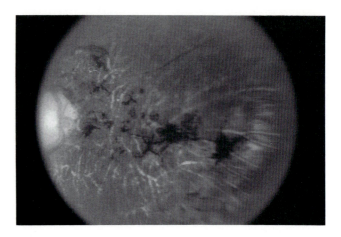

Figure 12–53. A more advanced stage of the second type of lesion of cone dystrophy with larger pigment clumps and more extensive atrophy.

show great variability in the rate of progression and ophthalmoscopic appearance. Their ultimate level of acuity can range from 20/60 to 20/400.

The second most frequent macular lesion consists of diffuse pigment stippling resulting in a "salt-and-pepper" appearance, which eventually spreads outside the macular area, on both sides of the optic nerve (Fig. 12–52). In time, larger clumps of pigment are noted (Fig. 12–53). Patients with this type of involvement have a more rapid progression and more severe functional impairment. Most of these patients have visual acuities of 20/200 or less by the end of their first decade.

The rarest form of the disorder is characterized by atrophy of the choriocapillaris, larger choroidal vessels, pigment epithelium, and photoreceptors (Fig. 12–54). Many patients with cone degenerations have flecks similar to fundus flavimaculatus (Fig. 12–55),

and in a few patients optic atrophy, particularly temporally, may be the most prominent finding.

The diagnosis of cone dystrophy is confirmed by specific findings on the ERG. The portions of the ERG related to cone function are always more abnormal than the portions related to rod function. Abnormalities include a smaller-than-normal, single-flash photopic response, a smaller-than-normal flicker response, and a reduced flicker fusion frequency. Subjective dark adaptation is either normal or only minimally abnormal even in advanced cases of cone dystrophy. In contrast, dark adaptation is markedly abnormal in retinitis pigmentosa. Fluorescein angiography may demonstrate an early bull's-eye lesion better than it can be appreciated on ophthalmoscopy. Color vision abnormalities in cone dystrophy usually occur only after the visual acuity has dropped to 20/40 or 20/60. Errors on the Farnsworth–Munsell 100 hue test occur most fre-

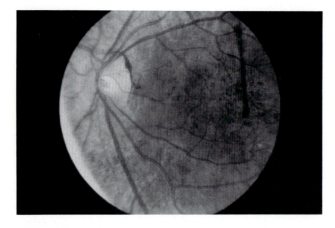

Figure 12–52. Diffuse pigment stippling form of cone dystrophy. The macular area is predominantly involved, but changes can be seen outside the macular area.

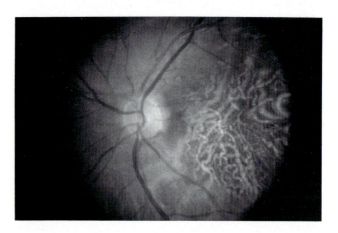

Figure 12–54. Rarest form of cone dystrophy, characterized by choroidal vascular atrophy in the macular region, and temporal optic atrophy.

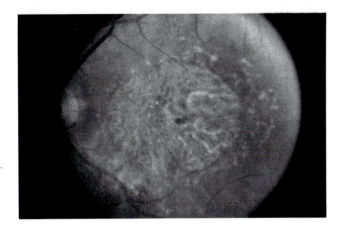

Figure 12–55. Another patient with cone dystrophy and choroidal vascular atrophy. Note also the presence of surrounding flecks, similar to the appearance of fundus flavimaculatus.

quently along the deutan axis. In other macular diseases, errors are usually distributed along the tritan axis.

The use of heavily tinted glasses or miotics may be helpful to some patients in whom visual acuity falls off at low levels of luminance. No treatment is available that can slow the progression of the disease.

Stationary Cone Disorders

Congenital achromatopsia or **rod monochromatism** is a rare, nonprogressive, autosomal recessive disorder characterized by the absence of functioning cones. It presents during the first few months of life with horizontal pendular nystagmus and photophobia (see Chapter 7). The macular and optic nerve appearance are normal. Vision is usually in the 20/200 to 20/400 range and remains stable throughout life. The diagnosis is confirmed by the presence of an abnormal ERG response to a flicker stimulus, an abnormal photopic ERG, and a normal scotopic ERG. These findings may be similar to those seen in patients with cone dystrophy. Achromatopsia, however, is stationary, with an onset at birth; cone dystrophy is progressive, and has characteristic macular changes.

Rod Dystrophies

Congenital Stationary Night Blindness (CSNB)

Congenital stationary night blindness (CSNB) is a nonprogressive disorder characterized by nyctalopia (night blindness) and mildly reduced vision in the 20/30 to 20/50 range. The visual fields and color vision are normal, and the fundus appears normal. Dark adaptometry shows an essentially intact cone system, but reduced retinal sensitivity, and the ERG demonstrates a deep normal a-wave with an absent b-wave on dark-adapted, bright flash (scotopic) testing. These findings

have been reported in both autosomal recessive and dominant pedigrees.

An X-linked variety of CSNB can be associated with high myopia, nystagmus, decreased visual acuity, and occasionally strabismus. Another feature of this form of CSNB is tilting of the optic nerves.

Oguchi's disease is a special form of CSNB. In this condition, the fundus assumes an unusual color, varying from shades of gray white to yellow. The abnormal color may involve a small area of the midperiphery or may extend throughout the entire fundus in a discontinuous or homogeneous pattern. A unique feature of Oguchi's disease is the Mizuo phenomenon, which is a change in the color of the fundus in the dark-adapted state. When light is prevented from entering the eye, the fundus color changes from the light shade seen initially to a reddish, more normal appearance. The time needed to elicit the change in fundus color varies. Patients with this condition have normal vision that remains stable, but their adaptation to dim illumination is prolonged. The ERG reveals a decreased scotopic response that may revert to normal during prolonged dark adaptation.

Fundus Albipunctatus

Fundus albipunctatus is another form of CSNB. Patients present with nyctalopia and essentially normal vision. Ophthalmoscopically, there are multiple, discrete, yellow-white spots at the level of the RPE, scattered throughout the posterior pole but sparing the macula and the peripapillary area (Fig. 12–56). Electroretinography initially reveals a reduced photopic ERG and an abnormal scotopic ERG. After 2 to 3 hours of dark adaptation, however, the ERG becomes normal. Psychophysical testing confirms this slow readaptation of both rod and cone thresholds over time.

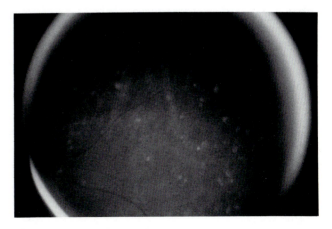

Figure 12–56. Fundus albipunctatus characterized by punctate white spots at the level of the retinal pigment epithelium in the peripheral fundus.

RPE Dystrophies

Stargardt's Disease (Fundus Flavimaculatus)

Stargardt's disease and fundus flavimaculatus are most likely manifestations of the same disease entity, believed to be caused by the accumulation of lipofuscin within the RPE. "Stargardt's disease" is the term used when the macula is predominantly involved and "fundus flavimaculatus" when the peripheral retina shows greater involvement. Inheritance is as an autosomal recessive trait. The electrooculogram is abnormal in 1 of 3 patients; the electroretinogram demonstrates a subnormal b-wave in one of 6 patients. Fluorescein angiography demonstrates a mottled hyperfluorescence in the macular area in Stargardt's disease, and poor visibility of the choroidal circulation ("silent choroid") in all cases. The "silent choroid" results from lipofuscin blockage of fluorescence.

Stargardt's disease is a bilateral, slowly progressive disorder characterized in the early stages by a loss of central vision out of proportion to the appearance of the macula. It presents between the ages of 8 and 14 years, and affected children are often initially misdiagnosed as having functional visual loss. Eventually an oval-shaped area of chorioretinal atrophy and depigmentation develops in the macula, sometimes in a bull's-eye pattern (Figs. 12–57 and 12–58). Rarely, subretinal neovascularization in the macula can develop (Fig. 12–59). Visual loss is progressive over a period of years, and generally deteriorates to the 20/200 range by age 30. No effective therapy is known.

Fundus flavimaculatus is characterized by irregular or pisciform-shaped yellow-white flecks at the level of the pigment epithelium in the posterior pole, occasionally extending anteriorly to the equator (Figs. 12–60 and 12–61). Unlike Stargardt's disease, this disorder is usually stationary and vision is unaffected unless there is macular involvement.

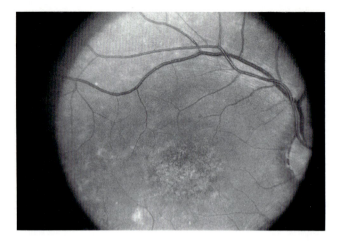

Figure 12–58. Another patient with Stargardt's disease, demonstrating an RPE disturbance in the central macular region. *(From Nelson LB, Brown GC, Arentsen JJ: Recognizing Patterns of Ocular Childhood Diseases. Thorofare, NJ, Slack, 1985, p 123, with permission.)*

Pattern Dystrophies

A multitude of central pigmentary disturbances, each with the retention of good central vision, have been described (Fig. 12–62). Different configurations are usually named after an object that they resemble (for example, fish net, spider-like, and butterfly). Salt-and-pepper and other distributions have also been described. Different configurations in different members of the same family suggests that a single underlying defect is likely present for all the various patterns.

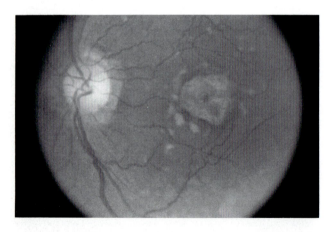

Figure 12–57. Stargardt's disease characterized by an oval-shaped area of atrophy in almost a "bull's-eye" pattern. Note also the surrounding flecks, which help confirm the diagnosis.

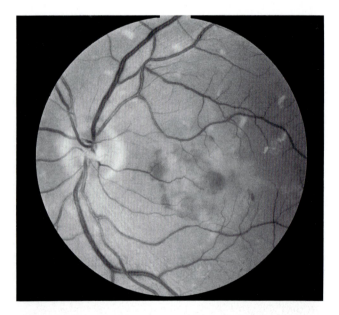

Figure 12–59. Hemorrhage from a subretinal neovascular membrane in an eye with Stargardt's disease. *(From Nelson LB, Brown GC, Arentsen JJ: Recognizing Patterns of Ocular Childhood Diseases. Thorofare, NJ, Slack, 1985, p 123, with permission.)*

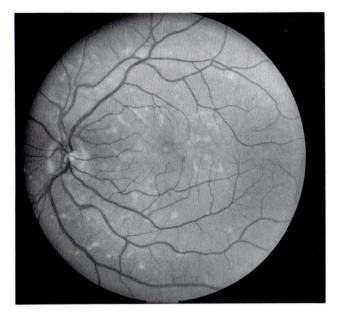

Figure 12–60. Fundus flavimaculatus characterized by irregular yellow-white lesions at the level of the RPE. *(From Nelson LB, Brown GC, Arentsen JJ: Recognizing Patterns of Ocular Childhood Diseases. Thorofare, NJ, Slack, 1985, p 123, with permission.)*

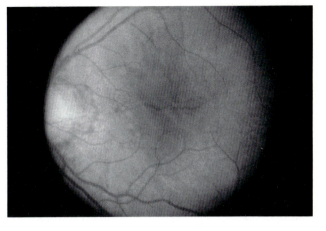

Figure 12–62. Pattern dystrophy of the RPE.

Familial Drusen

Drusen are excrescences of basement membrane material between the RPE and Bruch's membrane. They appear as small, yellow-white, round or oval lesions, and predominantly occur in the macular area (Fig. 12–63). Familial drusen is an autosomal dominant disorder in which drusen appear during childhood. Complications resulting in decreased central vision (such as hemorrhage from subretinal neovascularization) are rare before 40 years of age.

Aicardi's Syndrome

Aicardi's syndrome is a rare congenital disorder of females characterized by severe mental retardation, infantile spasms, defects of the corpus callosum, dorsal

vertebral anomalies, and chorioretinal lacunar infarcts. The latter appear as round, depigmented chorioretinal lesions clustered around the optic disc (Fig. 12–64). Optic nerve colobomas and microphthalmos can also occur. The disorder is thought to be X-linked dominant and lethal in males.

Best's Vitelliform Dystrophy

Best's disease is an autosomal dominant disorder distinguished by the appearance of a yellow, subretinal, "egg-yolk" lesion in the central macular area (Figs. 12–65 and 12–66). Initially, even with this appearance, the vision is usually normal. With time the yolk may "scramble," leading to a central cicatricial macular scar and a precipitous drop in visual acuity to the 20/200 range (vitelliruptive stage). The appearance at this stage is often indistinguishable from other forms of macular degeneration.

Best's disease is diagnosed by its ophthalmoscopic appearance, and is associated with a depressed electrooculogram. The ERG is normal. The condition is almost always bilateral, and multiple lesions may occur. It

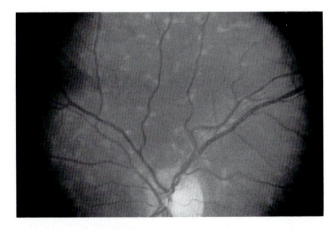

Figure 12–61. Pisciform (fish-like) flecks in fundus flavimaculatus.

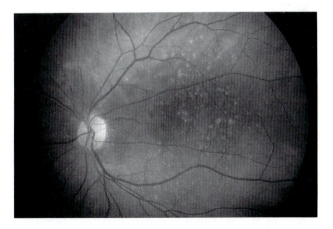

Figure 12–63. Familial drusen.

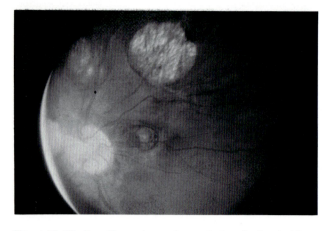

Figure 12–64. Aicardi's syndrome demonstrating chorioretinal lacunar infarcts, clustered around the optic disc.

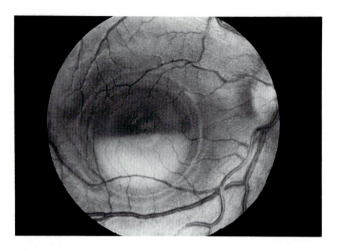

Figure 12–66. Variant of the vitelliform macular lesion of Best's disease, in which the "yolk" has partially settled. *(From Nelson LB, Brown GC, Arentsen JJ: Recognizing Patterns of Ocular Childhood Diseases. Thorofare, NJ, Slack, 1985, p 93, with permission.)*

usually manifests between 3 and 15 years of age, with a mean age of presentation of 6 years. Despite being dominantly transmitted, there is reduced penetrance and the disorder may skip generations. The EOG can be used to detect carriers, as it is abnormal in all bearers, even in the absence of fundus abnormalities. Pathologically, lipofuscin granules accumulate within the choroid and RPE. In some cases subretinal neovascularization may occur. No therapy has proven efficacious in preventing visual loss.

Dominant Cystoid Macular Edema

Dominant cystoid macular edema is characterized by the development of cystic changes in the macula, and an abnormal EOG, in the first decade of life. Fluid accumulates in the outer plexiform layer of the retina in a spoke-like pattern, due to the tangential orientation of this layer in the fovea. With fluorescein angiography, an abnormal permeability of perifoveal capillaries and the accumulation of dye in a characteristic pattern can

be demonstrated (Fig. 12–67). Visual acuity is usually good until the middle years of life, when atrophic changes develop. The EOG is usually abnormal.

Vitreoretinal Dystrophies

X-linked Recessive (Juvenile) Retinoschisis

Juvenile retinoschisis is a vitreoretinal dystrophy identified by vitreous degeneration and splitting of the sensory retina, predominantly within the nerve fiber layer. It affects only males, and can be observed as early as birth.

Schisis of the fovea is virtually pathognomonic and is found in almost 100% of patients. Ophthalmoscopically, this appears in early stages as small fine striae in the internal limiting membrane that radiate outward in a petaloid or spoke-wheel configuration (Fig. 12–68). This appearance may resemble cystoid macular edema, but fluorescein angiography reveals no cysts in this disorder. Peripheral retinoschisis also occurs in 50 per-

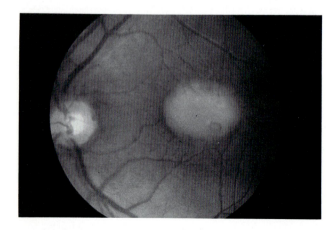

Figure 12–65. Eggyolk (vitelliform) lesion of Best's disease.

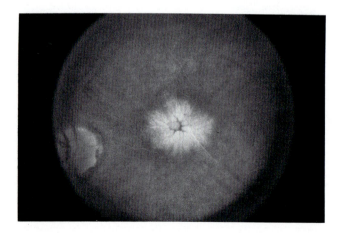

Figure 12–67. Fluorescein angiography demonstrating cystoid macular edema.

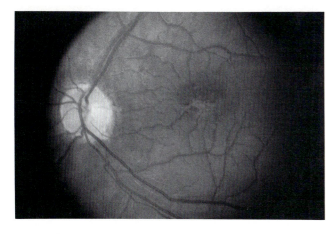

Figure 12–68. Foveal retinoschisis in juvenile retinoschisis. A finer, stellate pattern is appreciated in earlier stages.

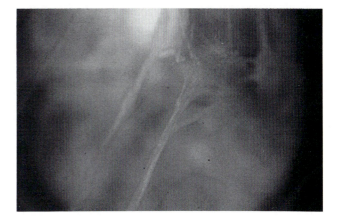

Figure 12–70. Prominent vitreous veils (separated nerve fiber layer) in juvenile retinoschisis.

cent of affected boys. When it occurs, this is always bilateral, but may be asymmetric. The inferior temporal quadrant is more commonly involved, and a secondary retinal detachment may occur in 5 to 20 percent of cases. Nerve fiber layer breaks, which appear as large round or oval holes, are also common (Fig. 12–69), and vitreous veils, which may contain branching retinal vessels, are sometimes prominent (Fig. 12–70). Tears in these vessels can result in vitreous hemorrhage.

Vision is variable and cannot be predicted ophthalmoscopically. As the disease progresses, there is a gradual deterioration of central vision to counting fingers or hand motion vision. The ERG often shows a subnormal scotopic b-wave in conjunction with a normal a-wave. Color vision abnormalities parallel the degree of foveal involvement. Visual field testing demonstrates central scotomas secondary to foveal changes, and absolute scotomas corresponding to areas of peripheral schisis.

The most important complications are vitreous hemorrhage and retinal detachment. No treatment is available for the foveal schisis; delimiting photocoagu-

lation has been tried with variable success in preventing encroachment of the fovea by peripheral schisis.

Wagner Vitreoretinal Dystrophy/Stickler Syndrome

The eponym "Wagner vitreoretinal dystrophy" is used to describe a constellation of vitreoretinal degeneration: radial perivascular lattice degeneration, optically empty vitreous, high myopia, cataracts, infantile glaucoma, ectopia lentis, strabismus, ptosis, and retinal detachment. Stickler syndrome is used when the above occurs in association with systemic findings of Marfanoid habitus, Pierre–Robin anomaly (flattened facies, small mandible, and cleft palate), progressive joint degeneration, arthritis, heart defects, and deafness. The disorder is transmitted as an autosomal dominant trait; great variability in the expression of the gene is seen even within a single family.

Goldmann–Favre Vitreoretinal Dystrophy

Goldmann–Favre dystrophy is distinguished by vitreoretinal degeneration associated with changes re-

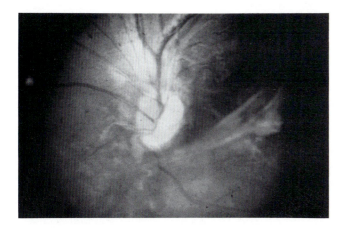

Figure 12–69. Nerve fiber layer tear in juvenile retinoschisis. *(Courtesy of the Wills Eye Hospital slide collection.)*

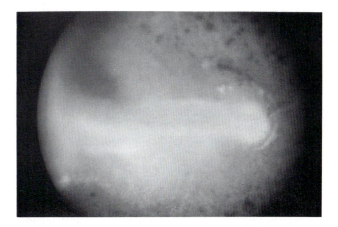

Figure 12–71. Preretinal membrane and retinal pigmentary changes in Goldmann–Favre disease.

sembling retinitis pigmentosa (Fig. 12–71). Foveal and peripheral retinoschisis, vitreous strands and veils, and an optically empty vitreous cavity are present. In addition, pigmentary changes in the peripheral retina occur, along with attenuation of retinal vessels and optic nerve pallor. These changes account for the presenting symptoms of decreased central acuity and night blindness. The ERG and EOG are both abnormal, differentiating this syndrome from juvenile retinoschisis, in which the EOG is normal. The disorder is transmitted as an autosomal recessive trait. Affected individuals have poor vision at birth, which deteriorates further in adulthood.

Familial Exudative Vitreoretinopathy

This autosomal dominant disorder has great variability of expression. In almost 75 percent of eyes the fundus abnormalities are subtle and the visual acuity is good. The remaining 25 percent of eyes are susceptible to retinal detachment subsequent to vitreoretinal traction or exudation. Over 90 percent of affected individuals have peripheral retinal nonperfusion (Fig. 12–72). Fifty to 60 percent develop temporal dragging of the retina secondary to traction from peripheral vitreous bands or membranes (Fig. 12–73). In severe cases, thick peripheral exudates develop in and under the retina, and can lead to total loss of vision if an exudative retinal detachment results. The disease presents in the neonate, and progresses in the school-age child. Progressive changes or visual loss rarely occur, however, beyond 20 years of age. The differential diagnosis includes retinopathy of prematurity when the disorder manifests as retinal traction, and Coats' disease when exudation occurs.

Incontinentia Pigmenti[*]

Incontinentia pigmenti, also known as Bloch–Sulzberger syndrome, is a rare X chromosome-linked disorder characterized by a triphasic dermopathy and variable malformations of the eyes, teeth, and central nervous system. The abnormal and dominant X chromosome, responsible for changes in females, causes death in male fetuses.

The first stage of the skin lesions occurs within days of birth and consists of a linear pattern of erythema and bullae on the extremities (Fig. 12–74). At approximately 2 months of age the vesicular lesions are superseded by verrucous lesions that last several months (Fig. 12–75). The final stage of irregular, whorled, marbled pigmentation occurs a few months later (Fig. 12–76). This pigmentation is most pronounced on the trunk. Dental anomalies include delayed dentition and missing and cone-shaped teeth (Fig. 12–77). Central

[*]Reprinted from Catalano RA: Incontinentia pigmenti. Am J Ophthalmol 110:696, 1990, with permission. Copyright by the Ophthalmic Publishing Company.

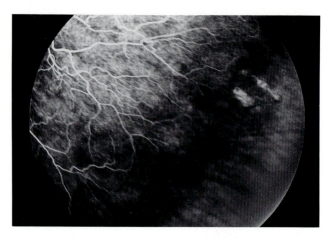

Figure 12–72. Fluorescein angiogram demonstrating peripheral nonperfusion in familial exudative vitreoretinopathy.

nervous system abnormalities include seizure disorders, microcephaly, and motor disturbances.

The initial retinal defect is avascularity of the peripheral temporal retina associated with intraretinal microvascular anomalies. In approximately one third of affected individuals, retinal fibrovascular proliferation and total retinal detachment develop. These changes resemble those seen in retinopathy of prematurity and familial exudative vitreoretinopathy. The eyes are often asymmetrically involved, and the affected eye is often microphthalmic. Ocular involvement occurs in approximately one third of affected individuals; if ocular abnormalities do not appear within the first year of life, the prognosis for normal vision is good.

Treatment of the peripheral retinopathy of incontinentia pigmenti with laser photocoagulation or cryotherapy is variably successful in arresting the vascular changes. The outcome may be more favorable if the abnormal vascular tissue is treated directly (unlike

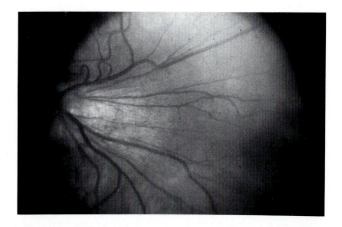

Figure 12–73. Temporal dragging of the retina in familial exudative vitreoretinopathy.

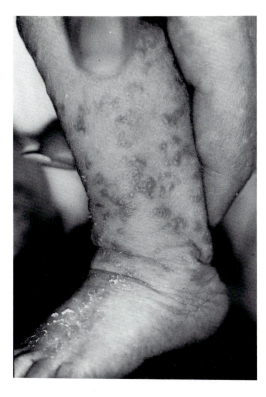

Figure 12–74. Stage 1, vesicular dermopathy of incontinentia pigmenti on the leg of a 15-day-old infant. *(Reprinted from Catalano RA: Incontinentia pigmenti. Am J Ophthalmol 110:696, 1990; copyright by the Ophthalmic Publishing Company, with permission.)*

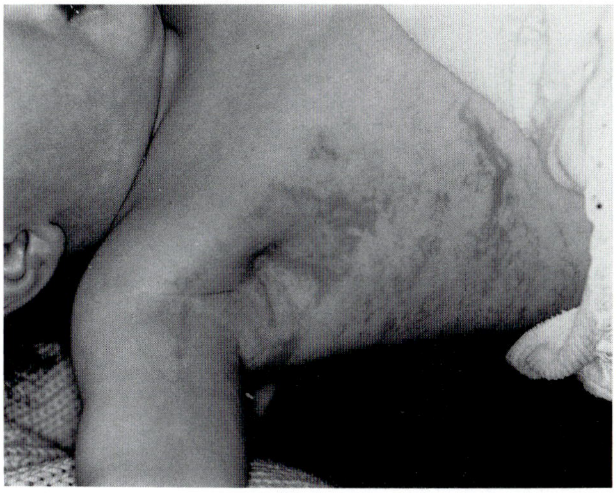

Figure 12–76. Stage 3, whorled pigmentary dermopathy on the trunk of the same infant as in Figures 12–74 and 12–75 at 6 months of age. *(Reprinted from Catalano RA: Incontinentia pigmenti. Am J Ophthalmol 110:696, 1990; copyright by the Ophthalmic Publishing Company, with permission.)*

retinopathy of prematurity). The indications and timing for intervention in individuals with proliferative changes remain undefined.

Diabetic Retinopathy

Diabetic retinopathy is categorized as either background or proliferative. In both types, retinal microaneurysms, hard and soft exudates, dot and blot hemorrhages, macular edema, and microangiopathy occur (Fig. 12–78). Hard exudates represent extravasated lipid; soft exudates (cotton-wool patches) are nerve fiber layer infarcts. Hemorrhages can occur within the retina or preretinally. If the internal limiting membrane

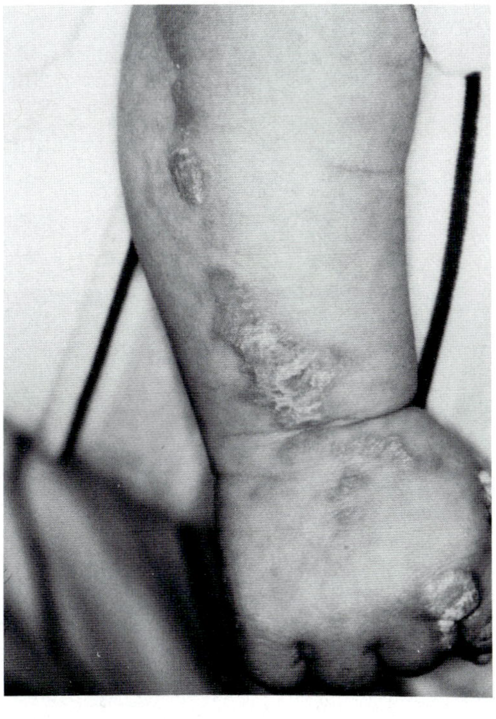

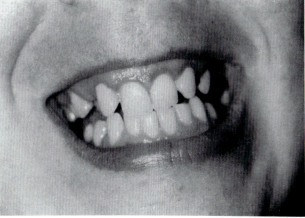

Figure 12–75. Stage 2, verrucous dermopathy on the hand of the same infant as in Figure 12–74 at 2 months of age. *(Reprinted from Catalano RA: Incontinentia pigmenti. Am J Ophthalmol 110:696, 1990; copyright by the Ophthalmic Publishing Company, with permission.)*

Figure 12–77. Missing and cone-shaped teeth in a 30-year-old woman with incontinentia pigmenti. *(Reprinted from Catalano RA: Incontinentia pigmenti. Am J Ophthalmol 110:696, 1990; copyright by the Ophthalmic Publishing Company, with permission.)*

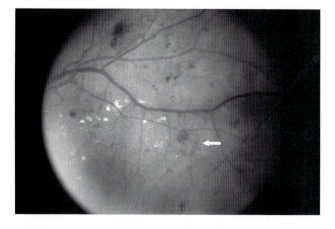

Figure 12–78. Diabetic retinopathy demonstrating dot-and-blot hemorrhages, hard exudates, and neovascularization (*arrow*).

were adolescents (Kimmel et al, 1985). Increased growth hormone levels during adolescence, however, may have an unfavorable effect on preexisting retinopathy. For this reason, teenage diabetics should be examined for the presence of retinopathy within 5 years after the initiation of treatment. The treatment of proliferative diabetic retinopathy is beyond the scope of this book, but involves laser photocoagulation of the retina.

Chorioretinal Degenerations

Choroideremia

Choroideremia is a progressive retinal degeneration, inherited in an X-linked recessive manner. Fundus changes may be seen as early as 2 years of age and are heralded by the onset of night blindness and visual field loss. In the young child there is initially widespread scattering of pigment in all quadrants of the retina. Occasionally, there may be areas of choroidal atrophy in the midperiphery. By age 10, areas of midperipheral choriocapillaris and RPE atrophy become obvious. By age 40, the atrophy extends to the periphery, and the affected area appears yellow-white (Fig. 12–80). Overlying this are dispersed clumps of pigment. An island of normal macula is retained until late in the disease. By age 60, nearly all affected individuals are blind.

Central visual acuity is good until late in the course of the disease. Visual field testing reveals a midperipheral scotoma early that breaks centrally and to the periphery with time. The ERG is usually extinguished, even when the patient is young and the fields are good. Female carriers uniformly show normal visual acuity, but may have pigment stippling or clumps of pigment in the midperiphery. Most have full fields or only a minimal midperipheral field loss. Carriers also have a normal to low-normal ERG.

contains the hemorrhage, it will appear boat-shaped (Fig. 12–79).

Proliferative retinopathy is characterized by the additional presence of new blood vessels in and anterior to the retina (see Fig. 12–78). These usually originate from a retinal vein near an arteriovenous crossing, or from the surface of the optic disc. Vitreous hemorrhage results when the vitreous detaches, and vessels growing on the surface of the retina rupture. At the time of occurrence the patient notices a shower of floaters, black strands, or sudden loss of vision, depending on the magnitude of hemorrhage. An examiner in turn will notice blurring of fundus details, or a black reflex on ophthalmoscopy. Traction by contracting vitreous can cause a tractional (nonrhegmatogenous) retinal detachment.

Although the frequency of proliferative retinopathy increases with the duration of diabetes, it rarely occurs under the age of 20 years. In one large study only 1 to 2 percent of diabetics with proliferative changes

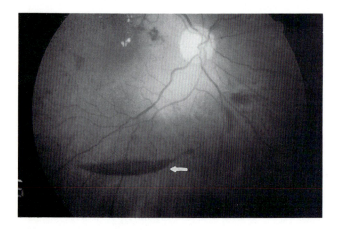

Figure 12–79. Diabetic retinopathy demonstrating a boat-shaped, preretinal hemorrhage (*arrow*).

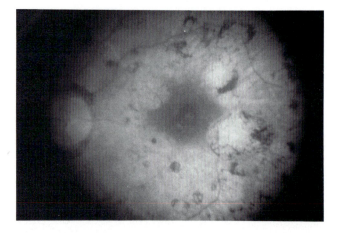

Figure 12–80. Choriocapillaris and RPE atrophy in choroideremia. Note the overlying clumps of pigment, and the island of normal macula.

Gyrate Atrophy

Gyrate atrophy of the choroid and retina is a rare, autosomal recessive, progressive, chorioretinal dystrophy that begins in childhood and leads to blindness in the fourth to seventh decade of life. The primary defect is deficiency of the mitochondrial enzyme, ornithine aminotransferase. This results in the accumulation of ornithine, which is believed to be toxic to the RPE. Blood ornithine levels of 10 to 20 times normal can be detected, confirming the diagnosis. Carriers can be detected by reduced levels of the enzyme in cultures of their skin fibroblasts.

During the late teens, sharply demarcated circular patches of chorioretinal atrophy appear in the retinal periphery (Fig. 12–81). Affected patients note night blindness and increasing visual field loss. Atrophic areas increase in size and number, and gradually coalesce to involve more of the posterior pole, until there is complete chorioretinal atrophy (Fig. 12–82). Unlike choroideremia, which involves only the choriocapillaris and RPE, gyrate atrophy results in widespread choroidal loss.

High myopia (5 to 10 diopters) develops in childhood and most patients have impaired peripheral and night vision by age 10 years. Visual field loss parallels the abnormalities of the fundus; eventually tunnel vision results. Posterior subcapsular lens changes begin in the late teens, and the ERG is usually decreased or not recordable. Dietary restriction of arginine and intake of pyridoxine have been tried, but no long-term data exist regarding their effectiveness.

Coats' Disease

Coats' disease, also known as Leber's miliary aneurysms, is a nonheritable retinal vascular disorder characterized by intraretinal and subretinal lipid exudation (Fig. 12–83). It is unilateral in 90 percent of cases, and is usually diagnosed between 18 months and 10 years of

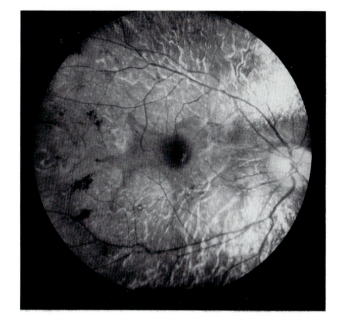

Figure 12–82. Progression of gyrate atrophy demonstrating scalloped areas of chorioretinal atrophy approaching the macula. *(From Nelson LB, Brown GC, Arentsen JJ: Recognizing patterns of ocular childhood diseases. Thorofare, NJ, Slack, 1985, p 103, with permission.)*

age. Boys are affected three times as often as girls. The most common presenting signs are leukocoria and strabismus.

The disorder is manifest by telangiectatic retinal vascular abnormalities that are best demonstrated with fluorescein angiography (Fig. 12–84). The abnormal vessels leak lipid that accumulates intraretinally and subretinally, giving an appearance that can be mistaken for retinoblastoma (see Figs. 12–35 and 12–85). Exudative retinal detachments occur in approximately two thirds of eyes. The anterior segment of the eye is usually normal, but neovascular glaucoma can ensue in advanced cases.

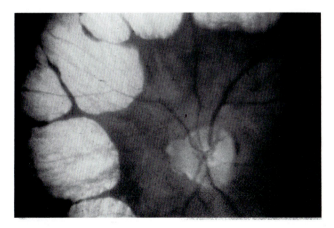

Figure 12–81. Sharply demarcated circular patches of chorioretinal atrophy in gyrate atrophy.

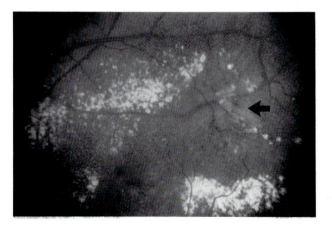

Figure 12–83. Exudation from saccular aneurysms *(arrow)* in Coats' disease. *(Courtesy of Calvin Mein.)*

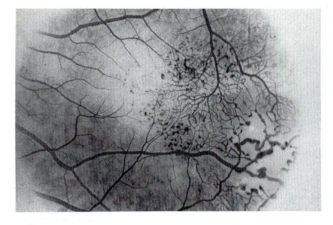

Figure 12–84. Fluorescein angiography in Coats' disease demonstrating a dilated capillary network and saccular aneurysms. *(Courtesy of Calvin Mein.)*

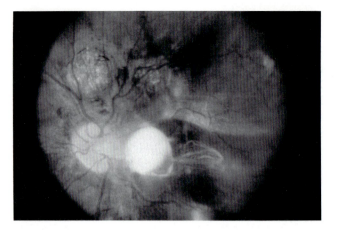

Figure 12–86. Toxocariasis. *(From Catalano RA: Ocular Emergencies. Philadelphia, Saunders, 1992, p 386, with permission.)*

Treatment modalities include photocoagulation or cryoablation of the abnormal telangiectatic vessels. Usually two or three treatment sessions at 4- to 6-week intervals are necessary. Without treatment all vision is usually lost; with treatment approximately one half of the eyes retain 20/70 to 20/400 vision. The disorder is more severe in those that show manifestations before the age of 4 years.

Ocular Toxocariasis

Ocular toxocariasis is caused by infestation of the eye with the wandering second-stage larvae of the dog ascarid worm, *Toxocara canis.* The larvae enter the child's eye following ingestion of ova that have been deposited in the soil through a puppy's stool. Systemically this organism causes visceral larva migrans, characterized by eosinophilia, leukocytosis, pulmonary infiltration, and hepatomegaly. Affected children present

with chronic cough, often paroxysmal and worse at night, wheezing, irritability, and fever.

The average age of affected patients is 7.5 years. The disorder is typically unilateral and may present as a vitreous abscess, a lesion of the posterior pole, an inflammatory mass in the peripheral retina, or an optic papillitis (Fig. 12–86). The lesion may be confused with retinoblastoma in younger children. An enzyme linked immunosorbent assay is available for *Toxocara* and may be useful in its diagnosis. No specific therapy is absolutely efficacious; antihelminthics that kill the worm may cause greater damage from the attendant inflammatory response.

Retinal Detachment

A retinal detachment is a separation of the outer layers of the retina from the underlying RPE (Fig. 12–87). A detachment can occur as a congenital anomaly, but

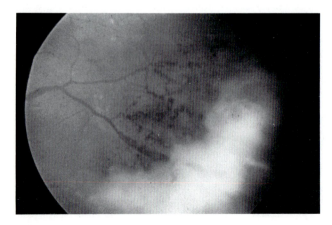

Figure 12–85. Massive intraretinal and subretinal exudate in Coats' disease.

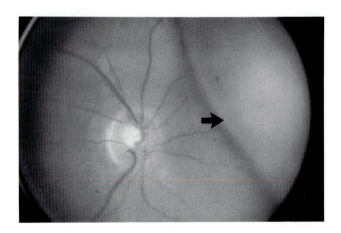

Figure 12–87. Retinal detachment (*arrow*).

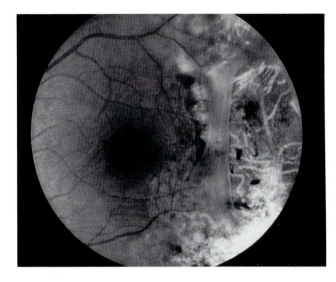

Figure 12–88. Peripheral retinal detachment (retinodialysis) secondary to trauma. *(From Catalano RA: Ocular Emergencies. Philadelphia, Saunders, 1992, p 171, with permission.)*

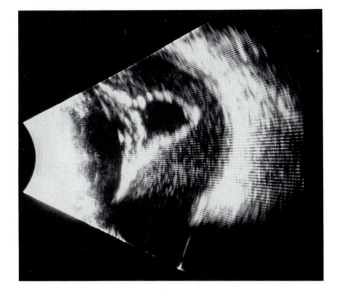

Figure 12–90. B-scan ultrasound demonstrating a funnel-shaped retinal detachment.

more commonly detachments arise secondary to other abnormalities or trauma.

Three types of detachment are described, each of which may occur in children. Rhegmatogenous detachments result from a break in the retina that allows fluid to enter the subretinal space (Fig. 12–88). In children these are usually the result of trauma (such as child abuse), but may occur secondary to myopia or retinopathy of prematurity, or following congenital cataract surgery. Tractional retinal detachments result when vitreoretinal membranes pull on the retina (see Fig. 12–20). They can occur in diabetes, sickle-cell disease, and retinopathy of prematurity. Exudative retinal detachments result when exudation exceeds absorption. This can be seen in Coats' disease (Fig. 12–89), retinoblastoma, and ocular inflammation.

When visualization of the retina is not possible because of cataract or vitreous hemorrhage, ultrasonography and neuroimaging can be used to detect retinal detachments (Figs. 12–90 and 12–91).

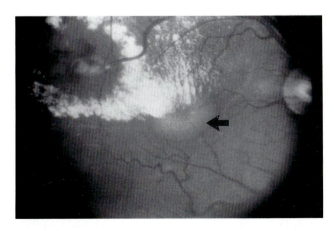

Figure 12–89. Exudative retinal detachment in the macular area *(arrow)* secondary to Coats' disease.

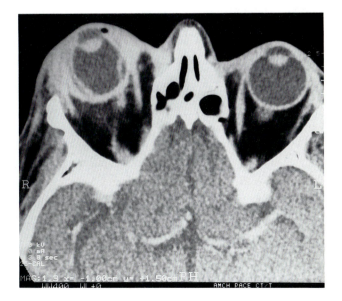

Figure 12–91. Computerized tomography demonstrating a retinal detachment in the left eye.

REFERENCES

Albinism

Creel, D, Witkop CJ, King RA: Asymmetric visual evoked potential in human albinos: Evidence for visual system anomalies. Invest Ophthalmol 13:430, 1974.

Kinnear PE, Jay B, Witkop CJ Jr.: Albinism. Surv Ophthalmol 30:75, 1985.

O'Donnell FE Jr, Green WR: The eye in albinism. In Tasman W, Jaeger EA (eds): Clinical Ophthalmology. Philadelphia, Lippincott, 1982.

O'Donnell FE Jr, King RA, Green WR, et al: Autosomal recessively inherited ocular albinism. Arch Ophthalmol 96:1621, 1978.

Choroideremia

Kurstjens JH: Choroideremia and gyrate atrophy of the choroid and retina. Doc Ophthalmol 19:79, 1965.

McCulloch C: Choroideremia: A clinical and pathologic review. Trans Am Ophthalmol Soc 67:142, 1969.

McCulloch C, Ashiinoff S: Choroideremia and gyrate atrophy. In Tasman W, Jaeger EA (eds): Duane's Clinical Ophthalmology. Philadelphia, Lippincott, 1990.

Coats' Disease

Ridley ME, Shields JA, Brown GC, et al: Coats' disease. Evaluation and management. Ophthalmology 89:1381, 1982.

Tasman W: Coats' disease. In Tasman W (ed): Retinal Diseases in Children. Hagerstown, MD, Harper & Row, 1971, pp 59–69.

Combined Hamartoma of the Retina and RPE

Ellis FD, Helveston EM, Plager DA: Combined hamartoma of the retina and retinal pigment epithelium. Paper presented at the American Association for Pediatric Ophthalmology and Strabismus annual meeting, 1991.

Palmer ML, Carney MD, Combs JL: Combined hamartomas of the retinal pigment epithelium and retina. Retina 10:33, 1990.

Sappenfield DL, Gitter KA: Surgical intervention for combined retinal–RPE hamartoma. Retina 10:119, 1990.

Cone Dystrophy

Berson EL, Gouras P, Gunkel RD: Progressive cone–rod degeneration. Arch Ophthalmol 80:68, 1962.

Franceschetti A, François J, Bobel J: Chorioretinal Heredodegenerations. Springfield IL, Thomas, 1974.

Goodman G, Rips H, Siegel IM: Cone dysfunction syndromes. Arch Ophthalmol 70:214, 1963.

Krill AE, Deutman AF: Dominant macular degenerations: The cone dystrophies. Am J Ophthalmol 73:352, 1972.

Krill AE, Deutman AF, Fishman M: The cone degenerations. Doc Ophthalmol 35:1, 1973.

Schroeder RP, Tasman W, Bensen WE: Diseases of the retina and vitreous. In Nelson LB, Calhoun JC, Harley RD: Pediatric Ophthalmology, ed 3. Philadelphia, Saunders, 1991, pp 292–309.

Congenital Stationary Night Blindness

Carr RE: Congenital stationary night blindness. Trans Am Ophthalmol Soc 72:448, 1974.

Carr RE, Margolis S, Siegel IM: Fluorescein angiography and vitamin A and oxalate levels in fundus albipunctatus. Am J Ophthalmol 82:549, 1976.

Krill AE: Hereditary retinal and choroidal diseases, vol 2. Clinical Characteristics. Hagerstown, MD, Harper & Row, 1977.

Levy NS, Toskes PP: Fundus albipunctatus and vitamin A deficiency. Am J Ophthalmol 78:926, 1974.

Mizuo A: On new discovery in dark adaptation in Oguchi's disease. Acta Soc Ophthalmol Jpn 17:1148, 1973.

Wilder H: Oguchi's disease. Am J Ophthalmol 36:718, 1953.

Diabetic Retinopathy

Frank RN, Hoffman WH, Podgor MJ, et al: Retinopathy in juvenile-onset type 1 diabetes of short duration. Diabetes 31:874, 1982.

Kimmel AS, Magargal LE, Annesley WH Jr, Donoso LA: Diabetic retinopathy under age 20. A review of 71 cases. Ophthalmology 92:1047, 1985.

Kingsley R, Ghosh G, Lawson P, Kohner EM: Severe diabetic retinopathy in adolescents. Br J Ophthalmol 67:73, 1983.

Malone JI, Van Cader TC, Edwards WC: Diabetic vascular changes in children. Diabetes 26:673, 1977.

Palmberg P, Smith M, Waltman S, et al: The natural history of retinopathy in insulin-dependent juvenile onset diabetes. Ophthalmology 88:613, 1981.

Gyrate Atrophy

Kaiser-Kupfer MI, Caruso RC, Valle D: Gyrate atrophy of the choroid and retina. Long-term reduction of ornithine slows retinal degeneration. Arch Ophthalmol 109:1939, 1991.

McClatchey AI, Kaufman DL, Berson EL, et al: Splicing defect at the ornithine amino-transferase locus in gyrate atrophy. Am J Hum Genet 47:790, 1990.

McCulloch JC, Arshinoff SA: Choroideremia and gyrate atrophy. In Tasman W, Jaeger EA (eds): Clinical Ophthalmology. Philadelphia, Lippincott, 1991.

McCulloch JC, Arshinoff SA, Marliss EB, et al: Hyperornithinemia and gyrate atrophy of the choroid and retina. Ophthalmology 85:918, 1978.

Simell O, Takki K: Raised plasma ornithine and gyrate atrophy of the choroid and retina. Lancet 1:1031, 1973.

Incontinentia Pigmenti

Catalano RA: Incontinentia pigmenti. Am J Ophthalmol 110:696, 1990.

Catalano RA, Lopatynsky M, Tasman WS: Treatment of proliferative retinopathy associated with incontinentia pigmenti. Am J Ophthalmol 110:701, 1990.

Migeon BR, Axelman J, Jan de Beur, et al: Selection against lethal alleles in females heterozygous for incontinentia pigmenti. Am J Hum Genet 44:100, 1989.

Nix RR, Apple DJ: Proliferative retinopathy associated with incontinentia pigmenti. Retina 1:156, 1981.

Raab EL: Ocular lesions in incontinentia pigmenti. J Pediatr Ophthalmol Strabismus 20:42, 1983.

Watzke RC, Stevens TS, Carney RG Jr: Retinal vascular

changes of incontinentia pigmenti. Arch Ophthalmol 94:743, 1976.

Juvenile (X-linked) Retinoschisis

Harris GS, Young JWS: Maculopathy of sex-linked juvenile retinoschisis. Can J Ophthalmol 11:1, 1976.

Krill AE, Deutman HF: Variations of juvenile macular degeneration. Trans Am Ophthalmol 70:220, 1972.

Manschot WA: Pathology of hereditary juvenile retinoschisis. Arch Ophthalmol 88:131, 1972.

Yanoff M, Rahn EK, Zimmerman LE: Histopathology of juvenile retinoschisis. Arch Ophthalmol 79:49, 1968.

Leber's Congenital Amaurosis

Dagi LR, Leys MJ, Hansen RH, Fulton AB: Hyperopia in complicated Leber's congenital amaurosis. Am J Ophthalmol 108:709, 1990.

Foxman SG, Wirtschafter FD, Letson RD: Leber's congenital amaurosis and high hyperopia: A discrete entity. In Henkind P (ed): ACTA: 24th International Congress of Ophthalmology. Philadelphia, Lippincott, 1983.

Lambert SR, Kress A, Taylor D, et al: Follow-up and diagnostic reappraisal of 75 patients with Leber's congenital amaurosis. Am J Ophthalmol 107:624, 1989.

Leber T: Über Retinitis pigmentosa and angeborene Amaurose. Grafes Arch Clin Exp Ophthalmol 15:1, 1869.

Nickel B, Hoyt CS: Leber's congenital amaurosis: Is mental retardation a frequent associated defect? Arch Ophthalmol 100:1089, 1982.

Noble KC, Carr RE: Leber's congenital amaurosis. Arch Ophthalmol 96:818, 1978.

Schroeder R, Mets MB, Maumenee IH: Leber's congenital amaurosis: Retrospective review of 43 cases and a new fundus finding in two cases. Arch Ophthalmol 105:356, 1987.

Steinberg A, Ronen S, Zlotogorski Z, et al: Central nervous system involvement in Leber congenital amaurosis. J Pediatr Ophthalmol Strabismus 29:224, 1992.

Sullivan TJ, Lambert SR, Buncic JR, Musarella MA: The optic disc in Leber congenital amaurosis. J Pediatr Ophthalmol Strabismus 29:246, 1992.

Wagner RS, Caputo AR, Nelson LB, Zanoni D: High hyperopia in Leber's congenital amaurosis. Arch Ophthalmol 103:1507, 1985.

Leukemia

Azkka KA, Yee RD, Shorr N, et al: Leukemic iris infiltration. Am J Ophthalmol 89:204, 1980.

Kincaid MC, Green WR: Ocular and orbital involvement in leukemia. Surv Ophthalmol 27:211, 1983.

Ridgway E, Jaffe N, Walton DS: Leukemic ophthalmology in children. Cancer 38:1744, 1976.

Rosenthal HR: Ocular manifestations of leukemia. Ophthalmology 90:899, 1983.

Schachat AP, Markowitz JA, Guyer DR, et al: Ophthalmic manifestations of leukemia. Arch Ophthalmol 107:697, 1989.

RPE Dystrophies

Bertoni JM, von Loh S, Allen RJ: The Aicardi syndrome: Report of 4 cases and review of the literature. Ann Neurol 5:475, 1979.

Bloome MA, Garcia CA: Manual of Retinal and Choroidal Dystrophies. New York, Appleton-Century-Crofts, 1982.

Krill AE: Hereditary Retinal and Choroidal Diseases. Hagerstown, MD, Harper & Row, 1972, vol 2.

Noble KG, Carr RE: Stargardt's disease and fundus flavimaculatus. Arch Ophthalmol 97:1281, 1979.

Retinitis Pigmentosa

Bloome MA, Garcia CA: Manual of Retinal and Choroidal Dystrophies. New York, Appleton-Century-Crofts, 1988.

Carr RE, Heckenlively JR: Hereditary pigmentary degenerations of the retina. In Tasman W, Jaeger EA (eds): Clinical Ophthalmology. Philadelphia, Lippincott, 1986.

Dryja TP, McGee TL, Reichel E, et al: A point mutation of the rhodopsin gene in one form of retinitis pigmentosa. Nature 343:364, 1990.

Heckenlively JR: The classification of retinitis pigmentosa. In Henkind P (ed): ACTA: 24th International Congress of Ophthalmology. Philadelphia, Lippincott, 1983, vol 1.

Mussoff RW, Finkelstein D: Subclassifications of retinitis pigmentosa from two-color scotopic static perimetry. Doc Ophthalmol Proc Ser 26:219, 1981.

Retinoblastoma

Dryja TP: DNA testing for retinoblastoma. Arch Ophthalmol 109:1210, 1991.

Lemieux J, Milot J, Barsoum-Homsy M, et al: First cytogenic evidence of homozygosity for the retinoblastoma deletion in chromosome 13. Cancer Genet Cytogenet 43:73, 1989.

Messmer EP, Heinrich T, Hopping W, et al: Risk factors for metastases in patients with retinoblastoma. Ophthalmology 98:136, 1991.

Pratt CB, Meyer D, Chenaille P, Crom DB: The use of bone marrow aspirations and lumbar punctures at the time of diagnosis of retinoblastoma. J Clin Oncol 7:140, 1989.

Scheffer H, te Meerman GJ, Kruize YC, et al: Linkage analysis of families with hereditary retinoblastoma: Nonpenetrance of mutation, revealed by combined use of markers within and flanking the RBI gene. Am J Hum Genet 45:252, 1989.

Shields JA, Augsburger JJ: Current approaches to the diagnosis and management of retinoblastoma. Surv Ophthalmol 25:347, 1981.

Shields JA, Augsburger JJ, Donoso LA: Recent developments related to retinoblastoma. J Pediatr Ophthalmol Strabismus 23:148, 1986.

Shields JA, Shields CL: Intraocular Tumors. A Text and Atlas. Philadelphia, Saunders, 1992.

Shields JA, Shields CL: Update on retinoblastoma. Semin Ophthalmol 5:183, 1990.

Shields JA, Shields CL, Shah P: Retinoblastoma in older children. Ophthalmology 98:395, 1991.

Yandell DW, Campbell TA, Dayton SH, et al: Oncogenic point mutations in the human retinoblastoma gene: Their application to genetic counseling. N Engl J Med 321:1689, 1989.

Retinopathy of Prematurity

American Academy of Pediatrics and American College of Obstetrics and Gynecology: Clinical considerations in the use of oxygen. In: Guidelines for perinatal care, ed 2. 1988.

Batton DG, Robert C, Trese M, Maisels MJ: Severe retinopathy of prematurity and steroid exposure. Pediatrics 90:534, 1992.

Ben-Sera I, Nessenkorn I, Kremer I: Retinopathy of prematurity. Surv Ophthalmol 33:1, 1988.

Biglan AW, Brown DR, Reynolds JD, Milley JR: Risk factors associated with retrolental fibroplasia. Ophthalmology 91:1504, 1984.

Brown GC, Tasman WS, Naidoff M, et al: Systemic complications associated with retinal cryoablation for retinopathy of prematurity. Ophthalmology 97:855, 1990.

Committee for the Classification of Retinopathy of Prematurity. An international classification of retinopathy of prematurity. Arch Ophthalmol 102:1120, 1984.

Cryotherapy for Retinopathy of Prematurity Cooperative Group: Multicenter trial of cryotherapy for retinopathy of prematurity. Three-month outcome. Arch Ophthalmol 108:195, 1990a.

Cryotherapy for Retinopathy of Prematurity Cooperative Group: Multicenter trial of cryotherapy for retinopathy of prematurity. One year outcome—structure and function. Arch Ophthalmol 108:1408, 1990b.

Dobson V: Visual acuity results at one year in treated versus untreated eyes in the cryotherapy for retinopathy of prematurity (CRYO-ROP) trial. Paper presented at the American Association for Pediatric Ophthalmology and Strabismus annual meeting, Lake George, NY, July, 1990.

Fielder AR, Robinson J, Shaw DE, et al: Light and retinopathy of prematurity: Does retinal location offer a clue? Pediatrics 89:648, 1992.

Flowers R, Blake DA, Waser SD: Retrolental fibroplasia: Evidence for a role of the prostaglandin cascade in the pathogenesis of oxygen-induced retinopathy in the newborn beagle. Pediatr Res 15:1293, 1982.

Flynn JT: Retinopathy of prematurity. In Nelson LB, Calhoun JC, Harley RD: Pediatric Ophthalmology, ed 3. Philadelphia, Saunders, 1991, pp 59–74.

Flynn JT, Bancalari E, Bawol R, et al: Retinopathy of prematurity: A randomized, prospective trial of transcutaneous oxygen monitoring. Ophthalmology 94:630, 1987.

Glass P, Avery GB, Subramanian KN, et al: Effect of bright light in the hospital nursery on the incidence of retinopathy of prematurity. N Engl J Med 333:401, 1985.

Hartnett ME, Gilbert MM, Richardson TM, et al: Anterior segment evaluation of infants with retinopathy of prematurity. Ophthalmology 991:122, 1990.

Hindle NW: Critical mass retinopathy of prematurity. What is it and what can you do about it? Doc Ophthalmol 74:253, 1990.

Hindle NW: Cryotherapy for retinopathy of prematurity. None, one, or both eyes. Arch Ophthalmol 108:1375, 1990.

International Committee for the Classification of Late Stages of Retinopathy of Prematurity. An international classification of retinal detachment. Arch Ophthalmol 105:906, 1987.

Kushner BJ: The sequelae of regressed retinopathy of prematurity. In Silverman WA, Flynn JT (ed): Retinopathy of Prematurity. Boston, Blackwell, 1986.

Lakatos L, Hatvani I, Oroszlan G, et al: Controlled trial of D-penicillamine to prevent retinopathy of prematurity. Acta Paediatr Hung 27:47, 1986.

McNamara JA, Moreno R, Tasman WS: Retinopathy of prematurity. In Tasman WS, Jaeger EA (eds): Clinical Ophthalmology. Philadelphia, Lippincott, 1990.

McNamara JA, Tasman WS: Retinopathy of prematurity. Ophthalmol Clin North Am 3:413, 1990.

McNamara JA, Tasman WS, Brown GC, Federman JL: Laser photocoagulation for stage 3+ retinopathy of prematurity. Ophthalmology 98:576, 1991.

Nissenkorn I, Ben-Sira I, Kremer I, et al: Eleven years experience with retinopathy of prematurity: Visual results and contribution of cryoablation. Br J Ophthalmol 75:158, 1991.

Repka MX, Parsa CF, Hudak ML: Surfactant prophylaxis and retinopathy of prematurity. Paper presented at the American Association for Pediatric Ophthalmology and Strabismus annual meeting, Hawaii, February, 1991.

Saunders RA, Miller KW: Does topical anesthesia reduce infant stress during eye examination? Paper presented at the American Association for Pediatric Ophthalmology and Strabismus annual meeting, Hawaii, February, 1991.

Schaffer DB: Update on retinopathy of prematurity: The examination guidelines. Semin Ophthalmol 5:100, 1990.

Schaffer DB, Metz HS, Palmer EA, et al: Prognostic factors in the natural course of retinopathy of prematurity. Paper presented at the American Association for Pediatric Ophthalmology and Strabismus annual meeting, Lake George, NY, July, 1990.

Sobel DP, Philip AGS: Prolonged dexamethasone therapy reduces the incidence of cryotherapy for retinopathy of prematurity in infants less than 1 kilogram with bronchopulmonary dysplasia. Pediatrics 90:529, 1992.

Sternberg P Jr, Lopez PF, Lambert HM, et al: Controversies in the management of retinopathy of prematurity. Am J Ophthalmol 113:198, 1992.

Tasman W: Multicenter trial of cryotherapy for retinopathy of prematurity. Editorial. Arch Ophthalmol 106:463, 1988.

Tasman W: Management of retinopathy of prematurity. Ophthalmology 92:995, 1985.

Tasman W: The natural history of retinopathy of prematurity. Ophthalmology 91:1499, 1984.

Tingley DH, Flynn JT: Perspectives on retinopathy of prematurity. Int Pediatr 5:232, 1990.

Valentine PH, Jackson JC, Kalina RE, et al: Increased survival of low birth weight infants: Impact on the incidence of retinopathy of prematurity. Pediatrics 84:442, 1989.

Vitreoretinal Dystrophies

Liberfarb R, Hirose T: The Wagner–Stickler's syndrome. Birth Defects 18:525, 1982.

Nielsen CE: Stickler's syndrome. Acta Ophthalmol (KGL) 59:286, 1981.

Regentogen L: Hereditary vitreoretinal degeneration, cleft lip and palate, deafness and skeletal dysplasia. Am J Ophthalmol 89:414, 1980.

Spallone A: Stickler's syndrome: A study of 12 families. Br J Ophthalmol 71:504, 1987.

Stickler GB, Belau PG, Farrell FJ, et al: Hereditary progressive arthro-ophthalmopathy. Mayo Clin Proc 40:433, 1965.

OPTIC NERVE
AND NEUROLOGICAL DISORDERS

ESSENTIAL INFORMATION FOR PRIMARY CARE PRACTITIONERS

Congenital Anomalies of the Optic Nerve

A number of developmental defects of the optic disc have been described. It is useful to categorize these (Table 13–1) as vascular anomalies (Fig. 13–1), colobomatous/excavated defects (Fig. 13–2 and 13–3), and size abnormalities (Fig. 13–4).

Vascular anomalies tend not to severely affect vision, with the exception of grade III arteriovenous malformations (racemose angiomas). Excavation or hypoplasia of the nerve, however, can result in severe visual disability. This disability is often compounded by the association of these disorders with a variety of other ocular abnormalities, ranging from microphthalmos (small eye with multiple defects) to ocular motor palsy.

Several neurological abnormalities have also been associated with colobomatous/excavated defects and hypoplastic discs. These include hydrencephaly, anencephaly, basal encephaloceles, and septo-optic dysplasia (deMorsier's syndrome). The latter is characterized by absence of the septum pellucidum, partial or complete agenesis of the corpus callosum, dysplasia of the anterior third ventricle, malformation of the optic chiasm, and pituitary dysfunction. Affected children have growth retardation, hypothyroidism, and other endocrine abnormalities. Early detection of this syndrome is important, because the endocrine deficiencies are treatable. Magnetic resonance imaging is, therefore, advised for any child with bilateral small or excavated discs and short stature, or signs of an encephalocele.

Further information regarding specific disorders is discussed under "Comprehensive Information" later in the chapter.

TABLE 13–1. CONGENITAL ANOMALIES OF THE OPTIC DISC

Category	Examples
Vascular	Prepapillary vascular loops
	Persistent hyaloid artery
	Persistent Bergmeister's papilla
	Enlarged blood vessels on the optic disc (arteriovenous malformations)
Colobomatous/ excavated defects	Congenital optic pits
	Optic nerve head coloboma
	Morning glory disc anomaly
	Peripapillary staphyloma
	Tilted disc syndrome
Size abnormalities	Optic nerve aplasia
	Optic nerve hypoplasia
	Megalopapilla

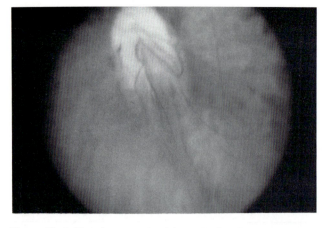

Figure 13–1. Vascular anomaly of the optic disc: Persistent hyaloid artery.

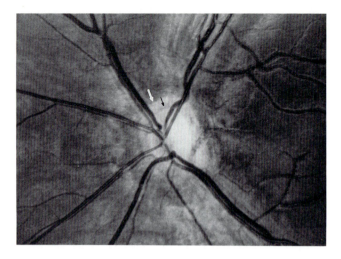

Figure 13–4. Size abnormality of the optic nerve head: Hypoplastic disc. The black arrow marks the limiting edge of the nerve, within a normal-sized scleral canal (*white arrow*). *(From Brown G, Tasman W: Congenital Anomalies of the Optic Disc. New York, Grune & Stratton, 1983, with permission.)*

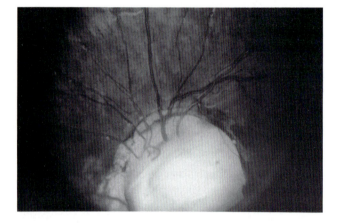

Figure 13–2. Colobomatous/excavated defect of the optic nerve: Optic nerve head coloboma.

Swelling and "Pseudo"-swelling of the Optic Disc

True swelling of the optic disc is a neurological emergency (Fig. 13–5). If it is due to an inflammatory disorder of the optic nerve head (such as optic neuritis), the child will present with reduced vision, leading to early detection. Optic nerve head swelling due to increased intracranial pressure (papilledema), however, does not result in early visual loss, and may not be detected until other signs of an intracranial disorder become evident (headache, vomiting, ataxia, seizure).

Table 13–2 lists the common causes of true and pseudo-papilledema in children. Each of these disorders is discussed later in the chapter. The primary care physician should know that it is difficult to differenti-

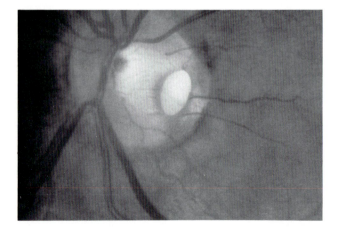

Figure 13–3. Colobomatous/excavated defect of the optic nerve: Optic nerve head pit.

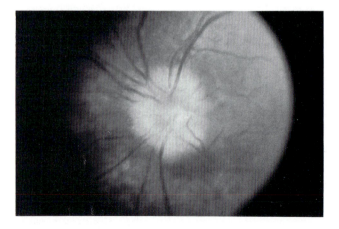

Figure 13–5. Papilledema. Notice the swelled optic nerve, and the loss of visibility of some retinal vessels within the disc and as they cross the disc margin.

TABLE 13–2. SWELLING AND PSEUDO-SWELLING OF THE OPTIC DISC: CHILDHOOD CAUSES

Category	Examples
True swelling	Optic neuritis
	Neuroretinitis
	Leber's optic neuropathy
	Papilledema
	Optic nerve glioma
Pseudo-swelling	Myelinated nerve fibers
	Optic disc drusen

ate between some of these disorders. A few signs of true disc swelling include obscuration of retinal vessels near the disc, hermorrhages on or near the disc, retinal vein dilation, nerve fiber layer infarcts ("cotton-wool spots"), and retinal exudates.

Because some of the disorders listed represent life-threatening as well as vision-threatening conditions, urgent ophthalmologic referral is suggested for any child believed to have true disc swelling.

Diplopia

Diplopia (double vision) is the illusion of one object appearing as two. Infants and young children have a very plastic visual system capable of preventing diplopia by inhibiting the image of one eye from reaching conscious regard. Because of this ability, called **suppression,** diplopia is rarely, if ever, encountered in a child less than 5 or 6 years of age. For this reason, diplopia is not a finding in children with infantile esotropia (crossed eyes) or exotropia (turned out eyes).

A few simple questions can narrow the differential diagnosis when a child presents with diplopia (Table 13–3). When a cranial nerve palsy is suspected, it is helpful to try to localize the disorder to a particular nerve or the extraocular muscle(s) it innervates. This can be achieved by asking the child several questions.

The first question is whether the images are separated horizontally or vertically. If the diplopia is horizontal, further localization to the muscles that turn the eyes out (lateral recti) or in (medial recti) is possible. Diplopia that is greater at distant fixation directs attention to the lateral recti and the sixth cranial nerves; diplopia greater at near fixation directs attention to the medial recti and the third cranial nerves.

In addition to an ophthalmologic examination, children who present with the sudden onset of diplopia should be tested for lymphocytosis with a peripheral blood count. In the absence of other signs, an elevated white blood cell count could suggest a benign postviral illness. In traumatized patients, a computed axial tomography (CAT) scan provides good visualization of soft tissues, bony structures, acute hematomas, and foreign bodies. Coronal or sagittal scans may be particularly useful to visualize entrapped extraocular muscles in patients with facial fractures. In nontraumatized children, CAT scan or magnetic resonance imaging (MRI) is indicated if there is an incomplete or nonresolving third-nerve palsy, or multiple cranial nerve abnormalities. MRI is superior in evaluating posterior fossa disease.

Pupillary Abnormalities

A variety of toxic, traumatic, infectious, and vascular disorders are accompanied by pupillary signs. The common involvement of the pupil is related to the dual innervation of the iris by both sympathetic and parasympathetic nerves. Often pupillary findings are incidental to the chief complaint, but they can be very useful diagnostically.

The most common presenting abnormality specific to the pupil is anisocoria, or asymmetric pupil size (Fig. 13–6). Most patients with anisocoria are otherwise asymptomatic. A few historical questions may help direct whether any investigation is necessary (Table 13–4).

A small pupil (miosis) that dilates poorly is consistent with Horner's syndrome. This syndrome occurs

TABLE 13–3. DIPLOPIA IN CHILDREN: DIFFERENTIATING QUESTIONS

Question	Comment
Is the diplopia monocular or binocular?	If diplopia persists with one eye occluded it is not neurological. Consider refractive error, corneal irregularity, dislocated lens, cataract, retinal disorder.
Is there associated pain?	Consider tumors, pseudotumor, infections. Pain that remits with the onset of third-nerve palsy suggests ophthalmoplegic migraine.
Is the pupil dilated?	The presence of a fixed dilated pupil and blurred vision suggests a compressive disorder affecting the third nerve.
Is the diplopia persistent or intermittent?	In children intermittent palsies are seen following viral-like illnesses, migraine, inflammation, and trauma.
Is more than one cranial nerve involved?	The involvement of multiple cranial nerves in children suggests an orbital or cavernous sinus syndrome, brainstem lesion, or Guillain-Barré syndrome.

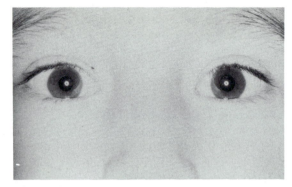

A

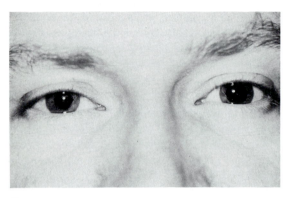

B

Figure 13–6. Physiological, familial anisocoria (inequality of pupil size). The left pupil is larger than the right pupil in both this girl (**A**) and her father (**B**).

due to any interruption along the sympathetic pathway from the hypothalamus to the iris. The duration of findings and any history of recent surgery that may have damaged the sympathetic chain should be asked. A long duration of miosis, without other signs or symptoms, suggests a benign etiology; a lighter color of the affected iris suggests a congenital origin. Further questioning should elicit hypothalamic symptoms such as diabetes insipidus or disturbed temperature regulation, evidence of a pulmonary tumor (hemopty-

sis), cervical trauma, brachial plexus abnormalities, enlarged gland or mass in the neck, associated sensory or motor deficits, or headache.

A large pupil that constricts poorly is suggestive of inadvertent instillation of a mydriatic (dilating) agent, a third-nerve palsy, or Adie's syndrome, which usually affects young women and occasionally occurs bilaterally.

Patients with neurological disorders who present with bilaterally large or small pupils usually have other localizing signs or symptoms. It is important to recognize, however, that many drugs and toxins can cause mydriatic (large) or miotic (small) pupils (discussed later in the chapter). It is also important to remember that the pupils are smaller in infancy, old age, and sleep. Hyperopes (farsighted) individuals tend to have smaller pupils than myopes (nearsighted). Additionally, the pupil is generally smaller with brown irides than blue, in men, and when fatigued.

The physician who incidentally notes an irregularly shaped pupil will usually find a history of ocular trauma, surgery, inflammation (iridocyclitis), or a congenital abnormality (such as an iris coloboma).

COMPREHENSIVE INFORMATION ON OPTIC NERVE AND NEUROLOGICAL DISORDERS

Congenital Anomalies of the Optic Nerve

Vascular Anomalies

Prepapillary Vascular Loops. Prepapillary vascular loops were first described by Lieblich in 1871. Although only approximately 100 additional cases have been reported in the literature, the anomaly likely occurs in 1 in every 2000 to 9000 individuals. The disorder is bilateral in 9 to 17 percent of patients. Approximately 95 percent of prepapillary loops are arterial; cilioretinal arteries are commonly associated with arterial loops. Venous loops are rare, and the presence of multiple venous loops suggests an acquired cause,

TABLE 13–4. PUPILLARY ABNORMALITIES: DIFFERENTIATING QUESTIONS

Question	Comment
Is the smaller pupil always on the same side?	A reversal of sides (sometimes right eye, other times left eye) within hours or days, suggests physiological anisocoria. This entity is familial and benign.
Was there previous trauma to the eye?	Damage to the pupillary sphincter can result in an enlarged pupil, to the dilator muscle a contracted pupil.
Does someone in the family use eyedrops for glaucoma?	Use of these eyedrops by a child may result in one or both pupils being smaller than normal.
Is the asymmetry greater in dim illumination	A disorder of the sympathetic system is likely (see Fig. 13–53).
Is the asymmetry greater in bright illumination?	A disorder of the parasympathetic system is likely (see Fig. 13–53).

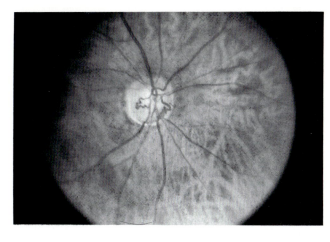

Figure 13–7. Multiple acquired prepapillary venous loops in an eye that had previously sustained a central retinal vein obstruction.

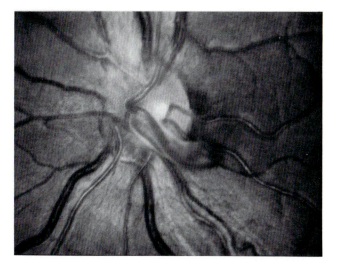

Figure 13–9. Congenital prepapillary arterial loop with a surrounding fibroglial sheath. *(From Brown GC, Tasman WS: Congenital Anomalies of the Optic Disc. New York, Grune & Stratton, 1983, p 36, with permission.)*

such as an optic nerve tumor or retinal venous obstruction (Fig. 13–7). Intravenous fluorescein angiography can differentiate arterial from venous loops in questionable cases.

Clinically, the vessels appear as loops that extend from the optic nerve into the vitreous cavity and then back to the nerve. They may have a corkscrew or spiral shape, a figure-eight twist, or a simple hairpin turn configuration (Fig. 13–8). Approximately 30 percent of loops are encased by a white, glial-appearing sheath (Fig. 13–9). Spontaneous pulsations synchronous with the heartbeat are present in approximately 50 percent of the cases. These vessels are probably unrelated to the hyaloid artery and there are no known predisposing factors for their development. Furthermore, there are no systemic associations.

Most patients with prepapillary loops have normal

visual acuity. The affected eye may, however, be predisposed to vitreous hemorrhage, amaurosis fugax, and/or branch retinal artery occlusion in the distribution of the retina supplied by the loop.

Persistent Hyaloid Artery. Hyaloid artery remnants are seen in 95 percent of premature infants and in approximately 3 percent of full-term infants. The prev-

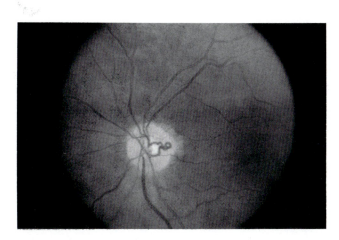

Figure 13–8. Congenital prepapillary arterial loop with a corkscrew configuration.

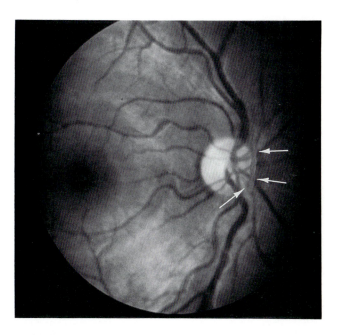

Figure 13–10. A collapsed hyaloid artery remnant originating on the optic disc (*inferior arrow*), and coursing anteriorly through Cloquet's canal. *(From Degenhart W, Brown GC, Augsburger JJ, et al: Congenital vascular anomalies of the optic nerve head. Trans PA Acad Ophthalmol Otolaryngol 34:152, 1981, with permission.)*

alence in otherwise normal adults is unknown, but is substantially lower.

A persistent hyaloid artery presents clinically as a circuitous vessel extending from the optic disc, through Cloquet's canal, to the posterior lens capsule (see Figs. 13–1 and 13–10). The point of attachment to the posterior capsule, most often located inferonasal to the visual axis, is known as a Mittendorf dot (Fig. 13–11).

A persistent hyaloid artery may be associated with persistent hyperplastic primary vitreous (see Chapter 11), colobomas of the optic nerve, optic nerve hypoplasia, and posterior vitreous cysts. There are no associated systemic abnormalities.

Although they may be filled with blood (see Fig. 13–1), most hyaloid arteries in children and adults are bloodless. A patent persistent hyaloid artery may rarely cause a vitreous hemorrhage, but the visual prognosis is generally good. In cases with vitreous hemorrhage, argon laser photocoagulation can be attempted. Severe bleeding may require vitrectomy.

Persistent Bergmeister's Papilla. Although this condition is not truly a vascular abnormality, its development is intricately related to the fetal hyaloid artery. It is, therefore, included in this section.

A persistent Bergmeister's papilla, also known as an epipapillary veil, is found in nearly 28 percent of autopsy eyes. The majority of these, however, are not visible ophthalmoscopically. This disorder occurs when the primitive epithelial papilla (forerunner of the optic disc) fails to involute during embryogenesis.

Clinically, this condition appears as glial tissue overlying the optic nerve head and adjacent retinal tissue (Figs. 13–12 and 13–13). The exuberant tissue is usually more pronounced nasally, and may obscure the physiological cup of the nerve. A variety of other congenital optic nerve abnormalities, including prepapil-

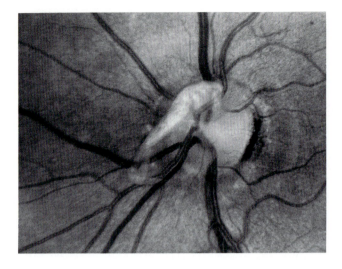

Figure 13–12. Persistent Bergmeister's papilla (epipapillary veil) overlying the nasal optic disc and peripapillary retina. *(From Brown GC, Tasman WS: Congenital Anomalies of the Optic Disc, New York, Grune & Stratton, 1983, p 68, with permission.)*

lary vascular loops, persistent hyperplastic primary vitreous, and the morning glory syndrome, may accompany a persistent Bergmeister's papilla. Generally, however, this is a benign congenital structure with little clinical significance. The visual acuity is seldom, if ever, affected, and there are no associated systemic abnormalities.

Enlarged Vessels on the Optic Nerve. Enlarged vessels emanating from the optic nerve head accompany a number of ocular conditions. These include arteriovenous malformations, retinal capillary hemangiomas (von Hippel tumors), and retinoblastoma (Fig. 13–14). The latter two conditions are discussed further in Chapters 4 and 12, respectively.

Arteriovenous malformations are anomalous con-

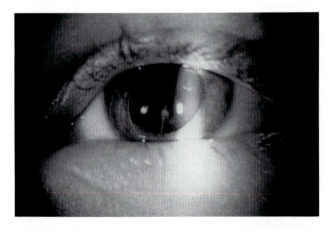

Figure 13–11. Mittendorf dot, the point of attachment of a hyaloid remnant to the posterior lens capsule, with attached hyaloid artery remnant inferiorly.

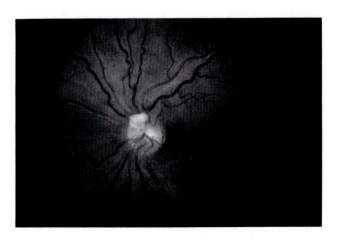

Figure 13–13. Another eye with a persistent Bergmeister's papillae.

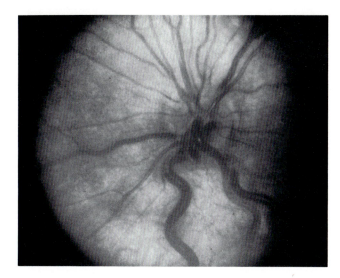

Figure 13–14. Enlarged blood vessels at the optic disc associated with an inferior, peripheral retinoblastoma (not visible).

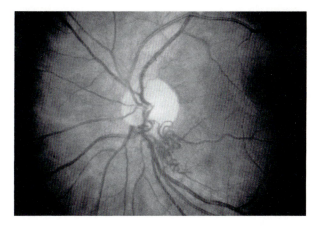

Figure 13–16. Grade II arteriovenous (racemose) malformation. *(Courtesy of the Albany Medical College slide collection.)*

nections between arteries and veins. Three grades are described. Grade I communications are mild malformations also known as congenital macrovessels. They are comprised of a single enlarged vessel, usually a vein, that may transverse both sides of the horizontal raphe (Fig. 13–15). The visual acuity is usually unaffected, even when these vessels cross the foveal avascular area. There are no known systemic associations with macrovessels.

Grades II and III arteriovenous communications are also referred to as racemose angiomas or racemose hemangiomas. The grade II variant is moderate, and visual acuity is usually unaffected by these malformations (Fig. 13–16). The grade III variant, however, may involve replacement of optic nerve tissue by enlarged

vascular elements, severely compromising vision (Fig. 13–17). The retina may be involved segmentally or totally with dilated, tortuous vessels. These vessels do not pulsate and do not leak fluid. If the abnormal vessels occur peripherally, however, vision may be unaffected. Both subtypes are present at birth, invariably nonprogressive, and usually unilateral. Because intraocular hemorrhage is rare, treatment is not advisable.

Grades II and III racemose angiomas of the eye have been associated with similar malformations in the mandible, central nervous system, and on the face. The eponym Wyburn–Mason syndrome is used when an angioma of the retina is associated with an ipsilateral angioma of the midbrain. The latter may become

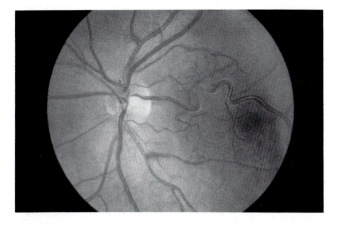

Figure 13–15. Grade I arteriovenous malformation (congenital retinal macrovessel). The enlarged vein drains both the superior and inferior retina. Visual acuity in this eye was 20/20. *(Courtesy of the Albany Medical College slide collection.)*

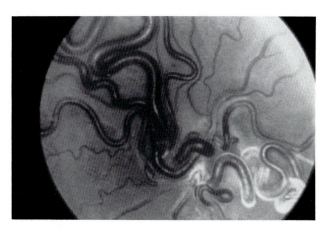

Figure 13–17. Grade III arteriovenous (racemose) malformation. *(Courtesy of the Albany Medical College slide collection.)*

symptomatic in the second or third decade of life, heralded by epilepsy. An acute intracranial hemorrhage should be suspected if mental status changes, hemiparesis, or papilledema develop. Approximately one fourth of individuals with a retinal angioma have an intracranial lesion.

Colobomatous and other Excavated Defects of the Optic Nerve

Congenital Optic Pits. First described by Wiethe in 1882, congenital optic pits are encountered with a frequency of 1 in 11,000 ophthalmic patients. Over 250 cases have been reported; 85 percent of these have been unilateral.

A congenital optic pit appears as a round or oval-shaped depression on the nerve head (see Figs. 13–3 and 13–18). They can be yellow-white, black, or gray in color. The defect ranges in size from 0.25 to 0.40 disc diameters, and in over 50 percent of cases is located temporally. Peripapillary chorioretinal atrophy adjacent to an optic pit occurs in 95 percent of noncentrally located anomalies. In unilateral cases, the nerve head with the pit is usually larger than the normal contralateral nerve head.

Approximately 40 percent of eyes with a congenital optic pit have an associated serous detachment of the sensory retina (Fig. 13–19). Retinal detachment is usually observed with larger, temporally located pits. The etiology of the subretinal fluid associated with congenital optic pits is uncertain. Although evidence in the collie dog model suggests that it originates from the vitreous cavity, other possible sources in humans include transudate from choroidal vessels or small vessels at the base of the pit, or leakage of cerebrospinal fluid from the subarachnoid space. Over 50 percent of

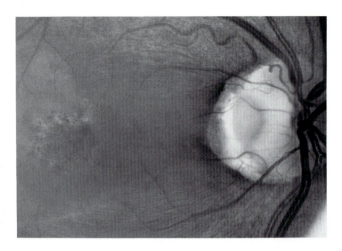

Figure 13–19. Gray congenital optic pit associated with a serous detachment of the sensory retina in the macula and a macular hole. *(From Nelson LB, Brown GC, Arentsen JJ: Recognizing Patterns of Ocular Childhood Disease. Thorofare, NJ, Slack, 1985, p 79, with permission.)*

eyes with an associated retinal detachment have an acuity of 20/100 or less, even after 1 year follow-up.

Congenital optic pits are not usually associated with other major ocular abnormalities. In rare patients, they occur concomitant with retinochoroidal and optic nerve colobomas. Systemic abnormalities are not usually seen with congenital optic pits.

Optic Nerve Coloboma. The term "coloboma" is used to describe any congenital notch, gap, or fissure of

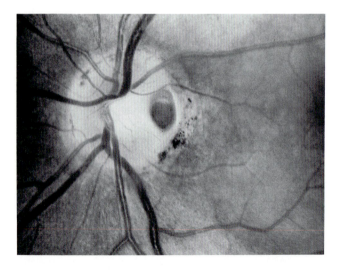

Figure 13–18. Congenital optic pit.

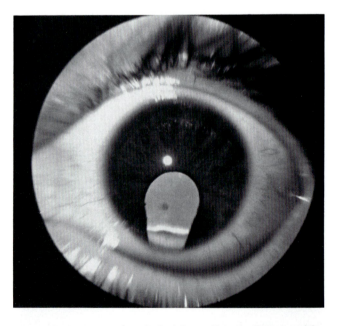

Figure 13–20. Iris coloboma in the left eye. Note the flattening of the edge of the lens and leukocoria secondary to a retinochoroidal coloboma. *(From Nelson LB, Brown GC, Arentsen JJ: Recognizing Patterns of Ocular Childhood Disease. Thorofare, NJ, Slack, 1985, p 9, with permission.)*

the ocular structure. Typical colobomas are located in the inferonasal eye, anywhere along a line extending from the optic disc to the inferonasal pupillary border. They result from incomplete closure of the embryonic fissure, and can be inherited as an autosomal dominant condition with incomplete penetrance.

The colobomatous defect may involve the iris, chorioretinal tissue, or the optic nerve individually, or in any combination. Iris colobomas are characterized by an inferonasal keyhole-shaped defect (Fig. 13–20). The exposed edge of the ocular lens may be flattened if a localized gap in the zonule coexists. Chorioretinal colobomas are glistening white and have distinct margins often outlined by irregular pigment clumps (Fig. 13–21). Individuals with large chorioretinal colobomas may have leukocoria (white pupils) due to reflection of light from the defect. Eyes with retinochoroidal colobomas are predisposed to develop nonrhegmatogenous retinal detachments. These usually present in the second to third decade of life.

An optic nerve coloboma occurs with a frequency of approximately 1 in 12,000 ophthalmic patients. It is characterized by an enlarged, frequently vertically oval optic nerve (Fig. 13–22). The nerve may be partially or totally excavated, especially inferiorly, with a glistening white surface. Retinal blood vessels enter and exit the nerve head from the border of the defect, and radiate outward in a spokelike fashion with fewer bifurcations than normal (Fig. 13–23).

Optic nerve colobomas may be unilateral or bilateral. Visual acuity is variable and ranges from normal to no light perception. They can accompany a variety of other ocular abnormalities including posterior lenticonus, posterior embryotoxin, congenital optic pit, optic nerve sheath cysts, and remnants of the hyaloid artery. Myopia is a commonly noted refractive error among patients with optic nerve coloboma.

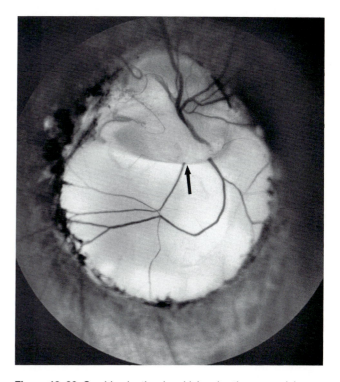

Figure 13–22. Combined retinochoroidal and optic nerve coloboma. Note how tissue from the disc itself (*arrow*) appears to extend inferiorly over the retinochoroidal defect. *(From Nelson LB, Brown GC, Arentsen JJ: Recognizing Patterns of Ocular Childhood Disease. Thorofare, NJ, Slack, 1985, p 9, with permission.)*

Systemic abnormalities seen with optic nerve coloboma may be part of the CHARGE association (*C*oloboma, *H*eart disease, choanal *A*tresia, *R*etarded growth, *G*enital anomalies, and *E*ar anomalies and/or

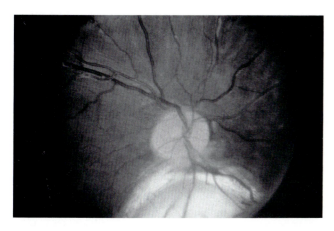

Figure 13–21. Retinochoroidal coloboma. The colobomatous defect is glistening white, and retinal blood vessels course over the defect. The well-delineated margins are marked by pigmentary changes.

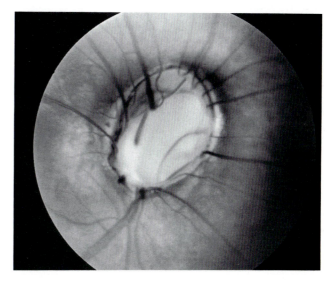

Figure 13–23. Optic nerve coloboma. The inferior aspect of the enlarged disc is more involved; blood vessels enter and exit largely through the borders of the defect. *(From Brown GC, Tasman WS: Congenital Anomalies of the Optic Disc. New York, Grune & Stratton, 1983, with permission.)*

deafness). Colobomas are also a feature of multiple chromosomal aberrations including triploidy; trisomies 13 and 18; duplications (4q+, 7q+, 9p+, 10q+, 13q+, and 22q+); deletions (3q−, 4p−, 7q−, 11q−, 13q−, and 18q−); and ring chromosomes (4r, 13r, and 18r). These eyes are usually also microphthalmic. Colobomas can also be a feature of multiple single gene disorders with multisystem involvement including Lenz's, Goltz, Warburg's, and Aicardi's, Rubenstein–Taybi, and Goldenhar's syndromes.

Morning Glory Disc Anomaly. The morning glory optic disc anomaly was first described by Kindler in 1970 and named after its resemblance to the morning glory flower. Characteristics of the morning glory disc anomaly include an enlarged and usually excavated optic disc, pink color with a central core of white gliotic tissue, a subretinal peripapillary annulus of variably pigmented tissue, straightened retinal vessels entering and exiting from the disc margins, and sheathed retinal vessels (Figs. 13–24 and 13–25).

Most cases are unilateral. The visual acuity usually ranges from 20/200 to hand motion. In approximately 30 percent of involved eyes a nonrhegmatogenous retinal detachment develops. Refractive errors are usually mildly to moderately myopic. Associated abnormalities in the involved eye include hyaloid artery remnant, persistent Bergmeister's papilla, strabismus, congenital cataract, vitreous cyst, and persistent pupillary membrane. Contralateral eyes can also be anomalous. Microphthalmos, microcornea, anterior chamber

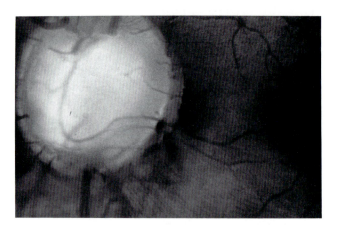

Figure 13–25. Morning glory optic disc anomaly.

cleavage syndrome, and Duane's retraction syndrome have all been reported in eyes contralateral to one with morning glory disc anomaly.

Several systemic abnormalities have been noted with the morning glory syndrome including basal encephalocele, hypertelorism, and radiological defects in the floor of the sella turcica. Any child with this syndrome, short stature, and pituitary hormone deficiencies should be evaluated for deMorsier's syndrome.

Peripapillary Staphyloma. Peripapillary staphyloma is a rare congenital anomaly characterized by posterior bulging of the sclera around the optic nerve. Clinically, a relatively normal appearing optic nerve is seen at the base of the outpouching (Fig. 13–26). Within the walls of the defect there are usually atrophic changes in the choroid and retinal pigment epithelium. The visual acuity varies, ranging from normal in mild cases to severe visual impairment with more pro-

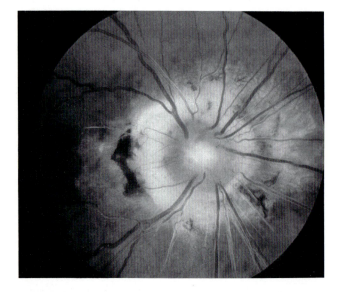

Figure 13–24. Morning glory optic disc anomaly characterized by an enlarged nerve head and a central core of tissue with a fibroglial appearance. A peripapillary pigmentary disturbance and sheathing of retinal vessels is evident. Note how the vessels enter and exit from the disc margin. *(From Brown GC, Tasman WS: Congenital Anomalies of the Optic Disc. New York, Grune & Stratton, 1983, p 158, with permission.)*

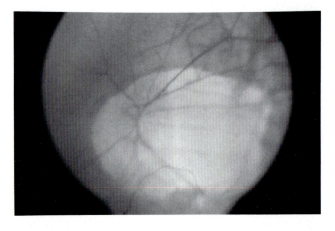

Figure 13–26. Peripapillary staphyloma. The normal appearing-optic nerve head appears out of focus, as it lies deep within the staphyloma.

TABLE 13–5. CLINICAL CHARACTERISTICS OF THE TILTED DISC SYNDROME

Visual acuity	Reduced to 20/25 to 20/50 in 75% of cases
Refraction	Myopia (> 1 diopter) in 85–90% of cases
	Astigmatism (> 1 diopter) in 70%
Bilaterality	Bilateral in 75% of cases
Visual field	Superotemporal field cut that crosses midline
Appearance	Inferonasally tilted optic disc
	Inferonasal or inferior crescent
	Situs inversus (nasal coursing of retinal vessels as they approach the optic disc)
	Fundus ectasia (inferiorly)
	Elevated appearance of superotemporal disc
External	May be exophthalmic if high myopia present

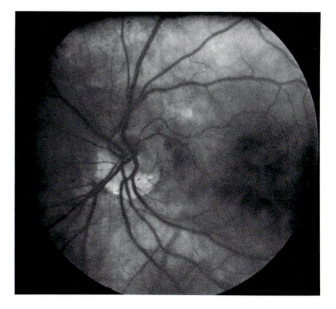

Figure 13–27. Tilted disc syndrome in the left eye. Note the inferior crescent, situs inversus of the retinal vessels, and lightening of the ectatic (stretched) inferior retina. *(From Nelson LB, Brown GC, Arentsen JJ: Recognizing Patterns of Ocular Childhood Disease. Thorofare, NJ, Slack, 1985, p 87, with permission.)*

nounced defects. Contraction within the walls of larger defects may be present. A peripapillary staphyloma is usually an isolated finding; there are typically no associated ocular or systemic abnormalities.

Tilted Disc Syndrome. Initially recognized by Fuchs in 1882, the tilted disc syndrome is also known as the nasal fundus ectasia syndrome or Fuchs' coloboma. It occurs in approximately 1 to 2 percent of the general population, and likely arises from partial nonclosure of the embryonic fissure, a variant of a colobomatous defect. The clinical features of the tilted disc syndrome are listed in Table 13–5.

The superior aspect of the nerve head can appear elevated because of the tilting effect (Fig. 13–27). This appearance often mimics papilledema. Most of the affected eyes with inferior fundus ectasia have superotemporal visual field defects that cross the midline, and reduced visual acuity of 20/25 to 20/50. Familial cases have been reported, but a hereditary pattern has not been defined.

Size Abnormalities of the Optic Nerve

Optic Nerve Aplasia. Optic nerve aplasia is a rare entity in which there is absence of the normally defined optic nerve head, macula, and central retinal vessels (Fig. 13–28). The latter features are of principal importance. An eye with an avascular white disc, or a deep cavity surrounded by a whitish area similar to the peripapillary cone, may still have optic nerve aplasia if central retinal vessels and macular differentiation are absent. The condition is usually unilateral, and the visual acuity in affected eyes is no light perception. The pathogenesis of the disorder is unknown; there are no known predisposing factors. A number of teratogenic agents, however, have been suggested, including maternal diabetes, fetal alcohol syndrome, maternal drug abuse, and intrauterine cytomegalovirus infection.

Microphthalmos, cataracts, and retinochoroidal colobomas are common ocular associations.

Optic nerve aplasia may occur as an isolated ocular anomaly. It has also been reported in association with cyclopia, partial agenesis of the central nervous system, Hallermann–Streiff syndrome, and absence of the radii.

Optic Nerve Hypoplasia. Optic nerve hypoplasia is a developmental anomaly in which there is a subnormal number of axons within the affected nerve, although the mesodermal elements and glial supporting tissue of the nerve are normal. The size of the optic

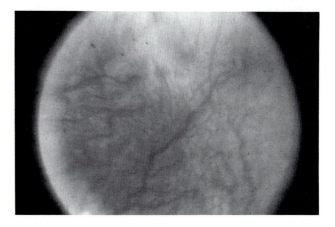

Figure 13–28. Optic nerve aplasia. Note the total absence of the optic nerve, and disarrayed vasculature.

nerve may vary from almost imperceptible hypoplasia to severe involvement. When the diagnosis is in doubt, the size of the optic nerve can be confirmed by ultrasonography or magnetic resonance imaging (Fig. 13–29).

The typical funduscopic appearance is that of a small and often pale optic nerve. Surrounding the nerve may be a yellow-white, variably pigmented ring. This appearance has been referred to as the "double ring" sign (Figs. 13–30 and 13–31). The outer ring, which has been shown histologically to correlate with the junction of the sclera and lamina cribosa, corresponds to the size of the normal nerve. Although the nerve head is small, the retinal vessels are usually of normal caliber and enter and exit centrally.

Unilateral and bilateral cases occur with almost equal frequency. Visual acuity ranges from normal to no light perception, but does not correlate well with the appearance of the nerve. The visual field may show generalized constriction. Children with unilateral hypoplasia and amblyopia may respond well or not at all to occlusion therapy. A 2- to 3-month trial of occlusion therapy is warranted if the disorder is discovered in young children. If the acuity improves, patching is continued until the acuity plateaus. The presence of a relative afferent pupillary defect (see Chapter 2) in unilateral cases is a poor prognostic sign.

A number of ocular anomalies are associated with optic nerve hypoplasia (Table 13–6). The disorder has also been associated with several central nervous system anomalies, including anencephaly, hydrencephaly,

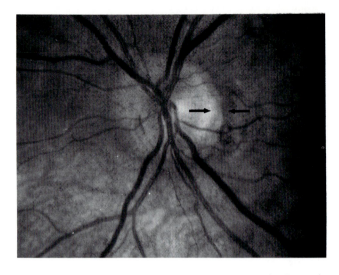

Figure 13–30. Optic nerve hypoplasia with double ring sign (*arrows*). *(From Nelson LB, Brown GC, Arentsen JJ: Recognizing Patterns of Ocular Childhood Disease. Thorofare, NJ, Slack, 1985, p 85, with permission.)*

and deMorsier's syndrome (see discussion on page 271). Nonocular congenital anomalies occur with a higher frequency in children with bilateral hypoplasia and poor vision. Neuroimaging should be strongly considered in these cases. It may not be necessary in unilateral cases unless other signs (such as delayed growth and hypopituitarism) are present.

Certain prenatal pharmacological insults may be associated with the development of optic nerve hypoplasia. Drug associations include exposure to pheny-

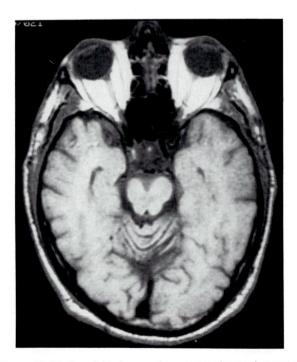

Figure 13–29. T$_1$-weighted magnetic resonance image demonstrating optic nerve hypoplasia in the left eye (compare with opposite optic nerve).

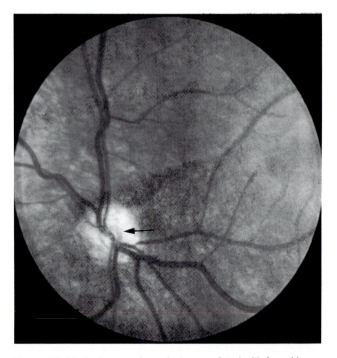

Figure 13–31. Optic nerve hypoplasia associated with foveal hypoplasia. Note the edge of the optic nerve (*arrow*) and the absence of a foveal reflex.

TABLE 13–6. OPHTHALMIC AND SYSTEMIC ASSOCIATIONS OF OPTIC NERVE HYPOPLASIA

Ophthalmic	Nystagmus (bilateral cases)
	Strabismus
	Foveal hypoplasia
	Pupillary light reaction slow or absent
Systemic	Anencephaly
	Hydrencephaly
	deMorsier's syndrome

toin, quinine, lysergic acid diethylamide, meperidine, diuretics, and corticosteroids. The presence of maternal diabetes mellitus has also been implicated in some cases.

Megalopapilla. Franceschetti and Bock first described megalopapilla in 1950. Clinically, megalopapilla is characterized by an enlarged but otherwise normal-appearing optic nerve (Figs. 13–32 and 13–33). A mild peripapillary retinal pigmentary epithelial disturbance is often present, but no other ocular abnormalities have been consistently associated with this condition.

Megalopapilla is usually unilateral, and the globe in most cases is normal in size. Visual acuity is usually normal, although mild to moderate loss has been noted. An enlarged blind spot is typically noted on visual field testing; rarely a partial superotemporal quadrantanopsia defect has been documented.

Systemic abnormalities associated with megalo-

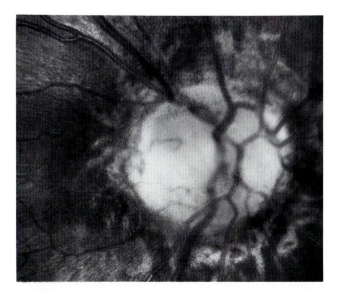

Figure 13–32. Enlarged optic disc (megalopapilla). *(From Nelson LB, Brown GC, Arentsen JJ: Recognizing Patterns of Ocular Childhood Disease. Thorofare, NJ, Slack, 1985, p 81, with permission.)*

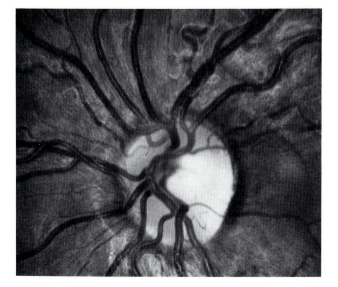

Figure 13–33. Opposite optic disc of the same patient as in Figure 13–32, at the same magnification, demonstrating a normal-sized optic nerve head. *(From Nelson LB, Brown GC, Arentsen JJ: Recognizing Patterns of Ocular Childhood Disease. Thorofare, NJ, Slack, 1985, p 81, with permission.)*

papilla include sphenoethmoidal encephalocele, cleft palate, and mandibulofacial dysostosis.

Acquired Anomalies of the Optic Nerve

Swelling and "Pseudo"-swelling of the Optic Disc

Optic Neuritis. Optic neuritis is an inflammatory disorder of the optic nerve. The typical presentation in children differs from that in adults (Table 13–7). In children, the disorder is more likely to be bilateral, and associated with systemic infections such as measles, mumps, chicken pox, pertussis, infectious mononucleosis, and immunizations. It almost always results in a severe loss of vision. In adults, the disorder is more likely to be unilateral and associated with demyelinating or autoimmune disease. Children typically present with a history of fever, malaise, and headaches, and their loss of vision is often associated with other neurological deficits including seizures or ataxia, implicating the possibility of an aseptic meningitis.

In both children and adults, acuity reaches its nadir 1 to 2 weeks after onset. Colors appear desaturated, and there is a reduced perception of light intensity. The majority of cases in children involve the anterior optic nerve (anterior optic neuropathy); in these cases, the optic disc appears swollen and surrounded by flame hemorrhages (Fig. 13–34).

A serological test for syphilis should be performed, and a lumbar puncture should be considered. Cerebro-

TABLE 13–7. DIFFERENTIAL CHARACTERISTICS OF OPTIC NEURITIS IN ADULTS AND CHILDREN

Characteristic	Adults	Children
Age of onset	18–50 years	3–16 years
Laterality	Unilateral > Bilateral	Bilateral > Unilateral
Etiology	Demyelinating, viral or autoimmune disease	Systemic viral infection or immunization; meningoencephalitis
Visual acuity	20/25 to no light perception	Usually severe; (20/200 or less)
Disc edema	Present in 30–40%	Present in 70–80%
Associations	Retrobulbar discomfort and flashes of light aggravated by movement of eyes, photophobia	+/– Neurological deficits, seizures, cerebellar dysfunction, headache, malaise, fever, rhinorrhea
Multiple sclerosis	Develops in 40–80%	Develops in < 20%

spinal fluid lymphocytic pleocytosis is a common finding in children with bilateral optic neuritis. Neuroimaging is controversial but should be performed if the history is atypical to rule out a neoplastic disorder. In optic neuritis, the optic nerve may appear thickened on magnetic resonance imaging. Demyelinating plaques are rarely, if ever, appreciated in the optic nerve, but multiple, enhancing, high-intensity signals in the subcortical white matter, consistent with demyelination, are often detected. Computed tomography typically demonstrates no abnormalities.

The usual outcome of optic neuritis in children is good, but the acuity may take several months to recover, and the child may be left with optic nerve pallor and residual visual field and acuity deficits. Treatment for the acute visual loss is controversial; there is little evidence that any treatment improves the long-term outcome. Intravenous methylprednisone 0.25 to 4.8 mg/kg every 6 hours for 5 days, however, may hasten the visual recovery in some children. Most investigators believe that bilateral optic neuritis in children is rarely associated with multiple sclerosis, but this asso-

ciation does appear to increase with the age of the affected child.

Optic neuritis in children may also develop secondary to lead poisoning, chronic chloramphenicol toxicity, and herpes zoster ophthalmicus. Rare systemic associations include Devic's and Schilder's diseases. Devic's neuromyelitis is characterized by bilateral optic neuritis and paraplegia secondary to transverse myelitis. Schilder's disease is a relentlessly progressive demyelinating disease that usually presents before age 10 years and leads to death within 1 to 2 years.

Neuroretinitis. The term "neuroretinitis" is usually reserved to describe an acute disc swelling caused by a local inflammatory process, characterized by the presence of deep retinal exudates in a "macular star" configuration (Fig. 13–35). Neuroretinitis is a nonspecific entity, but in many cases a viral etiology is suspected, particularly mumps or chicken pox. The condition may be unilateral, or bilateral and asymmetric. Vision is rapidly lost and asymmetric cases may demonstrate a relative afferent pupillary defect. Early in the course,

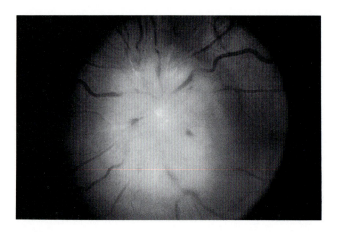

Figure 13–34. Diffusely edematous optic disc, with exudates and small, streak hemorrhages in the peripapillary area in optic neuritis.

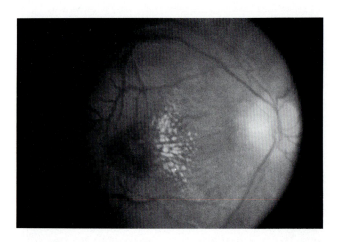

Figure 13–35. Neuroretinitis. Note the mild disc swelling and the deep retinal exudates in a stellate pattern involving only the nasal macula *(From Catalano RA: Ocular Emergencies. Philadelphia, Saunders, 1992, p 426, with permission.)*

cells in the vitreous, anterior to the optic disc, may occasionally be seen. Some vision usually recovers, but progressive optic atrophy may ensue, and the prognosis should remain guarded. Recurrences have been reported, but these are very rare.

Leber's Optic Neuropathy. Leber's optic neuropathy presents similar to optic neuritis. Affected individuals develop a sudden decrease in central vision, associated with optic nerve head swelling and hyperemia (Fig. 13–36). The disorder occurs more commonly between the ages of 18 and 23, but there have been many reports of its occurrence in adolescents and even children under the age of 10 years. Because it is transmitted through the mitochondria of the egg, it occurs nine times more often in males and is transmitted only through maternal lines. Affliction may begin unilaterally, but the second eye usually develops a similar disorder within days to weeks. If it does not become involved within 1 year, a different diagnosis should be suspected. Decreased visual acuity to less than 20/200 with a 20- to 30-degree central field defect is common. A peripapillary microangiopathy may be present premorbidly in asymptomatic eyes, and fluorescein angiography may show arteriovenous shunts at the disc without leakage of dye. Partial recovery may occur in 12 to 30 percent of those affected but may be delayed 1 to 20 years. Although a deficiency of cyanide detoxification has been noted, Phillips and Gosden (1991) report that treatment with intramuscular hydroxocobalamin and/or oral cystine, even in the acute phase, is unlikely to be of any value.

Myelinated Nerve Fibers. Myelination of nerve fibers is a benign clinical entity that arises when oligodendrites are aberrantly present within the retina and optic disc. This anomaly is observed in 1 percent of

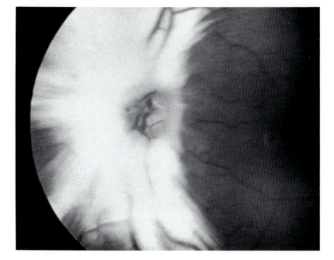

Figure 13–37. Myelinated nerve fibers completely encircling the optic disc, giving a pseudo-swelling appearance. *(From Brown GC, Tasman WS: Congenital Anomalies of the Optic Disc. New York, Grune & Stratton, 1983, with permission.)*

autopsy eyes, but is much less apparent clinically. Involvement of fibers on or near the nerve head can give an appearance that resembles optic nerve swelling (Fig. 13–37).

Clinically, myelinated nerve fibers appear as yellow-white patches in the retinal nerve fiber layer and/or optic nerve head. Most commonly they are noted to extend from the optic disc (Figs. 13–38 and 13–39), but they can occur peripherally, unassociated with the disc (Figs. 13–40 to 13–41). They often obscure retinal vessels and have feathery margins.

The anomaly typically presents at birth or early infancy and remains stationary. A relative or absolute visual field defect, smaller in size than the nerve fiber

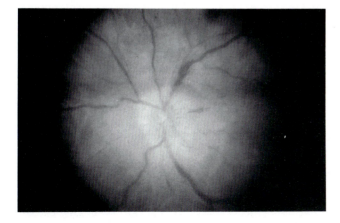

Figure 13–36. Swollen disc in Leber's optic neuropathy. Note the hyperemia of the disc.

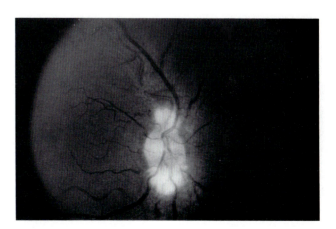

Figure 13–38. Myelinated nerve fibers at the superior and inferior poles of the optic nerve.

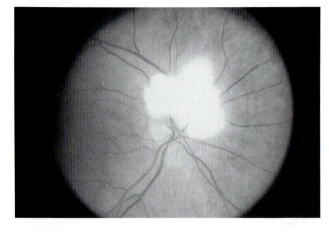

Figure 13–39. Myelinated nerve fibers at the superior pole of the disc obscuring underlying retina and retinal vessels.

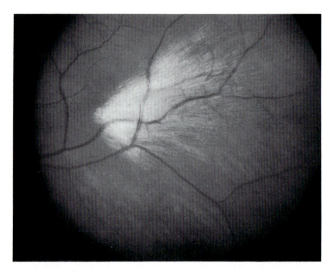

Figure 13–41. Peripheral cluster of myelinated nerve fibers demonstrating well the nerve fiber layer of the retina (optic radiations). *(From Brown GC, Tasman WS: Congenital Anomalies of the Optic Disc. New York, Grune & Stratton, 1983, with permission.)*

layer lesion, is usually the only associated abnormality. Extensive unilateral involvement, however, has been associated with ipsilateral myopia, amblyopia, and strabismus.

For unknown reasons, the disorder is more commonly encountered in patients with craniofacial dysostosis, oxycephaly, neurofibromatosis, and Down syndrome. Because the central macula is generally unaffected, the visual prognosis is good. If unilateral high myopia and amblyopia are present, appropriate optical correction and occlusion therapy should be instituted.

Papilledema. Papilledema is a sign of increased intracranial pressure (ICP). Because it is a sign, and not a diagnosis in itself, the discovery of papilledema should

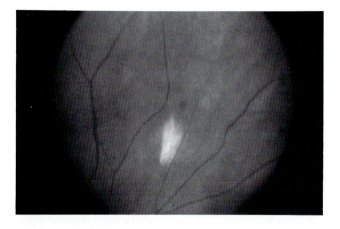

Figure 13–40. Isolated myelinated nerve fibers in the peripheral retina.

lead to a differential of the causes of increased ICP (Table 13–8). It is frequently necessary to distinguish papilledema from optic neuritis and pseudopapilledema (optic disc drusen); distinguishing features of each are presented in Table 13–9.

Papilledema often presents with repetitive, transient obscurations of vision. Described as a graying-out or dimming of vision, these episodes usually last only seconds, but can occur several times a day. They can often be incited by orthostatic changes. The visual acuity in acute papilledema is normal unless the macula is

TABLE 13–8. ETIOLOGIC CAUSES OF PAPILLEDEMA IN CHILDREN

Category	Entities
Tumor	Cerebral cortex (especially infratentorial)
	Cerebral hamartomas (neurofibromatosis)
	Cerebral teratoma
	Spinal cord ependymoma or neurofibroma
Vascular	Cerebral hematoma
	Subdural hematoma
	Epidural hematoma
	Subarachnoid hemorrhage
	Arteriovenous malformation
Infectious	Granuloma (sarcoid, tubercular, syphilitic)
	Paracytic lesion (*Cysticercus* cysts)
	Brain abscess (especially occipital lobe)
	Meningitis/encephalitis (due to diffuse cerebral edema)
	Lyme disease
Other	Guillain-Barré syndrome
	Craniostenoses
	Mucopolysaccharidoses

Modified from Catalano RA: Ocular Emergencies. Philadelphia, Saunders, 1992, Table 14–8, p 433, with permission.

TABLE 13–9. CHARACTERISTICS OF OPTIC NEURITIS, PAPILLEDEMA, AND PSEUDOPAPILLEDEMA

Feature	Optic Neuritis	Papilledema	Pseudopapilledema
Visual loss	Rapidly progressive loss of central and color vision, acuity diminished	No acuity loss until late, but transient obscurations of vision are common	+/– Enlarged blind spot, arcuate visual field defects
Bilaterality	Usually bilateral in children, but unilateral in adults	Almost always bilateral, may be asymmetric	Bilateral in 70% (those with drusen), may be asymmetric
Pupillary responses	Decreased reaction, afferent defect when unilateral	Normal	Normal
Optic nerve appearance	With anterior papillitis: variable disc swelling, cotton-wool spots, flame-shaped hemorrhages	Variable disc swelling and flame-shaped hemorrhages	Disc elevation, margin blurred, cup obliterated, no hemorrhages or edema, +/– hyaline bodies
Visual prognosis	Good, but optic atrophy may ensue	Good with lowering of intracranial pressure	Good, usually not progressive

Modified from Catalano RA: Ocular Emergencies. Philadelphia, Saunders, 1992, Table 14–6, p 417, with permission.

involved by exudate or edema. Rarely, an acute loss of vision can occur due to a superimposed ischemic optic neuropathy. The visual field usually shows only a mild enlargement of the blind spot; pupillary responses and color vision are also usually normal.

Signs of papilledema include hyperemia of the optic disc, obscuration of blood vessels near the optic disc (due to swelling of the peripapillary nerve fiber layer), circumferential retinal folds (Paton's lines), retinal vein dilation, and flame-shaped hemorrhages at the disc margin (Fig. 13–42). With chronicity, the hemorrhages, exudate, and venous dilation decrease, but the disc elevation persists (Fig. 13–43). The diagnosis of chronic papilledema may be quite difficult to make on ophthalmoscopic appearance alone. Testing to confirm visual field constriction may also not be possible in children. A heightened awareness of this possibility is, therefore, necessary in susceptible cases. Untreated, chronic papilledema can lead to optic pallor, constriction of the retinal vessels, and calcifications on the surface of the disc. Irreversible loss of vision and an inferior nasal or arcuate visual field defect can result.

Papilledema is a neurological emergency. It can be accompanied by other signs of increased ICP, including headaches, nausea, and vomiting. Neuroimaging should be performed; if no intracranial masses are detected, a lumbar puncture should follow. In children, posterior fossa tumors are often found. In adults, metastatic and primary cerebral neoplasms, and pseudotumor cerebri, are most common.

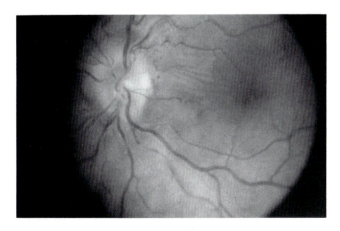

Figure 13–42. Acute papilledema demonstrating marked optic disc edema, dilation of the retinal venous system, and circumferential retinal folds (Paton's lines) extending to the macular area. *(From Catalano RA: Ocular Emergencies. Philadelphia, Saunders, 1992, p 377, with permission.)*

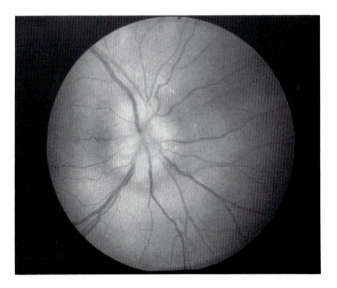

Figure 13–43. Chronic papilledema. The disc remains elevated but the peripapillary hemorrhages have resolved. The disc resembles that of pseudopapilledema. Note, however, the faint ring of exudate surrounding the disc, and the dilated nasal vessels.

Rare associations of increased ICP and papilledema in children include vitamin A, nalidixic acid, penicillin, and tetracycline toxicity; corticosteroid use or withdrawal; and lead or arsenic poisoning. ICP can also occur with chronic iron deficiency anemia, chronic lung disease (for example, cystic fibrosis due to polycythemia), and malignant hypertension (renal disorders).

Another rare association is Lyme disease, a tick-borne illness caused by the spirochete *Borrelia burgdorferi*. Optic neuritis, papilledema, and neuroretinitis can occur during the second or third stage of this disease. Neurological manifestations usually present approximately 4 weeks after the first-stage skin rash and are associated with signs of meningitis. Treatment involves intravenous cefriaxone, cefotaxime, or penicillin.

Pseudopapilledema (Optic Disc Drusen). The majority of cases of anomalous elevation of the optic disc (pseudopapilledema) are associated with hyaline bodies (concretions) of the nerve head called drusen. Drusen usually become visible with increasing age as they enlarge toward the disc margins and surface. In adolescents and adults they may be visible as crystalline bodies with a semitranslucent appearance (Fig. 13–44). In children less than 10 years of age, drusen may not be visible (Fig. 13–45), but are suspected based on other characteristic features of pseudopapilledema (Table 13–10).

Drusen are more commonly encountered in caucasians, especially those of fair complexion. They are inherited as an autosomal dominant trait with incomplete penetrance. In 70 percent of cases they occur bilaterally, but they may be very asymmetric. Notably, transient obscurations of vision, the most common presenting symptom of papilledema, may also occur with disc drusen. The presence of this symptom, therefore, has no differential significance. There is no relationship

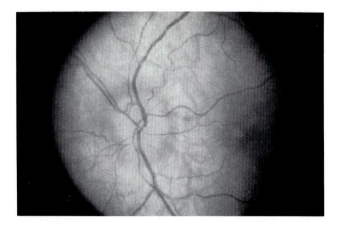

Figure 13–45. Pseudopapilledema in which disc drusen are not obvious. Note, however, the absence of retinal hemorrhages, or exudate, or obsuration of blood vessels at the optic disc.

between disc drusen and refractive error, or other ocular or neurological disorders.

Pseudopapilledema is usually asymptomatic, although an enlarged blind spot may be detected on visual field testing. Rare complications of optic nerve head drusen include other patterns of visual field loss and spontaneous hemorrhages. Rare field defects include nerve fiber bundle (arcuate) defects and irregular contraction of the peripheral field. Diminished central acuity occurs only with hemorrhagic complications.

Disc hemorrhages are a rare complication of optic nerve drusen. They are usually associated with the sudden onset of a nerve fiber bundle visual field defect. Vitreous and subretinal hemorrhages are even rarer complications. The latter usually present with a hemorrhagic elevation of the disc that may extend under the macula (Fig. 13–46).

Anomalous elevation of the optic nerve head has also been reported in young children with Down syn-

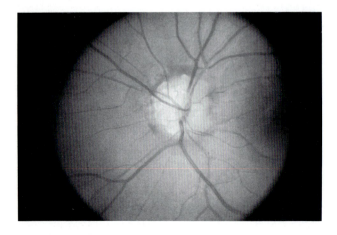

Figure 13–44. Pseudopapilledema due to disc drusen.

TABLE 13–10. OPHTHALMOSCOPIC FEATURES OF PSEUDOPAPILLEDEMA

Elevation of the optic nerve head
Absence of the physiological optic nerve head cup
Irregularity of the disc margins
Vessels arise from a central area of the disc
Anomalous branching of retinal vessels
Increased number of vessels crossing the disc
Derangement of retinal pigment surrounding the disc
Disc drusen may transilluminate or autofluoresce
No disc hemorrhages present (with rare exceptions)
No exudates or cotton-wool spots present
Superficial capillary telangiectasis absent
Spontaneous venous pulsations may be present

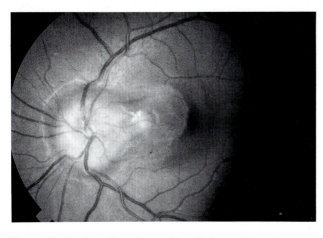

Figure 13–46. Complicated pseudopapilledema. This 10-year-old boy, followed for several years with disc drusen, developed a spontaneous subretinal hemorrhage extending into the macular area.

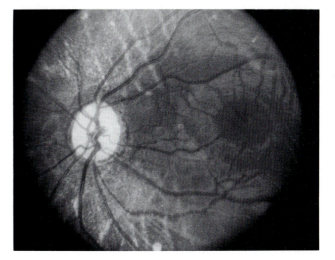

Figure 13–47. Optic atrophy.

drome, in the absence of an intracranial mass, disc drusen, or inflammation (Catalano & Simon, 1990). The elevation may be transient and recurrent, and it is not associated with apparent visual loss.

Optic Atrophy

Hereditary Optic Atrophy. **Dominant optic neuropathy (Kjer's disease)** presents insidiously between 4 and 8 years of age, with a moderately reduced visual acuity of between 20/30 and 20/80. In young children it may be heralded as a sudden loss of vision. The optic nerve often shows a wedge-shaped pallor temporally. Visual field testing reveals a central field loss connected to the blind spot, and color vision testing demonstrates a loss of blue-sensitive cones. The visual acuity may eventually diminish to 20/200. Examination of other family members may confirm a subtle abnormality.

Simple recessive optic neuropathy has an earlier onset, and is usually discovered by the age of 3 to 4 years due to severe visual impairment, with or without nystagmus. By the time of diagnosis, the disc is usually pale and the retinal vessels attenuated (Fig. 13–47). **Complicated recessive optic neuropathy (Behr's syndrome)** has an onset between 1 and 9 years of age and is complicated by the association of mild mental deficiency, hyperreflexia, hypertonia, and ataxia. Disc pallor is predominantly temporal; nystagmus and strabismus are present in more than half the affected children. Visual acuity may eventually be reduced to less than 20/300.

Acquired Optic Atrophy. Neuroradiological imaging of the afferent visual system, as well as the posterior fossa, has demonstrated that in the absence of a pedigree consistent with hereditary disorder, the most

frequent cause of unilateral or bilateral optic atrophy is a tumor (Repka & Miller, 1988). The most common tumor is a glioma of the optic nerve, chiasm, or both, followed by a craniopharyngioma. As a category, postinflammatory optic atrophy was the second most common cause of optic atrophy in children; traumatic causes ranked third. Acquired etiologies may be five times as prevalent as hereditary optic atrophy.

Diplopia

Diplopia can arise secondary to a host of ocular and neurological disorders. The ocular causes of diplopia (such as cataract, dislocated lens, uncorrected refractive error, and corneal irregularity) are rare in children. In this age group, diplopia is most often due to the sudden development of a muscle imbalance (misaligned eyes, or strabismus) secondary to a cranial nerve palsy. These, in turn, are manifestations of neoplastic, traumatic, and inflammatory disorders (Table 13–11).

The evaluation of children with diplopia can be greatly simplified if an isolated cranial nerve palsy can be differentiated. The discussion below reviews the characteristics of isolated palsies of the three cranial nerves that innervate extraocular muscles.

Isolated Sixth-nerve Palsies

The sixth nerve innervates only the lateral rectus muscle, which pulls the eye outward (see Fig. 13–54). Eyes with sixth-nerve palsies deviate inward; their ability to turn outward is diminished (Fig. 13–48).

The association of findings is helpful in localizing an isolated sixth-nerve palsy. Disorders in the area of the sixth nerve (abducens) nucleus cause an ipsilateral gaze paresis rather than an isolated sixth-nerve palsy. Lesions in the dorsal pons (Foville's syndrome) result in the associated findings of ipsilateral facial weakness,

TABLE 13–11. CAUSES OF CRANIAL NERVE PALSIES IN CHILDREN

Category	Examples	Comment
CNS tumor	Brainstem glioma Posterior fossa astrocytoma Medulloblastoma	Coexisting papilledema, decreased corneal sensation, nystagmus, bilateral; history of trauma often elicited because ataxia and falling are early manifestations of posterior fossa tumors.
Cavernous sinus tumor	Metastatic lymphoma and leukemia	Combined unilateral third-, fourth-, and sixth-nerve palsies with facial pain and numbness in the distribution of the fifth cranial nerve.
Head trauma	Generalized	Sixth, third, and fourth nerves affected in this order.
	Sudden deceleration	Bilateral fourth-nerve injuries due to their relationship to the tentorial edge.
	Severe crushing injury	With loss of consciousness and skull fracture: sixth- and seventh-nerve palsies.
	Carotid–cavernous fistula	Rapid onset of conjunctival redness, swelling, proptosis, diplopia, and bruit.
	Orbital apex syndrome	Same as carotid–cavernous fistula with the addition of optic neuropathy.
Inflammation	Pseudotumor	Lid erythema and swelling, ptosis, restricted eye movements, orbital pain, proptosis, conjunctival swelling and hyperemia, reduced corneal sensation; bilateral in one third, headache, fever, abdominal pain, and eosinophilia common.
Infection	Cavernous sinus thrombosis	Bacteremic spread from the face, nasal cavity, sinuses, orbit, or mouth.
	Orbital cellulitis	Proptosis, restricted motility, ocular pain, fever, leukocytosis, lid swelling, conjunctival swelling, facial numbness.
	Syphilis and tuberculosis	Basilar meningitis, bilateral third-nerve palsies and other brainstem findings.
	Lyme disease	Meningitis, papilledema, optic neuritis, neuroretinitis, sixth-nerve palsy.
	Postviral	Benign, recurrent sixth-nerve palsies, rarely follows an immunization.
Neurogenic	Guillain–Barré syndrome	Miller–Fisher bulbar variant: facial paralysis, pupillary involvement, inability to move the extraocular muscles, ataxia, areflexia.
	Ophthalmoplegic migraine	Children in their first decade, with a family history of migraine; pain around the eye, nausea, and vomiting; remits with the onset of third-nerve palsy (with pupil involvement); most resolve within 1 month.
Increased intracranial pressure		Inability to turn the eyes outward (sixth-nerve palsy) is an early sign, headache, vomiting, circulatory, respiratory, and psychic changes.

facial analgesia, deafness, and Horner's syndrome (small pupil, lid droop, and decreased sweating). If the lesion is in the ventral pons (Millard–Gubler syndrome), contralateral hemiplegia will accompany the abduction weakness. Meningiomas and acoustic neu-romas in the cerebellopontine angle result in sixth-nerve palsies in association with seventh- and eighth-nerve disorders, corneal hypesthesia, nystagmus, and cerebellar signs.

After leaving the brainstem, the sixth nerve travels

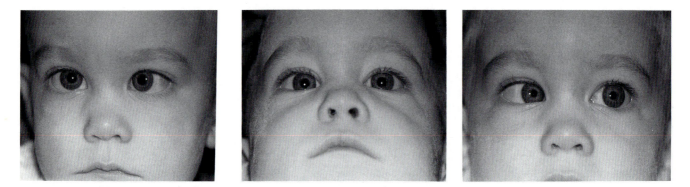

Figure 13–48. Congenital bilateral sixth cranial nerve palsy. Note that the eyes are only slightly turned in (esotropic) in the straight-ahead (primary) position, but there is marked inability to turn either eye outward.

TABLE 13–12. ETIOLOGY OF SIXTH-NERVE PALSY

Etiology	Children < 15 Years of Age (%)	Patients of All Age Groups (%)
Neoplasm	39	31
Head trauma	20	11
Inflammatory	17	—
Vascular disease	3	9
Aneurysm	—	3
Undetermined	9	12
Other	12	34

Modified from Catalano RA: Ocular Emergencies. Philadelphia, Saunders, 1992, p 349, with permission. Data from Harley RD: Paralytic strabismus in children. Ophthalmology 87:24, 1980.

in the basal cistern, where it is susceptible to tumors such as craniopharyngioma. Increased intracranial pressure from tumors or hydrocephalus can also stretch the sixth nerve between its exit from the brainstem and its attachment to the clivus. Farther anteriorly, the sixth nerve passes beneath the petroclinoid ligament. Mastoiditis, arising from middle ear infections, can cause a petrositis with involvement of the facial nerve (facial palsy), trigeminal ganglion (facial pain), and sixth nerve (Gradenigo's syndrome). The sixth nerve then traverses through the middle of the cavernous sinus, where in association with the third and fourth nerves, it is susceptible to traumatic, vascular, and inflammatory disorders. Lesions in the superior orbital fissure or orbital apex typically involve multiple cranial nerves and/or produce proptosis.

The cause of sixth-nerve paresis differs in pediatric and adult populations (Table 13–12). Tumors and trauma are encountered more frequently in the pediatric age range. Inflammatory disease as a cause of sixth-nerve palsy—including meningoencephalitis, Gradenigo's syndrome, and brain abscess—also occurs

almost exclusively in children. With the exception of congenital anomalies, vascular disease is essentially a nonexistent cause in children. Rare causes in either group include lumbar puncture or spinal anesthesia.

Congenital sixth-nerve palsies are rare. In newborns, a transient lateral rectus muscle palsy may rarely occur, which usually resolves within 6 months. Most infants with a significant inward deviation of the eyes (esotropia) are congenital esotropes who view their world by cross-fixating. Others may have Duane's retraction syndrome or Möbius syndrome (see Chapter 6).

A transient sixth-nerve palsy after an otherwise benign viral illness in children has also been described. The palsy develops 7 to 21 days following a fever or upper respiratory infection and usually resolves within 10 weeks. The age range of reported patients has been 18 months to the early teenage years. Hydrocephalus and leukemia comprise rarer causes of sixth-nerve paresis in children and young adults.

Although the prognosis is poor when the cause is neoplastic, complete spontaneous resolution usually occurs in over 50 percent of patients with traumatic sixth-nerve palsies. The prognosis is even better when the cause is inflammatory; greater than 90 percent of inflammatory pareses resolve completely and spontaneously.

Isolated Fourth-nerve Palsies

The fourth cranial nerve innervates only the superior oblique muscle (see Fig. 13–54). This muscle serves to rotate the eye inward, depress, and slightly turn the eye outward. An eye with a fourth-nerve palsy is higher than the contralateral eye, and this difference becomes greater upon tilting the head to the affected side (Fig. 13–49). Because of this, patients with a unilateral fourth-nerve palsy often present with torticolis

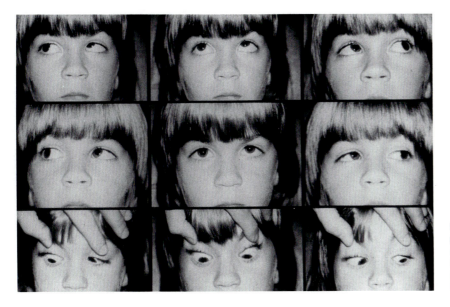

Figure 13–49. Left fourth cranial nerve palsy. Note the left hyperdeviation, worse in right gaze. Note also the underaction of the left superior oblique muscle (*lower left frame*) and overreaction of its antagonist, the left inferior oblique muscle (*upper left frame*).

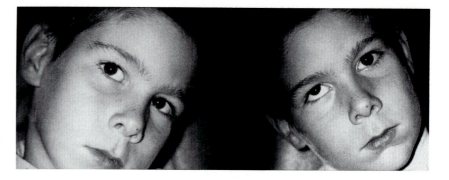

Figure 13–50. Right fourth cranial nerve palsy. Head tilt to the right increases the hyperdeviation.

(head tilt) to the contralateral side (Fig. 13–50). This reduces the ocular misalignment, and when present suggests that the child is maintaining binocular vision. The absence of head tilt is usually attributed to amblyopia or extremely large amplitudes of vertical fusion.

In most series, closed head trauma is the most common cause of fourth nerve palsy. In many cases, however, no definitive diagnosis is identified. Harley (1980) reviewed the causes of paralytic strabismus in 121 children from birth to age 16 years, and found 67 percent of fourth-nerve paralysis to be of undetermined origin. Herpes zoster ophthalmicus, inflammation, and injury to the trochlea (the fibrocartilagenous loop that suspends the superior oblique tendon) are rare causes of isolated fourth-nerve palsy in children.

Superior oblique palsies that present spontaneously in late childhood or early adulthood often represent "decompensated" congenital palsies that can no longer be controlled by fusional mechanisms. Increased vertical fusion amplitudes are indicative of congenital palsies that decompensated. Head tilts in old photographs also suggest a long-standing condition.

Isolated Third-Nerve Palsies

The third nerve functions to elevate, depress, and turn the eye in. In addition, the upper eyelid, pupil, and ciliary body are innervated by the third nerve (see Fig. 13–54). Signs of third-nerve palsy include an outward and downward deviation of the eye and ptosis (lid droop) of the eyelid(s) (Fig. 13–51). If the pupillary fibers are involved, the pupil is enlarged and responds poorly to light.

Similar to the sixth nerve, the association of findings is helpful in localizing an isolated third-nerve palsy. A lesion of the third-nerve nucleus should be suspected with bilateral total third-nerve palsy, bilateral ptosis, or bilateral pupillary involvement. Unilateral ptosis or pupillary involvement, and unilateral involvement of the extraocular muscles with sparing of the contralateral superior rectus muscle, cannot represent a nuclear lesion. Oculomotor palsy in association with contralateral hemiplegia (Weber syndrome) indicates involvement of the corticospinal tracts. If the red

nucleus is involved, the patient will also have contralateral ataxia and intention tremor (Benedikt syndrome). These brainstem syndromes usually result from vascular infarction, demyelination, or tumor.

Third-nerve palsies in children are more frequently congenital than acquired. Congenital palsies are characterized by variable involvement of the four extraocular muscles (medial rectus, inferior rectus, superior rectus, and inferior oblique) innervated by the third nerve, and variable limitations of ocular movement (Fig. 13–52). Variable degrees of ptosis may also be present. The intraocular musculature, however, is not usually affected in congenital third-nerve palsies.

Some children with congenital third-nerve palsy develop binocular vision by maintaining a compensatory head posture. In the absence of this, amblyopia may develop in either eye. These palsies are otherwise usually benign and isolated. Balkan and Hoyt (1984), however, reported other focal neurological findings in congenital third-nerve palsy, including hemiplegia, seizures, and developmental delays.

Perinatal trauma to the peripheral oculomotor nerve has been considered the primary pathogenic mechanism in the development of congenital third-

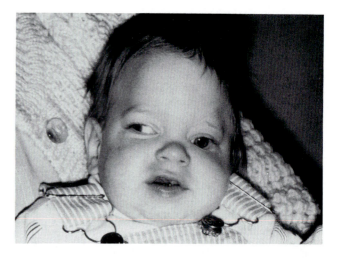

Figure 13–51. Bilateral congenital third cranial nerve palsies. Note that the eyes are deviated downward and outward, and the bilateral ptosis (drooping) and pupillary involvement.

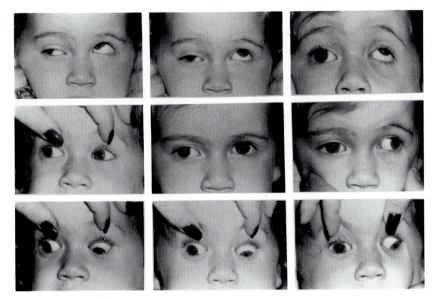

Figure 13–52. Right third cranial nerve palsy. Note the limited mobility of the right eye, larger right pupil, and associated ptosis of the right upper eyelid.

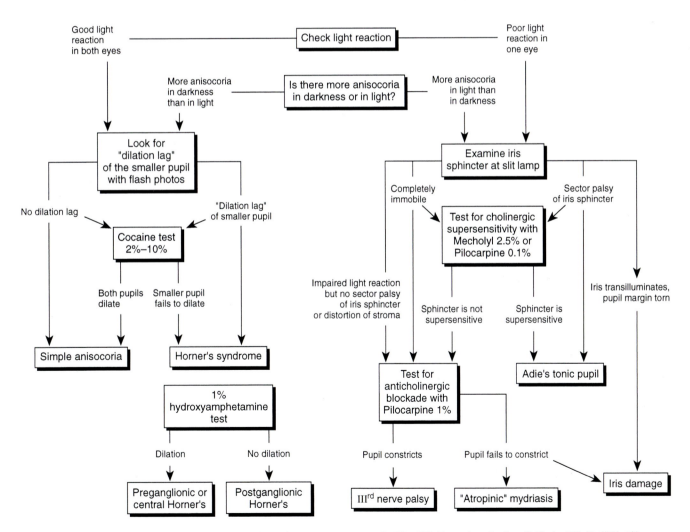

Figure 13–53. Flowchart for patients with anisocoria. *(From Thompson HS, Pilley SFJ: Unequal pupils. Surv Ophthalmol 21:45, 1976, with permission.)*

nerve palsy. The absence of other brainstem findings, and the presence of aberrant regeneration, supports this diagnosis. Ischemic and hypoxic insults to the brainstem in utero have been shown to produce unilateral or bilateral nuclear aplasia, and may be causative in infants with associated neurological abnormalities.

Pupillary Abnormalities

Figure 13–53 presents a flowchart that is useful in the evaluation of anisocoria (asymmetric pupil size). Disorders where the abnormal pupil is the smaller one (a problem with dilation—sympathetic nervous system) are separated from disorders with an enlarged pupil (a problem with constriction—parasympathetic nervous system). The first step asks whether the anisocoria changes depending on the degree of illumination. If there is no change in the anisocoria based on illumination and if both pupils constrict briskly to light without dilation lag in darkness, the patient likely has physiological or simple anisocoria. This common anomaly occurs in the absence of other visual or neuro-ophthalmologic deficits. The degree of pupillary inequality in physiological anisocoria varies with time, and usually reverses over a few hours or days.

If the anisocoria is accentuated in darkness and the smaller pupil fails to dilate with cocaine, the patient has Horner's syndrome. Greater anisocoria in light than darkness suggests a parasympathetic defect due to the instillation of an anticholinergic agent, a third-nerve palsy, or iris damage. The presence of ptosis (lid droop) associated with a large pupil suggests a third-nerve disorder, but ptosis associated with a small pupil suggests a sympathetic disorder (Horner's syndrome). Table 13–13 reviews common disorders that affect pupil size categorized by the size of the affected pupil and bilaterality of the findings.

Neurological Syndromes With Pupillary Abnormalities

The Parasympathetic Pathway. Light impulses are transmitted by the optic nerve to the optic chiasm, where decussation occurs. The first synapse for fibers carrying light impulses occurs in the midbrain in an area called the pretectum, near the superior colliculus. Fibers are sent from here to both the ipsilateral and contralateral accessory (Edinger–Westphal) nuclei, which form the parasympathetic centers of the third cranial nerve. From here, preganglionic efferent fibers travel with the extraocular motor fibers of the third cranial nerve, departing their company in the orbit to synapse in the ciliary ganglion (Fig. 13–54). Postganglionic fibers from the ciliary ganglion enter the eye and innervate the iris sphincter (controlling pupillary constriction) and ciliary body (controlling accommodation of the lens).

TABLE 13–13. COMMON DISORDERS THAT AFFECT PUPIL SIZE

Category	Disorder	Features
Unilateral small pupil	Horner's syndrome	Miosis, ptosis, anhydrosis, and enophthalmos (see text).
	Trauma	Damage to dilator muscle.
	Pharmacological	Cholinergic (e.g., pilocarpine) agents cause fixed small pupil.
Unilateral large pupil	Blindness	The pupil in a unilaterally blind eye is larger than the pupil in the seeing eye (amaurotic pupil).
	Trauma	Damage to sphincter muscle.
	Ciliary ganglion lesion	Destructive (e.g., herpes zoster, tumor) or traumatic.
	Pharmacological	Mydriatic (e.g., atropine) or adrenergic (e.g., neosynephrine) agents cause the pupil to be fixed and dilated.
	Tumor	Associated third-nerve signs and papilledema are usually present.
	Adie's syndrome	Irregularly dilated pupil that reacts poorly to light, and slightly to accommodation or convergence (see text).
Bilateral small pupils	Insecticide poisoning	Acts by inhibiting acetylcholinesterase; causes marked miosis.
	Pharmacological	Antipsychotics, barbiturates, injection and inhalation anesthetics, morphine, codeine, levodopa, and propranolol.
	Tumor	Pontine glioma (pupil may react poorly to light but better to accommodation).
	Inflammatory	Encephalitis, meningitis.
	Functional	Spasm of the near reflex, not sustainable, convergence, myopia.
	Syphilis	Argyll–Robertson pupils (pupils less than 2 mm in size, react poorly to light), iris atrophy.
Bilateral large pupils	Pharmacological	Digoxin, prednisone, quinine, reserpine, and thioridazine.
	Drug induced	Amphetamine, LSD, marijuana, and mescaline.
	Toxic	Clostridium, tetanus, lead, and carbon monoxide.
	Coma	Alcohol induced, or due to diabetes, uremia, meningitis, eclampsia, or epilepsy.
	Midbrain lesion	Parinaud's syndrome (see text).
	Hemorrhage	Midbrain, epidural or subdural.

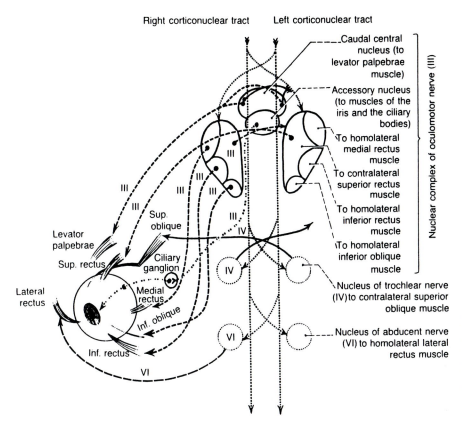

Right corticonuclear tract   Left corticonuclear tract

Caudal central nucleus (to levator palpebrae muscle)

Accessory nucleus (to muscles of the iris and the ciliary bodies)

To homolateral medial rectus muscle

To contralateral superior rectus muscle

To homolateral inferior rectus muscle

To homolateral inferior oblique muscle

Nucleus of trochlear nerve (IV) to contralateral superior oblique muscle

Nucleus of abducent nerve (VI) to homolateral lateral rectus muscle

Nuclear complex of oculomotor nerve (III)

Levator palpebrae
Sup. rectus
Sup. oblique
Ciliary ganglion
Medial rectus
Inf. oblique
Inf. rectus
Lateral rectus
VI

Figure 13–54. The cranial nerves that innervate the extraocular muscles. The preganglionic parasympathetic neuron originates in the accessory nucleus of the third cranial nerve and synapses in the ciliary ganglion. The postganglionic neuron travels to the eye. *(From Bossy J: Atlas of Neuroanatomy and Special Sense Organs. Philadelphia, Saunders, 1970, with permission.)*

The Sympathetic Pathway. Impulses from the hypothalamus travel via first-order neurons to the cervical spinal cord, where they synapse in the ciliospinal center of Budge in the lower cervical and upper thoracic spinal cord. Second-order (preganglionic) neurons then travel cephalad to synapse in the superior cervical ganglion. Third-order (postganglionic) neurons course various pathways without synapsing, to enter the eye and innervate the dilator muscle of the iris (Fig. 13–55).

Adie's Syndrome. Adie's syndrome is characterized by an irregularly dilated pupil that reacts minimally to light, and slowly to convergence and accommodation. With time, the pupil becomes suprasensitive to dilute concentrations of pilocarpine (0.1 percent). An associated finding is reduced deep tendon reflexes. Females are more commonly affected than males, and the condition is bilateral in 20 percent of patients. The etiology is unknown, but the condition is benign. Herpes zoster, varicella, temporal arteritis, syphilis, diabetes, and Guillain–Barré syndrome can produce similar findings, and should be ruled out.

The presence of Adie's pupil, with or without suprasensitivity, in an infant less than 1 year of age is suggestive of familial dysautonomia (Riley–Day syndrome). This syndrome of Ashkenazi Jews includes feeding difficulties, hypotonia, delayed development, labile body temperature and blood pressure, corneal hypesthesia, decreased tearing, and the absence of fungiform papillae on the tongue. Breath-holding episodes, recurrent pneumonias, and intractable vomiting crises also occur.

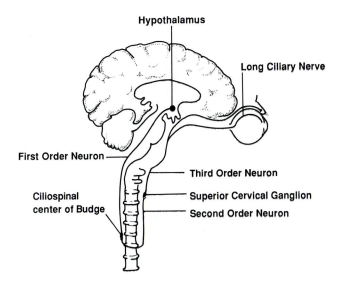

Hypothalamus

Long Ciliary Nerve

First Order Neuron

Third Order Neuron

Superior Cervical Ganglion

Ciliospinal center of Budge

Second Order Neuron

Figure 13–55. The oculosympathetic pathway. *(From Catalano RA: Ocular Emergencies. Philadelphia, Saunders, 1992, p 357, with permission.)*

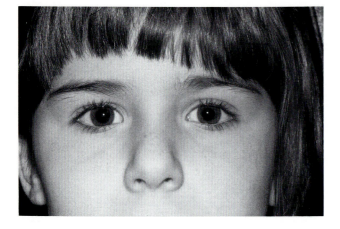

Figure 13–56. Horner's syndrome involving the left eye. Note the ptosis (lid droop) and miosis (small pupil).

TABLE 13–14. HORNER'S SYNDROME IN CHILDREN

Localization	Differential Diagnosis
First-order neuron	Hypothalamic syndrome
	Basal meningitis
	Brainstem infarction/hemorrhage
	Cerebral infarction/hemorrhage
	Pituitary or brainstem tumor
	Trauma (including surgery)
	Cervical spine: transection, tumor, meningitis, poliomyelitis, syringomyelia, syphilis, vascular malformation
	Cerebral palsy (rare)
Second-order neuron	Spinal birth injury (Klumpke's paralysis)
	Cervical rib
	Tumors of mediastinum, esophagus, sympathetic chain (neuroma), retropharynx, oral cavity
	Lymphadenopathy (Hodgkin's disease)
	Trauma (including surgery—tonsillectomy, corrective cardiac surgery)
	Thyroglossal duct surgery, thyroid adenoma
Third-order neuron	Otitis media
	Trauma (including surgery)
	Cavernous sinus/Tolosa–Hunt syndrome
	Herpes zoster ophthalmicus
	Orbital tumor/cyst
	Migraine/cluster headaches

Horner's Syndrome. Horner's syndrome results from an interruption in the sympathetic pathway. It is characterized by miosis (small pupil), ptosis (droopy eyelid), anhydrosis (decreased sweating on the ipsilateral face), and enophthalmos (less protrusion of the affected eye) (Figs. 13–56 and 13–57). The last is seldom clinically striking; usually the difference in protrusion between the eyes is less than 2 mm. The anisocoria is greater in dim illumination because the affected smaller pupil dilates poorly. The lower lid on the involved side is also 1 mm higher than the opposite side (upside-down ptosis).

Horner's syndrome can be congenital or acquired. When congenital, it is usually secondary to birth trauma. Trauma to the spine can be associated with injury to the lower brachial plexus (Klumpke's paralysis). Although less than 5 to 10 percent of infants with "congenital Horner's syndrome" have neuroblastoma, screening for this curable malignancy is appropriate in infants. All cases of true congenital Horner's syndrome will have heterochromia, with the affected iris being lighter.

Pharmacological testing is employed to diagnose and localize the lesion in acute acquired Horner's syndrome (see Fig. 13–53). The absence of iris dilation with cocaine diagnoses Horner's syndrome. The cocaine test, however, does not localize the lesion; other tests are used for this purpose. There is no reliable test to differentiate a first-order from a second-order neuron disorder. Hydroxyamphetamine 1 percent (Paredrine), however, will differentiate first- and second- from third-order neuron disorders. This is important be-

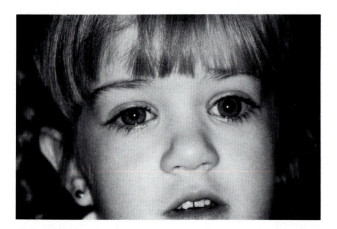

Figure 13–57. Horner's syndrome involving the right eye.

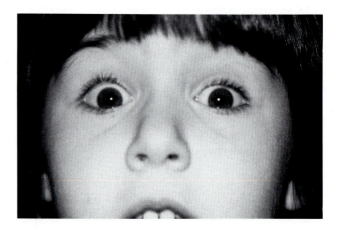

Figure 13–58. Eyelid retraction and retraction–convergence nystagmus on attempted upward gaze in a child with Parinaud's syndrome.

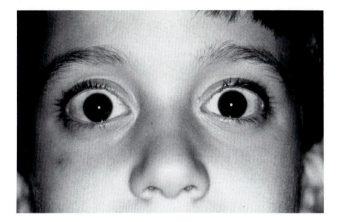

Figure 13–59. Eyelid retraction in another child with Parinaud's syndrome.

cause third-order (postganglionic) lesions are most often benign. In contrast, almost 50 percent of first- and second-order neuron defects result from neoplastic processes (Table 13–14). Lesions involving the postganglionic neuron result in an absence of iris dilation with paredrine. Lesions of the first- and second-order neurons do not interfere with the integrity of the third-order neuron; iris dilation still occurs. The cocaine and Paredrine tests should be done on separate days because they interfere with each other's actions. They should also not be done on the same day as other tests that disrupt the corneal epithelium, such as intraocular pressure testing.

Parinaud's Syndrome. Parinaud's syndrome is a midbrain lesion characterized by bilaterally mid-dilated pupils that respond poorly to light but react normally to accommodative effort. Upward gaze is reduced, but downward gaze is preserved. Although the eyes elevate with the doll's-head maneuver, or Bell's phenomenon, volitional attempts at upward gaze produce variable degrees of retraction-convergence nystagmus and widening of the palpebral fissures (Collier's sign) (Figs. 13–58 and 13–59). In children a pinealoma or craniopharyngioma should be sought. Other causes include stroke, multiple sclerosis, and hydrocephalus due to aqueductal stenosis.

REFERENCES

Bergmeister's Papilla

Bergmeister O: Beitrage zur Entwicklungsgeschichter des Saugethrerauges. Mittheil aus d Embryol Inst der KK in Wien, Shenk SL (ed), 1:63, 1877.
Brown G, Tasman WS: Congenital Anomalies of the Optic Disc. New York, Grune & Stratton, 1983.
Lloyd RI: Variations in the development and regression of Bergmeister's papilla and the hyaloid artery. Trans Am Ophthalmol Soc 38:326, 1940.
Roth AM, Foos RY: Surface structure of the optic nerve head: Epipapillary membranes. Am J Ophthalmol 74:977, 1982.

Coloboma of the Optic Nerve

Brown G, Tasman W: Congenital Anomalies of the Optic Disc. New York, Grune & Stratton, 1983.
Pagan RA: Ocular coloboma. Surv Ophthalmol 25:223, 1981.
Pagan RA, Graham JM, Zonana J, et al: Coloboma, congenital heart disease and chronic atresia with multiple anomalies: CHARGE association. J Pediatr 99:223, 1981.
Savell J, Cooke JR: Optic nerve colobomas of autosomal dominant heredity. Arch Ophthalmol 94:395, 1976.

Cranial Nerve Palsies

Balkan R, Hoyt CS: Associated neurologic abnormalities in congenital third nerve palsies. Am J Ophthalmol 97:315, 1984.
Buncic JR: Pediatric neuro-ophthalmology and ocular emergencies. Ophthalmic Prac 8:146, 1990.
Burger LJ, Kalvin NH, Smith JL: Acquired lesions of fourth cranial nerve. Brain 93:567, 1970.
Eyster EF, Hoyt WF, Wilson CV: Ocular motor palsy from minor head trauma: An initial sign of basal intracranial tumor. JAMA 220:1083, 1972.
Hamed LM: Associated neurologic and ophthalmologic findings in congenital oculomotor nerve palsy. Ophthalmology 98:708, 1991.
Harley RD: Paralytic strabismus in children. Etiologic incidence and management of the third, fourth and sixth nerve palsies. Ophthalmology 87:24, 1980.
Kahana E, Leibowitz U, Alter M: Brainstem and cranial nerve involvement in multiple sclerosis. Acta Neurol Scand 49:269, 1973.
Kirkham TH, Bird AC, Sanders MD: Divergence paralysis with raised intracranial pressure: An electrooculographic study. Br J Ophthalmol 56:776, 1972.
Lesser RL, Kornmehl EW, Pachner AR, et al: Neuro-ophthalmologic manifestations of Lyme disease. Ophthalmology 97:699, 1990.
Lewis MA, Goldstein S, Baker RS: Magnetic resonance imaging of the posterior fossa in ocular motility disorders. J Clin Neuro-ophthalmol 7:235, 1987.
Miller NR: Solitary oculomotor nerve palsy in childhood. Am J Ophthalmol 83:106, 1977.
Richards R: Ocular motility disturbances following trauma. Adv Ophthalmic Plast Reconstr Surg 7:133, 1987.
Robertson DM, Hines JD, Rucker CW: Acquired sixth nerve paresis in children. Arch Ophthalmol 83:574, 1970.
Rucker CW: The causes of paralysis of the third, fourth and sixth cranial nerves. Am J Ophthalmol 61:1293, 1966.
Schwartz BS, Goldstein MD, Riberio JMC, et al: Antibody testing in Lyme disease. JAMA 262:3431, 1989.
Smith JL: Lyme disease appears to have many ocular manifestations. Arch Ophthalmol 108:337, 1990.
Victor DI: The diagnosis of congenital unilateral third nerve palsy. Brain 99:711, 1976.
Weber RB, Daroff RB, Mackey EA: Pathology of oculomotor nerve palsy in diabetics. Neurology 20:835, 1970.

Werner BS, Savino PJ, Schatz NJ: Benign recurrent sixth nerve palsies in children. Arch Ophthalmol 101:607, 1983.

Winward KE, Smith JL, Culbertson WW, Paris-Hamelin A: Ocular Lyme borreliosis. Am J Ophthalmol 108:651, 1989.

Younge BR, Sutula F: Analysis of trochlear nerve palsies: Diagnosis, etiology and treatment. Mayo Clin Proc 52:11, 1977.

Enlarged Vessels on the Optic Nerve

Archer DB, Deutman A, Ernest JT, et al: Arteriovenous communication in the retina. Am J Ophthalmol 75:224, 1973.

Augsburger JJ, Goldberg RE, Shields JA, et al: Changing appearances of retinal arterial malformation. Albrecht von Graefes Arch Klin Exp Ophthalmol 215:65, 1980.

Brown GC: Congenital abnormalities of the optic disc. In Nelson LB, Calhoun JC, Harley RD (eds): Pediatric Ophthalmology, ed 3. Philadelphia, Saunders, 1991.

Brown GC, Donoso LA, Magargal LE, et al: Congenital retinal macrovessels. Arch Ophthalmol 100:1430, 1982.

Cameron ME, Green CH: Congenital arteriovenous aneurysm of the retina. Br J Ophthalmol 52:768, 1968.

Wyburn-Mason R: Arteriovenous aneurysm of midbrain and retina, optic nerve, chiasm and brain. Brain 66:165, 1943.

Leber's Optic Neuropathy

Nikoskelainen EK, Hoyt WF, Nummelin K, Schatz H: Fundus findings in Leber's hereditary optic neuropathy, III. Fluorescein angiographic studies. Arch Ophthalmol 102:981, 1984.

Nikoskelainen EK, Savountas ML, Wanne OP, et al: Leber's hereditary optic neuropathy, a maternally inherited disease. A genealogic study in four pedigrees. Arch Ophthalmol 105:665, 1987.

Phillips CI, Gosden CM: Leber's hereditary optic neuritis and Kearns–Sayre syndrome: Mitochondrial DNA mutations. Surv Ophthalmol 35:463, 1991.

Singh G, Lott MT, Wallace DC: A mitochondrial DNA mutation as a cause of Leber's hereditary optic neuropathy. N Engl J Med 320:1300, 1989.

Smith JL, Hoyt WF, Susac JO: Optic fundus in acute Leber optic neuropathy. Arch Ophthalmol 90:349, 1973.

Megalopapilla

Brown, G, Tasman W: Congenital Anomalies of the Optic Disc. New York, Grune & Stratton, 1983.

Franceschetti A, Bock RH: Megalopapilla: A new congenital anomaly. Am J Ophthalmol 33:227, 1950.

Goldhammer Y, Smith JL: Optic nerve anomalies in basal encephalocele. Arch Ophthalmol 63:115, 1975.

Merin S, Harwood-Nash DC, Crawford JS: Axial tomography of optic nerve defects. Am J Ophthalmol 72:1122, 1971.

Morning Glory Disc Anomaly

Brown G, Tasman W: Congenital Anomalies of the Optic Disc. New York, Grune & Stratton, 1983.

Hamada S, Ellsworth RM: Congenital retinal detachment and the optic disc anomaly. Am J Ophthalmol 71:460, 1971.

Kindler P: Morning glory syndrome: Unusual congenital optic disc anomaly. Am J Ophthalmol 69:376, 1970.

Pollack JA, Newton TH, Hoyt WF: Transphenoidal and transethmoidal encephaloceles. Radiology 90:442, 1968.

Steinkuller PG: The morning glory disc anomaly: Case report and literature review. Pediatr Ophthalmol 17:81, 1980.

Optic Atrophy

Costenbader FD, O'Rourk TR: Optic atrophy in children. J Pediatr Ophthalmol 5:77, 1968.

Hoyt CS: Autosomal dominant optic atrophy. A spectrum of disability. Ophthalmology 87:245, 1980.

Kline LB, Glaser JS: Dominant optic atrophy. Arch Ophthalmol 97:1680, 1979.

Repka MX, Miller NR: Optic atrophy in children. Am J Ophthalmol 106:191, 1988.

Optic Nerve Aplasia

Blanco R, Salvador F, Galan A, Gil-Gibernau JJ: Aplasia of the optic nerve: Report of three cases. J Pediatr Ophthalmol Strabismus 29:228, 1992.

Brown G, Tasman W: Congenital Anomalies of the Optic Disc. New York, Grune & Stratton, 1983.

Hotchkiss ML, Green WR: Optic nerve aplasia and hypoplasia. J Pediatr Ophthalmol 16:225, 1979.

Little LE, Whitemore PV, Wells TV: Aplasia of the optic nerve. J Pediatr Ophthalmol 13:84, 1976.

Weiter JS, MacLean IW, Zimmerman LE: Aplasia of the optic nerve and disc. Am J Ophthalmol 83:569, 1977.

Optic Nerve Hypoplasia

Acers TE: Optic nerve hypoplasia: Septo-optic pituitary dysplasia syndrome. Trans Am Ophthalmol Soc 79:425, 1981.

Brown G, Tasman W: Congenital Anomalies of the Optic Disc. New York, Grune & Stratton, 1983.

Costin G, Murphree AL: Hypothalamic–pituitary function in children with optic nerve hypoplasia. Am J Dis Child 139:249, 1985.

Frusen L, Holmegaard L: Spectrum of optic nerve hypoplasia. Br J Ophthalmol 62:7, 1978.

Margalith D, Jan JE, McCormick AQ, et al: Clinical spectrum of congenital optic nerve hypoplasia: Review of 51 patients. Dev Med Child Neurol 26:311, 1984.

Mosier MA, Lieberman MF, Green WR, et al: Hypoplasia of the optic nerve. Arch Ophthalmol 96:1437, 1978.

Salevetz MI, Nelson LB, Finnegan LP: Congenital and developmental ocular anomalies associated with maternal drug use during pregnancy. Semin Ophthalmol 5:117, 1990.

Skarf B, Hoyt CS: Optic nerve hypoplasia in children: Association with anomalies of the endocrine and CNS. Arch Ophthalmol 102:62, 1984.

Optic Neuritis

Beck RW: The optic neuritis treatment trial. Arch Ophthalmol 106:1051, 1988.

Cohen MM, Lessell S, Wolf PA: A prospective study of the risk of developing multiple sclerosis in uncomplicated optic neuritis. Neurology 11:324, 1979.

Cox TA: Prognostic factors in optic neuritis. Ann Neurol 42:702, 1985.

Ebers GC: Optic neuritis and multiple sclerosis. Arch Neurol 42:702, 1985.

Farris BK, Pickard DJ: Bilateral postinfectious optic neuritis and intravenous steroid therapy in children. Ophthalmology 97:339, 1990.

Gebarski SS, Gabrielson TO, Gilman S, et al: The initial diagnosis of multiple sclerosis: Clinical impact of magnetic resonance imaging. Ann Neurol 17:469, 1985.

Perkins GD, Rose FC: Optic Neuritis and its Differential Diagnosis. Oxford, Oxford Medical Publications, 1979.

Rizzo JF, Lessell S: Risk of developing multiple sclerosis after uncomplicated optic neuritis. A long term prospective study. Neurology 38:185, 1988.

Slamovits TL, Rosen CE, Cheng KP, Striph GC: Visual loss in patients with optic neuritis and visual loss to no light perception. Am J Ophthalmol 111:209, 1991.

Spoor TC, Rockwell DL: Treatment of optic neuritis with intravenous megadose corticosteroids: A consecutive series. Ophthalmology 95:131, 1988.

Weiss AH, Beck RW: Neuroretinitis in childhood. J Pediatr Ophthalmol Strabismus 26:198, 1989.

Optic Pits

Brown GC: Congenital abnormalities of the optic disc. In Nelson LB, Calhoun JC, Harley RD (eds): Pediatric Ophthalmology, ed 3. Philadelphia, Saunders, 1991.

Brown GC, Shields JA, Goldberg RE: Congenital pits of the optic nerve head, II. Clinical studies in humans. Ophthalmology 87:51, 1980.

Brown GC, Shields JA, Patty BE, Goldberg RE: Congenital pit of the optic nerve head, I. Experimental studies in collie dogs. Arch Ophthalmol 87:1341, 1979.

Kranenburg EW: Crater-like holes in the optic disc and central serous retinopathy. Arch Ophthalmol 64:912, 1960.

Van Nouhuys JM, Bruyn GW: Nasopharyngeal transphenoidal encephalocele, crater-like hole in the optic disc and agenesis of the corpus collosum, pneumoencephalographic visualization in a case. Psychiatr Neurol Neurochir 67:243, 1964.

Papilledema and Pseudopapilledema

Catalano RA, Simon JW: Optic disc elevation in Down's syndrome. Am J Ophthalmol 110:28, 1990.

Cohen DN: Drusen of the optic disc and the development of field defects. Arch Ophthalmol 85:224, 1971.

Miller NR, Fine SL: The Ocular Fundus in Neuro-ophthalomologic Diagnosis. St. Louis, Mosby, 1977.

Sanders TE, Gay AJ, Newman M: Hemorrhagic complications of drusen of the optic nerve. Am J Ophthalmol 71:204, 1971.

Wirtschafter JD, Rizzo FJ, Smiley BC: Optic nerve axoplasm and papilledema. Surv Ophthalmol 20:157, 1975.

Persistent Hyaloid Artery

Brown G, Tasman W: Congenital Anomalies of the Optic Disc. New York, Grune & Stratton, 1983.

Delaney WV: Prepapillary hemorrhage and persistent hyaloid artery. Am J Ophthalmol 90:419, 1980.

Jones HE: Hyaloid remnants in the eyes of premature babies. Br J Ophthalmol 47:39, 1963.

Prepapillary Loops

Brown GC: Congenital abnormalities of the optic disc. In Nelson LB, Calhoun JC, Harley RD (eds): Pediatric Ophthalmology, ed 3. Philadelphia, Saunders, 1991.

Brown GC, Magargal LE, Augsburger JJ, Shields JA: Preretinal arterial loops and retinal arterial occlusion. Am J Ophthalmol 87:646, 1979.

Brown G, Tasman W: Congenital Anomalies of the Optic Disc. New York, Grune & Stratton, 1983.

Degenhart W, Brown GC, Augsburger JJ, Magargal LE: Prepapillary vascular loops: A clinical and fluorescein angiographic study. Ophthalmology 88:1126, 1981.

Shakin EP, Shields JA, Augsburger JJ, Brown JC: Clinicopathologic correlation of a prepapillary vascular loop. Retina 8:55, 1988.

Pupillary Abnormalities

Axelrod FB: Familial dysautonomia. In Gellis SS, Kagan BM (eds): Current Pediatric Therapy 10. Philadelphia, Saunders, 1982, pp 80–82.

Corbett JJ, Thompson HS: Pupillary function and dysfunction. In Asbury AK, McKhann GM, McDonald WI (eds): Diseases of the Nervous System: Clinical Neurobiology. Philadelphia, Saunders, 1986, pp 606–617.

Grimson BS, Thompson HS: Raeder's syndrome. A clinical review. Surv Ophthalmol 24:199, 1980.

Grimson BS, Thompson HS: Drug testing in Horner's syndrome. In Glaser JS, Smith JL (eds): Neuro-ophthalmology. St. Louis, Mosby, 1974, Ch 8, pp 265–270.

Kase M, Nagata R, Yoshida A, et al: Pupillary light reflex in amblyopia. Invest Ophthalmol Vis Sci 25:467, 1984.

Loewenfeld IE: "Simple, central" anisocoria: A common condition, seldom recognized. Trans Am Acad Ophthalmol Otolaryngol 83:832, 1977.

Miller NR: Disorders of pupillary function, accommodation and lacrimation. In Miller NR (ed): Walsh and Hoyt's Clinical Neuro-ophthalmology, ed 4. Baltimore, Williams & Wilkins, 1985, vol 2, pp 469–528.

Plum F, Posner JB: The Diagnosis of Stupor and Coma. Philadelphia, Davis, 1972.

Portnoy JZ, Thompson SH, Lennarson L, et al: Pupillary defects in amblyopia. Am J Ophthalmol 96:609, 1983.

Thompson HS: The pupil. In Lessell S, van Dalen JTW (eds): Current Neuro-ophthalmology. Chicago, Year Book, 1988, pp 201–216.

Thompson HS: Adie's syndrome. Some new observations. Trans Am Ophthalmol Soc 75:587, 1977.

Thompson HS, Pilley SFJ: Unequal pupils: A flowchart for sorting out the anisocorias. Surv Ophthalmol 21:45, 1976.

Thompson HS, Zackon DH, Czarnecki JSC: Tadpole-shaped pupils caused by segmental spasm of the iris dilator muscle. Am J Ophthalmol 96:467, 1983.

Trobe JD: Third nerve palsy and the pupil. Arch Ophthalmol 106:602, 1988.

Van der Wiel HL, van Ginj J: Localization of Horner's syndrome: Use and limitations of the hydroxyamphetamine test. J Neurol Sci 59:229, 1983.

Weinstein JM, Zweifel TJ, Thompson HS: Congenital Horner's syndrome. Arch Ophthalmol 98:1074, 1980.

Staphyloma (Peripapillary)

Brown G, Tasman W: Congenital Anomalies of the Optic Disc. New York, Grune & Stratton, 1983.

Kral K, Svarc D: Contractile peripapillary staphyloma. Am J Ophthalmol 71:1090, 1971.

Wise JB, MacLean JL, Gass JDM: Contractile peripapillary staphyloma. Arch Ophthalmol 75:626, 1966.

Tilted Disc Syndrome

Brown GC: Congenital abnormalities of the optic disc. In Nelson LB, Calhoun JC, Harley RD (eds): Pediatric Ophthalmology, ed 3. Philadelphia, Saunders, 1991.
Dorrell D: The tilted disc. Br J Ophthalmol 62:16, 1978.

Riise D: The nasal fundus ectasia. Acta Ophthalmol 126 (suppl):5, 1975.
Riise D: Visual field defects in optic disc malformation with ectasia of the fundus. Acta Ophthalmol 44:906, 1966.
Rucker CW: Bitemporal defects in the visual fields resulting from developmental anomalies of the optic discs. Arch Ophthalmol 35:546, 1946.
Young SE, Walsh FB, Knox DL: The tilted disc syndrome. Br J Ophthalmol 82:16, 1976.

CHAPTER

14

INFECTIONS AND INFLAMMATION OF THE EYE

ESSENTIAL INFORMATION FOR PRIMARY CARE PRACTITIONERS

Infection in the Newborn (Ophthalmia Neonatorum)

"Ophthalmia neonatorum" is a term used to describe redness, swelling, and discharge of the eye and eyelids during the first few weeks of life. Etiologic agents include bacteria, viruses, and Chlamydia, and the differential includes chemical irritation from silver nitrate used to prevent *Neisseria gonorrhoeae* infection (Table 14–1). Although the time of onset and appearance of the ophthalmia often suggest the cause, special tests and cultures are usually obtained to confirm clinical suspicions.

Most neonatal ocular infections are acquired when the infant passes through the birth canal. Chlamydia is the most common infectious cause and is characterized by swelling of the eyelids and a watery or filmy discharge (Fig. 14–1). Although this infection rarely causes a severe ocular problem, infected infants may develop chlamydial pneumonia 2 to 3 months after birth. Because of this possibility, oral antibiotics are

used in conjunction with topical agents when the causative agent is Chlamydia. The infant's parents should also be examined and treated.

Neisseria gonorrhoeae infections usually present 2 to 4 days after birth, involve both eyes, and are characterized by marked injection and copious yellow discharge (Fig. 14–2). The development of a corneal ulcer and/or infection of the entire eye can result in blindness. Treatment consists of topical and systemic antibiotics. Prophylaxis involves instilling two drops of 1% silver nitrate solution, or a 1- to 2-cm ribbon of 0.5% erythromycin or 1% tetracycline ointment to the eyes, after wiping the eyelids with sterile cotton.

Other bacteria, principally *Staphylococcus*, can also infect the newborn eye. The time of onset for these infections is usually later than *N. gonorrhoeae* and their damage less severe. Cultures of the discharge direct specific topical antibiotic therapy.

Herpes virus infection is a very rare cause of ophthalmia neonatorum. Herpetic infections arise from 2 to 15 days after birth, and are characterized by swollen, red eyelids and a filmy discharge. Small blisters containing clear fluid often appear on the eyelids before the eyes become red. Corneal infection as well as a disseminated infection of multiple organ systems can occur. Topical and systemic antivirals are used.

Two other causes of red eyes in infants need to be differentiated from ophthalmia neonatorum. These are

Sections of this chapter have been modified and reprinted from Catalano RA: Ocular Emergencies. Philadelphia, Saunders, 1992; and Catalano RA, Nelson LB: Conjunctivitis. In Dershewitz RA (ed): Ambulatory Pediatric Care. Philadelphia, Lippincott, 1993, pp 366–369.

301

TABLE 14–1. COMMON CAUSES OF OPHTHALMIA NEONATORUM

Cause	Time of Onset	Course	Treatment
Neisseria gonorrhoeae	2–4 days	Severe and rapid	Antibiotics
Other bacteria	3–7 days	Moderate to severe	Antibiotics
Chlamydia	5–12 days	Moderate/pneumonia	Antibiotics
Herpes simplex	2–15 days	Moderate/generalized	Antivirals
▪ OTHER CAUSES OF RED EYES IN INFANTS			
Silver nitrate	< 24 hours	Mild and limited	Observation
Blocked tear duct (+/– infection)	> 2 weeks (usually)	Mild to moderate	Antibiotics

chemical conjunctivitis from the administration of silver nitrate, and infected blocked tear ducts. Silver nitrate mildly irritates the eyes of some children who develop mild redness and swelling. This appears within 24 hours of administration, resolves within 3 to 5 days, and requires no treatment. Conjunctivitis can also result when bacteria residing within a blocked tear duct spill over into the eye. Treatment is directed at opening the blocked tear duct (see Chapter 8).

Laboratory investigations are usually performed when infants present with red, swollen eyes and discharge (see "Laboratory Tests," later in the chapter.) Examination of the infant's parents for the presence of infection may also be helpful. Early treatment is usually effective for most types of conjunctivitis in the newborn.

Conjunctivitis

Signs and Symptoms

Infection of the conjunctival coat of the eye ("pink eye") is characterized by tearing, discharge, conjunctival injection, conjunctival swelling (chemosis), papillae, lymphoid follicles, membranes, pseudomembranes, and/or regional adenopathy. Papillae are thickened, polygonal elevations of the conjunctiva that form a mosaic pattern. A fibrovascular core is present at the center of each papilla, which erupts on the surface of the conjunctiva in a spoke-like pattern. Papillae occur in bacterial and allergic conjunctivitis; in the latter, giant papillae (> 1 mm in size) are found (Fig. 14–3). Lymphoid follicles represent active germinal centers and occur in adenoviral, herpetic, and toxic conjunctivitis. They appear as translucent, dome-shaped protuberances, 0.2 to 2.0 mm in diameter, with a lacy vascularization between the elevations (Fig. 14–4). Transudation of inflammatory cells and fibrin through the conjunctival blood vessels produces pseudomembranes and membranes (Fig. 14–5). The difference between these two is one of degree. True membranes are more adherent and cause bleeding when stripped from the conjunctiva. They occur in bacterial and viral (particularly adenoviral) infections.

History and Physical Exam

The workup of conjunctivitis includes a detailed history and conjunctival cultures. A history of recent exposure to a friend or family member with conjunctivi-

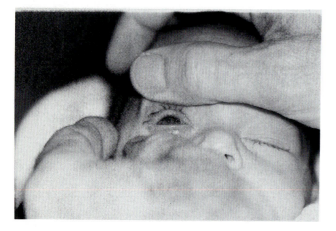

Figure 14–1. Red, swollen eyelids and watery (serous) discharge in an infant with chlamydial conjunctivitis. *(From Catalano RA: Ocular Emergencies. Philadelphia, Saunders, 1992, p 462, with permission.)*

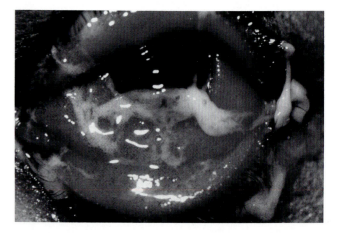

Figure 14–2. Adult with gonococcal conjunctivitis. Note the profuse purulent discharge. *(From Catalano RA: Ocular Emergencies. Philadelphia, Saunders, 1992, p 465, with permission.)*

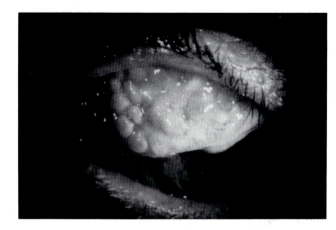

Figure 14–3. Giant papillary reaction in vernal conjunctivitis. *(From Catalano RA: Ocular Emergencies. Philadelphia, Saunders, 1992, p 29, with permission.)*

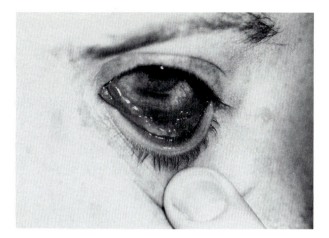

Figure 14–5. Membrane in adenoviral epidemic keratoconjunctivitis.

tis or an upper respiratory infection suggests a viral etiology. Itching is a prominent sign of allergy. Chronic itching in a boy with a ropy discharge (worse during the summer) is consistent with vernal conjunctivitis. Chronic injection and mucopurulent discharge in a sexually active adolescent is characteristic of chlamydial infection. A community epidemic of painful conjunctivitis characterized by conjunctival hemorrhages, pseudomembranes, and photophobia suggests adenoviral epidemic keratoconjunctivitis. Corneal involvement is suggested by severe pain and photophobia. The term used for this is keratoconjunctivitis, "kerato" meaning corneal.

The physical exam should characterize the discharge, presence of preauricular adenopathy, visual reduction, papillae, follicles, and (pseudo)membranes. Lesions on the lid margin should be sought (for example, molluscum contagiosum; Fig. 14–6), and skin vesicles should be noted (such as herpes simplex; Fig. 14–7). Examination with a hand-held magnifier under good illumination may demonstrate follicles or papil-

lae. Phenylephrine 2.5 percent eyedrops can be instilled to determine the depth of the hyperemic vessels. The hyperemia of conjunctivitis and secondary conjunctival reactions will be significantly blanched by phenylephrine, but the deeper hyperemic injection of iritis, scleritis, or glaucoma will not. If there is a question of corneal involvement, the instillation of one drop of fluorescein dye and examination with a Wood's lamp will vividly demonstrate any corneal involvement as a bright green defect.

Etiology

The cause of conjunctivitis can be narrowed by evaluating the patient's signs and symptoms (Table 14–2). It is important to differentiate conjunctivitis from ocular inflammation (iritis). Although acute glaucoma is very rare in childhood, it is usually included in the differential diagnosis (Table 14–3). Other causes of conjunctival irritation and inflammation include exposure, trichiasis (malpositioned eyelashes), eyelid infections (described later), blocked tear ducts, and trauma.

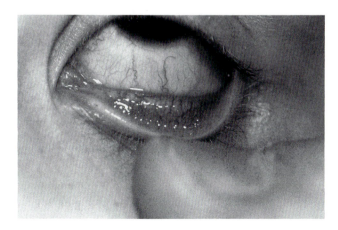

Figure 14–4. Follicular conjunctival reaction in viral conjunctivitis.

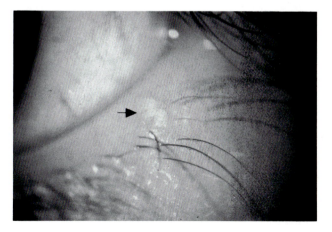

Figure 14–6. Molluscum contagiosum at eyelid margin *(arrow)*.

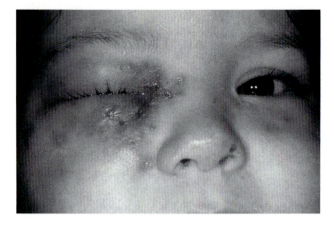

Figure 14–7. Primary herpetic conjunctivitis.

Additional information regarding etiologic agents is presented in the second half of this chapter.

Laboratory Tests

When the history and clinical findings are insufficient to render a definitive diagnosis, or when the infection is severe and recalcitrant to treatment, conjunctival cultures are indicated. The most widely used media for bacterial infections are blood and chocolate agar. Thayer–Martin medium is useful when gonococcus is suspected, and thioglycollate is used to isolate micro-aerophilic species. Chlamydial cultures have been nearly supplanted by immunologic tests for *Chlamydia* (described later), and viral cultures, which require special media and facilities, are usually not indicated.

Treatment

Topical antibiotics are used for bacterial infections. Ten to 15% sulfacetamide drops, 0.5 percent erythromycin ointment, and neomycin–polymixin–bacitracin combinations are equally efficacious, but allergic reactions to neomycin are common. The aminoglycosides are best reserved for severe infections caused by organisms that are especially sensitive to these drugs (such as *Pseudomonas* and *Proteus*). Steroids are contraindicated in bacterial conjunctivitis.

Viral conjunctivitis is self-limiting and usually does not require more than symptomatic treatment. If molluscum is present at the lid margin (Fig. 14–6), excision or curretage of the lesion may be necessary to cure the conjunctivitis. Removing the central core, which produces bleeding within the lesion, is usually necessary to prevent recurrence. Cryotherapy can be used, but may cause depigmentation of the surrounding skin. Mild herpetic vesicular eruption of the eyelids (Fig. 14–7) without involvement of the eyelid margins or conjunctiva requires no treatment. If vesicles are present on or near the lid margin, 1 percent trifluridine solution should be used six times per day until resolution. If conjunctival inflammation is present, referral to an ophthalmologist for a corneal examination is indicated. Presently available antivirals are ineffective against adenoviral conjunctivitis. Cold or hot compresses and artificial tears can provide some comfort. Topical corticosteroids for adenoviral disease should only be used sparingly and under careful ophthalmologic supervision. Some authorities believe that subepithelial infiltrates are actually worsened and prolonged with the use of steroids. Patients with adenovirus often have positive cultures for herpes simplex, and the latter can be made disastrously worse with the use of steroids.

Chlamydial infections in neonates are discussed later in the chapter. Infections in adolescents should be treated with oral erythromycin 250 mg four times daily for 2 weeks, or oral tetracycline 500 mg four times daily

TABLE 14–2. CONJUNCTIVITIS DIFFERENTIATED BY SIGNS AND SYMPTOMS

	Bacterial	Viral	Chlamydial	Allergic/Atopic
Discharge	Purulent	Serous	Mucopurulent	Serous
Cells on smear	PMN	Mononuclear	PMN/mononuclear	Eosinophil/PMN
Inclusions on stain (stain)	—	Herpes simplex (Papanicolaou stain)	+ (Giemsa stain)	—
Follicles	—	+	+	—
Papillae	+/–	—	+/–	+
Membrane	*Staphylococcus pyogenes* *Corynebacterium diphtheriae*	Adenovirus	—	+/– (Vernal)
Injection	+	+		+
Chemosis	+	+/–	+/–	+
Hemorrhage	Haemophilus	Adenovirus	—	—
Lymphadenopathy	—	+	+/–	—
Itching	—	—	—	+
Photophobia	—	Adenovirus	—	+/– (Vernal)
Bilaterality	+/–	Within days	+/–	+
Skin vesicles	—	Herpes simplex	—	—

PMN = polymorphonuclear neutrophil leukocytes.

TABLE 14–3. DIFFERENTIAL DIAGNOSIS OF CONJUNCTIVITIS

	Conjunctivitis	Acute Iridocyclitis	Angle-closure Glaucoma
■ *HISTORY*			
Onset	Gradual	Gradual	Sudden
Bilaterality	Often bilateral	Unilateral	Unilateral
Pain	Burning, itching	Moderate	Severe, boring
Photophobia	Absent except in keratoconjunctivitis (see text)	Severe	Moderate
■ *EXAMINATION*			
Vision	Normal	Decreased	Markedly decreased
Site of injection	Near cul-de-sac	Near limbus (ciliary flush)	
Injected vessels	Bright red, move with the conjunctiva	Diffuse violaceous color, do not move when the conjunctiva is moved with a cotton-tipped applicator	
Phenylephrine test	Vessels blanch	Vessels do not blanch	
Discharge	Watery or purulent	Watery	Watery
Cornea	Clear	Usually clear, +/– posterior deposits	Cloudy if prolonged
Pupil size	Normal size	Small	Mid-dilated
Pupil reaction	Normal	Slow or absent	Unreactive
Intraocular pressure	Normal	Normal or low	Increased
Anterior chamber angle	Open	Open	Closed

for 7 to 10 days. Concomitant topical therapy is unnecessary. Chlamydial infections in young children should be viewed as highly suspicious of sexual abuse.

The itching and discomfort of allergic conjunctivitis can be treated with cold compresses and oral antihistamines. If the patient remains symptomatic, the judicious use of topical antihistamines and vasoconstrictors can be tried. Sodium cromoglycolate (Cromolyn) 4 percent prevents the release of histamine and other biochemical mediators from mast cells and has been shown to be efficacious when used four times per day in atopic conjunctivitis. It may also be valuable as adjunctive therapy in vernal conjunctivitis. Topical corticosteroids are the mainstay of therapy in this disorder, but are associated with an increased incidence of cataracts and glaucoma. Iced compresses, dark glasses, and oral antihistamines may also be of some benefit. The surgical removal of papillae and desensitization to inhalant allergens have not generally been found effective in the treatment of vernal disease.

Eyelid Infections

The many terms used to describe different infections of the eyelids are often confused and used inappropriately. **Blepharitis** simply means inflammation of the eyelids. **Squamous blepharitis** is characterized by hypertrophy and desquamation of the epidermis near the lid margin (Fig. 14–8). The affected eyelid is erythematous and scaly. **Ulcerative blepharitis** occurs when glands at the eyelid margin become purulently inflamed and ulcerate. Chronic blepharitis can result in loss of eyelashes (madarosis), secondary conjunctivitis, thickening of the eyelid margin, and chalazia (described below). Individuals with Down syndrome or immune deficiency are at greatest risk. Commonly isolated organisms include *Staphylococcus* and *Streptococcus*, and management involves lid hygiene (lid scrubs with diluted baby shampoo) and topical antibiotics three or four times daily until resolution. Individuals susceptible to recurrence should continue lid scrubs indefinitely.

Infections of the glands of the eyelid are called **hordeola.** An abscess of one of the sweat or sebaceous glands of a lash follicle (glands of Moll and Zeiss) is called an **external hordeolum,** or **stye.** These present superficially at the margin of the eyelid as red, swollen, tender pustules (Fig. 14–9). The pathogenic organism is

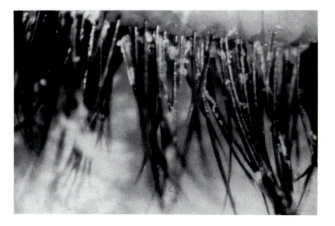

Figure 14–8. Squamous blepharitis.

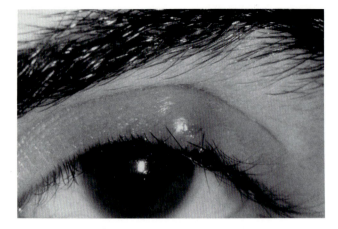

Figure 14–9. External hordeolum or stye. *(From Catalano RA: Ocular Emergencies. Philadelphia, Saunders, 1992, p 469, with permission.)*

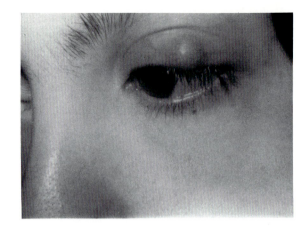

Figure 14–11. Chalazion in the left upper eyelid.

commonly *Staphylococcus.* An infection of the large sebaceous gland inside the tarsus of the eyelid (the meibomian gland) is called an **internal hordeolum,** or **meibomianitis.** These infections occur deep in the eyelid, and are usually larger than styes (Fig. 14–10). Eversion of the eyelids may demonstrate elevation and injection of the overlying conjunctiva, and pointing of a pustule to the surface. Hordeola are treated with a topical antibiotic ointment (such as erythromycin or Polysporin) into the conjunctival sac. Warm compresses may also be helpful by increasing blood flow to the eyelid. Incision and drainage is indicated if the infection does not begin to resolve within 48 hours. Systemic antibiotics are indicated only if cellulitis develops (cellulitis is described later in the chapter under "Orbital Infections").

A **chalazion** results from chronic inflammation of a meibomian gland of the eyelid. It arises from obstruction of the gland duct, often subsequent to chronic blepharitis, meibomianitis, or a hordeola. Usually the midportion of the gland (and therefore eyelid) is in-

volved (Fig. 14–11). Chalazia are palpably firm, nontender nodules. Histologically they are composed of sterile lipogranulomatous inflammation. Warm compresses may be all that is needed to cause small chalazia to spontaneously rupture and resolve. Many clinicians prescribe a topical antibiotic four times per day, but the efficacy of an antibiotic in a sterile inflammation is questionable. Larger chalazia may require incision and curettage, or topical injection with a short-acting steroid (0.2 to 0.5 mL of triamcinolone 40 mg/mL). Steroid injections should be performed from the conjunctival side. Complications of steroid injection include skin depigmentation, atrophy of the overlying skin, and granuloma formation.

A **pyogenic granuloma** is a fleshy-appearing and often pedunculated mass on the conjunctival surface of the eyelid (Fig. 14–12). They result from chronic inflammation due to an eyelid infection or foreign body. They are highly vascularized, can enlarge rapidly, and bleed spontaneously. Surgical excision is usually required.

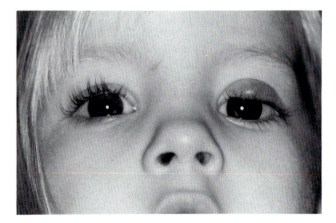

Figure 14–10. Internal hordeolum or meibomianitis.

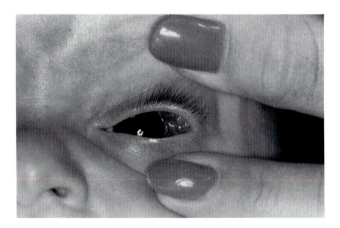

Figure 14–12. Pyogenic granuloma.

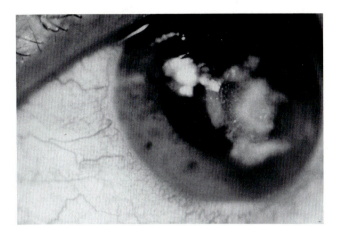

Figure 14–13. Corneal ulcer.

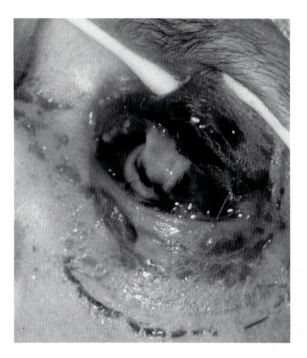

Figure 14–15. Untreated corneal ulcer resulting in corneal perforation and endophthalmitis. *(From Catalano RA: Ocular Emergencies. Philadelphia, Saunders, 1992, p 484, with permission.)*

Ocular Infections

Corneal Ulcers

Patients with corneal infections present with pain, injection, photophobia (light sensitivity), mucopurulent discharge, and decreased vision. The term **corneal ulcer** describes an infiltrate in the corneal stroma associated with an overlying corneal epithelial defect (Fig. 14–13). Additional signs of inflammation include folds in Descemet's membrane and inflammatory cells within the anterior chamber of the eye (uveitis), which may layer to form a hypopyon (Fig. 14–14). Untreated, a corneal ulcer can lead to corneal perforation and endophthalmitis (intraocular infection; Fig. 14–15).

Although the ocular history and examination may suggest an etiology, corneal scrapings for Gram stain and culture are mandatory prior to initiating therapy. Treatment regimens differ based on the clinical severity and potential pathogens encountered in the patient's geographic area. Antibiotics are chosen based upon the results of cultures and sensitivities, and the patient's response. Frequent (hourly) antibiotic use is often required. To increase compliance and monitor progress, hospitalization is usually required.

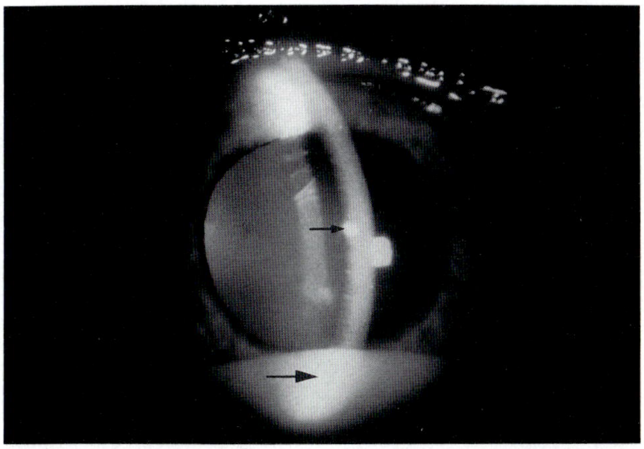

Endophthalmitis

Endophthalmitis is most commonly seen following intraocular surgery. Patients present with conjunctival injection and swelling (chemosis), increasing pain, and decreasing vision beginning 1 to 2 days after surgery. Marked eyelid edema and inflammatory cells within the eye are common (Figs. 14–16 and 14–17). The cellular reaction in the eye usually obscures the red reflex. The most common source of bacteria is normal flora of the periocular area. Management includes culture of aqueous and vitreous aspirates, and intravitreal, topical, and intravenous antibiotics.

Disseminated candidiasis is becoming an increasingly important pathogen in the premature nursery. Up to 3 percent of very-low-birthweight infants develop systemic candidiasis associated with the use of broad-spectrum antibiotics, parenteral alimentation, and indwelling catheters (Johnson et al, 1985). *Candida* endophthalmitis occurs in as many as 50 percent of these infants (Baley et al, 1981). Oral ketoconazole or fluconazole may be the most appropriate systemic agents for sensitive organisms. Therapeutic vitreous concentrations have been demonstrated with oral administration of ketoconazole. The side effects of this therapy include gastrointestinal distress and a tran-

Figure 14–14. Folds in Descemet's membrane and hypopyon (*large arrow*) from corneal ulcer (*small arrow*). *(From Catalano RA: Ocular Emergencies. Philadelphia, Saunders, 1992, p 490, with permission.)*

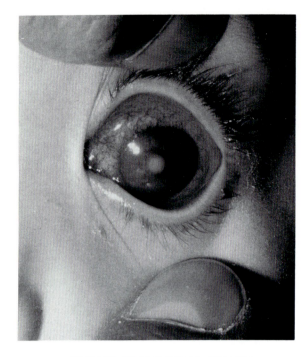

Figure 14–16. Bacterial endophthalmitis.

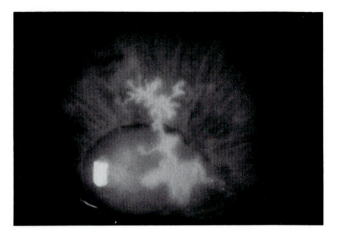

Figure 14–18. Dendritic herpetic keratitis. *(From Catalano RA: Ocular Emergencies. Philadelphia, Saunders, 1992, p 480, with permission.)*

sient rise in serum liver enzymes. Amphotericin B, however, is still recommended for intraocular use. Intravenous amphotericin B is less frequently used due to its associated side effects of anemia and azotemia, and *Candida* isolates resistant to flucytosine have been reported (Pflugfelder et al, 1988). Vitrectomy and surgical excision of visibly infected ocular tissues in the infected premature infant are controversial. Surgical intervention should be based on the response to systemic antifungals (Annable et al, 1990).

Herpes Simplex Keratitis
Primary infections with herpes simplex virus present with unilateral eyelid vesicles and follicular conjunctivitis (see Figs. 14–7 and 14–89). Following the primary

infection, the herpes virus can remain dormant in the trigeminal ganglion until a precipitating factor (such as stress, trauma, fever, or bright sunlight) reactivates the virus. Recurrent infections present as epithelial keratitis.

Herpetic epithelial keratitis presents with a unilateral red eye, pain, photophobia, tearing, and decreased vision. The most common manifestation is an epithelial branching "dendritic" ulcer, which can be easily visualized using a Wood's lamp after staining with fluorescein dye (Fig. 14–18). Although not helpful on skin lesions, several antiviral agents are active against herpetic corneal lesions. Trifluridine ointment every 2 hours while awake (maximum six doses per day) is recommended. An alternate treatment is simple mechanical debridement of the dendritic ulcer with a cotton-tipped swab. If inflammation of the anterior eye is also present, the addition of a topical cycloplegic agent (such as Cyclogel 1%) three times daily is useful to relieve pain from spasm of the ciliary muscle. The differential diagnosis includes herpes zoster virus infection

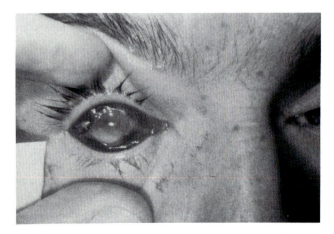

Figure 14–17. Fungal endophthalmitis.

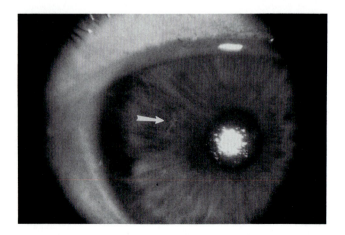

Figure 14–19. Pseudodendrite of a healing corneal abrasion (*arrow*).

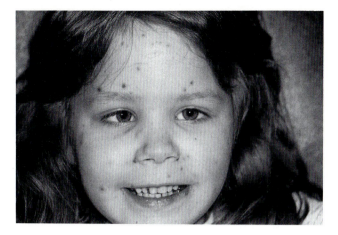

Figure 14–20. Chickenpox.

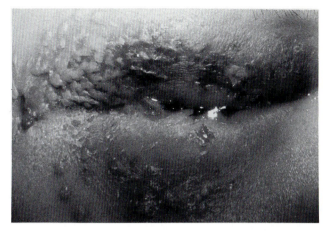

Figure 14–22. Confluent pustular skin lesions of herpes zoster infection.

(described below) and a healing epithelial defect from a corneal abrasion (Fig. 14–19). Less common clinical forms of herpes simplex keratitis are discussed in the latter half of this chapter.

Herpes Zoster Ophthalmicus

Herpes zoster ophthalmicus (HZO) is caused by the varicella-zoster virus. The initial infection results in chickenpox (Fig. 14–20). Similar to herpes simplex the virus remains dormant in the trigeminal ganglion until reactivated by stress, concurrent infection, or malignancy. Reactivation involves any of the branches of the trigeminal ganglion; when the ophthalmic nerve is in-volved, the term "ophthalmicus" is used. Involvement of the tip of the nose suggests that the eye will be involved (Hutchinson's sign; Fig. 14–21).

HZO is most commonly encountered in young children and older adults. It presents with a prodrome of fever, malaise, chills, and a burning or tingling sensation in the involved dermatome. Erythematous skin lesions appear within 2 days and gradually progress to vesicular lesions. Skin lesions can become confluent and form pustules and crusted lesions (Fig. 14–22). Additional ocular findings include conjunctivitis, keratitis, and inflammation of any region of the eye including the retina, choroid, sclera, and optic nerve (Fig. 14–23).

Oral acyclovir 800 mg five times per day for 7 to 10 days is the recommended treatment. Cool compresses and artificial tears may be symptomatically helpful. A topical cycloplegic agent (for example, Cyclogel 1 percent) and corticosteroid (such as prednisolone acetate 1 percent) three times daily are warranted if intraocular inflammation is present.

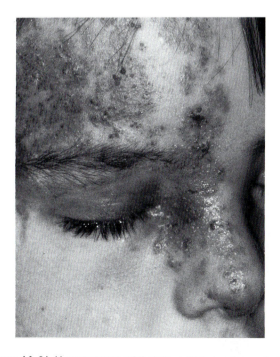

Figure 14–21. Herpes zoster ophthalmicus. Note involvement of the tip of the nose (Hutchinson's sign). (From Catalano RA: Ocular Emergencies. Philadelphia, Saunders, 1992, p 486, with permission.)

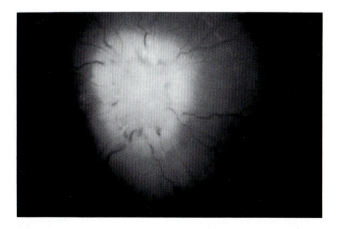

Figure 14–23. Herpes zoster optic neuritis in an immunocompromised child.

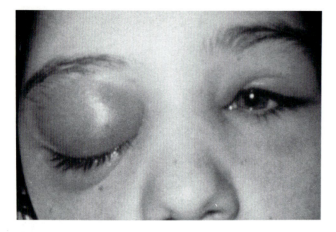

Figure 14–24. Preseptal cellulitis. *(From Catalano RA: Ocular Emergencies. Philadelphia, Saunders, 1992, p 467, with permission.)*

Orbital Infections

An infectious process that involves only the subcutaneous tissue of the eyelid, brow, or forehead is called **preseptal cellulitis** (Fig. 14–24). Involvement deeper than the orbital septum is called **orbital cellulitis** (Fig. 14–25).

Preseptal cellulitis is often preceded by local skin infections, facial trauma, and upper respiratory or middle ear infections. The patient presents with erythema, swelling, and tenderness of the eyelids and periorbital area. Conjunctivitis and conjunctival swelling (chemosis) may also be present. Orbital cellulitis presents with all of the signs of preseptal cellulitis with the addition of reduced visual acuity, decreased ocular motility, diplopia, pain on ocular movement, and abnormal pupillary reaction. It is the most common cause of sudden protrusion of the eye (proptosis) in childhood, and can

be accompanied by fever, leukocytosis, lid edema, and rhinorrhea. Table 14–4 differentiates the clinical findings in preseptal and septal cellulitis.

The pathogenic organism in preseptal cellulitis resulting from hordeola is almost always *Staphylococcus aureus,* or *Streptococcus pyogenes* or *pneumoniae.* Anaerobic infections (as from *Clostridium* or *Bacillus*) can occur in contaminated traumatic wounds. The management of preseptal cellulitis involves culturing any purulent material, draining any fluctuant abscesses, and instituting systemic antibiotics. In children over 5 years of age a 48- to 72-hour course of a penicillinase-resistant oral penicillin (such as nafcillin 150 mg/kg per day in four to six doses) or cephalosporin (such as Augmentin 20 to 40 mg/kg per day in three divided doses) is generally acceptable. In penicillin-allergic children, Bactrim (8/40 mg/kg per day in two divided doses), or erythromycin 30 to 50 mg/kg per day in four divided doses) can be used. If the patient is under 5 years, intravenous therapy is required. Cefuroxime is suggested because of the possibility of *Haemophilus influenzae* infection (see discussion later in the chapter). Intravenous therapy is also required if the preseptal cellulitis is not responding to oral antibiotics, or if signs of orbital cellulitis develop.

Orbital cellulitis usually results from the spread of infection in the paranasal sinuses. In children, the ethmoid is the most commonly involved sinus (Fig. 14–26). Other causes include puncture wounds deep to the orbital septum, surgical trauma, acute dacryocystitis (infection of the lacrimal sac), extension from intracranial or dental abscesses, and endogenous bacteremia. *H. influenzae* type B is the most common bacteremic cause in children.

Uncontrolled orbital cellulitis can thrombose the blood supply of the retina and choroid, leading to in-

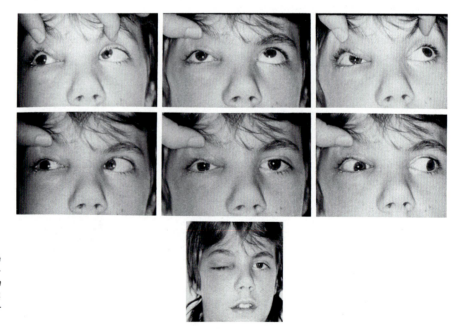

Figure 14–25. Orbital cellulitis involving the right eye. Note the restriction of ocular movement outward, inward, and upward. *(From Nelson LB, Catalano RA: Atlas of Ocular Motility. Philadelphia, Saunders, 1989, p 201, with permission.)*

TABLE 14–4. DIFFERENTIAL CLINICAL FINDINGS IN PRESEPTAL AND ORBITAL CELLULITIS

Sign or Symptom	Preseptal Cellulitis	Orbital Cellulitis[a]
Visual acuity	Normal	Reduced
Proptosis	Absent	Marked
Ocular motility	Normal	Restricted
Pain	Absent or minimal	Moderate to severe
Fever	Absent or minimal	High
Leukocytosis	Absent to moderate	Marked
Lid swelling	Mild to moderate	Marked
Chemosis	Absent to moderate	Marked
Sensation over V_1, V_2	Normal	May be reduced
Mean age	2 years	7 to 9 years

[a]Cavernous sinus involvement is suggested by the progressive involvement of multiple cranial nerves, diminished pupillary response, optic disc edema, congestion of the retinal veins, infarction of the retina or choroid, and bilaterality.

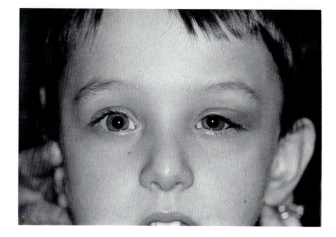

Figure 14–27. Acute dacryoadenitis of the left eye. Note "S"-shaped deformity of the upper eyelid.

farction. It can also extend to the cavernous sinus, orbital apex, or cranium. Orbital and subperiosteal orbital abscesses can result, and are suggested by the lack of response to adequate antibiotic therapy. Orbital cellulitis always requires intravenous antibiotics, and orbital abscesses require surgical drainage (see later discussion).

Lacrimal Infections

Acute dacryoadenitis is an infection of the lacrimal gland. It presents with unilateral swelling, erythema, and localized tenderness of the gland. Chemosis and conjunctival injection, as well as an "S"-shaped deformity of the gland, may be present (Fig. 14–27). The globe may be proptotic and displaced inferiorly and nasally. Fever, leukocytosis, and preauricular lymphadenopathy are usually found. The etiology may be viral (mumps, influenza, Epstein–Barr virus) or bacterial (*Staphylococcus*, *Streptococcus*, and *Neisseria gonorrhoeae*). Management includes culture of any discharge, complete blood count, and when proptosis or ophthalmoplegia are present, computed tomography of the orbit. Bacterial causes usually respond to Augmentin 20 to 40 mg/kg per day in three divided doses for 7 to 10 days. If an abscess develops, surgical drainage is necessary.

Congenital nasolacrimal duct obstruction (NLDO) occurs in nearly 5 percent of otherwise healthy infants. It is usually the result of a failure of the distal end of the lacrimal duct to fully canalize into the nose. Infants with congenital NLDO present with unilateral or bilateral overflow tearing onto the cheeks (Fig. 14–28). Some patients present with a dilated lacrimal sac filled

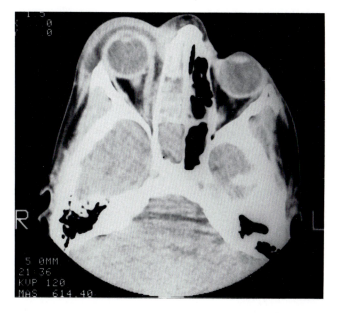

Figure 14–26. Computed tomography demonstrating ethmoid involvement in orbital cellulitis.

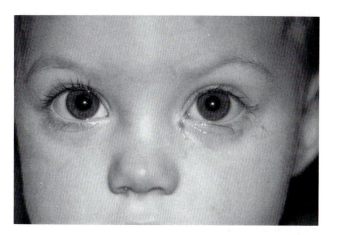

Figure 14–28. Congenital nasolacrimal duct obstruction without infection. Note the wet-appearing eye and overflow tearing onto the face.

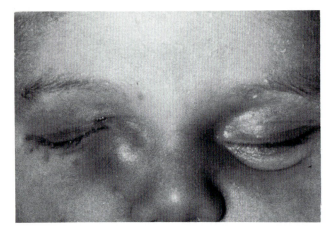

Figure 14–29. Lacrimal sac mucocele.

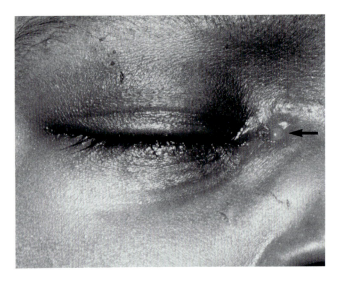

Figure 14–31. Lacrimal sac fistula. Note the teardrop at the openning of the fistula (*arrow*). (*From Catalano RA: Ocular Emergencies. Philadelphia, Saunders, 1992, p 223, with permission.*)

with mucous (lacrimal sac mucocele; Fig. 14–29). Others present with an indolent infection characterized by mucopurulent discharge and crusting of the lid margins on the affected side (chronic dacryocystitis) and/or chronic conjunctivitis (Fig. 14–30). A few children present with acute dacryocystitis requiring urgent treatment.

A **lacrimal sac mucocele** (amniocele, amniotocele, dacryocystocele) presents within the first few days of life as a firm, cystic, bluish mass inferior to the medial canthal angle (Fig. 14–29). It results from a combined obstruction of the nasolacrimal system distal and proximal to the lacrimal sac. Mucous is unable to reflux onto the eye and continues to accumulate until pressure within the sac prevents further production. Occasionally, an infected dilated lacrimal sac spontaneously decompresses with the development of a fistula be-

tween the lacrimal sac and overlying skin (Fig. 14–31). Warm compresses should be tried as the initial therapy. If unsuccessful after 2 days, or if any sign of inflammation develops, probing of the lacrimal duct should be performed. Untreated mucoceles usually become infected, often with a fulminant course. If acute dacryocystitis or cellulitis develops, intravenous antibiotics will be required (see discussion later in the chapter).

Chronic dacryocystitis is an indolent infection characterized by tearing (epiphora), blepharitis, and a mild chronic conjunctivitis (see Fig. 14–30). Mucopurulent discharge can often be expressed from the inferior punctum (Fig. 14–32). These children require early probing and irrigation to relieve the obstructed nasolacrimal duct. While awaiting this, one drop of a topical antibiotic (such as sulfacetamide 10 or 15%; Poly-

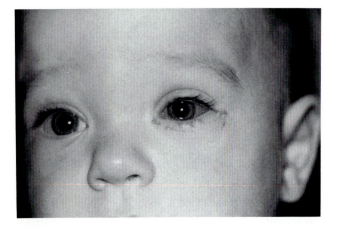

Figure 14–30. Congenital nasolacrimal duct obstruction with infection. Note discharge and crusting about the eyelids and the secondary conjunctivitis.

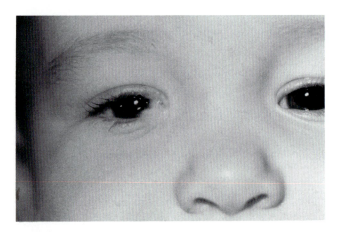

Figure 14–32. Mucopurulent discharge expressed from the inferior punctum in a child with chronic dacryocystitis.

trim) can be used on a daily basis to reduce pathogenic flora.

Acute dacryocystitis is a bacterial infection of the lacrimal sac. In newborns, it arises secondary to obstruction of the nasolacrimal duct. Affected infants can present with the rapid development of erythema and swelling over the lacrimal sac. Treatment includes massage, topical erythromycin ointment, and oral Augmentin or Ceclor (20 to 40 mg/kg per day in three divided doses). If systemic signs (such as fever) are present, however, hospitalization and treatment with Cefuroxime 50 to 100 mg/kg per day in three divided doses is recommended.

The differential diagnosis of congenital NLDO in infancy includes infantile glaucoma, primary infectious conjunctivitis, keratitis (corneal inflammation or irritation), uveitis (intraocular inflammation), and eyelid anomalies that cause the eyelids or eyelashes to touch the cornea. Infantile glaucoma is characterized by corneal edema or haze, increased corneal diameter, enlarged cup-to-disc ratio, and myopia. It also presents with photophobia, as do keratitis and uveitis. Conjunctivitis is characterized by discharge more than tearing. Older children with conjunctivitis will also have papillae or follicles. The presence of mucopurulent discharge from the puncta upon palpation of the lacrimal sac is diagnostic of lacrimal duct obstruction. The absence of this sign, however, does not preclude this diagnosis.

The differential diagnosis of a lacrimal sac mucocele includes encephalocele, ethmoid mucocele, hemangioma, and dermoid. These disorders should be considered when the mass extends above the medial canthal tendon. Neuroradiological imaging should be obtained if the diagnosis is uncertain, especially if an encephalocele is a possibility.

Intraocular Inflammation (Uveitis)

Uveitis is a general term meaning inflammation of the uvea (one of the three coats of the eye). More specific terms describe inflammation of the iris (iritis), ciliary body (cyclitis), iris and ciliary body (iridocyclitis), pars plana (pars planitis), and choroid (choroiditis). Additional terms describe inflammation in nonuveal ocular structures including the retina (retinitis), vitreous (vitritis), the vasculature of the retina (vasculitis, periphlebitis), the retinal pigment epithelium (epitheliitis), sclera (scleritis), and episclera (episcleritis).

Over 100 disease syndromes can be associated with inflammation within the eye. Although a complete description of these is beyond the scope of this chapter, the workup for certain common entities, based on the patient's sex, race, and location of the primary inflammation, is presented in Table 14–5. Syphilis and tuberculosis are two disorders that should always be considered in the patient with uveitis because they are common and can be specifically treated. An FTA-ABS serologic test can confirm whether the patient ever had syphilis, and a VDRL can determine its state of activity. Both should be ordered if syphilis is under consideration. Any previous systemic infection with tuberculosis is diagnosed with a tuberculin PPD-#2 skin test and chest x-ray.

TABLE 14–5. SUGGESTED UVEITIS WORKUP

Primary Site	Sex	Race	Potential Disorder	Suggested Tests
Iridocyclitis	M/F	B/W	Syphilis	FTA-ABS, VDRL
	M/F	B/W	Tuberculosis	PPD, chest x-ray, ESR
	F	B/W	Juvenile rheumatoid arthritis	ANA, knee x-ray, ESR
	F	B	Sarcoidosis	Chest x-ray, skin test anergy, gallium scan, serum ACE level, serum calcium level, Kveim test
	M	W	Ankylosing spondylitis, Reiter's syndrome	Sacroiliac joint x-ray, HLA-B27, ESR
Chorioretinitis	M/F	B/W	Toxocariasis	ELISA for toxocara, ESR, CBC (for eosinophilia)
	M/F	B/W	Toxoplasmosis	Serological tests, indirect FA test, hemagglutination test
	M/F	B/W	Histoplasmosis	Histoplasma skin test, chest x-ray, HLA-B7
	M/F	B/W	Cytomegalovirus, herpes zoster ophthalmicus, acute retinal necrosis	Serological tests for acquired immune deficiency syndrome (AIDS)
	M/F	B/W	Tuberculosis	As above
	M/F	B/W	Syphilis	As above
	F	B	Sarcoidosis	As above

Abbreviations: M/F = male or female; M = male; F = female; B/W = black or white; B = black; W = white; FTA-ABS = fluorescent treponemal antibody absorption test; VDRL = venereal disease research lab test; PPD = purified protein derivative (tuberculin skin test); ANA = antinuclear antibody test; ESR = erythrocyte sedimentation rate; HLA = human leukocyte antigen; FA = fluorescent antibody test; ELISA = enzyme-linked immunosorbent assay; CBC = complete blood count; ACE = angiotensin-converting enzyme.

TABLE 14–6. GRANULOMATOUS VERSUS NONGRANULOMATOUS UVEITIS

Characteristic	Granulomatous	Non-granulomatous
Onset	Insidious	Acute
Pain	Minimal to moderate	Moderate to marked
Injection	None to minimal	Marked ciliary flush
Photophobia	Minimal to moderate	Moderated to marked
Keratic precipitates[a]	Medium to large	Small to medium
Presence of fibrin	None to minimal	Minimal to marked
Iris nodules	May be present	None

[a]Focal collections of inflammatory cells and cellular debris on the posterior surface of the cornea.

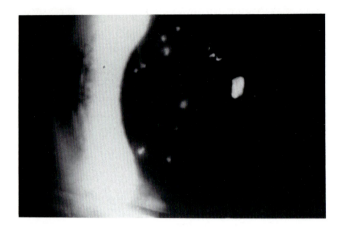

Figure 14–34. Large "mutton-fat" keratic precipitates in granulomatous uveitis.

Uveitic entities are commonly divided into two groups: granulomatous and nongranulomatous. The differences between the two are presented in Table 14–6. This classification does not help to establish etiology, because several organisms can cause both types of reaction. Nonetheless, it is useful for descriptive purposes.

The symptoms of uveitis include decreased vision, pain, and photophobia. Signs include ocular injection and inflammatory cells, fibrin, and nodules within the eye. Ocular injection in uveitis is characterized by the predominant involvement of the circumcorneal blood vessels. These radially arranged blood vessels are deep to the conjunctiva and give the eye a violaceous color centered around the cornea (ciliary flush; Fig. 14–33). In contrast to conjunctivitis, the injected vessels do not move on pressure with a cotton applicator, and do not blanch with phenylephrine (see Table 14–3). Inflammatory cells within the eye create the photophobia. They

can be detected by slit-lamp examination. Collections of inflammatory cells and debris on the posterior surface of the cornea are called keratic precipitates. Keratic precipitates in granulomatous uveitis are large and greasy appearing ("mutton-fat" keratic precipitates; Fig. 14–34). They are smaller in nongranulomatous uveitis (Fig. 14–35). Intraocular nodules are associated with granulomatous uveitis. They are commonly located within the iris (Fig. 14–36), choroid, or retina.

Granulomatous uveitis has an insidious onset. An affected child may be unaware of its onset, and complain only when vision becomes very blurred. There is characteristically minimal redness or pain. "Mutton-fat" keratic precipitates and inflammatory nodules may be seen. Long-standing granulomatous uveitis can be associated with the development of calcific band keratopathy. This occurs secondary to the deposition of calcium salts in the anterior layers of the cornea, and is characteristically associated with juvenile rheu-

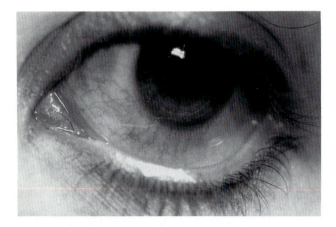

Figure 14–33. Ocular injection in uveitis. Note the predominant involvement of the radially arranged blood vessels surrounding the cornea (ciliary flush).

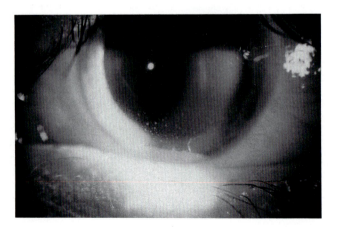

Figure 14–35. Smaller keratic precipitates in nongranulomatous uveitis. Also note the hypopyon.

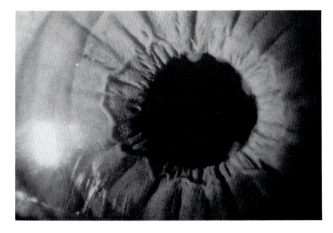

Figure 14–36. Inflammatory iris nodules at the pupillary margin in a patient with sarcoidosis (Koeppe nodules).

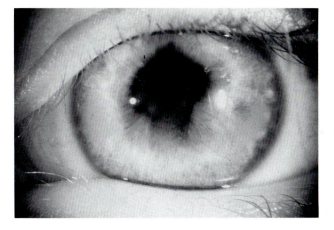

Figure 14–38. Inflammatory adhesions of the posterior iris to the anterior lens capsule (posterior synechiae) in juvenile rheumatoid arthritis.

matoid arthritis, sarcoidosis, and leprosy (Fig. 14–37). Band keratopathy is usually limited to the interpalpebral area.

Nongranulomatous uveitis has a much more acute onset. It is characterized by marked pain, photophobia, tearing, and blurred vision. Injection of the scleral and episcleral vessels surrounding the cornea (limbal flush) is common. Additional findings of nongranulomatous uveitis include a small (miotic) pupil and the presence of inflammatory cells and protein flare on slit-lamp examination.

With severe inflammation, adhesions of the iris to the cornea (anterior synechiae), or of the posterior iris to the anterior lens capsule (posterior synechiae) can develop, regardless of the type of uveitis (Fig. 14–38).

Common uveitic entities are reviewed in the "Uveitic Entities in Children" section later in the chapter.

Episcleritis

Episcleritis is a transient, usually self-limited inflammation of the outermost layers of the white of the eye. The term is derived from "epi" (meaning on, near, or over) the sclera. It presents as either a diffuse (Fig. 14–39) or sectoral (Fig. 14–40) inflammation.

Most cases of episcleritis are idiopathic and many affected patients are asymptomatic. Bilateral involvement occurs in 30 percent. Examination reveals prominent, inflamed, radial, superficial, episcleral vessels. The episcleral tissue is usually salmon pink to red, and is movable with a cotton-tipped applicator over the underlying sclera. Episcleritis can be differentiated from scleritis with the use of a topical vasoconstrictor (such as phenylephrine 2.5%). This will decrease the redness of episcleritis, but not scleritis. In the latter disease, the deeper scleral vessels remain engorged. These are also not movable with a cotton-tipped applicator. As op-

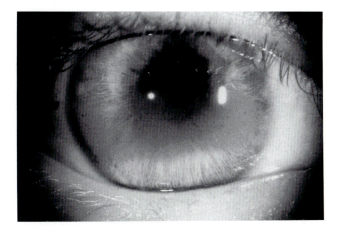

Figure 14–37. Calcific band keratopathy in long-standing uveitis associated with juvenile rheumatoid arthritis.

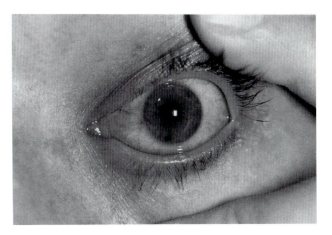

Figure 14–39. Diffuse episcleritis.

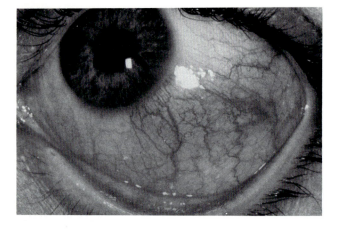

Figure 14–40. Sectoral episcleritis. Only the inferotemporal quadrant of the eye is involved. *(From Catalano RA: Ocular Emergencies. Philadelphia, Saunders, 1992, p 487, with permission.)*

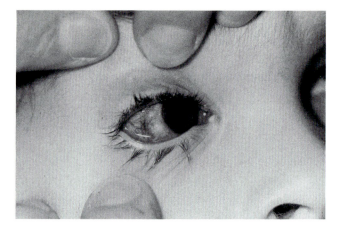

Figure 14–42. Nodular scleritis. Note elevated inflammatory nodules near the cornea. *(From Catalano RA: Ocular Emergencies. Philadelphia, Saunders, 1992, p 488, with permission.)*

posed to episcleritis and scleritis, the involved vessels in conjunctivitis are not radially arranged.

Laboratory tests should be performed only in recurrent or prolonged cases. Suggested studies are FTA-ABS, rheumatoid factor, antinuclear antibody, and serum uric acid. Treatment is supportive as most cases resolve in a few weeks without sequelae. In recurrent or severe cases associated with moderate discomfort, topical steroids (for example, FML three times daily) or topical or systemic anti-inflammatory agents (such as oral indomethacin 25 to 50 mg two or three times per day) can be used.

Scleritis

Scleritis is a severe inflammatory disease of the sclera and episclera. It is most commonly associated with collagen vascular disease, especially rheumatoid arthritis,

and therefore rarely occurs in children. It can occur, however, in association with syphilis, herpes simplex, herpes zoster, and tuberculosis.

Scleritis is bilateral in more than half of all cases. More than 95 percent involve the anterior sclera; the remainder present as posterior scleritis. Anterior scleritis presents as diffuse (Fig. 14–41), nodular (Fig. 14–42), or necrotizing (Fig. 14–43) inflammation. Diffuse episcleritis presents as a widespread area of inflammation without nodules or necrosis. It is the most common and benign form of scleritis. Nodular episcleritis is characterized by red, tender, immobile nodules that do not blanch with phenylephrine. Necrotizing episcleritis is the most destructive form. It results in the destruction of sclera, with potential exposure of the underlying uveal tissue. A rare form, scleromalacia perforans, presents with progressive scleral thinning without inflammation. This form is usually associated

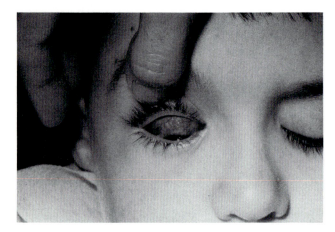

Figure 14–41. Diffuse scleritis.

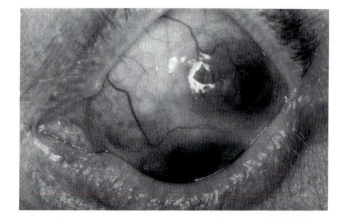

Figure 14–43. Necrotizing scleritis. Discoloration is uvea visible through thinned overlying sclera. *(From Catalano RA: Ocular Emergencies. Philadelphia, Saunders, 1992, p 489, with permission.)*

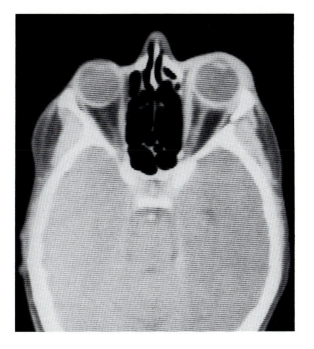

Figure 14–44. Scleral enhancement of the right eye on computed tomography in a patient with pseudotumor and posterior scleritis. *(From Catalano RA: Ocular Emergencies. Philadelphia, Saunders, 1992, p 302, with permission.)*

with severe rheumatoid arthritis, and as such is very unusual in children. Posterior scleritis is characterized by pain, proptosis (outward displacement of the eye), edema of the optic nerve head, and serous retinal detachments (secondary to exudated fluid). Scleral enhancement on computed tomography is a characteristic finding (Fig. 14–44).

Patients with scleritis usually present with deep throbbing pain localized to the forehead or periocular area. The sclera is edematous, and the scleral and episcleral vessels are engorged, giving the eye a purplish red color. Complications can include cataracts, intraocular inflammation, and glaucoma. Laboratory investigation should include sedimentation rate, FTA-ABS, rheumatoid factor, antinuclear antibody, PPD skin test, and chest x-ray. Topical corticosteroids can be used as adjunctive therapy, but are usually inadequate to treat scleritis. Oral nonsteroidal agents (for example, indomethacin or flurbiprofen) are often adequate, but oral prednisone (60 to 100 mg daily) may be necessary for severe non-necrotizing cases, and is mandatory for necrotizing episcleritis. Other immunosuppressive agents (cyclophosphamide, azathioprine, methotrexate, and cylcosporine A) have had limited reported success.

Referral Criteria and Precautions

Ophthalmia neonatorum is best managed using a team approach, involving the primary care practitioner, ophthalmologist, and infectious disease specialist. Neonates with gonococcal and herpetic infections require

hospitalization, isolation, and intravenous antibiotics or antivirals. Infants with other infections can usually be managed on an outpatient basis, unless systemic infection is suspected. Parents of infants infected with venereal-type diseases should be treated concomitantly. It is mandatory to report venereal disease in most states.

The primary care practitioner should be able to treat most cases of conjunctivitis. Referral to an ophthalmologist is appropriate if the conjunctivitis is hyperacute or recalcitrant, or if intraocular inflammation cannot be ruled out. Children with eyelid infections should be referred if there is no improvement after 48 hours of treatment with hot packs and topical antibiotics. Orbital infections are treated by a team approach, similar to ophthalmia neonatorum. When the sinuses are involved, an otolaryngologist should be consulted. Children with severe preseptal cellulitis and orbital cellulitis require hospitalization for intravenous antibiotics, and close monitoring of their ocular and neurological status.

Any ocular infection that involves the cornea or intraocular structures should be promptly referred to the ophthalmologist. Corneal ulcers usually require hospitalization and frequent applications of enriched antibiotics or antifungal agents. Intraocular inflammation warrants a complete ocular examination.

Although ophthalmic steroid preparations are beneficial for many conditions, they are not without significant adverse effects. Steroid induced cataracts and glaucoma are well-recognized entities. If increased intraocular pressure persists in steroid users, the optic nerve may be damaged, resulting in severe or total loss of vision. In the presence of herpes simplex infections, steroid use can lead to fulminant corneal infection and loss of the eye. For these reasons, ophthalmic steroids should be used only by those specifically trained in recognizing and treating their complications. Any ocular condition severe enough to necessitate steroid treatment is best referred to an ophthalmologist.

The indications for referral are reviewed in Table 14–7.

COMPREHENSIVE INFORMATION ON INFECTIONS AND INFLAMMATION OF THE EYE

Infection in the Newborn (Ophthalmia Neonatorum)

Factors that predispose an infant to ophthalmia neonatorum include the presence of virulent organisms within the birth canal, premature membrane rupture, local injury to the eyes during delivery, and postnatal exposure to microorganisms. Cesarean section can reduce the incidence of ophthalmia neonatorum in the

TABLE 14–7. INDICATIONS FOR REFERRING CHILDREN WITH OCULAR INFECTIONS AND INFLAMMATION

- Reduced visual acuity
  Corneal involvement
  Intraocular involvement
- Tearing and light sensitivity
  Corneal involvement
  Infantile glaucoma
- Severe pain
  Corneal involvement
  Intraocular inflammation
  Scleritis
  Infantile glaucoma
- Eyelid infection/inflammation
  No improvement in infection after 48 hours of treatment
  Severe atopic disease (vernal)
- Lacrimal infection
  Acute dacryocystitis
  Lacrimal sac mucocele
  Chronic dacryocystitis unresponsive to massage and topical antibiotics
- Orbital infection
  Orbital cellulitis (proptosis, restricted ocular motility, decreased vision, severe pain, and/or reduced sensation in the distribution of cranial nerve V_1 or V_2)
  Sinus involvement requires otolaryngology consultation
- Conjunctival injection
  Hyperacute or recalcitrant conjunctivitis
  Deep, circumcorneal, radially oriented, and violaceous injection (glaucoma, iritis, or scleritis)

- Absence of vascular blanching with topical 2.5% phenylephrine (iritis, scleritis)
- Corneal changes
  Herpes simplex or adenovirus infection
  Corneal ulcer
  Enlarged, cloudy cornea (infantile glaucoma)
  Presence of keratic precipitates (intraocular inflammation)
- Restriction in ocular movement
  Orbital cellulitis
  Cavernous sinus/orbital apex disease/pseudotumor
- Asymmetric pupillary size
  Small and irregular (iritis)
  Mid-dilated and fixed (glaucoma)
- Abnormal intraocular pressure
  Elevated (glaucoma)
  Reduced (iritis, trauma)
- Retinal abnormalities
  Intraocular inflammation
  Intraocular infection (endophthalmitis)
- Optic nerve
  Intraocular inflammation
  Optic neuritis
- Other
  Age (neonate)
  Disorder necessitating steroid use
  Any inflammation or infection associated with trauma
  Any inflammation or infection associated with immunosuppression (e.g., AIDS)

presence of maternal infection (particularly active herpetic infections). This protection is diminished, however, if the membranes have ruptured prematurely. With membrane rupture, herpes simplex virus and bacteria can ascend and infect the neonate while still in utero. Infants are also susceptible to infection upon contact with infected medical personnel and family members. Congenital nasolacrimal duct obstruction and the immature immune system of infants add to this susceptibility.

Salient points regarding the causes of ophthalmia neonatorum are reviewed in the beginning of this chapter. The workup and management of this entity are summarized in Tables 14–8 and 14–9, respectively.

Gonococcal infection presents as a hyperacute conjunctivitis with marked lid swelling and copious purulent exudate (Figs. 14–2 and 14–45). It begins 1 to 2 days after birth. Without treatment, corneal ulceration, perforation, endophthalmitis, and blindness can result. Extraocular infections of the oropharynx, upper gastrointestinal tract, and rectum, are not infrequent. Bacteremia, arthritis, and rarely, meningitis, can also occur. A presumptive diagnosis is made upon Gram stain findings of gram-negative diplococci within polymorphonuclear cells (Fig. 14–46). Cultures using chocolate agar and Thayer–Martin media, and biochemical testing, are necessary for confirmation. The organism should be promptly inoculated and incubated at 35 to 37°C, in

3 to 5% carbon dioxide, as it rapidly dies at room temperature.

Hospitalization and isolation are required. Treatment involves aqueous penicillin G (50,000 U/kg body weight) divided in two intravenous doses for 7 days. Higher doses may be necessary in children with extraocular infections. Because of the increased incidence of penicillinase-producing *N. gonorrhoeae*, single intra-

TABLE 14–8. WORKUP OF OPHTHALMIA NEONATORUM

- **STAIN CONJUNCTIVAL SCRAPINGS**

  Gram (bacteria)
  Giemsa (Chlamydia)
  Papanicolaou (herpes)
  Immunologic (Chlamydia)

- **CULTURE CONJUNCTIVAL SWABS**

  Chocolate agar (Neisseria)
  Thayer–Martin (Neisseria)
  Blood agar (bacteria)
  Chlamydial transport medium
  Viral transport medium

- **OTHER**

  Chest x-ray (Chlamydia)
  Blood culture (septic infants)
  Spinal tap (herpes)

TABLE 14–9. TREATMENT OF OPHTHALMIA NEONATORUM

Etiologic Agent	Treatment
Prophylaxis	1% silver nitrate; or 0.5% erythromycin; or 1% tetracycline ointment
Chemical conjunctivitis	Observation
Gonococcal conjunctivitis	
With extraocular manifestations	Ceftriaxone 25–50 mg/kg/day IV or IM × 7 days; or cefotaxime 25 mg/kg IV or IM every 12 hours
Without extraocular manifestations	Ceftriaxone 50–125 mg/kg in a single dose
With known susceptibility	Penicillin G 50,000 U/kg/day divided in 2 IV doses × 7 days
In severe infections **ADD**	Bacitracin ointment 500 U/g every 2 hours for 2 days, and 5 times daily thereafter
Bacterial conjunctivitis	
Gram-positive cocci	0.5% erythromycin ointment every 2–4 hours
Gram-negative rods	0.3% gentamicin or tobramycin ointment every 1–3 hours; may need subconjunctival injections and/or systemic therapy
Gram-negative coccobacilli	0.5% erythromycin ointment every 2–4 hours
Chlamydial conjunctivitis	Oral erythromycin ethylsuccinate 50 mg/kg/day in 4 divided doses for 2 weeks; plus topical 0.5% erythromycin or 1% tetracycline ointment 4 times per day
Herpetic conjunctivitis	Systemic acyclovir plus topical 1% trifluridine, 6 times per day × 5–14 days

muscular doses of cefotaxime 100 mg/kg (LePage et al, 1988) and ceftriaxone 125 mg (Laga et al, 1987) may be more efficacious than penicillin G. In September 1989, the Centers for Disease Control recommended treatment for 7 days with ceftriaxone 50 to 100 mg/kg per day intravenously (IV) in two divided doses, or a single dose of 125 mg intramuscularly (IM), or cefotaxime 25 mg/kg IV or IM every 12 hours. A single injection of ceftriaxone 50 to 125 mg/kg in cases without extraocular infection, and penicillin G in cases of known susceptibility, are suitable alternatives. Concurrent use of topical antibiotics may not be necessary, but the eyes should be irrigated with buffered saline until the discharge has stopped. For severe infections, topical bacitracin ointment 500 U/g may be instilled every 2 hours for 2 days, and five times daily thereafter until resolution.

Infants born to mothers with known gonococcal infections should be prophylaxed with penicillin G (20,000 U to 50,000 U IV or IM), or ceftriaxone 125 mg IM. Concurrent infection with Chlamydia is common in infants with *N. gonorrhoeae* conjunctivitis; these infants and their mothers should be tested for Chlamydia, and affected infants should be treated with systemic erythromycin (see later discussion).

The etiologic agent in **nongonococcal bacterial conjunctivitis** may be difficult to isolate. *Staphylococcus aureus* may be the most common pathogen in this group, but this organism is also a common nonpathogenic isolate of the skin and conjunctiva of the neonate. Staphylococcal infection is usually mild with minimal injection and discharge. Rarely, corneal infiltrates and ulcers may occur, and a rare systemic complication is the staphylococcal scalded skin syndrome. This results when an exotoxin produced by certain strains cleaves the epidermis beneath the stratum granulosum. It is manifest by a faint yellow-orange discoloration of the

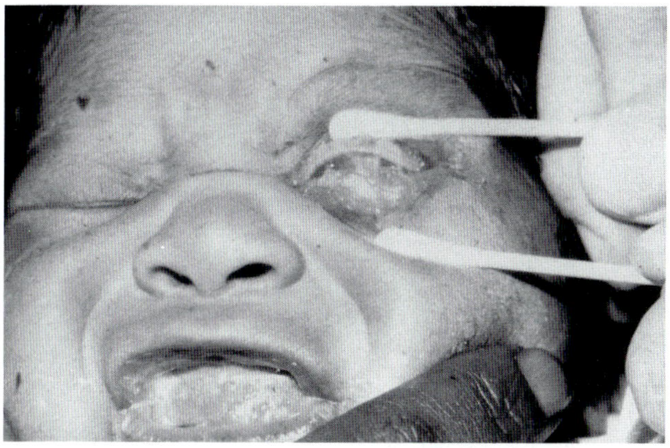

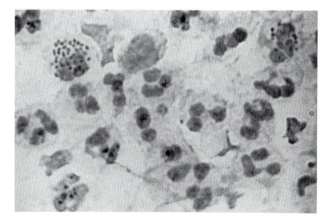

Figure 14–45. Hyperacute gonococcal conjunctivitis with marked lid swelling and copious purulent exudate. *(From Catalano RA: Ocular Emergencies. Philadelphia, Saunders, 1992, p 465, with permission.)*

Figure 14–46. Gram stain of intracellular gram-negative diplococci of *N. gonorrhoeae.* *(From Catalano RA: Ocular Emergencies. Philadelphia, Saunders, 1992, p 465, with permission.)*

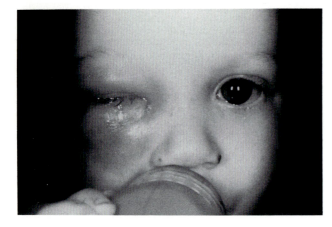

Figure 14–47. Orbital cellulitis secondary to *Haemophilus influenzae.*

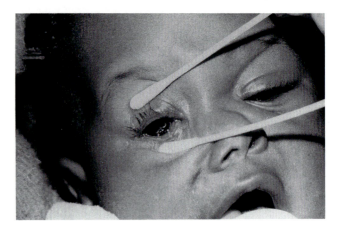

Figure 14–48. Neonatal chlamydial conjunctivitis.

skin, followed by large areas of exfoliation. Clinically it appears similar to the scalding caused by a burn. Parenteral antibiotics are indicated.

Other gram-positive pathogenic causes of ophthalmia neonatorum include *Streptococcus pneumoniae* and *S. viridans.* These respond well to erythromycin. *Branhamella catarrhalis* is a gram-negative diplococcus that may resemble *N. gonorrhoeae* on Gram stain. The two are differentiated by biochemical testing. *B. catarrhalis* can cause systemic disease and responds well to topical and oral erythromycin.

Haemophilus influenzae is the most common gram-negative cause of ophthalmia neonatorum. Because this is rarely cultured in maternal reproductive tracts, most infections likely occur from postnatal contact with an infected individual. The infection may be mild to severe, and may progress to orbital cellulitis (Fig. 14–47) or systemic infection (such as meningitis, mastoiditis, pericarditis, pneumonia, osteomyelitis, or sepsis). Other gram-negative pathogens include *Escherichia coli, Proteus mirabilis,* and *Pseudomonas aeruginosa.* The latter is capable of causing blinding eye disease, disseminated infection, and death in premature infants. Hourly topical antibiotics are required; subconjunctival and systemic antibiotics may be necessary. Gentamycin or tobramycin is suggested.

Chlamydia trachomatis is the most common infectious cause of ophthalmia neonatorum. Chlamydial conjunctivitis develops in as many as 18 percent of infants who pass through infected cervical tracts (Schacter et al, 1986), and as many as 12.7 percent of pregnant women have a culture-proven chlamydial cervical infection (Hammerschlag et al, 1989). The onset of conjunctivitis is usually between 5 and 14 days after birth, and is characterized by serous drainage that becomes copious, and marked lid swelling (Fig. 14–48). Unlike chlamydial infections in adults, a follicular response of the conjunctiva does not occur. The diagnosis can be confirmed by the demonstration of intracytoplasmic

inclusions in conjunctival epithelial cells by Giemsa stain (Fig. 14–49) or by tissue culture. Cultures should be obtained with cotton- or rayon-tipped swabs, because calcium-alginate and wood are believed toxic for Chlamydia. Direct fluorescent antibody (Micro Trak; Syva Co., Palo Alto, CA), and enzyme immunoassay testing (Chlamydiazyme; Abbott Laboratories Diagnostic Division, Abbott Park, IL) are also available. The latter are more sensitive than Giemsa staining. They are also less expensive, and give a more rapid result than Chlamydia cultures.

Sequelae of chlamydial conjunctivitis in the neonate include conjunctival scarring and symblepharon formation (adhesion between the conjunctival folds; Fig. 14–50). Topical antibiotics have a high failure rate and leave the infant at risk for chlamydial pneumonitis. The American Academy of Pediatrics currently recommends orally administered erythromycin (50 mg/kg per day in four divided doses for 14 days). An

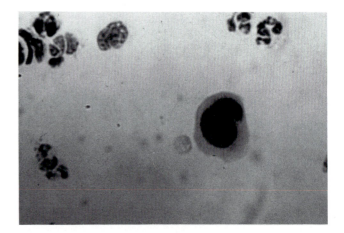

Figure 14–49. Giemsa stain of intracytoplasmic inclusion in conjunctival epithelial cell in neonatal chlamydial conjunctivitis. *(From Catalano RA: Ocular Emergencies. Philadelphia, Saunders, 1992, p 81, with permission.)*

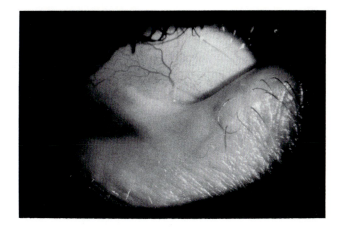

Figure 14–50. Symblepharon (adhesion between the conjunctival folds) secondary to chlamydial conjunctivitis.

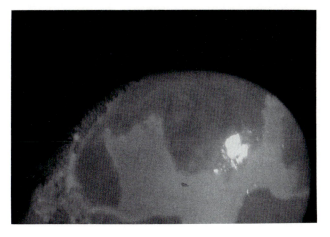

Figure 14–52. Geographic corneal ulcer in herpetic ophthalmia neonatorum.

alternative treatment is trimethoprimsulfamethoxaxole pediatric suspension (0.5 mL/kg per day in two divided doses) for 14 days, with topical tetracycline four times per day for 1 week. Both parents should also be treated.

Herpes simplex virus may cause a generalized systemic infection involving the central nervous system (CNS), localized CNS disease, or localized disease of the mouth, skin, and/or eyes. CNS disease can result in severe neurological damage or death. Ocular disease can result in conjunctivitis, keratitis (corneal infection), cataracts, optic neuritis, chorioretinitis (infection of the choroid and retina), or microphthalmia (small malformed eye). Approximately 50 percent of infants born to mothers with a primary herpetic infection contract the virus, as compared to only 5 percent of infants of mothers with recurrent herpes (Prober et al, 1987). Active genital disease is an indication for cesarean section, unless the membranes have been ruptured for more than 4 to 6 hours.

The most common manifestation of herpetic infection in the neonate is skin vesicles (Fig. 14–51). These

can be the presenting sign in as many as 70 percent of affected infants (Whitley et al, 1980). In over 70 percent of these neonates, the disease progresses within days to other sites, including the eye and central nervous system (Nahmias et al, 1976) Conjunctival involvement usually appears between 2 days to 15 days, and is characterized by a moderate injection without follicle formation. Herpetic infection should be suspected in the presence of herpetic skin lesions, dendritic keratitis, or a history of maternal herpetic infection. Corneal involvement occurs in 10 percent of infants with conjunctivitis. Geographic ulcers with large areas of denuded epithelium are most frequently seen (Fig. 14–52), but dendritic and punctate staining can occur. Retinal involvement may occur within the first week of life, but is more commonly noted between 30 and 90 days after birth. It is characterized by large areas of massive yellowish-white exudates with an associated perivasculitis and vitreous reaction (Fig. 14–53). Healing results in punched out circumscribed scars, similar to those seen with toxoplasmosis (Fig. 14–54).

Intranuclear inclusions and multinucleated giant

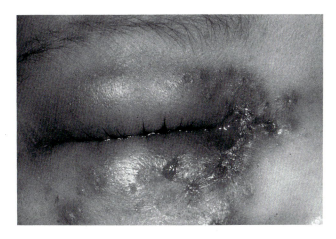

Figure 14–51. Skin vesicles in herpetic ophthalmia neonatorum.

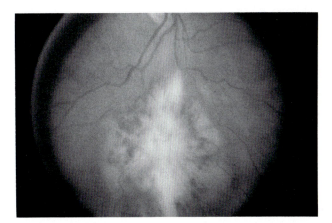

Figure 14–53. Neonatal herpetic retinitis (massive yellowish-white exudative lesion with an associated perivasculitis).

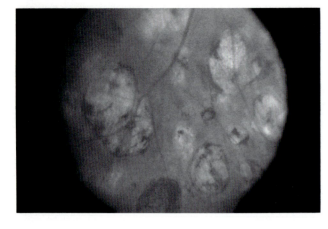

Figure 14–54. Healed neonatal herpetic retinitis characterized by punched-out circumscribed scars.

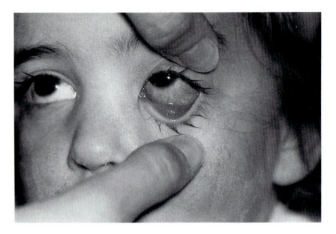

Figure 14–56. Viral conjunctivitis. Note the injection of fine reticulated vessels on the surface of the eye, and the follicular response of the conjunctiva.

cells on Papanicolaou stain, and tissue cultures, are diagnostic. Fluorescent antibody and electron microscopy techniques are also available. Infected infants should be hospitalized and isolated. Systemic antiviral chemotherapy, regardless of the extent of infection at the time of diagnosis, is necessary. Parenterally administered acyclovir is the treatment of choice; infants with conjunctivitis should also have 1 percent trifluridine instilled into the conjunctival sac six times per day for 5 to 14 days.

Chemical conjunctivitis occurs within 3 to 6 hours in up to 90 percent of neonates who receive 1% silver nitrate prophylaxis against *N. gonorrhoeae.* Protein within the conjunctival epithelial cells reacts to the chemical, resulting in conjunctival edema, injection, and discharge (Fig. 14–55). The reaction is self-limited and typically resolves within 24 hours. Nonetheless, alternate prophylactic agents (such as erythromycin and tetracycline), and flushing the eye after administration of silver nitrate, have been advocated. Flushing the eye may reduce the efficacy of the prophylaxis, and currently the American Academy of Pediatrics does not recommend this. A comparison of silver nitrate drops, erythromycin, and tetracycline ointments indicated that there was no significant difference in their efficacy against gonorrhea (Ridgway, 1986). Although the latter agents also have some effect against Chlamydia, their preferential use to silver nitrate does not reduce the incidence of chlamydial conjunctivitis. Some clinicians have postulated that silver nitrate may be a cause of nasolacrimal duct obstruction. Hick and associates (1985), however, found a similar incidence of obstruction in infants who received silver nitrate or 1% tetracycline prophylaxis.

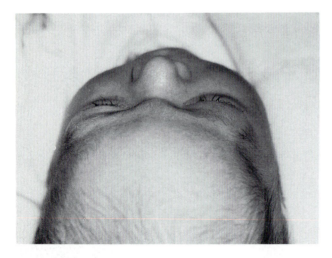

Figure 14–55. The differential diagnosis of this neonate with neuroblastoma and proptosis includes chemical conjunctivitis and pseudoproptosis due to eyelid swelling.

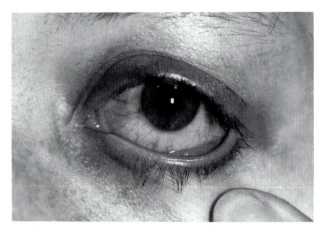

Figure 14–57. Iritis. Note the predominance of injection surrounding the cornea (ciliary flush).

Conjunctivitis

Salient points regarding the diagnosis and treatment of conjunctivitis are reviewed in the beginning of this chapter; additional information regarding common signs and pathogenic organisms is presented below.

Differentiating Signs

The first sign of conjunctivitis is hyperemia of the superficial conjunctival vessels. Intraocular inflammations such as iritis (uveitis) and acute glaucoma can cause hyperemia of the tissues of the globe itself with secondary conjunctival hyperemia. Determination of the primary site of inflammation is required to differentiate these disorders. Conjunctival vessels are fine and reticulated, and become bright red when inflamed (Fig. 14–56). They can be moved with a cotton-tipped applicator and blanch with topical 2.5% phenylephrine. This is in contrast to the ocular injection of iritis (Fig. 14–57), scleritis (Fig. 14–58), and glaucoma. In the latter disorders, vessels within the substance of the globe are involved. These run radially from the cornea, become a darker violaceous color when inflamed, and do not move with a cotton-tipped applicator. The injection of iritis predominantly involves the vessels surrounding the cornea (ciliary flush).

The discharge seen in conjunctivitis is a mixture of transudated fluid, inflammatory cells, desquamated epithelial cells, mucin, and tears. Additional findings of conjunctivitis include follicles, papillae, membranes, and pseudomembranes. Follicles are translucent, dome-shaped elevations (Fig. 14–59), whereas papillae are thickened polygonal elevations (Fig. 14–60). Lacy blood vessels course around the base of follicles, but a fibrovascular core runs through the center of each papilla and erupts into fine vessels on the surface of the conjunctiva. Follicles are lymphoid germinal centers. They occur in viral and toxic conjunctivitis. Papillae

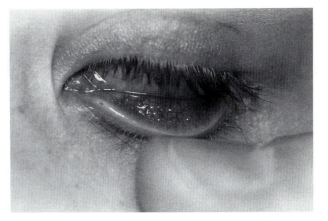

Figure 14–59. Follicular response in viral conjunctivitis.

are a nonspecific reaction of the conjunctiva to inflammation and occur in bacterial and allergic conjunctivitis. The accumulation of fibrin and inflammatory cells results in the formation of pseudomembranes in the conjunctival cul-de-sac (Fig. 14–61). Pseudomembranes are easily removed by swabbing without inducing bleeding. With chronicity, adherence of the coagulin to the epithelium and the proliferation of blood vessels creates a true membrane that bleeds upon scraping. The presence of follicles, papillae, and membranes or pseudomembranes is of differential importance in the diagnosis of conjunctivitis (Table 14–10).

Bacterial Conjunctivitis

Bacterial conjunctivitis is characterized by an acute purulent or mucopurulent discharge, mattering of the eyelashes, and papillary reaction (Fig. 14–62). Between the ages of 3 months and 8 years, staphylococcal, pneumococcal, and *Haemophilus* conjunctivitis predominate.

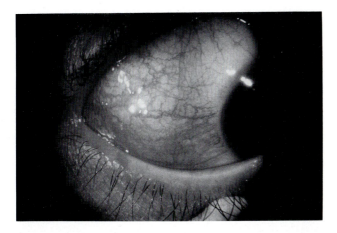

Figure 14–58. Nodular scleritis. Note the injection of deeper, radially directed vessels. *(From Catalano RA: Ocular Emergencies. Philadelphia, Saunders, 1992, p 488, with permission.)*

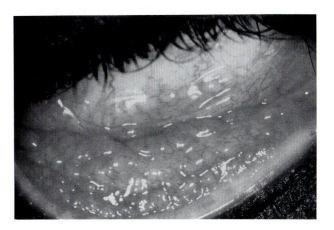

Figure 14–60. Papillary response in allergic conjunctivitis.

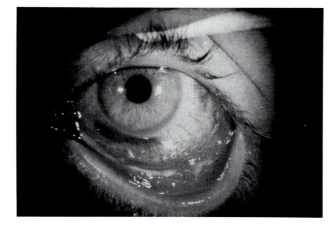

Figure 14–61. Pseudomembrane in adenovirus infection. *(From Catalano RA: Ocular Emergencies. Philadelphia, Saunders, 1992, p 474, with permission.)*

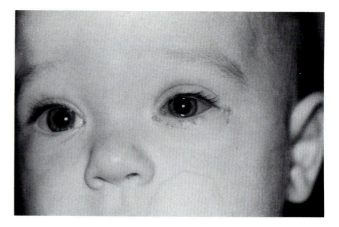

Figure 14–62. Bacterial conjunctivitis characterized by purulent discharge and mattering of the eyelashes in a child with a congenital nasolacrimal duct obstruction.

Whereas *S. aureus* shows no seasonal or geographic predilection, pneumococcus is typically seen in colder regions during the winter, and *Haemophilus* in warmer regions between May and October. Secondary bacterial conjunctivitis can also complicate nonbacterial conjunctivitis following compromise of the ocular defense mechanisms.

Acute bacterial conjunctivitis usually runs a self-limited course of approximately 10 days. Exceptions include *Haemophilus, Streptococcus, Neisseria,* and *Staphylococcus. Haemophilus* conjunctivitis can be a forerunner of more ominous periorbital cellulitis and bacteremia (described under "Orbital Infections" later in the chapter). It is toxogenic and can cause patchy conjunctival hemorrhages (Fig. 14–63). *Streptococcus* is an invasive bacteria capable of causing pseudomembranes. Small petechial subconjunctival hemorrhages, commonly involving the superior conjunctiva, are characteristic of *S. pneumoniae* conjunctivitis.

Neisseria is an aggressively invasive bacteria. A rapidly evolving, copiously exudative conjunctivitis associated with marked conjunctival and lid edema is suggestive of *Neisseria* conjunctivitis (see Fig. 14–2). Infection with this organism can rapidly proceed to corneal perforation and loss of the eye. *Neisseria* is the only bacteria that commonly causes preauricular lymphadenopathy. Systemic and topical therapy is necessary (see earlier discussion).

TABLE 14–10. DIFFERENTIAL DIAGNOSIS BASED ON CONJUNCTIVAL FINDINGS

- *PAPILLARY RESPONSE*

  Nonspecific (any type of inflammation)

- *GIANT PAPILLARY RESPONSE*

  Vernal conjunctivitis
  Atopic keratoconjunctivitis
  Contact lens giant papillary conjunctivitis
  Ocular prostheses giant papillary conjunctivitis

- *FOLLICULAR RESPONSE*

  Adult chlamydial infection
  Toxic (antivirals, miotics, atropine, adrenergics)
  Molluscum contagiosum
  Primary herpes simplex keratoconjunctivitis
  Adenovirus
  Benign lymphoid hyperplasia

- *PSEUDOMEMBRANES AND MEMBRANES*

  Adenovirus
  Herpes simplex virus
  Beta-hemolytic streptococcus
  Neisseria gonorrhoeae
  Neonatal chlamydial infection
  Corynebacterium diphtheriae
  Candida albicans
  Vernal conjunctivitis
  Ocular pemphigoid
  Stevens–Johnson syndrome
  Ligneous conjunctivitis

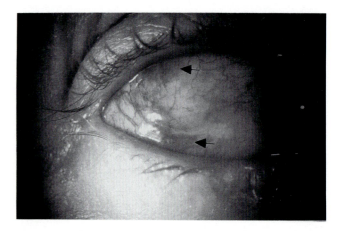

Figure 14–63. *Haemophilus* conjunctivitis characterized by patchy conjunctival hemorrhages (*arrows*).

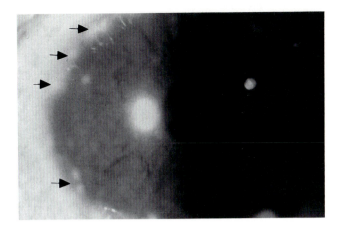

Figure 14–64. Staphylococcal marginal infiltrates (*arrows*).

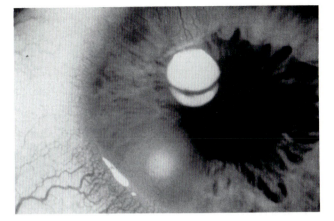

Figure 14–66. Recurrent staphylococcal phlyctenule on the cornea.

Staphylococcal blepharoconjunctivitis (infection of the eyelids and conjunctiva) can be a chronic disorder in individuals with Down syndrome or other immunologic sensitivity. Infection resides at the lash margins, upon which debris and secretions accumulate. Exotoxins contribute to the chronic injection of the lid margin and conjunctiva. This disorder is treated with lid scrubs (using a cotton-tipped applicator dipped in baby shampoo), and the judicious use of topical antibiotics (such as erythromycin ointment). Untreated, superficial punctate corneal erosions and marginal infiltrates on the conjunctiva, limbus, or cornea and phlyctenules can arise. Marginal infiltrates are round focal lesions that occur at the corneal limbus (Fig. 14–64). The overlying epithelium can ulcerate, but heals as the lesions resolve. Phlyctenules are similar round, elevated, focal infiltrates. They usually occur first at the limbus (Fig. 14–65), but with recurrence can march across the cornea or conjunctiva (Fig. 14–66). Both marginal infiltrates and phlyctenules are sterile. They occur due to type IV (T-lymphocyte mediated) hypersensitivity to microbial antigens. Those second-

ary to staphylococcus are treated with a mild antibiotic–steroid combination (such as Blephamide or Vasocidin) four times per day for several days. Antibiotic ointment is also applied to the lash margin to decrease the colonization of *Staphylococcus*. Rarer causes of phlyctenules include tuberculosis, lymphogranuloma venereum, coccidiomycosis, and candidiasis.

Viral Conjunctivitis

Viral conjunctivitis is characterized by a watery discharge, irritation, hyperemia, follicular response, and preauricular adenopathy. In children, adenovirus is the most common pathogen, causing both **pharyngoconjunctival fever (PCF)** (serotypes 3 and 7) and **epidemic keratoconjunctivitis (EKC)** (serotypes 8 and 19). An incubation period of 5 to 12 days is typical for both conditions. PCF is characterized by pharyngitis, fever, and follicular conjunctivitis. It occurs primarily in children under 10 years of age and is self-limited, lasting at most 4 to 14 days. EKC is more commonly observed in individuals between 20 and 40 years of age, but can occur in children. It begins unilaterally, but spreads to involve both eyes. The second eye is usually less severely affected than the first, but both may show conjunctival hemorrhages and membrane formation (see Fig. 14–61). Severe cases can cause corneal erosions and subepithelial infiltrates (Fig. 14–67). Affected individuals have protracted photophobia and decreased vision. Adenovirus conjunctivitis remains infectious for 14 days after onset; care is required to prevent transmission of this highly contagious disease.

Primary infections with herpes simplex virus occur in childhood in approximately 90 percent of the population (O'Day & Jones, 1987). Primary ocular infection may be subclinical, but more commonly presents as an acute unilateral follicular conjunctivitis with regional lymphadenopathy (Fig. 14–68). Vesicular ulcerations of the eyelids are common and corneal involvement not unusual. The initial infection is self-limited, but the

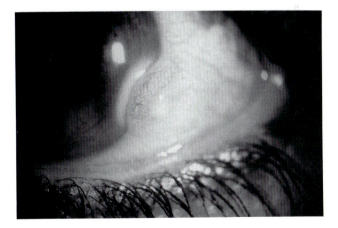

Figure 14–65. Staphylococcal phlyctenule occurring at the limbus.

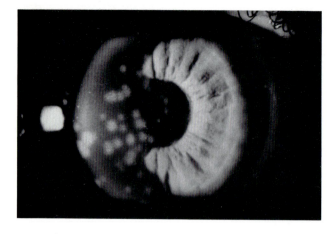

Figure 14–67. Corneal subepithelial infiltrates due to adenovirus infection. *(From Catalano RA: Ocular Emergencies. Philadelphia, Saunders, 1992, p 474, with permission.)*

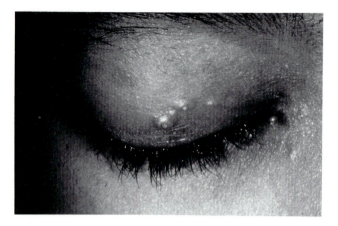

Figure 14–69. Molluscum contagiosum. Note the umbilicated appearance of the lesions.

virus remains latent in the trigeminal ganglion. Recurrent disease is manifest by dendritiform or geographic staining of the damaged corneal epithelium (see discussion later in the chapter).

Molluscum contagiosum can be responsible for a chronic follicular conjunctivitis due to shedding of viral particles from eyelid lesions onto the conjunctiva. It often, but not always, appears umbilicated, with a central concavity (Figs. 14–6 and 14–69). *Papillomavirus* can cause sessile, fleshy, vascularized growths on the eyelid margin, conjunctiva, or caruncle (Fig. 14–70). Spontaneous remission and exacerbation is common with this organism. Excision of the lesion can be attempted, but regrowth is common. Cryotherapy, radi-

ation, cautery, carbon dioxide laser, immunotherapy with chlorobenzene, and interferon therapy have been successful in ablating and inhibiting recurrence in some cases (Lass et al, 1987; Wilson, 1990).

Conjunctivitis occurs in up to 70 percent of children infected with rubella and rubeola. It occurs concomitant with the rash, and is generally mild. Corneal involvement (keratitis) probably occurs in all children with measles, but is symptomatic in only 50%.

Acute hemorrhagic conjunctivitis is a recently described entity that has caused several pandemics during the past 20 years. It is due to enterovirus 70, adenovirus, or coxsackievirus A24. Its incubation is only 1 to 2 days, and its course is likewise short, with improvement starting on the third day and resolution by the tenth day. Manifestations include a watery discharge, preauricular adenopathy, chemosis, and extensive subconjunctival hemorrhages ranging from small petechiae to large blotches (Fig. 14–71). Hemorrhages are most severe in the upper bulbar conjunctiva. Respira-

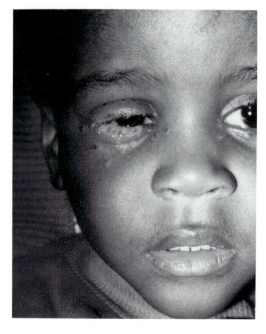

Figure 14–68. Primary herpes simplex conjunctivitis.

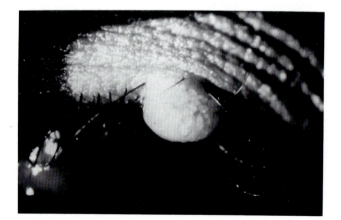

Figure 14–70. Papillomavirus on upper eyelid.

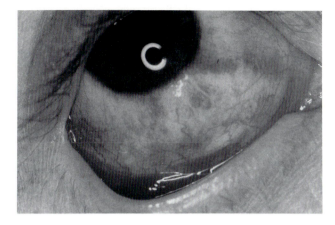

Figure 14–71. Blotchy hemorrhage in acute hemorrhagic conjunctivitis.

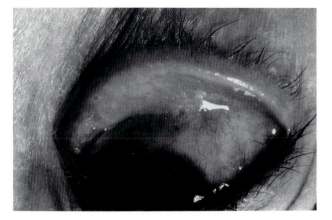

Figure 14–73. Scarring of the superior conjunctiva in trachoma.

tory and gastrointestinal disturbances can accompany the conjunctivitis, and neurological complications of palatal paresis and Bell's palsy have been reported in a few individuals.

Chlamydial Conjunctivitis

Chlamydial organisms cause a variety of disorders depending on the age of the affected individual and subgroup involved. Neonatal disease is discussed earlier. **"Adult" inclusion conjunctivitis** presents as an acute follicular conjunctivitis in sexually active adolescents, which progresses to a chronic follicular conjunctivitis. Keratitis involving the superior cornea can occur, and is characterized by a micropannus (infiltration of the superficial cornea with blood vessels) of up to 3 mm (Fig. 14–72). The latter is an important distinguishing characteristic, as it does not occur with adenoviral infections. Untreated, the disease may last 6 to 18 months. Systemic treatment is indicated because cervicitis or urethritis is always associated. **Trachoma** is the result of repeated chlamydial infections transmitted by vectors, with superimposed bacterial infections. In the early stages, trachoma and inclusion conjunctivitis appear similar. With recurrent attacks of trachoma, scarring of the conjunctiva becomes prominent, leading to eyelid abnormalities and corneal damage (Fig. 14–73).

Allergic/Atopic Conjunctivitis

Atopic conjunctivitis is characterized by itching, redness, and swelling of the eyelids and conjunctiva (Fig. 14–74). It is chronic and recurrent and tends to wax and wane with or without treatment. In sensitive individuals, hay, ragweed, pollen, and/or other airborne antigens cause an immediate type I (IgE-mediated) hypersensitivity. Antigenic stimulation results in mast cell degranulation and increased conjunctival vasculature permeability.

Contact dermatitis can be associated with conjunctival chemosis, hyperemia, and papillae. Medications including aminoglycoside antibiotics, sulfonamides,

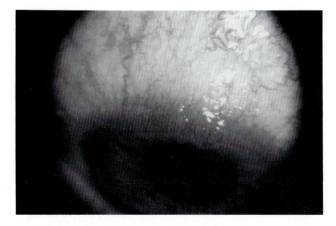

Figure 14–72. Micropannus of the superior limbus in chronic "adult" inclusion conjunctivitis.

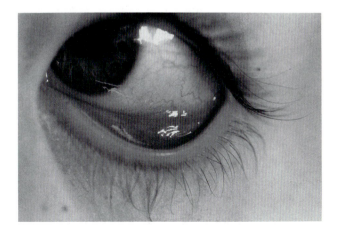

Figure 14–74. Atopic conjunctivitis. Note the watery appearance, conjunctival swelling (chemosis), and the absence of follicles.

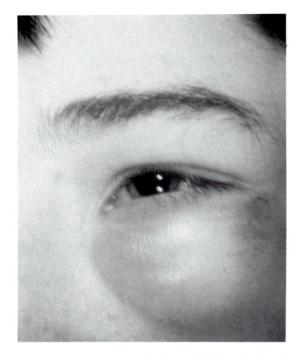

Figure 14–75. Contact dermatitis from topically applied eyedrops. Note the principal involvement of the lower eyelid.

chloramphenicol, adrenergic agents, atropine, and timolol are common causes. Patients can also be sensitive to the preservatives used in ocular medications or artificial tears. Cosmetics and poison ivy can cause a similar reaction. Symptoms include blurred vision and itching. Signs include swollen, erythematous eyelids. The skin may take on a leathery consistency. Contact dermatitis secondary to eyedrops principally involves the lower eyelids and cheeks due to spillage of medica-

tions from the lower cul-de-sac (Fig. 14–75). Moderate edema and papillae of the conjunctiva and superficial punctate erosions of the cornea may be present.

Vernal conjunctivitis is a bilateral, recurrent eye disease occurring mostly in boys, with exacerbations in the spring and summer. Although the etiology is unknown, there is a strong association with other atopic diseases. Affected children may also suffer from asthma, eczema, and hay fever. The conjunctiva of the upper eyelid is preferentially affected. Numerous, confluent, large (5- to 8-mm) papillae gives the upper palpebral conjunctiva a cobblestone appearance (Fig. 14–76). Over 80 percent of the children have itching, photophobia, and blepharospasm, and several times a day the child may pull a ropy, tenacious mucoid strand from under the upper eyelid. Severe cases are complicated by the development of poorly healing corneal ulcers and limbal excrescences with overlying white dots called **Trantas dots.** Corneal ulcers in vernal conjunctivitis are typically shallow, shaggy, and "shield"-shaped. They are usually oval or pentagonal in shape and involve the superior third of the cornea (Fig. 14–77). Trantas dots are collections of eosinophils that occur at the apices of the limbal excrescences (Fig. 14–78); they are more common in black patients. Superficial punctate keratopathy and pannus formation also occur. In most patients the disease remits after a few years of seasonal attacks, without causing serious sequelae.

Parinaud's Oculoglandular Syndrome

An uncommon disorder, **Parinaud's oculoglandular syndrome** is characterized by unilateral conjunctivitis and ipsilateral enlargement of the preauricular and submaxillary nodes. The conjunctivitis can have a follicular or nodular appearance (Figs. 14–79 and 14–80),

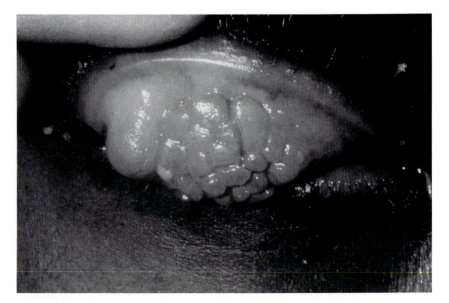

Figure 14–76. Giant papillae in vernal conjunctivitis. *(Courtesy of the Wills Eye Hospital slide collection.)*

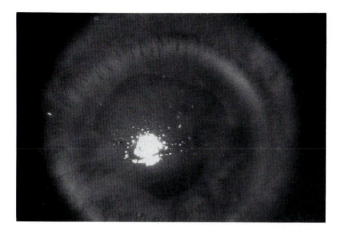

Figure 14–77. Shield-shaped superior corneal ulcer in vernal conjunctivitis.

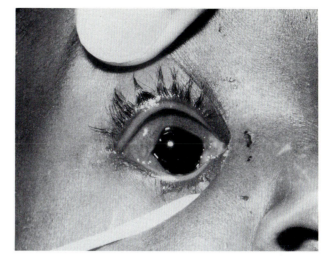

Figure 14–79. Nodular-appearing conjunctivitis of cat-scratch fever.

and the lymphadenopathy can be massive (Fig. 14–81). Because the causes are numerous (Table 14–11), the workup should include conjunctival scrapings for Gram, Giemsa, acid-fast, and fungal stains. Cultures for acid-fast and other bacteria, fungi, and microaerophilic species should be obtained. Serological tests for tularemia, sporotrichosis, syphilis, rickettsiae, infectious mononucleosis, and a cat-scratch skin test can be confirmatory in select cases. The most common cause is cat-scratch disease.

Cat-scratch disease is caused by a pleomorphic gram-negative rod. It is usually benign and self-limited, but can last several months. It begins 3 to 5 days after inoculation; the host reservoir is usually a kitten. The first sign is a small pink papule. This progresses to become a vesicle filled with opaque fluid. Over the ensuing 2 to 3 days, the vesicle ruptures to form a crusty

skin lesion. Several days to weeks later, painful, regional lymphadenopathy develops. Infected lymph glands are firm and conspicuously enlarged; lymphadenopathy may progress to lymphadenitis, suppuration, or dissemination. Systemic findings include mild generalized aching, malaise, anorexia, nausea, and abdominal pain. Temperature elevations are mild (<39°C) or nonexistent.

Ocular involvement occurs in less than 5 percent of cases. It results when the inoculation is confined to the eyelids. In many ocular cases, the organism is transmitted by the patient's hands (Carithers, 1985). Symptoms of photophobia, irritation, and foreign body sensation arise 7 to 14 days after inoculation. The palpebral conjunctiva is principally involved with soft, nodular granulations. Chemosis and intense inflammation of the conjunctiva may be present, but the surrounding

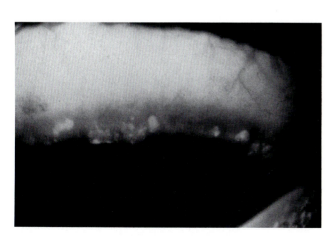

Figure 14–78. Trantas dots at the superior limbus in vernal conjunctivitis.

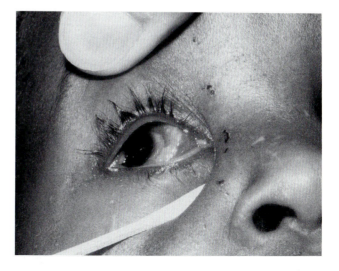

Figure 14–80. Nodular-appearing conjunctivitis of cat-scratch fever. Note that the conjunctival swelling slides over the cornea.

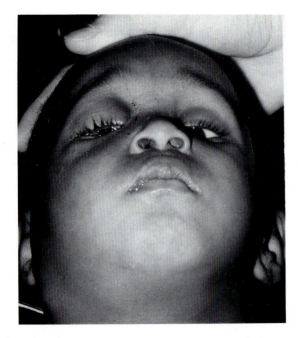

Figure 14–81. Massive preauricular and submandibular lymphadenopathy in cat-scratch fever.

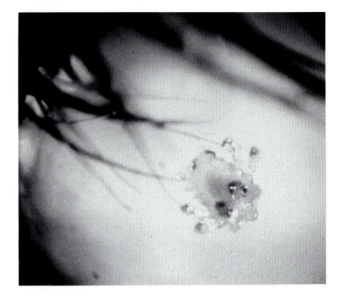

Figure 14–82. Crab louse attached to the end of an eyelash. *(Courtesy of Richard Cunningham.)*

tissues may be only minimally erythematous. Purulent discharge is not seen unless secondary infection occurs, which is rare. Resolution slowly occurs over several months, but may be protracted over 2 years in rare cases. Conjunctival scarring does not occur.

A skin test for cat-scratch disease is available to confirm the diagnosis. A recent study has suggested that oral ciprofloxacin (500 mg twice daily for 10 days) may be efficacious (Holley, 1991).

Crab Louse Conjunctivitis

Crab louse infestation (*Phthirus pubis* palpebraru) is an uncommon cause of chronic conjunctivitis. Lice attach to the base of the eyelashes (Fig. 14–82), where they

may deposit egg capsules (nits; Fig. 14–83). Follicular conjunctivitis results from a toxic reaction to lice products. Management includes manually removing the lice, and locally applying a pediculocide twice daily for 7 to 10 days. Agents that can be used include yellow mercuric oxide N.F. 1% ophthalmic ointment, physostigmine (Eserine) 0.25% ointment, gamma benzene hexachloride 1% ointment (Qwell), and concentrated sodium fluorescein solution (Couch et al, 1982). Medications should be applied carefully to avoid ocular toxicity. Repeated applications of a bland ophthalmic ointment may kill the organisms by smothering them, but do not kill the nits. Infested body hair should be treated by a one-time shampoo with gamma benzene

TABLE 14–11. PRESUMED CAUSES OF PARINAUD'S OCULOGLANDULAR SYNDROME

Cat-scratch disease
Tularemia
Tuberculosis
Syphilis
Yersinia
Chancroid
Listerellosis
Lymphogranuloma venereum
Sporotrichosis
Inclusion conjunctivitis
Infectious mononucleosis
Rickettsia
Actinomycosis

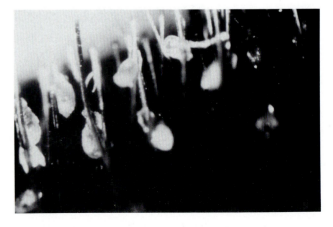

Figure 14–83. Egg capsules (nits) of the crab louse deposited on the eyelashes.

hexachloride 1% (Qwell). Excessive use of this agent should be avoided because of possible central nervous system toxicity. Clothing, linen, and personal items should be disinfected with heat of 50°C for 30 minutes.

Ocular Infections

Corneal Ulcers

The corneal epithelium is an effective barrier to microbial penetration. It can be penetrated by only three species of bacteria: *Neisseria*, *Corynebacterium diphtheriae*, and *Shigella*. Deep infections with other organisms must be preceded by an epithelial defect. Risk factors include trauma, contact lens wear, viral infection, and surgery.

A Kimura spatula, or sterile 23 gauge needle, is used to obtain material from the floor of a corneal ulcer for Gram stain and culture (Fig. 14–84), prior to the initiation of therapy. The spatula should be sterilized between cultures by flaming over an alcohol lamp. Microbiological stains (Figs. 14–85 and 14–86) and culture media useful in the diagnosis of corneal infections are reviewed in Table 14–12. Fresh media must always be used and taken directly to the microbiology laboratory.

Treatment regimens are based upon culture and sensitivity results. While awaiting sensitivities, small superficial infiltrates without epithelial disruption can be treated with a broad-spectrum topical antibiotic (for example, polytrim, gentamicin, tobramycin, or neosporin) four to six times daily. Corneal ulcers are treated with fortified cefazolin (33 to 50 mg/mL) alternating with a fortified aminoglycoside (such as gentamicin 10 to 15 mg/mL) hourly. Vancomycin (33 to 50 mg/mL) should be considered in geographical locations endemic for resistant Gram-positive organisms.

Fungal corneal ulcers are most commonly encountered in the southern and southwestern United States.

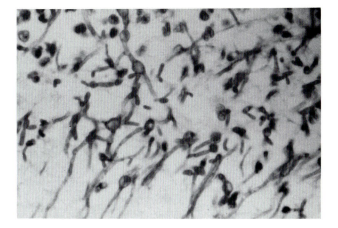

Figure 14–85. Gomori–methenamine–silver stain of *Fusarium solanae*, a filamentous fungus with fine septae (× 1000). *(From Catalano RA: Ocular Emergencies. Philadelphia, Saunders, 1992, p 83, with permission.)*

Often there is a history of trauma with vegetable matter. Septate fungi (such as *Fusarium* or *Aspergillus*) are the usual pathogens. Nonfilamentous fungi (for example, *Candida*) are more commonly encountered in northern climates and in immunocompromised hosts. Risk factors for fungal keratitis include corneal injury, soft contact lens wear, immunosuppression, and prolonged use of topical antibiotics. The ulcer usually presents as a primary infiltrate with satellite lesions (Fig. 14–87). A hypopyon (layering of inflammatory cells in the anterior chamber) may also be present. Cultures should include fungal media and blood agar incubated at room temperature. The laboratory must be informed of the suspected fungal etiology, so as not to disregard a saprophytic fungus as a contaminant. The treatment of choice for filamentous fungi is natamycin administered hourly. Amphotericin B 0.15% is more ef-

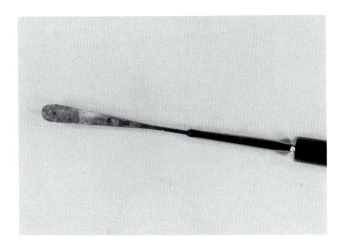

Figure 14–84. Kimura spatula used to obtain culture material from the bed of a corneal ulcer. *(From Catalano RA: Ocular Emergencies. Philadelphia, Saunders, 1992, p 478, with permission.)*

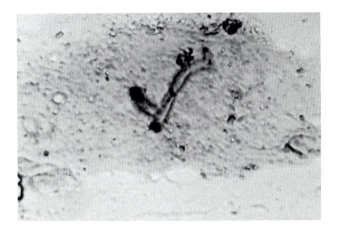

Figure 14–86. Gridley stain of Aspergillus, a septate fungus.

TABLE 14–12. MICROBIOLOGICAL STAINS AND CULTURE MEDIA FOR INFECTIOUS AGENTS

Agent	Stain	Culture Media
General bacteria	Gram	Blood, general nutrient
Neisseria species	Gram	Chocolate, Thayer–Martin
Anaerobes	Gram	Thioglycolate
Hemophilus	Gram	Blood, chocolate
Mycobacteria/Nocardia	Ziehl-Neelson	Lowenstein–Jensen
Fungi	Giemsa (hyphae) Gram (yeasts) Periodic acid–Schiff (PAS) with Gridley modification Gomori–methenamine–silver	Sabouraud, brain–heart
Viruses	Papanicolaou	Viral cultures
Chlamydia	Giemsa	McCoy cell
Acanthamoeba	Calcofluor white	Non-nutrient agar with *Escherichia coli* overlay

fective against *Candida* and other yeasts. Other topical and oral antifungals (for example, miconozole or clotrimazole) may be effective in resistant cases.

Acanthamoeba Keratitis

Acanthamoeba species can cause potentially blinding corneal infections. This protozoan has been recovered from drinking water, swimming pools, and hot tubs. A common history in contact lens wearers with *Acanthamoeba* keratitis is the use of homemade saline.

Early signs of *Acanthamoeba* infection include corneal ulceration, conjunctivitis, inflammation of the anterior eye (iridocyclitis), and severe pain. Epithelial and subepithelial infiltrates can progress to a ring-like corneal infiltrate (Fig. 14–88). Corneal scraping should be performed, as the diagnosis requires positive identification of the organism. A Giemsa stain may demonstrate the cystic form of the disease; the calcofluor white stain demonstrates both the trophozoite and cysts, but requires a fluorescent microscope. Culture

requires a nonnutrient agar with an overlay of *Escherichia coli*. A corneal biopsy may be needed if scrapings fail to yield the organism in suspected cases. Propamidine isethionate 0.1% (Brolene) hourly is recommended, but is available in the United States only through the Centers for Disease Control. Other antivirals may be effective, but some cases progress relentlessly to corneal perforation and loss of vision despite treatment.

Herpes Simplex Keratitis

Primary herpes simplex keratitis presents within 2 days to 2 weeks (mean 1 week) of contact with a patient with a recurrent herpes simplex infection (often a cold sore on the mouth). Systemic signs are usually mild, but occasionally generalized malaise and fever may herald the onset of ocular disease. Eye involvement is frequently mild. Marked eyelid swelling, vesicles, and crusting can occur (see Figs. 14–7 and 14–89), but it is often necessary to search the eyelashes and canthal

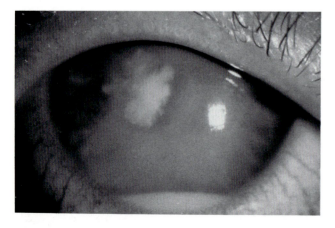

Figure 14–87. Fungal corneal ulcer with hypopyon. *(From Catalano RA: Ocular Emergencies. Philadelphia, Saunders, 1992, p 477, with permission.)*

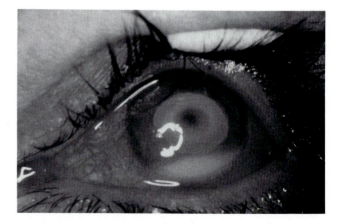

Figure 14–88. Ring-like infiltrate and hypopyon in Acanthamoeba keratitis. *(From Catalano RA: Ocular Emergencies. Philadelphia, Saunders, 1992, p 483, with permission.)*

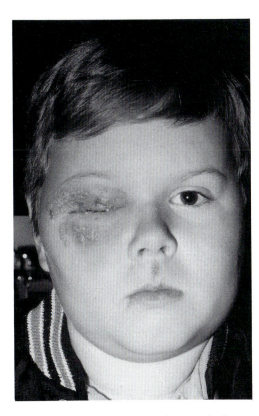

Figure 14–89. Primary ocular herpes simplex infection marked by eyelid swelling, grouped vesicles, and crusting lesions, as well as perioral lesions.

area for skin lesions. Ipsilateral preauricular nodes may be slightly swollen and tender. In most cases, acute unilateral redness, irritation, and watery discharge are present. Examination reveals follicular conjunctivitis, conjunctival edema and injection, and occasionally small conjunctival ecchymoses. Corneal involvement occurs within 2 weeks in half of the children with primary herpetic conjunctivitis. With rare exception, corneal involvement is confined to the epi-

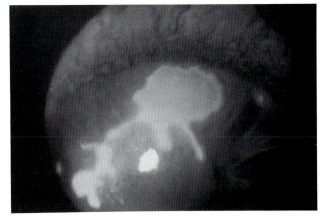

Figure 14–91. Geographical herpes simplex keratitis.

thelium; superficial punctate and dendritic epithelial keratitis (Fig. 14–90) are the usual manifestations. Topical antiviral therapy should be instituted if lesions occur on the cornea, conjunctiva, or adjacent skin. Topical antivirals include idoxuridine, vidarabine, and trifluridine. A cycloplegic agent (scopolamine hydrobromide 0.25 percent or cyclopentolate hydrochloride 1.0 percent, two to three times per day) may be comforting if ciliary spasm and photophobia occur due to secondary iritis.

Recurrent herpes simplex keratitis usually presents as a branching epithelial dendrite (Fig. 14–90); other presentations, however, are not uncommon. One variant is **geographical ulceration** (Fig. 14–91). These ulcers are especially likely to occur with corticosteroid enhancement of epithelial keratitis or in immunocompromised patients. Another variant is **indolent ulcers.** These are round or oval in shape, with smooth, rolled edges that stain poorly with rose bengal (Fig. 14–92). Indolent ulcers result when epithelial healing is retarded, usually due to the excessive use of antivirals or underlying stromal inflammatory disease.

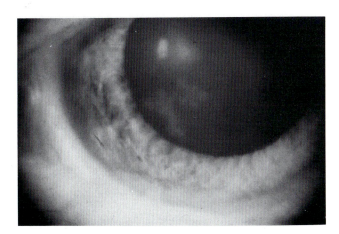

Figure 14–90. Dendritic herpes simplex keratitis.

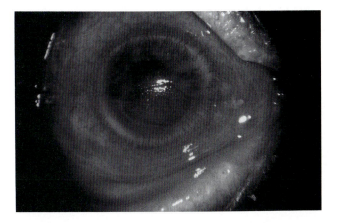

Figure 14–92. Oval-shaped indolent corneal ulcer due to excessive use of antivirals following geographic herpes simplex keratitis.

The herpes virus replicates little, if at all, within the corneal stroma. Virus particles, soluble antigens, and antigenically altered keratocytes, however, can penetrate the stroma following an attack of epithelial disease. Rarely, stromal disease occurs as part of the initial attack. In contrast to epithelial disease, where direct injury occurs due to viral replication, inflammation is the destructive force in stromal keratitis. Blurred vision is almost invariably the initial symptom; photophobia, tearing, pain, and blepharospasm are variably present.

Corneal edema and fine folds in Descemet's membrane signify active stromal inflammation. Edema results from endothelial destruction, presumably secondary to an accompanying anterior uveitis. In the early stages, the stroma has a finely granular appearance. With progressive disease, localized stromal edema, Descemet's folds, keratic precipitates, and iridocyclitis occur. This variant of stromal disease is often disc shaped and central or paracentral in location without epithelial involvement (Fig. 14–93). Called **disciform keratitis**, it is believed to represent a cell-mediated immune response to viral antigens. Another variant of stromal disease is called **infiltrative stromal keratitis.** This presents with diffuse corneal edema, with or without overlying epithelial ulceration. In chronic cases, lipid or cholesterol crystals may be deposited in the cornea. Additional findings include corneal vascularization, adhesions of the iris to the lens capsule, and inflammation of the trabecular meshwork. The latter results in elevated intraocular pressure. **Metaherpetic keratitis** is characterized by indolent stromal and epithelial edema. It is oval in shape and without epithelial involvement. Iridocyclitis, hypopyon, thinning and erosion of the corneal stroma (descemetocele), and corneal perforation can all occur in metaherpetic disease.

The treatment of stromal keratitis consists of topical antivirals (trifluridine ointment six times daily). The concomitant use of corticosteroids is controversial. Whereas steroids reduce the amount of inflammation and discomfort, recurrences following steroid use may be more frequent and severe. Systemic acyclovir (200 mg five times daily) has been advocated for the treatment of stromal keratitis in adults, but its efficacy and toxicity in children have not been evaluated.

The **acute retinal necrosis syndrome** is a specific clinical presentation of herpes simplex or zoster infection of the posterior eye. It consists of arteritis and phlebitis of the retinal and choroidal vasculature, a confluent, necrotizing peripheral retinitis, and a moderate to severe vitritis. Anterior segment inflammation, optic neuritis, and retinal detachment are common accompaniments (Fig. 14–94). The differential diagnosis includes CMV retinitis, toxoplasmosis, and syphilis. CMV retinitis produces significantly less vitreous cellular reaction, is posterior and perivenous in location, and is more likely to be associated with immunocompromise. Serum titers for toxoplasmosis and serological studies for syphilis (VDRL, FTA-ABS) are useful in differentiating these other disorders. The recommended treatment is intravenous acyclovir and oral corticosteroids (Duker & Blumenkranz, 1991).

Orbital Infections

Orbital infections include preseptal cellulitis and orbital cellulitis. **Preseptal cellulitis** involves only the subcutaneous tissue of the eyelid, brow, or forehead (see Figs. 14–24 and 14–95). Involvement deeper than the orbital septum is called **orbital cellulitis.** The latter is characterized by reduced visual acuity, decreased ocular motility, diplopia, pain on ocular movement, and abnormal pupillary reaction (see Fig. 14–25).

Children with *H. influenzae* orbital infection present with markedly swollen, violaceous eyelids, irritability, and coryza (Fig. 14–96). They may also have high fever,

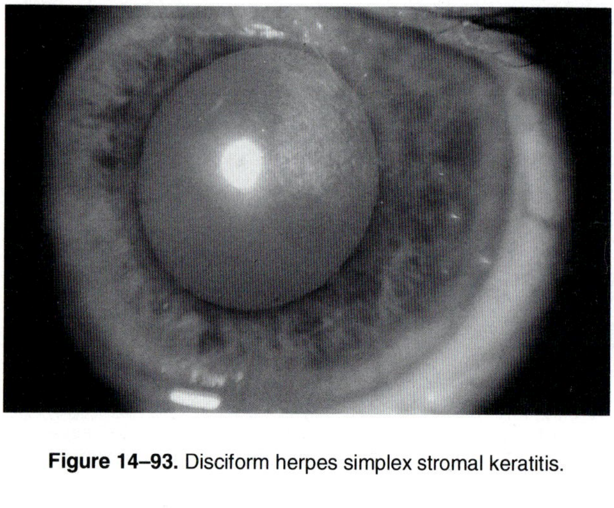

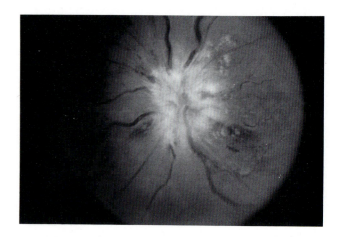

Figure 14–93. Disciform herpes simplex stromal keratitis.

Figure 14–94. Optic neuritis in the acute retinal necrosis syndrome.

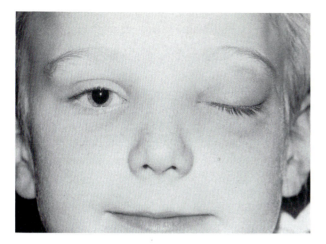

Figure 14–95. Preseptal cellulitis of the left eyelids and periorbital area.

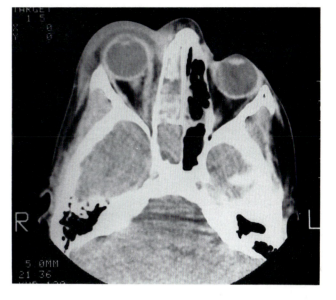

Figure 14–97. Computed tomography demonstrating periocular inflammation and ipsilateral ethmoiditis in a child with orbital cellulitis.

leukocytosis, and positive blood cultures. The presence of any of these, however, is not useful in differentiating *H. influenzae* preseptal from orbital cellulitis. Urgent treatment is necessary because bacteremia, meningitis, epiglottitis, and pneumonia can rapidly develop. The treatment of choice is cefuroxime 100 to 150 mg/kg per day intravenously, in three divided doses, for 10 to 14 days. An alternate choice is intravenous nafcillin or oxacillin (150 mg/kg per day in four divided doses) with ceftazidime (90 to 150 mg/kg per day in three divided doses). Strains resistant to ampicillin are common, and chloramphenicol is generally avoided in children because it can suppress the bone marrow.

Gram stain and culture material is often difficult to obtain in deep orbital cellulitis. Occasionally, material for culture is present on the nasal or nasopharyngeal mucosa. Urine antigen studies, which identify fractions of the infecting organism's cell wall polysaccharides excreted in the urine, may be helpful if available. Sinus x-rays are not generally helpful because the sinuses are not well developed in young children. Computed tomography (CT), however, may be useful in delineating the extent of orbital disease and demonstrating orbital (but not subperiosteal) abscesses (Fig. 14–97). CT is also helpful in differentiating a cellulitis-simulating tumor such as rhabdomyosarcoma (Fig. 14–98) or neuroblastoma. Bone destruction suggests tumor involvement.

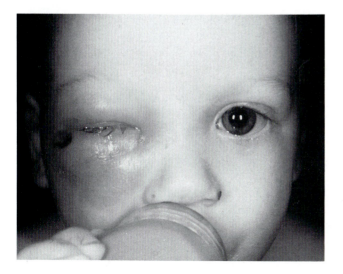

Figure 14–96. *Haemophilus influenzae* orbital cellulitis.

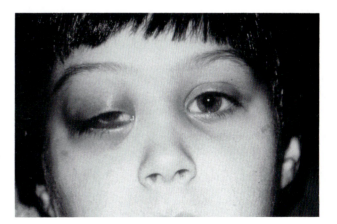

Figure 14–98. Orbital rhabdomyosarcoma.

The pathogens in orbital cellulitis are the same as in preseptal cellulitis, with the addition of *Pseudomonas aeruginosa, Escherichia coli,* Bacteroides, and Peptococcus. The latter two are more commonly encountered in animal or human bites. In children over 5 years of age, the treatment of choice is intravenous nafcillin pending culture results. Cefuroxime is used for children less than 5 years of age to cover *H. influenzae* (discussed earlier). Penicillin G, cefuroxime, or chloramphenicol (100 mg/kg per day in four divided doses) is recommended for human and animal bites, or other possible anaerobic infections. Ceftazidine (150 mg/kg per day in four divided doses) is useful against gram-negative bacteria. Topical or systemic sinus decongestants should also be considered. After an appropriate course of intravenous therapy dictated by clinical findings, outpatient treatment with oral cloxacillin or cefaclor (for staphylococcal and streptococcal infections), or Augmentin 40 mg/kg per day in three doses (for nonresistant strains of *H. influenzae*) can be instituted. Antibiotic treatment should continue for 5 to 7 days, or until there is complete clinical resolution; streptococcal infections require a minimum of 10 days of treatment.

The presence of an orbital abscess, suspected by lack of improvement and corroborated by CT, is an indication for surgical drainage. CT findings and surgical treatment for subperiosteal orbital abscesses (SOA) in children, however, are controversial (Fig. 14–99). Several reports have documented CT evidence of an SOA that was not found at surgery, and have suggested that SOA in children may be successfully managed by medical treatment alone (Catalano & Smoot, 1990; Rubin et al, 1989). We suggest that clinical findings govern whether surgical intervention is indicated in children with a radiographically detected subperiosteal mass. CT scanning can be useful in preventing surgical intervention in children who clearly show no radiographic signs of SOA, and scanning should be performed when there is evidence of clinical deterioration to delineate the extent of disease.

Inflammation of the Eye (Uveitis)

When a child presents with inflammation within the eye (uveitis), a directed approach, dependent upon historical and clinical findings, is suggested. Extensive laboratory testing is reserved for bilateral or severe recurrent uveitis.

The first step in the evaluation of uveitis is to obtain an accurate history. It is important to understand whether the uveitis is acute, chronic, or recurrent, and if it is unilateral or bilateral. The history should also determine whether there are any associated systemic conditions, particularly arthritis, gastrointestinal disorders, dermatologic disorders, and venereal diseases. Finally, the personal history should detail the patient's sex, age, race, geographical background, illicit drug use, and association with pets. The uveitic entities that should be considered based on historical information are reviewed in Table 14–13.

The second step is to establish the anatomic location of the primary inflammation, and identify any particular findings by clinical examination. Although certain disorders (such as sarcoidosis, syphilis, and tuberculosis) have a propensity to involve more than one region of the eye, others primarily involve the anterior eye (ankylosing spondylitis, herpes simplex, herpes zoster, and lens-induced uveitis) or posterior eye (toxoplasmosis, toxocariasis, and histoplasmosis). Iris

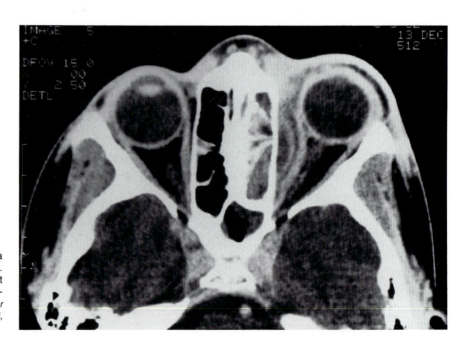

Figure 14–99. Computed tomography in a child with orbital cellulitis and ethmoiditis. The subperiosteal collection may represent reactive inflammatory edema or a subperiosteal abscess. *(From Catalano RA: Ocular Emergencies. Philadelphia, Saunders, 1992, p 74, with permission.)*

TABLE 14–13. HISTORICAL ASSOCIATIONS OF UVEITIS

Historical Information	Potential Uveitic Entities
▪ AGE	
Childhood/youth (0–21 years)	Juvenile rheumatoid arthritis, toxocariasis, pars planitis
Middle age (21–60 years)	Histoplasmosis, toxoplasmosis, pars planitis, Vogt–Koyanagi–Harada syndrome, Behçet's syndrome, acute multifocal posterior pigment epitheliopathy (AMMPE)
Elderly (over 60 years)	Masquerade syndrome, reticulum cell sarcoma, malignant melanoma, herpes zoster
▪ RACE	
Black	Sarcoidosis, sickle-cell disease
Caucasian	Reiter's syndrome, ankylosing spondylitis
Oriental	Vogt–Koyanagi–Harada syndrome, Behçet's syndrome
Mediterranean	Behçet's syndrome
▪ SEX	
Male	Ankylosing spondylitis, Reiter's syndrome, Behçet's syndrome, Eales disease
Female	Juvenile rheumatoid arthritis, sarcoidosis
▪ GEOGRAPHICAL BACKGROUND	
Ohio and Mississippi Valleys	Ocular histoplasmosis
Southeastern United States	Sarcoidosis
Mediterranean	Behçet's syndrome
Japan	Vogt–Koyanagi–Harada syndrome
San Joaquin Valley	Coccidioidomycosis
▪ PETS	
Cat	Toxoplasmosis
Dog	Toxocariasis
Birds	Psittacosis
▪ PERSONAL HISTORY	
Drug abuse	*Candida* retinitis
Venereal disease	Syphilitic iritis or chorioretinitis
AIDS	Cytomegalovirus retinitis, toxoplasmosis, herpes zoster ophthalmicus, tuberculosis, *Candida* retinitis, acute retinal necrosis, *Cryptococcus*
▪ ONSET/COURSE	
Insidious/chronic	Juvenile rheumatoid arthritis, *Candida* and toxoplasmosis retinitis, pars planitis
Sudden (pain and injection)	Ankylosing spondylitis; Vogt–Koyanagi–Harada, Behçet's, and Reiter's syndromes

Modified from Nozik RA: Laboratory testing in uveitis. Focal points: Clinical modules for ophthalmologists, vol 1, no. 8. American Academy of Ophthalmology, 1983, p 2, with permission.

nodules are most typical of sarcoidosis, and a hypopyon suggests HLA-B27 related anterior uveitis (D'Alessandro et al, 1991).

The third step is selected laboratory testing based on a presumed diagnosis (see Table 14–5). All patients with granulomatous uveitis should undergo serological testing for syphilis and skin testing for tuberculosis, as these are readily treatable conditions. Other laboratory tests are only used in selected severe, bilateral, or recurrent cases that present diagnostic dilemmas. Human leukocyte antigen (HLA) testing identifies the presence of cell-surface markers called histocompatability antigens. Several uveitic entities are associated with specific HLA antigens. These include B27 (ankylosing spondylitis, Reiter's syndrome, juvenile rheumatoid arthritis); B5 (Behçet's syndrome); B7 (histo-

plasmosis); DRW2 (macular histoplasmosis); BW22J (Vogt–Koyanagi–Harada syndrome); and B29 (birdshot choroiditis). HLA typing is expensive and often nonspecific; it should be performed only when one of the above disorders is being considered and other tests have been inconclusive. Invasive procedures should also be used judiciously. An anterior chamber tap in childhood can be considered when the differential includes bacterial or fungal endophthalmitis, iris or ciliary body tumor, leukemia, sarcoidosis (angiotensin-converting enzyme level), and toxocariasis (ELISA test). A vitreous tap should be performed in all cases of suspected bacterial or fungal endophthalmitis.

A few salient points regarding common uveitic entities in children are presented at the beginning of this chapter. Additional details are provided below.

Uveitic Entities in Children

Approximately 6 percent of all cases of uveitis occur in patients under 16 years of age (Kanski & Shun-Shin, 1984). By far the most common systemic association is **juvenile rheumatoid arthritis** (JRA; Still's disease). This predominantly affects girls. Characteristic findings include *chronic* anterior uveitis (duration longer than 3 months) and nongranulomatous inflammation. Complications include secondary cataracts, secondary glaucoma, posterior synechiae, and band keratopathy (Figs. 14–37, 14–38, and 14–100). Uveitis is more common when the onset of the JRA is confined to fewer than five joints (pauciarticular). The knees are most commonly affected, followed by the ankles (Fig. 14–101). Many of these children will subsequently develop polyarticular disease. The *onset* of pauciarticular disease is the important prognostic indicator; the subsequent involvement of more joints does not reduce the risk of ocular complications. The presence of antinuclear antibodies (ANA) is an additional risk factor, but the presence of rheumatoid factor (RF) suggests that the disease is similar to its adult counterpart, without an increased risk of developing uveitis. Additional extraocular manifestations include fever, secondary amyloidosis, ulcerative colitis, and psoriasis.

Because of the indolent onset of uveitis and common occurrence of complications, girls with pauciarticular onset and positive ANA titers should be screened by an ophthalmologist every 3 months. Patients who present with systemic symptoms and those with a positive RF have a negligible risk of uveitis and do not require repeated slit-lamp examination. The risk of uveitis diminishes by 5 years after onset. Topical corticosteroids are usually efficacious in treating the ocular disease, but some children are recalcitrant to steroids. Systemic steroids do not appear to offer any benefit in these cases, and the efficacy of immunosuppressive therapy is inconclusive.

In contrast to JRA, **juvenile ankylosing spondylitis**

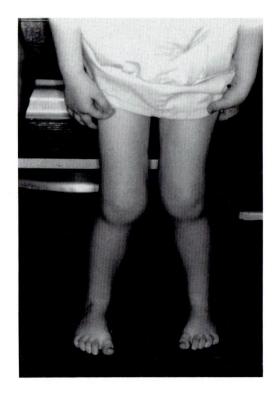

Figure 14–101. Arthritic involvement of both knees in juvenile rheumatoid arthritis.

occurs predominantly in boys with a mean age between 10 and 12 years. Rheumatoid factor testing is negative, but as many as 95 percent of affected boys test positive for HLA-B27. In further distinction to JRA, most boys present with *acute* anterior uveitis, as well as a peripheral arthropathy. Unlike ankylosing spondylitis in adults, symptoms of backache are infrequent and x-rays of the sacroiliac joints may initially show no abnormality. Bilaterality, hypopyon, secondary cataracts, regional ileitis, and chronicity can all develop. In most affected children, the inflammation can be controlled with topical corticosteroids.

Reiter's syndrome is rare in children. When present, it is usually associated with *Salmonella* or *Shigella* infection. Manifestations include a nonspecific urethritis and recurrent unilateral or bilateral anterior uveitis. Occasionally, the anterior chamber inflammation is severe, resulting in the formation of a hypopyon. Painless, bilateral conjunctivitis that resolves spontaneously without sequelae is common.

Behçet's syndrome is a rare uveitic entity that primarily affects men between the ages of 20 and 40 years. It is characterized by recurrent aphthous stomatitis (round, pearly specks found in the mouth; Fig. 14–102), genital ulcers, systemic vascular lesions, skin lesions, polyarthritis, and occasionally sacroiliitis and poliomyelitis. Acute or chronic anterior uveitis with the development of hypopyon is common (Fig. 14–103). Additional ocular findings include retinal vasculitis and

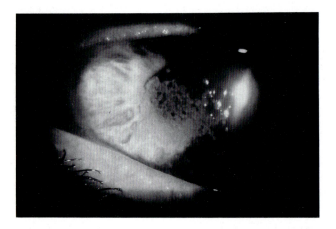

Figure 14–100. Band keratopathy in juvenile rheumatoid arthritis.

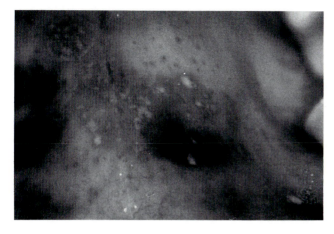

Figure 14–102. Aphthous stomatitis in Behçet's syndrome. Note the round pearly specs on the hard palate.

ischemia, vitreous hemorrhage, and ischemic optic neuropathy. Large, white areas of retinal infarction may appear similar to toxoplasmic retinitis, but are distinguished by the absence of exudation. Treatment requires systemic corticosteroids; in recalcitrant cases, chlorambucil can be tried.

Vogt–Koyanagi–Harada syndrome is another rare cause of uveitis. It predominantly affects individuals between 30 and 50 years of age of Asian (particularly Japanese) or American Indian descent. Adolescents can very rarely be affected. Characteristic signs include vitiligo (Fig. 14–104), poliosis (Fig. 14–105), deafness, tinnitus, vertigo, headache, and bilateral chronic uveitis. Less frequent symptoms include headache, stiff neck, paralysis, seizures, and coma. Anterior ocular findings include inflammation with seclusion of the pupil and ocular hypotony. Posterior ocular findings include multifocal exudative choroiditis, peripapillary edema, serous retinal detachment with mottled scarring, macular edema, and retinal phlebitis. Depigmen-

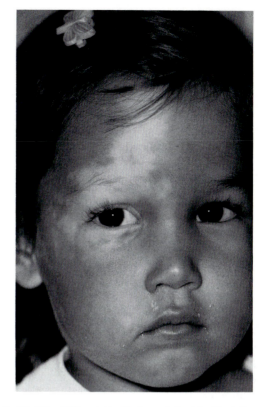

Figure 14–104. Vitiligo (skin depigmentation) in Vogt–Koyanagi–Harada syndrome.

tation of the skin and hair (vitiligo and poliosis) usually occurs weeks to months after the onset of ocular findings; occasionally the two systems are involved concurrently. The etiology is believed to be a viral infection or allergic reaction to uveal pigment; histopathology reveals a diffuse granulomatous uveitis resembling sympathetic ophthalmia, but with involvement of the choriocapillaris. Systemic, topical, and periocular steroids are indicated.

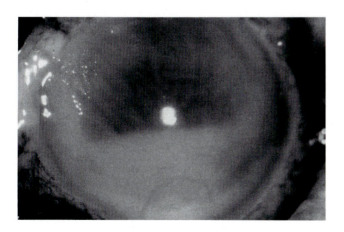

Figure 14–103. Uveitis with hypopyon in Behçet's syndrome.

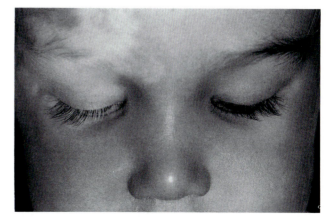

Figure 14–105. Poliosis (depigmentation of the eyelashes and eyebrows) in Vogt–Koyanagi–Harada syndrome.

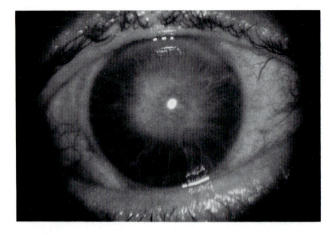

Figure 14–106. Interstitial keratitis and glaucoma in syphilis. *(From Catalano RA: Ocular Emergencies. Philadelphia, Saunders, 1992, p 265, with permission.)*

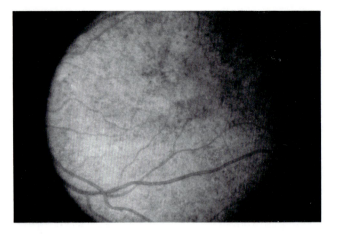

Figure 14–108. "Salt-and-pepper" chorioretinitis secondary to congenital syphilis.

Syphilis is transmitted by the spirochete *Treponema pallidum*. It can affect children as a congenital disorder, and adolescents as an acquired infectious disease.

Congenital syphilis results from transplacental transmission of the organism. It can become clinically apparent in utero, perinatally, or between late childhood and early adolescence.

The most common ocular manifestation of congenital syphilis is binocular interstitial keratitis. This usually presents between 7 and 17 years of age with anterior uveitis, superficial and deep corneal neovascularization, and secondary glaucoma (Fig. 14–106). With resolution, a characteristic sheath of translucent tissue remains near Descemet's membrane and linear "ghost vessels" remain from the neovascularization (Fig. 14–107). Inner ear inflammation may occur simultaneously or subsequent to interstitial keratitis and result in bilateral deafness. Other ocular findings include a chorioretinitis that leaves the fundus with a "salt-and-pepper" appearance (Fig. 14–108) or a "bone-cor-

puscular" pigmented and atrophic midperipheral retinopathy resembling retinitis pigmentosa (Fig. 14–109). Interstitial keratitis is not considered to be contagious; rather, it represents an inflammatory response to treponemal antigens.

Infants with congenital syphilis should always be treated for neurosyphilis, regardless of the cerebrospinal fluid serology. Penicillin G 50,000 U/kg in two divided doses intramuscularly or intravenously for 10 days is recommended. Oral erythromycin 30 to 50 mg/kg in four divided doses for 15 days can be used in penicillin-allergic individuals, but studies do not exist that verify that this is effective in eradicating neurological disease. Older children with interstitial keratitis should be treated with topical corticosteroids, topical cycloplegics, and systemic antibiotics. Oral ampicillin 1.5 g in combination with probenecid (500 mg every 6 hours) for 30 days is usually recommended.

Acquired syphilis can be encountered in sexually active adolescents and sexually abused children. The

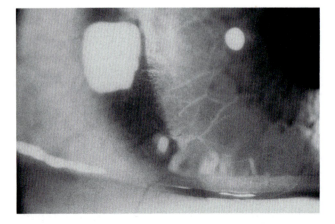

Figure 14–107. "Ghost vessels" following syphilitic interstitial keratitis.

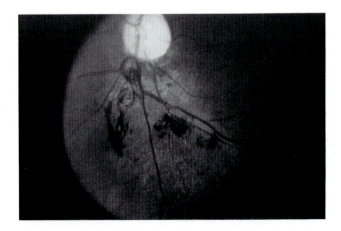

Figure 14–109. Sectoral "bone-corpuscular" chorioretinitis secondary to congenital syphilis, resembling retinitis pigmentosa.

first stage is characterized by a chancre and regional lymphadenopathy. The second stage begins weeks to months after infection, during which hematogenous dissemination occurs. Symptoms of tertiary syphilis may not occur until 20 years after the infection.

Ocular disease can occur during any stage; a conjunctival chancre can occur as the first stage. Second-stage findings include interstitial keratitis, conjunctivitis, anterior or posterior uveitis, scleritis, episcleritis, dacryoadenitis, dacryocystitis, retinochoroiditis, optic neuritis, papilledema, and vitritis. Tertiary findings include gummas of the extraocular muscles, sclera, iris, or optic nerve; optic atrophy; miotic pupils that constrict to accommodation but not light stimulation (Argyll–Robertson pupils); visual field defects; and an intense sectoral retinal pigmentary degeneration which can be mistaken for malignant melanoma (Fig. 14–110).

Primary and secondary acquired syphilis is treated with 2.4 million units of benzathine penicillin G administered by intramuscular injection in a single dose. Oral tetracycline 500 mg or erythromycin 500 mg four times daily for 15 days can be used in penicillin-allergic individuals. For latent syphilis of indeterminate duration, three consecutive weekly injections of penicillin G should be administered. Neurosyphilis requires 2 to 4 million units of crystalline penicillin G intravenously every 4 hours for 10 days, followed by 2.4 million units of benzathine penicillin G intramuscularly each week for a subsequent three weeks. Individuals with ocular syphilis should be treated in the same manner as those with neurosyphilis. A non-treponemal serological test for syphilis should be obtained 4 to 6 weeks after treatment to determine the adequacy of treatment.

Toxoplasmosis is a disease caused by the protozoan *Toxoplasma gondii*. This parasite has a predilection for the brain, lung, heart, nerve fiber layer of the retina, and muscle. Most infections are congenital in origin. An infection that occurs during the first trimester of gestation can result in microphthalmos, posterior uve-

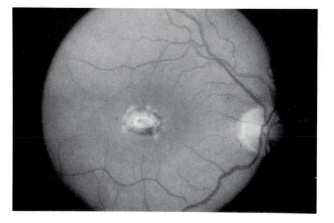

Figure 14–111. Congenital toxoplasmosis lesion involving the macula.

itis, optic atrophy, strabismus, nystagmus, and reduced visual acuity. The latter findings are due to the propensity of the organism to involve the macula (Fig. 14–111). Infection later in pregnancy is usually mild and subclinical, but may result in ocular sequelae later in life. Reactivation occurs when Toxoplasma cysts rupture, stimulating the host's immune response, and resulting in inflammation at or near the site of infection. It is recognized by the development of an exudative retinochoroiditis with a prominence of vitreous cells, in an eye that appears quiet externally (Fig. 14–112). Focal, necrotizing lesions are often observed juxtaposed to old pigmented scars (Fig. 14–113) from previous involvement. Acute retinitis is seen as a circumscribed white or yellow-white lesion with fluffy or indistinct edges. It may be as small as one-tenth disc diameter in size to as large as five or six disc diameters. Massive exudation of cells into the overlying vitreous gives the impression of "looking at a headlight through the fog." Lesions can occur near the optic nerve, and

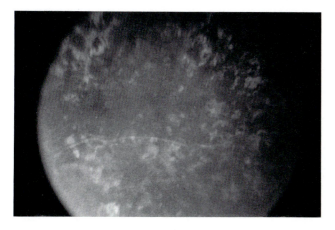

Figure 14–110. Profound retinal pigmentary changes in acquired syphilis, resembling malignant melanoma.

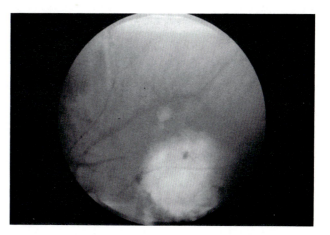

Figure 14–112. Active toxoplasmosis.

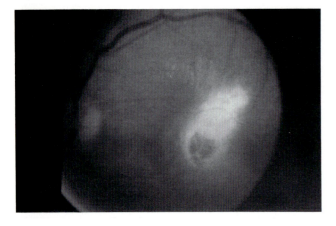

Figure 14–113. Reactivation of toxoplasmosis juxtaposed to an old toxoplasmosis chorioretinal scar.

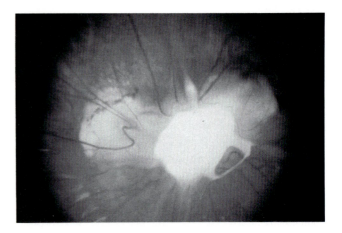

Figure 14–114. Toxocariasis near the optic nerve head. Note the vitreous strands creating retinal traction. *(Courtesy of the Wills Eye Hospital slide collection.)*

within the macular area, resulting in a profound loss of vision.

Peripheral lesions may be observed, but vision-threatening disease should be treated. The recommended treatment is sulfadiazine and pyrimethamine with folinic acid as first-line therapy (Table 14–14). An alternate antibiotic choice is clindamycin. Prednisone can be added if the lesion is threatening the macula or optic nerve.

Toxocariasis is a parasitic infection acquired by ingesting the ova of usually the dog roundworm, *Toxocara canis*, but occasionally the cat roundworm, *Toxocara cati*. The larva hatch in the intestine and migrate throughout the body (visceral larva migrans). The organs most commonly involved are the liver, lungs, brain, heart, eye, and orbit. Visceral larva migrans usually presents around age 2 to 3 years, but ocular findings usually occur or are discovered several years later. Toxocara ocular lesions are white in color and elevated (pseudoglioma). Vitreous strands can adhere to the granuloma and distort the retina (Fig. 14–114). This differs from toxoplasmic lesions, which are flat and without glial adhesions. A second presentation of tox-

ocariasis is endophthalmitis, which can present as leukocoria.

Diagnosis is made with a serological enzyme-linked immunosorbent assay test. Occasionally, serum titers are normal, in which case aqueous titers should be considered. The prognosis for visual acuity in ocular toxocariasis is poor; 80 percent of untreated cases will eventually have less than 20/200 vision. Treatment should include both an antihelminthic and corticosteroid, because the inflammatory response to the dead nematode is often more destructive than the roundworm itself. The suggested treatment is thiabendazole 25 to 50 mg in two divided doses daily for 7 to 10 days, with oral prednisone 2 mg/kg tapered over 3 weeks. Surgical excision can be attempted, but may be complicated by retinal detachment.

Although rare individuals with active choroiditis and endophthalmitis secondary to histoplasmosis infection have been described, the typical individual diagnosed with this disease does not have active disease. In these instances the term "presumed" is used for patients with retinal findings of multiple, small, punched-out lesions that often occur near the optic

TABLE 14–14. RECOMMENDED TREATMENT FOR OCULAR TOXOPLASMOSIS

Drug	Loading Dose	Maintenance	Duration (weeks)
Pyrimethamine[a]	50 mg every 12 hours × 2	25 mg 2 times/day	3–4
Sulfadiazine[b]	2 g	1 g 4 times/day	3–4
Prednisone[c]	—	20–40 mg/day	3–4
Folinic acid	—	3–5 mg every third day	3–4
Clindamycin[d]	—	300 mg 4 times/day	3

[a]White blood cells and platelets should be monitored weekly.
[b]Fluid intake should be maximized to decrease sulfadiazine renal crystallization.
[c]Contraindicated if tuberculosis, AIDS, or systemic infection suspected.
[d]Observe for pseudomembranous colitis.

nerve and macula. Inactive scars resemble toxoplasmic retinitis, except that they are smaller (Fig. 14–115). Furthermore, the vitreous is clear, because these lesions are secondary to a choroiditis, not a retinitis. The importance of this diagnosis is that presumed ocular histoplasmosis can be associated with the development of a subretinal neovascular membrane, which can rupture, resulting in a marked reduction of vision (Fig. 14–116).

Sarcoidosis is a multisystem granulomatous inflammatory disease that occurs rarely in children. Affected organs include the lungs, mediastinal and hilar lymph nodes, liver, spleen, phalangeal bones, parotid gland, skin, and eyes. Anergy is common, as is a reduction in circulating T lymphocytes, hypercalciuria, and hypergammaglobulinemia. Biopsy of focal lesions demonstrate noncaseating epitheliod granulomas. In the very young it rarely involves the lungs, and typically presents with joint, skin, and eye findings. Ocular involvement can present with either an acute or chronic anterior uveitis. Additional ocular findings include iris nodules (see Fig. 14–36), retinal vasculitis, "snowball" opacities in the vitreous (Fig. 14–117), and conjunctival nodules. Biopsy of the latter, which typically occur in the lower cul-de-sac, may be diagnostic.

Tuberculosis infection of the eye is rare. It may occur as a primary conjunctivitis, but more commonly represents a secondary infection due to hematogenous spread. Allergic manifestations (phlyctenules) and ocular symptoms from involvement of adjacent sinuses, the orbit, or intracranial optic pathways are more common than intraocular infection. External ocular manifestations include follicular, granulomatous, papillary, or purulent conjunctivitis; phlyctenules; subconjunctival nodules; blepharitis; cellulitis; chronic dacryoadenitis; and dacryocystitis. Internal ocular findings include disseminated choroiditis, interstitial keratitis, granulomatous anterior uveitis with mutton-fat keratic precipitates, exudative retinitis, scleritis, optic neuritis, and tuberculous panophthalmitis. Central nervous system

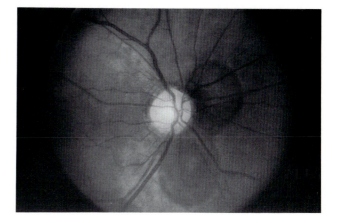

Figure 14–116. Subretinal hemorrhage from a subretinal neovascular membrane secondary to presumed ocular histoplasmosis.

involvement can cause internuclear ophthalmoplegia, gaze palsies, and optic nerve atrophy.

A reactive skin test in conjunction with ocular inflammation should prompt a systemic evaluation and consideration of full-dose antituberculous treatment. When active systemic disease cannot be confirmed, a trial of isoniazid before the use of high-dose corticosteroids has been advocated (Abrams & Schlaegel, 1982). Oral steroids in patients with unrecognized ocular tuberculosis can precipitate miliary tuberculosis. Topical steroids (with cycloplegics) can control inflammation and prevent corneal scarring due to keratitis or iritis.

Lyme disease is a tick-borne illness caused by the spirochete *Borrelia burgdorferi*. It is most common in the Eastern United States, Pacific Northwest, and Midwest. The illness usually begins in the summer, following a tick bite. The first stage includes a localized blotchy red skin rash, known as erythema chronicum migrans, stiff neck, fever, headache, fatigue, malaise, myalgias, and/or arthralgias. Not all patients, however, develop a fever or rash. The second stage, occurring in up to 15 percent of patients, includes meningitis

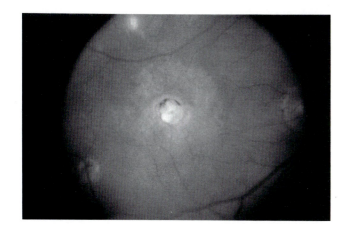

Figure 14–115. Presumed ocular histoplasmosis.

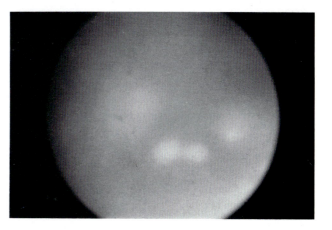

Figure 14–117. "Snowball" vitreous opacities in sarcoidosis.

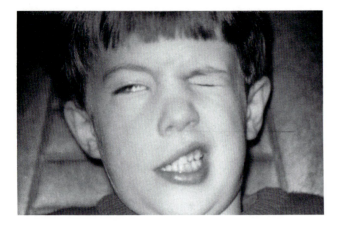

Figure 14–118. Seventh-nerve palsy affecting the right side of the face secondary to Lyme disease.

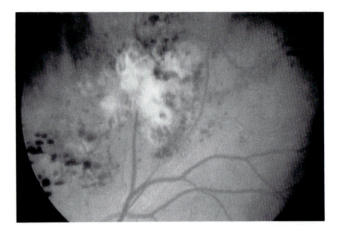

Figure 14–120. Cytomegalovirus retinitis in acquired immune deficiency syndrome (AIDS).

with or without facial nerve palsy (Fig. 14–118) and carditis. The third stage, occurring months to years later in up to 60 percent of these patients, is characterized by an oligoarticular arthritis. Central nervous system manifestations can occur during either the second or third stage; cranial neuropathies usually occur during the second stage, approximately 4 weeks after the onset of the rash.

Neuro-ophthalmologic findings include meningitis with papilledema, optic neuritis, neuroretinitis (Fig. 14–119), and sixth- and seventh-nerve paresis. Additional findings include other cranial nerve neuropathies, radiculopathy, conjunctivitis, episcleritis, keratitis, and iridocyclitis. Most patients with neurological manifestations also have headache, spinal fluid lymphocytic pleocytosis, and occasionally elevated CSF protein, but normal CSF glucose and opening pressure.

An enzyme-linked immunosorbent assay, immunofluorescent tests, Lyme Western blot, and lymphocyte stimulation tests are available for diagnosis (Mi-

crobiology Reference Laboratory, Cypress, CA). The recommended treatment for children is penicillin 50 mg/kg per day in four divided doses (not < 1 g or > 2 g/day) or erythromycin 30 mg/kg per day in three to four divided doses, for 15 to 20 days. If the central nervous system is involved, intravenous ceftriaxone (2 g every 12 hours for 14 days), or penicillin G (2 to 4 million units every 4 hours for 10 days) is recommended.

Cytomegalovirus (CMV) retinopathy is the most common, vision-threatening opportunistic infection in the acquired immune deficiency syndrome (AIDS). It is recognized as one to several areas of granular, ischemic, white retina intermixed with retinal hemorrhages ("crumbled cheese" or "pizza pie" appearance). The overlying vitreous is clear, distinguishing this from acute retinal necrosis and toxoplasmosis (Fig. 14–120). Several antivirals have been shown to have activity in halting or slowing the progression of CMV retinopathy. These include ganciclovir and foscarnet (Holland, 1990). Bone marrow suppression can occur with the former and renal toxicity with the latter. Both must be given as maintenance therapy to prevent reactivation. Steroids have no role, because the retinal destruction is due to viral infection of retinal cells, not inflammation.

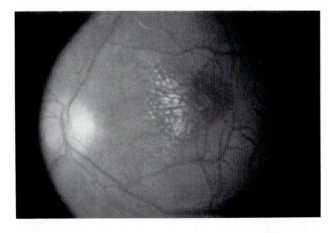

Figure 14–119. Neuroretinitis secondary to Lyme disease. *(From Catalano RA: Ocular Emergencies. Philadelphia, Saunders, 1992, p 426, with permission.)*

REFERENCES

Allergic Conjunctivitis

Abelson MB, Madiwale N, Weston JE: Conjunctival eosinophils in allergic ocular disease. Arch Ophthalmol 101:555, 1983.

Allansmith MR, Baird RS, Greiner JV: Vernal conjunctivitis compared and contrasted. Am J Ophthalmol 87:544, 1979.

Aswad MI, Tauber J, Baum J: Plasmapheresis treatment in patients with severe atopic keratoconjunctivitis. Ophthalmology 95:444, 1988.

Easty DL: External ocular disease in atopic patients. In Easty DL, Smolin G (eds): External Eye Disease. London, Butterworths, 1985, pp 239–271.

Foster CS: Evaluation of topical cromolyn sodium in the treatment of vernal conjunctivitis. Ophthalmology 95:194, 1988.

Jones BR: Allergic disease of the outer eye. Trans Ophthalmol Soc UK 91:441, 1989.

Kray KT, Squire EN, Tipton WR, et al: Cromolyn sodium in seasonal allergic conjunctivitis. J Allergy Clin Immunol 76:623, 1985.

Morgan G: The pathology of vernal keratoconjunctivitis. Trans Ophthalmol Soc UK 91:476, 1971.

Neumann E, Gutmann J, Blumenkrantz N, Michaelson IC: A review of 400 cases of vernal conjunctivitis. Am J Ophthalmol 47:166, 1957.

Syrbopoulos S, Gilbert D, Easty DL: Double-blind comparison of a steroid (prednisolone) and a nonsteroid (tolmetin) in vernal keratoconjunctivitis. Cornea 5:35, 1986.

Endophthalmitis

Affeldt JC, Flynn HW Jr, Forster RK, et al: Microbial endophthalmitis resulting from ocular trauma. Ophthalmology 94:407, 1987.

Annable WL, Kachmer ML, DiMarco M, DeSantis D: Long-term follow-up of Candida endophthalmitis in the premature infant. J Pediatr Ophthalmol Strabismus 27:104, 1990.

Baley JE, Annable WL, Kliegman RM: Candida endophthalmitis in the premature infant. J Pediatrics 98:458, 1981.

Clinch TE, Duker JS, Eagle RC, et al: Infantile endogenous Candida endophthalmitis presenting as a cataract. Surv Ophthalmol 34:197, 1989.

Forster RK: Etiology and diagnosis of bacterial postoperative endophthalmitis. Ophthalmology 85:320, 1978.

Johnson DE, Thompson TR, Green TP, Ferrieri P: Systemic candidiasis in very-low-birth-weight infants (<1500 grams). Pediatrics 73:138, 1985.

Pflugfelder SC, Flynn HW Jr, Zwickey TA, et al: Exogenous fungal endophthalmitis. Ophthalmology 95:19, 1988.

Puliafito CA, Baker AS, Haff J, Foster CS: Infectious endophthalmitis: Review of 36 cases. Ophthalmology 89:921, 1982.

Rowsey JJ, Newsome DL, Sexton DJ, Harms WK: Endophthalmitis: Current approaches. Ophthalmology 89:1055, 1982.

Eyelid Infections

Committee on Infectious Diseases, American Academy of Pediatrics: Herpes simplex. In: AAP 1990 Red Book. Elk Grove Village, IL, AAP, 1988, pp 230–239.

Jeffers JB, Bedrossian EH Jr; Medical and surgical treatment of chalazia. In Reinecke RD (ed): Ophthalmology Annual. East Norwalk, CT, Appleton-Century-Crofts, 1985, vol 1, pp 97–116.

Overall JC: Herpes simplex virus. In Behrman RE, Vaughan VC, Nelson WE (eds): Nelson Textbook of Pediatrics. Philadelphia, Saunders, 1987, pp 434–435.

Weiss A, Friendly D, Eglin K, et al: Bacterial periorbital and orbital cellulitis in childhood. Ophthalmology 90:195, 1983.

Winterkorn J: Lyme disease: Neurologic and ophthalmic manifestations. Surv Ophthalmol 35:191, 1990.

Zwaan J: Styes and chalazia. In Dershewitz RA (ed): Ambulatory Pediatric Care. Philadelphia, Lippincott, 1988, pp 419–423.

Infection in the Newborn (Ophthalmia Neonatorum)

American Academy of Pediatrics: Prevention of neonatal ophthalmia. In American Academy of Pediatrics, American College of Obstetricians and Gynecologists: Guidelines for perinatal care. Elk Grove Village, IL, AAP, 1988, pp 299–301.

Bell TA, Sandstrom KI, Gravett MG, et al: Comparison of ophthalmic silver nitrate solution and erythromycin for prevention of neonatally acquired chlamydial trachomatis. Sex Trans Dis 14:195, 1987.

Centers for Disease Control: 1989 Sexually transmitted diseases guidelines. MMWR 38 (suppl 8):1, 1989.

Cohen KL, McCarthy LR: Haemophilus influenzae ophthalmia neonatorum. Arch Ophthalmol 98:1214, 1980.

Doraiswamy B, Hammerschlag MR, Pringle GF, et al: Ophthalmia neonatorum caused by beta-lactamase producing Neisseria gonorrhea. JAMA 250:790, 1983.

Flach AJ: Ophthalmia neonatorum. In Tabbara KF, Hundiuk RA (eds): Infections of the Eye. Boston, Little, Brown, 1986, pp 437–460.

Fransen L, van den Berghe P, Mertens A, et al: Incidence and bacteriologic aetiology of neonatal conjunctivitis. Eur J Pediatr 146:152, 1987.

Friendly DS: Ophthalmia neonatorum. Pediatr Clin North Am 30:1033, 1983.

Haimovici R, Roussel TJ: Treatment of gonococcal conjunctivitis with a single-dose intramuscular ceftriaxone. Am J Ophthalmol 107:511, 1989.

Hammerschlag MR, Cummings C, Roblin PM, et al: Efficacy of neonatal ocular prophylaxis for the prevention of chlamydial and gonococcal conjunctivitis. N Engl J Med 320:769, 1989.

Harrison JR, English MG, Lee CK, et al: Chlamydia trachomatis infant pneumonitis. N Engl J Med 298:702, 1978.

Hick JF, Block DJ, Ilatrup DM; A controlled study of silver nitrate prophylaxis and the incidence of nasolacrimal duct obstruction. J Pediatr Ophthalmol Strabismus 22:92, 1985.

Hook EW, Holmes KK: Gonococcal infections. Ann Intern Med 102:229, 1985.

Isenberg SJ, Apt L, Yishimori R, et al: Source of the conjunctival bacterial flora at birth and implications for ophthalmia neonatorum prophylaxis. Am J Ophthalmol 106:458, 1988.

Kibrick S: Herpes simplex infection at term, what to do with mother, newborn, and nursery personnel. JAMA 243:157, 1980.

Koskiniemi M, Happonen JM, Javenpaa AA, et al: Neonatal herpes simplex virus infection: A report of 43 patients. Pediatr Infect Dis J 8:30, 1989.

Laga M, Plummer FA, Piot P, et al: Prophylaxis of gonococcal and chlamydial ophthalmia neonatorum. A comparison of silver nitrate and tetracycline. N Engl J Med 318:653, 1987.

LePage P, Bogaerts J, Kestelyn P, et al: Single dose cefotaxime intramuscularly cures gonococcal ophthalmia neonatorum. Br J Ophthalmol 72:518, 1988.

Nahmias AJ, Visintine AM, Caldwell DR, et al: Eye infections with herpes simplex virus in neonates. Surv Ophthalmol 21:100, 1976.

Pierce JM, Ward ME, Seal DV: Ophthalmia neonatorum in the 1980s: Incidence, aetiology and treatment. Br J Ophthalmol 66:728, 1982.

Prober CG, Sullender WM, Yasukawa LL, et al: Low risk of herpes simplex virus infections in neonates exposed to the virus at the time of vaginal delivery to mothers with recurrent genital herpes simplex virus infections. N Engl J Med 316:241, 1985.

Rapoza PA, Quinn TC, Kiessling LA, et al: Assessment of neonatal conjunctivitis with a direct immunofluorescent monoclonal antibody stain for chlamydia. JAMA 255:3369, 1986.

Rapoza PA, Quinn TC, Kiessling LA, Taylor HR: Epidemiology of neonatal conjunctivitis. Ophthalmology 93:456, 1986.

Ridgway GL: A fresh look at ophthalmia neonatorum. Trans Ophthalmol Soc UK 105:41, 1986.

Rotkis WM, Chandler JW: Neonatal conjunctivitis. In Tasman W, Jaeger EA (eds): Duane's Clinical Ophthalmology. Philadelphia, Lippincott, 1989, vol 4, pp 1–7.

Sandstrom KI, Bell TA, Chandler JW, et al: Microbial causes of neonatal conjunctivitis. J Pediatr 105:706, 1984.

Schacter J, Grossman M, Sweet RL, et al: Prospective study of perinatal transmission of Chlamydia trachomatis. JAMA 255:3374, 1986.

Schnall BM, Nelson LB: Ophthalmia neonatorum. Semin Ophthalmol 5:107, 1990.

Stenson S, Newman R, Fedukowicz H: Conjunctivitis in the newborn: Observations on incidence, cause, and prophylaxis. Ann Ophthalmol 13:329, 1981.

Traboulsi EI, Shamman IV, Ratl HE, et al: Pseudomonas aeruginosa ophthalmia neonatorum. Am J Ophthalmol 98:801, 1984.

Whitley RJ, Nahmais AJ, Visintine AM, et al: The natural history of herpes simplex virus infection of mother and newborn. Pediatrics 66:489, 1980.

Zwaan J: Ophthalmia neonatorum. In Dershewitz RA (ed): Ambulatory Pediatric Care. Philadelphia, Lippincott, 1988, pp 419–423.

Infectious Conjunctivitis

Aaberg TM: The expanding ophthalmologic spectrum of Lyme disease. Am J Ophthalmol 107:77, 1989.

Abu El Asrar AM, Geboes K, Maudgal PC, et al: Immunocytological study of phlyctenular eye disease. Int Ophthalmol 10:33, 1987.

Balfour HH Jr, Bean B, Laskin OL, et al: Acyclovir halts the progression of herpes zoster in immunocompromised patients. N Engl J Med 308:1448, 1983.

Beauchamp GR, Gillette TE, Friendly DS: Phlyctenular keratoconjunctivitis. J Pediatr Ophthalmol Strabismus 18:22, 1981.

Beauchamp GR, Meisler DM: Disorders of the conjunctiva. In Nelson LB, Calhoun JH, Harley RD (eds): Pediatric Ophthalmology, ed 3. Philadelphia, Saunders, 1991, pp 181–185. ·

Bron AJ, Mengher LS, Davey CC: The normal conjunctiva and its response to inflammation. Trans Ophthalmol Soc UK 104:424, 1985.

Carithers HA: Cat-scratch disease. An overview based on a study of 1,200 patients. Am J Dis Child 139:1124, 1985.

Chin GN, Hyndiuk RA: Parinaud's oculoglandular conjunctivitis. Clin Ophthalmol 4:1, 1987.

Chopra JS, Sawhney IMS, Dhand UK, et al: Neurological complications of acute hemorrhagic conjunctivitis. J Neurol Sci 73:177, 1986.

Couch JM, Green WR, Hirst LW, De La Cruz ZC: Diagnosing and treating Phthirus pubis palpebrarum. Surv Ophthalmol 26:219, 1982.

DeLuise VP: Viral conjunctivitis. In Tabbara KF, Hundiuk RA (eds): Infections of the Eye. Boston, Little, Brown, 1986, pp 437–460.

English CK, Wear DJ, Margileth AM, et al: Cat-scratch disease: Isolation and culture of the bacterial agent. JAMA 259:1347, 1988.

Gerber MA, Rapacz P, Kalter SS, Ballow M: Cell-mediated immunity in cat-scratch disease. J Allergy Clin Immunol 78:887, 1986.

Hammerschlag MR: Chlamydial infections. J Pediatr 114:727, 1989.

Holland GN: Infectious diseases. In Isenberg SJ (ed): The Eye in Infancy. Chicago, Year Book, 1989, pp 458–462.

Holley HP Jr: Successful treatment of cat-scratch disease with ciprofloxacin. JAMA 265:1563, 1991.

Kincaid MC: Pediculosis and phthiriasis. In Fraunfelder FT, Roy FH (eds): Current Ocular Therapy, ed 3. Philadelphia, Saunders, 1990, pp 115–117.

Lass JH, Foster CS, Grove AS, et al: Interferon-alpha therapy of recurrent conjunctival papillomas. Am J Ophthalmol 103:294, 1987.

Limberg MB: A review of bacterial keratitis and bacterial conjunctivitis. Am J Ophthalmol 112:2S, 1991.

Matoba A: Ocular viral infections. Ped Infect Dis 3:358, 1984.

Nelson LB, Catalano RA: Conjunctivitis. In Dershewitz RA (ed): Ambulatory Pediatric Care. Philadelphia, Lippincott, 1988, pp 419–423.

O'Day DM, Jones BR: Herpes simplex keratitis. In Duane TD, Jaeger EA (eds): Clinical Ophthalmology. Philadelphia, Harper & Row, 1987, vol 4, chapter 19.

Schwab IR: Oral acyclovir in the management of herpes simplex ocular infections. Ophthalmology 95:423, 1988.

Seal DV, Barrett SP, McGill JI: Aetiology and treatment of acute bacterial infection of the eye. Br J Ophthalmol 66:357, 1982.

Simon JW, Longo F, Smith RS: Spontaneous resolution of herpes simplex blepharoconjunctivitis in children. Am J Ophthalmol 102:598, 1986.

Steinert RF: Current therapy for bacterial keratitis and bacterial conjunctivitis. Am J Ophthalmol 112:10S, 1991.

Ullman S, Roussel TJ, Culbertson WW, et al: Gonococcal conjunctivitis. Surv Ophthalmol 32:199, 1987.

Ullman S, Roussel TJ, Culbertson WW, et al: Neisseria gonorrhea keratoconjunctivitis. Ophthalmology 94:525, 1987.

Wiley L, Springer D, Kowalski RP, et al: Rapid diagnostic test for ocular adenovirus. Ophthalmology 95:431, 1988.

Wilson FM: Papilloma. In Fraunfelder FT, Roy FH (eds): Current Ocular Therapy, ed 3. Philadelphia, Saunders, 1990, pp 286–288.

Inflammation of the Eye (Uveitis)

Abrams J, Schlaegel TF: The role of the isoniazid therapeutic test in tuberculosis uveitis. Am J Ophthalmol 94:511, 1982.

BenEzra D: Immunosuppressive treatment of uveitis. Int Ophthalmol Clin 30:291, 1990.

Cochereau-Massin I, Lehoang P, Lautier-Frau M, et al: Efficacy and tolerance of intravitreal ganciclovir in cytomegalovirus retinitis in acquired immune deficiency syndrome. Ophthalmology 98:1348, 1991.

Cohen KL, Peiffer RL Jr, Powell DA: Sarcoidosis and ocular disease in a young child. A case report and review of the literature. Arch Ophthalmol 99:422, 1981.

D'Alessandro LP, Forster DJ, Rao NA: Anterior uveitis and hypopyon. Am J Ophthalmol 112:317, 1991.

Duker JS, Blumenkranz MS: Diagnosis and management of the acute retinal necrosis (ARN) syndrome. Surv Ophthalmol 35:327, 1991.

Goto H, Rao NA: Sympathetic ophthalmia and Vogt–Koyanagi–Harada syndrome. Int Ophthalmol Clin 30:279, 1990.

Hemady R, Tauber J, Foster CS: Immunosuppressive drugs and inflammatory ocular disease. Surv Ophthalmol 35:369, 1991.

Holland GN: Acquired immune deficiency syndrome. In Fraunfelder FT, Roy FH (eds): Current Ocular Therapy. ed 3. Philadelphia, Saunders, 1990, pp 72–76.

Kanski JJ: Juvenile arthritis and uveitis. Surv Ophthalmol 34:253, 1990.

Kanski JJ: Anterior uveitis in juvenile rheumatoid arthritis. Arch Ophthalmol 95:1794, 1977.

Kanski JJ, Shun-Shin A: Systemic uveitic syndromes in childhood: An analysis of 340 cases. Ophthalmology 91:1247, 1984.

Mayers M: Ocular sarcoidosis. Int Ophthalmol Clin 30:257, 1990.

Nozik RA: Laboratory testing in uveitis. Focal points: Clinical Modules for Ophthalmologists. San Francisco, American Academy of Ophthalmology, 1983.

O'Connor GR: Tests in uveitis. In Duane TD, Jaeger EA (eds): Clinical Ophthalmology. vol 4, Philadelphia, Lippincott, 1981, chapter 34.

Pavesio CE, Nozik RA: Anterior and intermediate uveitis. Int Ophthalmol Clin 30:244, 1990.

Perkins ES: Pattern of uveitis in children. Br J Ophthalmol 50:169, 1966.

Regillo CD, Shields CL, Shields JA, et al: Ocular tuberculosis. JAMA 266:1490, 1991.

Rosen PH, Spalton DJ, Graham EM: Intraocular tuberculosis. Eye. 4:486, 1990.

Rosenbaum JT, Wermick R: Selection and interpretation of laboratory tests or patients with uveitis. Int Ophthalmol Clin 30:238, 1990.

Singsen BH, Bernstein BH, Koster-King KG, et al: Reiter's syndrome in childhood. Arthritis Rheum 20:402, 1977.

Smith RE, Nozik RA: Uveitis, A Clinical Approach to Diagnosis and Management, ed 2. Baltimore, Williams & Wilkins, 1989.

Tabbara KF, O'Connor GR: Treatment of ocular toxoplasmosis with clindamycin and sulfadiazine. Ophthalmology 87:129, 1980.

Tessler HH: Diagnosis and treatment of ocular toxoplasmosis. Focal points: Clinical modules for ophthalmologists. San Francisco, American Academy of Ophthalmology, 1985.

Winterkorn JMS: Lyme disease: Neurologic and ophthalmic manifestations. Surv Ophthalmol 35:191, 1990.

Ocular Infections

Auran JD, Starr MB, Jakobiec FA: Acanthomoeba keratitis. A review of the literature. Cornea 6:2, 1987.

Driebe WT, Stern GA, Epstein RJ: Acanthomoeba keratitis. Potential role for topical clotrimazole in combination therapy. Am J Ophthalmol 106:1196, 1988.

Jabs DA: Ocular toxoplasmosis. Int Ophthalmol Clin 30:264, 1990.

Pepose JS: Herpes simplex keratitis: Role of viral infection versus immune response. Surv Ophthalmol 35:345, 1991.

Tabbara KF, O'Connor GR: Treatment of ocular toxoplasmosis with clindamycin and sulfadiazine. Ophthalmology 87:129, 1980.

Orbital Infections

Catalano RA, Smoot C: Subperiosteal orbital abscesses in children with orbital cellulitis: Time for a reevaluation? J Pediatr Ophthalmol Strabismus 27:141, 1990.

Eustis HS, Armstrong DC, Buncic JR, et al: Staging of orbital cellulitis in children: Computerized tomography characteristics and treatment guidelines. J Pediatr Ophthalmol Strabismus 23:246, 1986.

Ferry AP, Abedi S: Diagnosis and management of rhino-orbitocerebral mucormycosis (phycomycosis). Ophthalmology 90:1096, 1983.

Gold SC, Arigg PG, Hedges TR III: Computerized tomography in the management of acute orbital cellulitis. Ophthalmic Surg 18:753, 1987.

Goodwin WJ Jr, Weinshall M, Chandler JR: The role of high resolution computerized tomography and standardized ultrasound in the evaluation of orbital cellulitis. Laryngoscope 92:728, 1982.

Harris GJ, Beatty RL: Acute proptosis in childhood. In Linberg JV (ed): Oculoplastic and Orbital Emergencies. Norwalk, CT, Appleton & Lange, 1990, pp 87–103.

Hornblass A, Herschorn BJ, Stern K, Grimes C: Orbital abscess. Surv Ophthalmol 29:169, 1984.

Israele V, Nelson JD, Periorbital and orbital cellulitis. Pediatr Infect Dis 6:404, 1987.

Jones DB: Microbial preseptal and orbital cellulitis. In Duane TD, Jaeger EA (eds): Clinical Ophthalmology. Philadelphia, Harper & Row, 1985, vol 4.

Kennerdel JS, Dresner SC: The nonspecific orbital inflammatory syndromes. Surv Ophthalmol 29:93, 1984.

Lawless M, Martin F: Orbital cellulitis and preseptal cellulitis in children. Aust NZ J Ophthalmol 14:211, 1986.

Leone CR Jr, Lloyd WC III: Treatment protocol for orbital inflammatory disease. Ophthalmology 92:1325, 1985.

Rubin SE, Garber PF: Orbital infections in childhood. Semin Ophthalmol 5:138, 1990.

Rubin SE, Rubin LG, Zito J, et al: Medical management of orbital subperiosteal abscesses in children. J Pediatr Ophthalmol Strabismus 26:21, 1989.

Schramm VL, Myers EN, Kennerdell JS: Orbital complications of acute sinusitis: Evaluation, management, and outcome. Trans Am Acad Ophthalmol Otolaryngol 86:221, 1978.

Schwartz JN, Donnelly EH, Klintworth GK: Ocular and orbital phycomycosis. Surv Ophthalmol 22:3, 1977.

Spires JR, Smith RJH: Bacterial infections of the orbital and periorbital soft tissues in children. Laryngoscope 96:763, 1986.

Steinkuller PG, Jones DB: Preseptal and orbital cellulitis and orbital abscess. In Linberg JV (ed): Oculoplastic and Orbital Emergencies. Norwalk, CT, Appleton & Lange, 1990, pp 51–66.

Tanenbaum M, Tanzel J, Byrne SF, et al: Medical management of orbital abscess. Surv Ophthalmol 30:211, 1985.

Weiss A, Friendly D, Eglin K, et al: Bacterial periorbital and orbital cellulitis in childhood. Ophthalmology 90:195, 1983.

ESSENTIAL INFORMATION FOR THE PRIMARY CARE PHYSICIAN

Children and adolescents account for a disproportionate share of ocular trauma. Boys aged 11 to 15 years are the most vulnerable; their injuries outnumber those of girls by a ratio of about 4 to 1. The majority of injuries are related to sports, toy darts, other projectiles, sticks, stones, and air-powered BB guns. The latter cause particularly devastating ocular and orbital injuries.

Evaluation of Ocular and Orbital Injuries

The following points are especially helpful in evaluating ocular and orbital injuries in children. In addition to detailed notes and sketches, photographic documentation is suggested, when possible.

The **history** details the mechanism and time of injury. A penetrating injury should be suspected if a projectile or pointed object was involved. Any symptoms—such as diplopia, decreased vision, visual floaters, or flashing lights—should be recorded. Treatments already given should be noted, and associated injuries described.

It is worth noting that the traumatically injured

child and/or the guardian may give an inaccurate or misleading history. The child may fear punishment for participating in a forbidden activity; the parent may try to conceal or deny improper or inadequate supervision. The physician should also be aware that adults guilty of child abuse will fabricate or misrepresent the history. Occasionally, abusing parents will not be aware that their action resulted in injury; this is common with parents who shake their babies.

The **past ocular history** notes any previous need for spectacles, ocular injuries, inflammation, or poor vision in an eye. Current medications, drug allergies, and the patient's tetanus immunization status should be recorded during the **medical history.**

The **visual acuity** should always be measured, even if only a gross estimate of vision (for example, able to detect hand motion at a distance of 5 feet) is possible. This is often forgotten in infants and toddlers. Illiterate eye charts, with tumbling "E's," Allen pictures, or "Landolt C" optotypes, are available for use in cooperative, preschool children (Fig. 15–1). The ability to fixate and follow objects is tested in younger children.

During the **external examination** any lid lacerations and/or potential orbital fractures are explored. Particular attention is directed toward potential injury of the lacrimal drainage system (Fig. 15–2). Palpation of the orbital rim can detect any interruptions, step-offs, or depressions suggesting an orbital rim fracture.

Modified in part from Catalano RA: Ocular Emergencies. Philadelphia, Saunders, 1992, with permission.

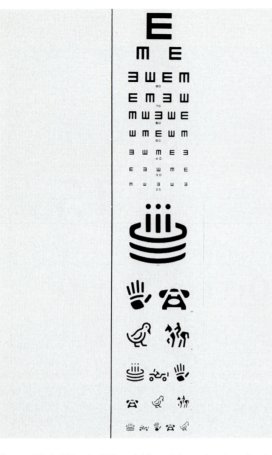

Figure 15–1. Illiterate "E" and Allen picture visual acuity charts for preverbal children.

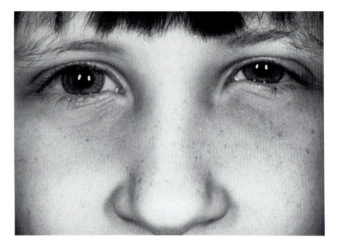

Figure 15–3. Enophthalmos of the left eye following a traumatic orbital floor fracture and herniation of orbital tissue into the maxillary sinus.

tance suggests either a medial canthal tendon injury or nasal fracture. The appearance of a sunken or depressed eye (enophthalmos) suggests an orbital fracture with herniation of tissue into either the maxillary or ethmoid sinus (Fig. 15–3). The appearance of a protruding eye (exophthalmos) suggests an orbital hemorrhage (Fig. 15–4). Skin elevation and crepitus (orbital emphysema) suggests a fracture through the ethmoid sinus or orbital floor (Fig. 15–5). Hypesthesia in the region of the infraorbital or supraorbital nerve suggests orbital floor or roof fracture, respectively. The presence of hemorrhage into the upper eyelid and conjunctiva is indicative of an orbital roof fracture (Fig. 15–6). Rhinorrhea suggests an orbital roof or basilar skull fracture.

An **ocular motility examination** is performed by asking the child to gaze in nine different positions as demonstrated in Figure 15–7. Any limitation of movement suggests either entrapment of an extraocular

Because much greater forces are necessary to fracture the orbital rim than the medial wall or orbital floor, an orbital wall fracture should be suspected if the orbital rim is discontinuous. Displacement of a globe to one side is suggestive of an orbital wall fracture to the side of the displacement. An increased intercanthal dis-

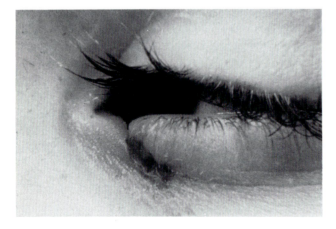

Figure 15–2. Eyelid laceration involving the eyelid margin and inferior lacrimal drainage apparatus.

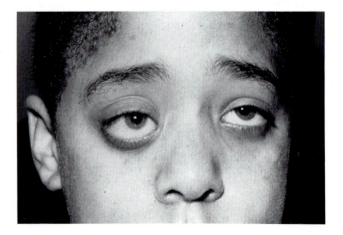

Figure 15–4. Exophthalmos of the right eye following a traumatic retrobulbar hemorrhage.

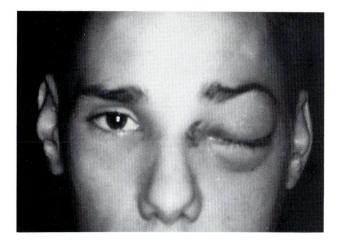

Figure 15–5. Orbital emphysema resulting from a fracture through the ethmoid sinus.

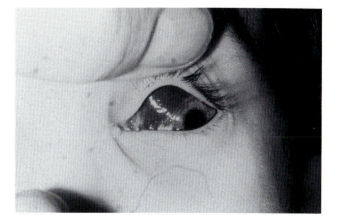

Figure 15–6. Hemorrhage under the superior conjunctiva in a child with an orbital roof fracture.

muscle or ocular motor paresis. Forced duction testing can help differentiate the two (Fig. 15–8). Inability to move an eye in a given direction (a positive test) suggests extraocular muscle entrapment, but restriction can also occur simply due to orbital edema or hemorrhage. Free rotation of the eye (a negative test) indicates an ocular motor paresis. Laceration or disinsertion of an extraocular muscle is extremely rare. When reported it is usually associated with either a high-impact motor vehicle accident or an atypical penetrating orbital injury.

Examination of the eye itself is more difficult. If the child is frightened or crying, this should only be performed with great care to avoid aggravating any preexisting injury. A papoose board may be helpful in restraining infants for examination and minor treatments

(Fig. 15–9). A useful position to restrain toddlers is demonstrated in Figure 15–10. The parent sits facing the physician's assistant. Both should be at the same level, and their knees should be close or touching. The child lies supine in the parent's and assistant's lap with the legs wrapped around the parent's waist and the head in the assistant's lap. The parent holds the child's hands folded across the child's waist. The physician's assistant, using both hands, immobilizes the child's head. In this position corneal abrasions can be easily detected with the ultraviolet illumination of a handheld Wood's lamp, after the installation of fluorescein dye (Fig. 15–11). A portable slit lamp can also be brought close to the child for examination of the external eye and eyelids (see Fig. 2–16).

If at any time during the examination suspicion of a

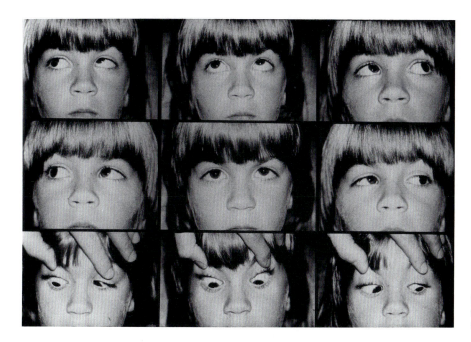

Figure 15–7. The nine positions of gaze used to detect any restriction of ocular movement.

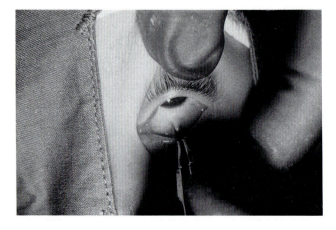

Figure 15–8. Forced duction testing. The conjunctiva and underlying extraocular muscle insertion are grasped with forceps and the eye is rotated in the direction of apparent restriction. In children, this test is only performed under general anesthesia.

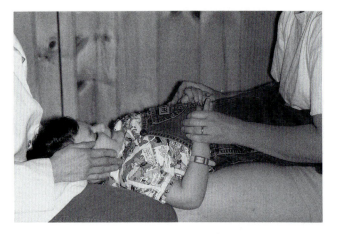

Figure 15–10. Two-person technique useful in restraining a toddler to examine the eye. *(From Catalano RA: Ocular Emergencies. Philadelphia, Saunders, 1992, p 93, with permission.)*

ruptured globe develops, no further diagnostic examinations should be performed. A protective eye shield that fits entirely over the bony orbit, completely encasing the eye (without a pressure patch), should be taped to the face (Fig. 15–12). Further examination and treatment should be carried out only under general anesthesia. Factors that portend a significant ocular injury are noted in Table 15–1.

Use of Sedation in Examination and Treatment

The injured child may be anxious and uncooperative in the physician's office or emergency room. Sedation or general anesthesia may be necessary to complete an examination that would be routine in an adult. Several options for sedation exist (Table 15–2). No drug has all of the desired characteristics of rapid onset, short duration, reversibility, and absolute safety. Infant death (presumably from respiratory depression) has been reported even with chloral hydrate (Jastak & Pallasch, 1988). When sedation is used, the radial pulse rate and the respiratory rate should be monitored at least every 15 minutes until the child is fully awake. A stethoscope should be used for the latter.

Chloral hydrate has been used for sedation for over 30 years. Although the manufacturer (E.R. Squibb &

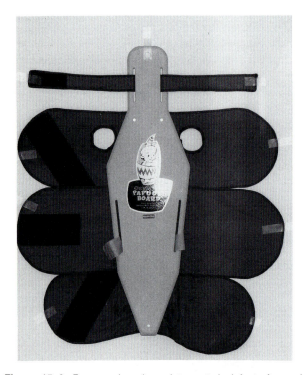

Figure 15–9. Papoose board used to restrain infants for ocular examination and minor treatments. *(From Catalano RA: Ocular Emergencies. Philadelphia, Saunders, 1992, p 93, with permission.)*

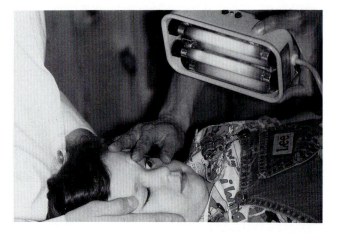

Figure 15–11. Use of a Wood's lamp to examine an eye for a corneal abrasion after the installation of fluorescein dye. *(From Catalano RA: Ocular Emergencies. Philadelphia, Saunders, 1992, p 93, with permission.)*

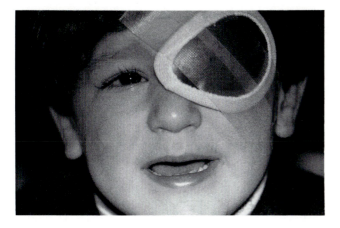

Figure 15–12. Protective eye shield used when a ruptured globe is suspected. *(From Catalano RA: Ocular Emergencies. Philadelphia, Saunders, 1992, p 112, with permission.)*

TABLE 15–1. FACTORS THAT PORTEND A SIGNIFICANT OCULAR INJURY

1. Markedly reduced visual acuity (< 5/200)
2. A relative afferent pupillary defect (see Chapter 2)
3. Shallowing of the anterior chamber
4. Irregularity of the pupil
5. Conjunctival chemosis (clear fluid under the conjunctiva)
6. Blood in the anterior eye (hyphema) or posterior eye (vitreous hemorrhage)
7. Markedly reduced or elevated intraocular pressure

Sons) recommends that 50 mg/kg be used, three groups of investigators (Fox et al, 1990; Judisch et al, 1980; Whitacre & Ellis, 1984) have suggested using a higher dose of 80 to 100 mg/kg. The total dose should not exceed 3 g, and supplemental administration, when required, should be one half of the original dose. Vomiting is a common side effect, and idiosyncratic reactions of excitement or delirium are occasionally encountered.

Children should fast for 4 hours prior to the administration of chloral hydrate to reduce the chance of aspiration should they vomit. In infants the medication can be given by slow injection into the mouth with a needleless syringe. It should not be diluted with fruit juice or water. The onset of sedation occurs variably between 30 and 60 minutes after administration. Even using the maximum dose of 3 g, there is a risk of un-

dersedation in heavier children. Undersedation results in arousal and unmanageability as soon as manipulations occur, requiring eventual conversion to another agent or general anesthesia. In practicality, using 100 mg/kg as a guideline, the maximum dose of 3 g is exceeded in most children over 5 years of age. For this reason another anesthetic agent is usually required in uncooperative children older than 5 years of age.

Alternate options for sedation are listed in Table 15–2. At many institutions the DPT or "pedi cocktail" of demerol, phenergan, and thorazine has lost favor to reversible agents such as morphine, demerol, and fentanyl. The latter, however, require intravenous administration. Valium and brevital have a rapid onset, but valium provides no analgesia and may require large doses, and brevital may cause apnea. Chloral hydrate also does not provide analgesia. Uncomfortable procedures generally require an alternate agent or general anesthesia. Occasionally, however, a local anesthetic (lidocaine 1%) can be used concomitantly with chloral hydrate for minor lid procedures.

The physician treating children should be aware of conditions that place the child at a higher general anesthetic risk (Table 15–3). Most of these are related to

TABLE 15–2. SEDATIVES USEFUL IN CHILDREN

Drug	Dose	Route	Comment
■ *CHLORAL HYDRATE*	80–100 mg/kg; maximum 3g	Oral	Safest, onset 30–60 minutes, no reversal, no analgesia
■ *DPT "COCKTAIL"*			
Demerol 25 mg/mL Phenergan 6.25 mg/mL Thorazine 6.35 mg/mL	1 mL of cocktail per 15 kg weight; maximum 2 mL	IM	Onset 30–60 minutes, no reversal
■ *ANALGESIC/NARCOTIC*			
Meperidine (Demerol)	1 mg/kg	IM/IV	Can give every 2–4 hours, reversible with naloxone
Morphine	0.1 mg/kg	IM/IV/SC	(Narcan) 0.01 mg/kg
Fentanyl	5–10 µg/kg	IV	
	5–40 µg/kg/hr	IV drip	
Valium	0.05–0.2 mg/kg	IV	Rapid onset, no analgesia
Methohexital (Brevital)	1–2 mg/kg	IV	Rapid onset, duration 5–10 minutes
	10–15 mg/kg	Rectal	Onset 5–10 minutes, duration 30 minutes, may cause apnea

Modified from Catalano RA: Ocular Emergencies. Philadelphia, Saunders, 1992, p 103, with permission.

TABLE 15–3. CONDITIONS WITH INCREASED GENERAL ANESTHETIC RISK

- **OPHTHALMOLOGIC**

  Strabismus
  Congenital ptosis

- **SYNDROMES**

  Down syndrome
  Sturge–Weber syndrome
  Marfan syndrome
  Homocystinuria
  Craniofacial syndromes

- **HEMOGLOBINOPATHIES**

  Sickle-cell disease
  Sickle thalassemia

- **NEUROMUSCULAR**

  Muscular dystrophy
  Myotonic dystrophy

Modified from Catalano RA: Ocular Emergencies. Philadelphia, Saunders, 1992, p 104, with permission.

cardiovascular abnormalities, but children with neuromuscular disorders, including strabismus and congenital ptosis, have a higher risk of malignant hyperthermia.

COMPREHENSIVE INFORMATION ON OCULAR AND ORBITAL TRAUMA

Eyelid and Orbital Injuries

History

All children with eyelid injuries should be questioned regarding the method, nature, and time of their injury. Careful attention should be given to the possibility of foreign bodies or organic contamination. A history of an animal bite should be reported to the local or state health department, and rabies prophylaxis should be considered when the animal cannot be captured. The status of tetanus immunization should also be ascertained and prophylaxis should be given as necessary (Table 15–4).

Eyelid Abrasions and Avulsed Skin

Eyelid abrasions should be cleaned of foreign and necrotic debris to reduce the risk of infection and skin tattooing. This is often best accomplished with vigorous irrigation. A prophylactic topical antibiotic (bacitracin, neomycin–bacitracin–polysporin, or erythromycin ointment four times daily) is indicated to protect against periorbital cellulitis due to staphylococci or streptococci. Tetanus immunization should be updated if devitalized tissue or deep wounds are present. Large abrasions should be kept moist with antibiotic ointment, and if dressings are necessary, they should be changed wet to avoid denuding the healing epithelium. Alternatively, Telfa strips can be used.

Eyelid Ecchymosis

If the force of impact crushes subcutaneous tissue, hemorrhage and edema (a **black eye**) results (Fig. 15–13). Blunt injuries can be associated with blowout or other orbital fractures, hyphema, angle recession, iridodialysis, retinal edema, and retinal breaks. Deep orbital bleeding can cause compression of the optic nerve or ophthalmic artery. Evaluation of orbital contusions, therefore, requires a complete ocular examination. Examination of the peripheral retina may have to wait until orbital edema subsides, but should not be delayed in patients symptomatic for a retinal break. Eyelid ecchymoses are treated with ice packs for the initial 48 hours, followed by warm compresses to reduce swelling and relieve discomfort.

Orbital Hemorrhage

Orbital hemorrhage is defined as bleeding into the orbital space behind the globe and orbital septum. Blunt and penetrating trauma are the most common causes, but orbital hemorrhage can also occur spontaneously. When the latter occurs, the bleeding time, prothrombin and partial thromboplastin time, as well as platelet

TABLE 15–4. TETANUS PROPHYLAXIS IN EYELID AND ORBITAL TRAUMA

	Clean/Nonpuncture Wounds		All Other Wounds	
Immunization History (Doses)	*Tetanus Toxoid*	*Human Immune Globulin*	*Tetanus Toxoid*	*Human Immune Globulin*
≥ 3	No[a]	No	No[b]	No
2	Yes	No	Yes	No[c]
0 to 1	Yes	No	Yes	Yes
Unknown	Yes	No	Yes	Yes

[a]Unless greater than 10 years since last booster.
[b]Unless greater than 5 years since last booster.
[c]Unless wound is more than 24 hours old.
Modified from Deutsch TA, Feller DB: Paton and Goldberg's Management of Ocular Injuries, ed 2. Philadelphia, Saunders, 1985, p 145, with permission.

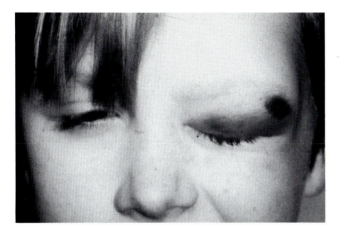

Figure 15–13. Orbital ecchymosis (black eye) left eye.

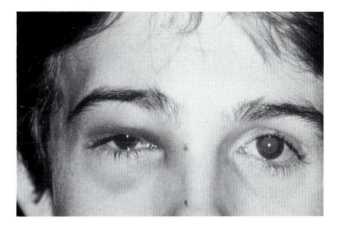

Figure 15–15. Ring-like distribution of periorbital blood associated with a basilar skull fracture.

count, should be investigated. Young children with spontaneous orbital hemorrhages should also be evaluated for metastatic neuroblastoma and leukemia (Fig. 15–14).

The distribution of hemorrhage can occasionally foretell a serious orbital injury. Blood under the superior conjunctiva suggests an orbital roof fracture (see Fig. 15–6). Basilar skull fractures are sometimes associated with a ringlike distribution of periorbital blood (Fig. 15–15). Hemorrhage into the lower lid and inferior orbit may signal an orbital floor fracture (Fig. 15–16). Unless there is an orbital fracture, optic nerve compression, or elevated intraocular pressure, orbital hemorrhages are treated conservatively with head elevation, ice to the orbit, and avoidance of aspirin.

Ophthalmoplegia

Ophthalmoplegia is defined as paralysis of extraocular muscle movement. Unless visual acuity is reduced in one eye, ophthalmoplegia will be accompanied by diplopia in at least one position of gaze. The differential diagnosis of restricted ocular motility following blunt orbital trauma is presented in Table 15–5. Axial, coronal, and/or sagittal 2-mm CT scanning (Fig. 15–17) and forced duction testing (see Fig. 15–8) will help differentiate extraocular muscle entrapment or other restriction from ocular motor nerve palsy. Ocular restriction due only to orbital edema or hemorrhage will resolve in a few weeks. Paresis due to an extraocular muscle hematoma may take several months to resolve. Traumatic ocular motor nerve palsies can take 6 to 9 months

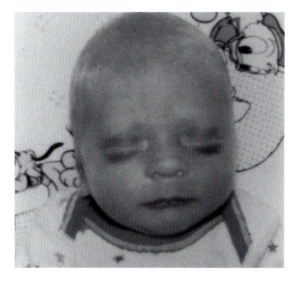

Figure 15–14. Spontaneous bilateral orbital ecchymoses ("raccoon eyes) in an infant with metastatic neuroblastoma. *(From Catalano RA: Ocular Emergencies. Philadelphia, Saunders, 1992, p 309, with permission.)*

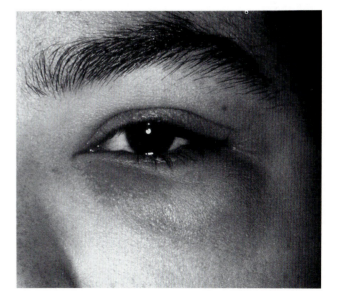

Figure 15–16. Hemorrhage in the left lower eyelid associated with a traumatic orbital floor fracture.

TABLE 15–5. CAUSES OF OPHTHALMOPLEGIA FOLLOWING ORBITAL TRAUMA

Orbital	Extraocular Muscle	Other
Edema	Entrapment	Brainstem injury
Hemorrhage	Avulsion	Carotid–cavernous fistula
Emphysema	Contusion/ hematoma	Decompensated phoria

to resolve, and full recovery of a paretic muscle occurs in less than 50 percent of cases.

In the absence of extraocular muscle entrapment, the treatment of ophthalmoplegia consists simply of observation and alleviation of diplopia. The latter can occasionally be achieved with ocular prisms, but more commonly occlusion of one eye is necessary. Should prolonged occlusion in children be necessary (greater than 1 week per year of age), the eyes should be alternately occluded to prevent the development of amblyopia. Botulinum injection of the affected muscle's antagonist should be considered to reduce its unopposed action.

Foreign Bodies Embedded in Eyelid and Orbit

Irrigation and scraping of tissue is usually sufficient to remove superficial foreign bodies in the eyelid. The treatment of deeper foreign bodies is based on associated infectious or ocular problems. Inorganic foreign bodies—such as glass, stone, plastic, and metal (with the exception of copper)—are essentially inert. Unless they are protruding from the skin, superficial, or causing optic nerve compression, they may be best left un-

disturbed. Removal is also necessary if they interfere with ocular motility, or cause a secondary reactive edema in the sclera and retina. Wood is a particularly difficult foreign body to effectively remove. If all wood fragments are not completely removed, chronic suppuration and further extrusion of retained foreign material may ensue for months.

The evaluation of a child with an orbital foreign body requires localization of the foreign body and examination of the eye for occult injury. Indirect ophthalmoscopy is mandatory. Any findings of vitreous hemorrhage, localized cataract, localized conjunctival and/or scleral injection, iris perforation, or hyphema suggests that the intraorbital foreign body may have traversed the globe. Intraorbital foreign bodies can also be associated with intracranial extension.

Deep metallic foreign bodies are easily recognized on plain-film radiography. This is the ideal imaging technique to outline the shape and number of metallic foreign bodies (Fig. 15–18). Plain-film radiography, however, does not delineate the relationship of foreign bodies to the globe (Fig. 15–19). Axial and coronal computed tomography, performed with attenuation of the beam to allow only bone visualization, is necessary for this purpose (Fig. 15–20). Magnetic resonance imaging can not be used when there is suspicion of a metallic foreign body, but may be the technique of choice in localizing wooden foreign bodies.

Even if it is decided not to remove the intraorbital foreign body, the patient should be hospitalized and treated with intravenous antibiotics. A commonly used combination is gentamicin 1.75 mg/kg as a loading dose, followed by 1 mg/kg every 8 hours with cefazolin 1 g or clindamycin 600 mg every 8 hours. A 14-

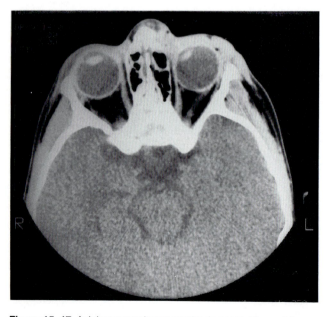

Figure 15–17. Axial computed tomography demonstrating soft tissue swelling and an inturning right eye, but no orbital fractures.

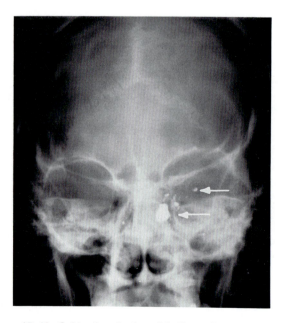

Figure 15–18. Caldwell projection plain-film radiography demonstrating multiple metallic foreign bodies (*arrows*).

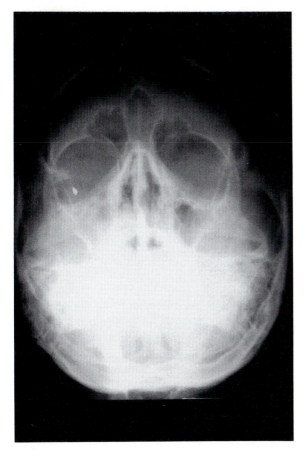

Figure 15–19. Waters view plain-film radiography demonstrating a single orbital foreign body in the right orbit, but poorly delineating its relationship to the globe. A right orbital floor fracture is also present.

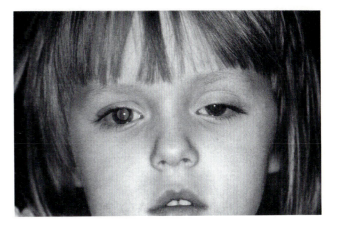

Figure 15–21. Traumatic ptosis of the left eye.

day course is recommended, but the patient can be switched to oral antibiotics and discharged on day 5 if no complications become apparent. Tetanus prophylaxis is given as needed.

Traumatic Ptosis

A hemorrhage in the levator muscle can occur with a contusion injury to the upper eyelid, causing traumatic ptosis (droopy eyelid). This generally resolves within 6 to 9 months, and surgical correction is, therefore, initially temporized. A permanent ptosis can result if the aponeurosis is stretched or torn (Fig. 15–21). A readily apparent traumatic disinsertion, or laceration, of the levator aponeurosis should be repaired at the time of eyelid suturing. Fingers or hooks caught under the upper eyelid often result in this type of injury.

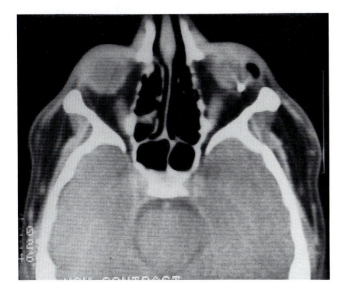

Figure 15–20. Computed tomography of same patient as Figure 15–19, demonstrating that the foreign body is located within the eye.

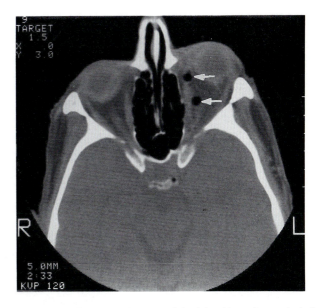

Figure 15–22. Orbital emphysema of the left orbit as demonstrated on axial computed tomography scan (*arrows*). (*From Catalano RA: Ocular Emergencies. Philadelphia, Saunders, 1992, p 67, with permission.*)

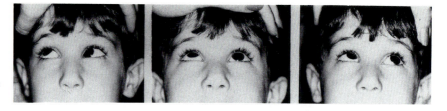

Figure 15–23. Limitation of upward gaze of the left eye following orbital floor fracture.

Orbital Emphysema

Orbital fractures involving the ethmoid bone or orbital floor can result in the expulsion of air from the ethmoid or maxillary sinus into the orbit. This can be grossly apparent clinically as orbital emphysema (see Fig. 15–5), or evident only on imaging studies (Fig. 15–22). Additional signs include subcutaneous crepitus, subconjunctival air, and proptosis. Orbital emphysema can dramatically increase with sneezing, coughing, or blowing the nose, all of which cause a sudden rise in paranasal sinus pressure. It is not unusual for this to occur several hours after injury. To prevent this, patients with orbital fractures should be forewarned against blowing their nose, and coughing episodes should be vigorously treated with antitussives (including codeine phosphate 10 to 20 mg every 4 to 6 hours if necessary).

Orbital Fractures

The term **direct orbital floor fracture** describes a floor fracture associated with an orbital rim fracture. The term **indirect orbital floor fracture** describes an isolated floor fracture, and is more commonly known as a "blowout fracture." Floor fractures are common when objects larger than the orbital opening, such as a ball,

fist, or the dashboard of an automobile, impact the orbit, particularly the inferior lateral orbit.

The most apparent clinical sign of an orbital floor fracture is a limitation of upward gaze (Fig. 15–23). A concomitant limitation of downward gaze, however, is a more certain indication of inferior rectus or oblique muscle entrapment. Additional signs include lower eyelid ecchymosis (See Fig. 15–16), nosebleed, orbital emphysema, and hypesthesia of the ipsilateral cheek and upper lip. The latter results from disruption of the infraorbital nerve as it traverses the orbital floor. Enophthalmos results from expansion of the orbital volume and is an overt sign of orbital floor fracture (see Fig. 15–3). It is more common with direct orbital floor fractures, but may not become apparent until orbital edema resolves.

A **fracture of the medial wall of the orbit** can be caused by the same forces that cause orbital floor fractures. Medial wall fractures can also occur with blows to the bridge of the nose. Signs of a medial wall fracture include orbital emphysema, epistaxis, a depressed bridge of the nose, and enophthalmos. If the nasal septum is also fractured, the nose will be deviated and nasal breathing impaired. Medial canthal tendon injuries are commonly associated with medial wall frac-

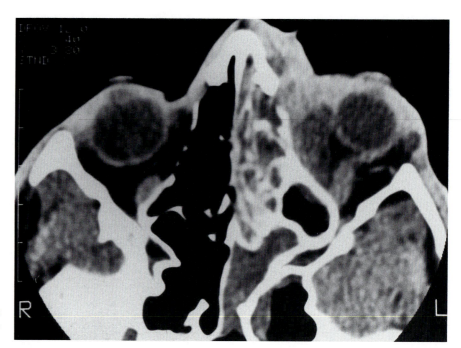

Figure 15–24. Medial wall fracture of the left orbit without entrapment of the medial rectus muscle.

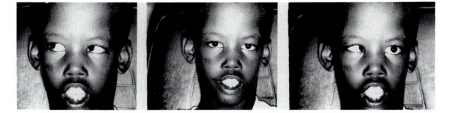

Figure 15–25. Limitation of adduction (turning inward) and abduction (turning outward) of the left eye following a medial wall fracture with entrapment of the medial rectus muscle. The abduction deficit is more profound.

tures. These should be suspected if the intercanthal distance is increased. The nasolacrimal drainage system can also be disrupted, resulting in epiphora, lacrimal sac mucocele, or dacryostenosis.

Entrapment of the medial rectus muscle is a rare consequence of medial wall fracture. Entrapment is difficult to demonstrate on plain-film radiography because of the multitude of overlying structures. CT scanning is recommended if there is suspicion of entrapment (Fig. 15–24). Clinically, both adduction and abduction of the affected eye are restricted, but the limitation of abduction is usually more profound (Fig. 15–25).

Superior wall (orbital roof) fractures are less common than inferior or medial wall fractures, but more life threatening (Fig. 15–26). The possibility of CNS injury, pneumocephalus, and/or an intracranial foreign body should be considered. Late complications include brain abscess and infectious meningitis. For these reasons, neurosurgical evaluation and management is recommended.

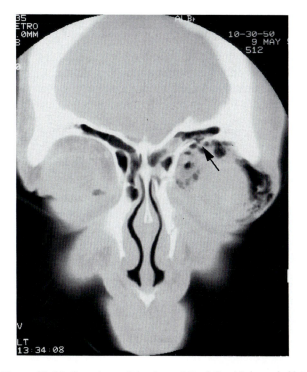

Figure 15–26. Superior wall fracture of the left orbit (*arrow*). Note also the orbital emphysema.

Signs of an orbital roof fracture include cerebrospinal fluid leakage (rhinorrhea) and superior and lateral subconjunctival hemorrhage (see Fig. 15–6). Rhinorrhea is usually transient because dural tears are usually self-sealing. Entrapment of the superior rectus or oblique muscles is very rare, but hemorrhage into these muscles may limit their action. A hematoma in the levator palpebrae muscle is more common, and results in a traumatic ptosis. An additional complication is disruption of the frontonasal duct that drains the frontal sinus, resulting in the development of a frontal sinus mucocele. An optic nerve injury can also occur (see discussion later in this chapter).

A **tripod (trimalar) fracture** is a three-part zygomatic fracture, which involves the zygomatic arch and its lateral and inferior orbital rim articulations. These articulations form the frontozygomatic and zygomaticomaxillary sutures, respectively. Because fractures of the inferior orbital rim often extend into the orbital floor, signs similar to a blowout fracture are common. If the zygoma is displaced inferiorly, there may be increased scleral show laterally, but usually edema obscures this finding in the acute setting. Of greater importance is limitation of mandibular movement and inability to open the mouth (trismus).

A **LeFort fracture** is a midfacial fracture that results from severe blunt trauma that separates facial structures. LeFort classified these into three categories, but asymmetry, overlap, and variations are common.

The best imaging techniques to visualize orbital fractures are plain-film radiography and computed tomography. The Waters view best demonstrates the orbital floor and maxillary sinus (see Fig. 15–19). A floor fracture is suggested by the prolapse of orbital contents into the maxillary sinus, an air–fluid level in the sinus, or orbital emphysema. Whereas plain-film radiography is suggested for screening, should surgical repair be contemplated, 1.5- to 2.0-mm CT scanning should be obtained. The latter provides more soft tissue and bone fragment detail (Fig. 15–27).

Additional therapeutic measures for children with acute orbital fractures include antibiotic prophylaxis, nasal decongestants, and ice packs. A broad-spectrum oral antibiotic (cephalexin 250 to 500 mg or erythromycin 250 to 500 mg four times a day; or cefaclor 40 mg/kg per day divided every 8 hours) for 10 to 14 days is appropriate. Should preseptal or orbital cellulitis de-

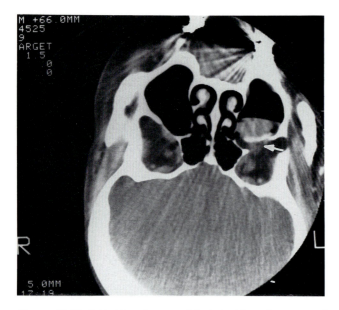

Figure 15–27. Orbital floor fracture of the left orbit as demonstrated by computed tomography (*arrow*).

velop, appropriate cultures and directed antibiotic therapy should be instituted. Ice packs are used for the initial 48 hours, and Afrin 0.05 percent nasal spray twice a day for 10 to 14 days.

Conjunctival Injuries

Subconjunctival Hemorrhage

The conjunctiva, a loose vascular tissue, covers the globe (bulbar conjunctiva) and lines the inside of the eyelids (palpebral conjunctiva). Blunt trauma, forceful sneezing, and eye rubbing can result in breakage of the fragile conjunctival blood vessels. The resultant subconjunctival hemorrhage presents as a painless, bright red accumulation of blood, usually limited to one section or quadrant of the eye (Fig. 15–28).

Whenever a traumatic subconjunctival hemorrhage occurs, a more severe underlying ocular injury should be ruled out. Accumulated blood can hide a retained foreign body or an occult scleral laceration. In the absence of other injury an affected patient is treated with reassurance alone. The patient should be told that the hemorrhage may appear to become larger over the first several days. This is because gravity and the weight of the eyelid smooth out blood clots, which can dissect under normal conjunctiva. Rarely, if ever, does a subconjunctival hemorrhage rebleed. The blood gradually resorbs over 2 to 3 weeks.

Conjunctival Edema (Chemosis)

Chemosis can likewise accompany a minor injury, but when present should raise the suspicion of scleral rupture (see later discussion), or a retained foreign body. Air under the conjunctiva (**emphysema**) suggests fracture through the ethmoid or maxillary sinus. Emphysema appears cystic and causes crepitus on palpation.

Conjunctival Lacerations

A conjunctival laceration is common when a sharp object such as a fingernail or glass strikes the eye. Small isolated conjunctival lacerations rarely require treatment (Fig. 15–29). Their identification is important, however, because they often indicate a deeper, more severe injury to the globe. It is imperative to examine the underlying sclera to rule out an accompanying scleral laceration (Fig. 15–30). Because these lacerations are usually accompanied by subconjunctival hemorrhage, examination of the deeper sclera may be difficult. When there is a high index of suspicion that the globe has been severely traumatized, an examination under anesthesia should be performed.

Conjunctival Foreign Bodies

The conjunctiva should be inspected for the presence of a foreign body when individuals present with pain

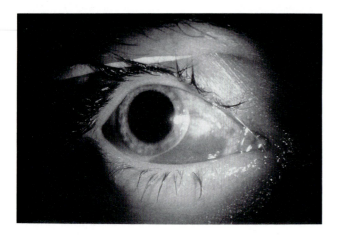

Figure 15–28. Subconjunctival hemorrhage.

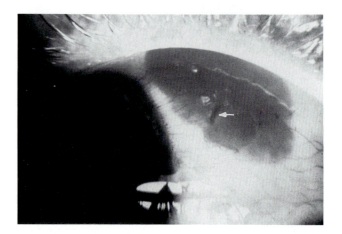

Figure 15–29. Small conjunctival laceration (*arrow*).

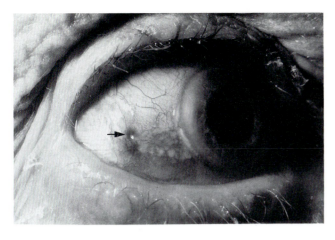

Figure 15–30. Small perforating injury of the globe surrounded by a subconjunctival hemorrhage (*arrow*).

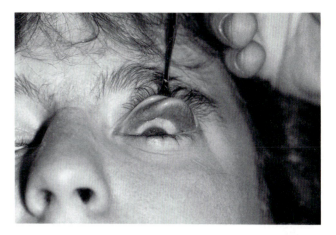

Figure 15–32. "Double eversion" of the upper eyelid to examine the entire upper palpebral conjunctiva and upper cul-de-sac. *(From Catalano RA: Ocular Emergencies. Philadelphia, Saunders, 1992, p 200, with permission.)*

and an ocular foreign body sensation. The palpebral conjunctiva of the lower eyelid and the inferior cul-de-sac can be examined by pulling down the lower eyelid and having the patient look upward (Fig. 15–31). Examination of the palpebral conjunctiva of the upper eyelid and the upper cul-de-sac is more difficult. The upper eyelid can be everted by gently grasping the eyelid at the lash line and pulling it down while placing minimal counter pressure at the upper border of the eyelid with a cotton-tipped applicator. The patient should be instructed to look down during the procedure. "Double" eversion of the upper eyelid is accomplished by substituting a Desmarre retractor for the cotton-tipped applicator, and pulling the eyelid forward as it is rolled around the retractor (Fig. 15–32). A careful search is then made of both the palpebral conjunctiva as well as the cul-de-sac. If a foreign body is found it can usually be easily removed (Fig. 15–33). Anesthesia is obtained with topical anesthetics (pro-

paracaine 0.5% or tetracaine 0.5%). One drop is usually adequate, but additional applications at 3- to 5-minute intervals may be necessary. Prior to removal of the foreign body, the underlying sclera should be examined to rule out a penetrating injury. If the conjunctiva as well as the retained foreign body is not easily movable over the underlying sclera, or if the foreign body appears fixed to deeper structures of the globe, an accompanying scleral injury should be suspected. Further manipulations and treatment should be carried out in the operating room, under the operating microscope.

Corneal Injuries

Corneal Abrasions

When the corneal epithelium is scratched, abraded, or denuded it exposes the underlying epithelial basement layer and superficial corneal nerves. This is accompa-

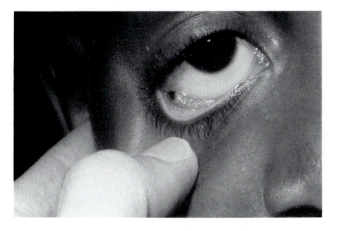

Figure 15–31. Examination of the lower palpebral conjunctiva and cul-de-sac, revealing a conjunctival foreign body.

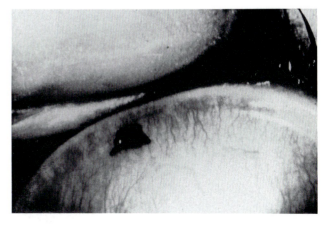

Figure 15–33. Easily removed foreign body located under the upper eyelid.

nied by pain, tearing, photophobia, and decreased vision. Corneal abrasions are detected by instilling fluorescein dye (Fig. 15–34) and inspecting the cornea using a blue-filtered light (Fig. 15–35). The slit lamp is ideal for this examination, but a hand-held Wood's lamp is adequate for young children (see Fig. 15–11).

The treatment of a corneal abrasion is directed at promoting healing and relieving pain. Very small abrasions can be treated with frequent applications of a topical antibacterial ointment four times daily. Larger abrasions require a semipressure patch to immobilize the eyelids and protect the healing epithelium from the constant trauma of repeated blinking. The patch should not be removed for 24 hours, even to instill antibiotics. Patients with larger abrasions should be followed until the epithelium has completely healed.

The intact corneal epithelium is an important barrier to bacterial infection. Abrasions should, therefore, be treated with prophylactic antibiotics. An antibiotic with good Gram positive coverage, which is not substantially toxic (such as sulfacetamide, erythromycin, or Polysporin ointment), is suggested. Although topical anesthetics result in an almost immediate relief of pain, they should be used only to complete the examination. An individual with an anesthetized cornea may inadvertently further injure their cornea. A topical cycloplegic agent (such as cyclopentolate hydrochloride 1%) can relieve the pain from ciliary spasm in patients with large corneal abrasions.

Corneal Foreign Bodies

Corneal foreign bodies can be removed with either a foreign body spud, fine forceps (jewelers or tying forceps), or the edge of a large-bore needle (22 gauge). This is best done at the slit lamp with the physician's hand resting on the patient's cheekbone. This position lessens the chance of striking the globe with a sharp object; any movement of the patient is automatically fol-

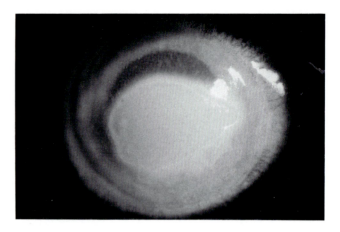

Figure 15–35. Corneal abrasion dyed with fluorescein.

lowed by the physician's hand. The foreign body is approached obliquely (Fig. 15–36). Many foreign bodies can also be removed by simply swabbing the cornea with the end of a cotton-tipped applicator upon which a bland ophthalmic ointment (Lacrilube, Duratears) has been applied. This is a safe approach to use when a slit lamp is not available, but is ineffective when the foreign body has been present for longer than several hours.

After the foreign body is removed, the guidelines outlined above for corneal abrasions should be followed. Iron-containing corneal foreign bodies often

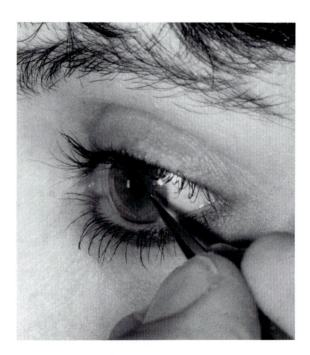

Figure 15–36. Oblique approach to removing a corneal foreign body. *(From Catalano RA: Ocular Emergencies. Philadelphia, Saunders, 1992, p 202, with permission.)*

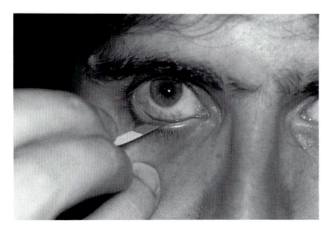

Figure 15–34. Fluorescein dye instilled in the eye using an impregnated strip to rule out a corneal abrasion.

leave a deposit of rust that may leech into the deeper layers of the cornea (Fig. 15–37). The rust ring can be either scraped with a foreign body spud or removed with a mechanical corneal burr (a battery-operated, low-speed drill).

Traumatic Corneal Hydrops

More severe corneal contusion can rupture Descemet's membrane and disrupt the corneal endothelium. This results in massive corneal edema (acute hydrops), characterized by cloudiness of the cornea and folds in Descemet's membrane. Numerous treatments have been advocated for this type of injury including patching, soft contact lenses, hypertonic eye drops, and topical intraocular-pressure-reducing medications, but none have been proven to hasten corneal repair. Obstetrical forceps injuries cause a similar injury (Fig. 15–38). These are distinguished from the Haab striae of congenital glaucoma by their vertical orientation and the absence of an enlarged globe (buphthalmos). The physician should be aware that a forceps injury can create a large irregular astigmatism, which can be amblyogenic in this age group.

Corneal Lacerations

A corneal laceration can be either full or partial thickness. A laceration should be suspected when the Seidel test is positive. This test is performed by applying a dry strip of fluorescein over the wound while observing the cornea at the slit lamp with the cobalt blue light. A slow leak of aqueous humor from the eye is visible as progressive dilution of the green fluorescein dye.

The treatment of corneal lacerations is beyond the scope of this book. A shield should be placed over an eye suspected of having a corneal laceration until the patient can be examined by an ophthalmologist (see Figure 15–12). A pressure patch should *never* be applied to a potentially lacerated eye.

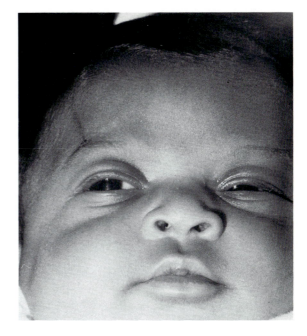

Figure 15–38. Forceps injury to the cornea. Note the oblique orientation of the Descemet's rupture and the contiguous skin marking from the applied forceps. *(From Catalano RA: Ocular Emergencies. Philadelphia, Saunders, 1992, p 156, with permission.)*

Injuries to the Iris

Traumatic Iritis

Blunt ocular contusion can injure the iris sphincter muscle, resulting in pupillary constriction (**traumatic miosis**) during the first several hours, followed by dilation (**traumatic mydriasis**). Patients present with pain, photophobia, perilimbal conjunctival injection, and anisocoria (asymmetry in pupil size). An accommodative spasm or paralysis may be associated, resulting in blurred vision and difficulty with near tasks. Signs include inflammatory or pigment cells in the anterior chamber (**traumatic iritis**) and iris sphincter tears (Fig.

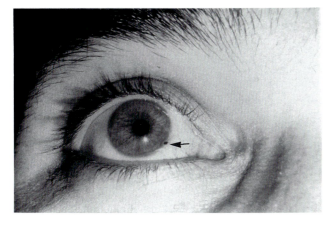

Figure 15–37. Rust ring from a foreign body located at the edge of the cornea (*arrow*).

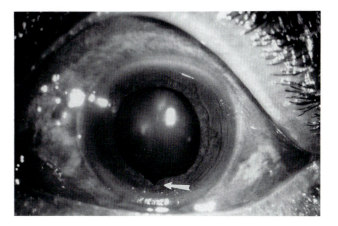

Figure 15–39. Traumatic iris sphincter tear (*arrow*).

15–39), both of which are recognizable on slit-lamp examination. Additionally, the pupil does not constrict to light stimulation as briskly as the unaffected eye, or dilate as rapidly when the illumination is reduced.

It may be difficult to distinguish traumatic iritis from traumatic microhyphema. A hyphema is characterized by red blood cells in the anterior chamber, as opposed to the white blood cells of iritis. Allowing the patient to sit quietly for several minutes will allow red blood cells that may have been dispersed with patient movement to layer, confirming the diagnosis of hyphema (Fig. 15–40). Other disorders in the differential of traumatic iritis include long-standing, untreated corneal abrasions and traumatic retinal detachments, both of which can result in a secondary anterior chamber reaction.

The treatment of traumatic mydriasis or miosis is supportive. Cyclopegia alone (for example, scopalamine 0.25 percent three times a day or cyclopentolate hydrochloride 1 to 2 percent four times a day) may be sufficient in relieving spasm and pain. More severe iritis should also be treated with a topical corticosteroid (such as prednisolone acetate ⅛ to 1 percent three or four times a day). Corticosteroids reduce the formation of anterior and posterior synechiae (abnormal adhesions of the iris to the cornea and lens, respectively). Both medications are tapered over several days.

Iridodialysis

Disinsertion of the iris at its root (iridodialysis) is characterized by polycoria (the appearance of multiple pupils) and a D-shaped pupillary aperture (Fig. 15–41). Patients with iridodialysis often experience glare and photophobia, and may have diplopia. Its occurrence is usually accompanied by hyphema, lens dislocation, and/or traumatic cataract (Fig. 15–42). Rare iris injuries include iris atrophy and iridoschisis (a split within the iris stroma). An iris abnormality should be clearly

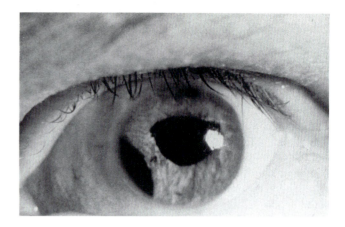

Figure 15–41. Iridodialysis. *(Courtesy of the Wills Eye Hospital slide collection; from Catalano RA: Ocular Emergencies. Philadelphia, Saunders, 1992, p 158, with permission.)*

documented, as other physicians may mistake pupillary asymmetry or irregularity as a sign of third-nerve dysfunction, related to uncal herniation.

Traumatic Horner's Syndrome

Traumatic Horner's syndrome results from injury of the carotid plexus, cervical ganglion, cervical spine, or brainstem. Features of this syndrome include miosis, ipsilateral ptosis (lid droop), anhidrosis (decreased sweating), and relative enophthalmos (recession of the eye within the orbit) (Fig. 15–43).

Traumatic Hyphema

Blunt ocular injury can tear the face of the anterior ciliary body, resulting in **hyphema** (bleeding into the anterior chamber) (see Fig. 15–40). If a history of trauma is not elicited in a child with hyphema, one should suspect leukemia, hemophilia, juvenile xanthogranuloma,

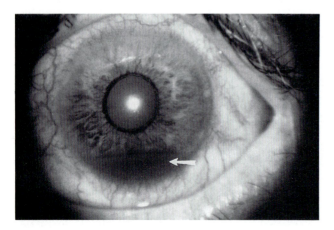

Figure 15–40. Traumatic hyphema. *(From Catalano RA: Ocular Emergencies. Philadelphia, Saunders, 1992, p 159, with permission.)*

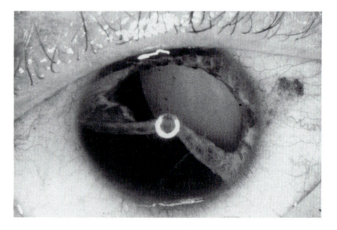

Figure 15–42. Iridodialysis, traumatic cataract, and lens dislocation. *(Courtesy of the Wills Eye Hospital slide collection.)*

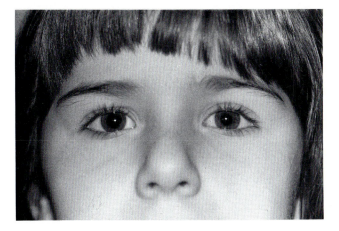

Figure 15–43. Traumatic Horner's syndrome of the left eye. Note the miosis, ptosis, and enophthalmic appearance.

retinoblastoma, a fictitious history by the child, or child abuse.

Children with hyphema have pain, and may be somnolent. The history should elicit the mechanism of injury, and any complicating factors such as a bleeding disorder, anticoagulant therapy, kidney or liver disease, and sickle-cell disease or trait. Hyphemas are graded at presentation based on the amount of blood present in the anterior chamber (Table 15–6). Grading should also be recorded as the height in mm of layered blood.

The management of traumatic hyphema is variable and controversial. There is no consensus as to whether patients should be at strict bedrest or allowed limited ambulation, and whether they can watch television or read. There is also no agreement as to the efficacy of ocular occlusion, patching of the traumatized eye, cycloplegics, topical corticosteroids, and antifibrinolytic agents. Children with hyphema are usually hospitalized.

Antifibrinolytic agents (aminocaproic acid, tranexamic acid) should be considered in populations with high rebleed rates (urban, younger age, delayed time from injury to admission). The side effects of nausea, vomiting, postural hypotension, tinnitus, lethargy, and hematuria, as well as the cost of treatment should be

taken into account when making this decision. Absolute contraindications of antifibrinolytic therapy include a cardiac, hepatic, renal, or intravascular clotting disorder. Relative contraindications include sickle-cell disease or trait and total hyphema. Suggested treatment of traumatic hyphema is presented in Table 15–7. Indications for surgical evacuation of the clot are reviewed in Table 15–8.

Rebleeding of a hyphema usually occurs from the second to fifth day following injury. Rebleeds are frequently of greater magnitude than the original hemorrhage, and more likely to be associated with elevated intraocular pressure. An increase in size of the hyphema, particularly the presence of bright red blood over darker, clotted blood confirms this occurrence. If rebleeding does not occur, cycloplegic agents and steroids should be tapered beginning on the sixth day after injury. The rapidity of tapering is based on the presence of anterior chamber inflammation. Antiglaucoma medication may have to be continued indefinitely. The child should continue to refrain from strenuous exercise and wear an eye shield at night for an additional 2 weeks. Normal activities can resume 1 month after injury, but polycarbonate eye protection for sports or hazardous labor should be used for the rest of the patient's life. A dilated fundus examination with scleral depression and gonioscopy should be performed 1 month after injury. Patients with **recession of the anterior chamber angle** should be informed of the necessity of yearly eye examinations to detect the onset of glaucoma, which can occur years after the injury.

Injuries to the Lens

Dislocation of the Ocular Lens
Trauma is the most common cause of dislocation of the ocular lens. Other causes include congenital dislocation, systemic syndromes (such as Marfan syndrome or homocystinuria), inflammation, and congenital glaucoma with buphthalmos (See Fig. 10–27).

Traumatic dislocation results when contusion induced equatorial expansion of the eye disrupts the zonule. A complete rupture results in a free-floating ("luxated") lens (Figs. 15–44 to 15–46), partial severance results in a "subluxated" lens. Symptoms of dislocation include fluctuating vision, glare, monocular diplopia, and decreased vision.

A partial dislocation is occasionally difficult to diagnose. The pupil should be dilated, and the lens examined using retroillumination at the slit lamp, to detect ruptured zonules (Fig. 15–47). Visualization of vitreous between broken zonules, or the edge of the lens within the pupil, confirms the diagnosis. Additional signs include shallowing (or deepening) of the anterior chamber, iridodonesis (movement of the iris with ocular movement), and phacodonesis (fine movement of the lens on ocular movement). Patients with a

TABLE 15–6. GRADING OF HYPHEMA

Grade	Percentage of Anterior Chamber Filled With Blood
Microscopic	Circulation of red blood cells only, no layering
I	< 33%
II	33–50%
III	50–95%
IV	100% (total or "eight-ball" hyphema)

Modified from Catalano RA: Ocular Emergencies. Philadelphia, Saunders, 1992, p 160, with permission.

TABLE 15–7. TREATMENT OF HYPHEMA

Suggested Orders	Comment
1. Hospitalization	All children; all patients with rebleeds.
2. Bed rest	Elevate the head of the bed 30 degrees; bathroom privileges with assistance.
3. Sedation as needed	Adolescents: Lorazepam (Ativan) 2–3 mg/day every 8–12 hours by mouth. Children: Chloral hydrate 50 mg/kg 3 or 4 times daily.
4. Shield involved eye	Patch only if there is an associated corneal abrasion.
5. Eye rest	May watch television at a distance, no prolonged reading or near visual tasks.
6. Cycloplegia	Atropine 1% topically, 3 or 4 times per day.
7. Topical steroids	Prednisolone acetate 1% every 2–6 hours if a fibrinous anterior chamber reaction develops.
8. No aspirin products	Use acetaminophen with or without codeine for analgesia.
9. Antiemetic as needed	Prochloroperazine (Compazine) 0.06 mg/lb body weight intramuscularly, or 2.5 mg suppository 2 or 3 times per day; or promethazine hydrochloride (Phenergan) 0.5 mg/lb body weight (maximum dose 25 mg) every 4–6 hours. The safety of these medications in children less than 20 pounds in weight or 2 years in age has not been established.
10. Antiglaucoma medications	For elevations of intraocular pressure > 40 mm Hg at presentation, or > 30 mm Hg for 2 weeks or more subsequently (20 mm Hg in those with sickle-cell trait or disease): Topical beta-blocker (e.g., levobunolol or timolol ¼% 2 times per day.) Acetazolamide 250 mg by mouth 4 times per day. (In sickle cell anemia, use Neptazane 50 mg 2–3 times per day.) Mannitol 1–2 g/kg intravenously over 45 minutes once every 24 hours.
11. Aminocaproic acid (Amicar)	Use based on community standards and patient presentation (see text); initial dose is 50 mg/kg by mouth every 4 hours (maximum 30 g/day).
12. Laboratory studies	Complete blood count; clotting studies, platelet count, and liver function tests if there is a history of bleeding disorder. Baseline creatinine and blood urea nitrogen (BUN) if aminocaproic acid is to be used. Sickle-cell prep, hemoglobin electrophoresis in black patients.
13. Surgical evacuation	See Table 15–8 for the indications for surgical evacuation of blood clot.

Modified from Catalano RA: Ocular Emergencies. Philadelphia, Saunders, 1992, pp 161–162, with permission.

dislocated lens should always be evaluated for other signs of ocular injury.

Complications of dislocated lenses include refractive disorders, pupillary-block glaucoma, and lenticular–corneal touch. Pupillary block occurs when the pupillary aperture is occluded by the dislocated lens. An anteriorly dislocated lens can also touch the posterior cornea, damaging the endothelial cells.

A noncataractous, dislocated lens may be stable and asymptomatic for years. Children and their families should, however, be forewarned of the symptoms of pupillary-block and glaucoma and advised to wear eye protection for sports and hazardous labor. The surgical considerations for removal of a dislocated lens include pupillary-block glaucoma, corneal touch, inflammation, and decreased vision uncorrectable by other means.

Traumatic Cataract

Any penetrating or perforating injury to the anterior eye may be complicated by damage to the ocular lens. Lens damage can vary from a small rent in the anterior

TABLE 15–8. INDICATIONS FOR SURGICAL EVACUATION OF CLOT IN HYPHEMA

Indication	Comment
Elevated intraocular pressure (IOP) unresponsive to medical therapy	IOP > 50 mm Hg for 5 days IOP > 35 mm Hg for 7 days IOP > 25 mm Hg for 1 day in patients with sickle-cell disease or trait, or preexisting glaucoma
Corneal bloodstaining	At first sign of bloodstaining, regardless of IOP or grade of hyphema If IOP > 25 mm Hg and total hyphema (to prevent bloodstaining)
Prolonged clot duration	Persistent total hyphema > 5 days Persistent small hyphema > 10 days

Modified from Catalano RA: Ocular Emergencies. Philadelphia, Saunders, 1992, p 162, with permission.

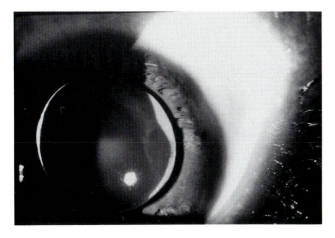

Figure 15–44. Traumatic dislocation of the lens into the anterior chamber of the eye.

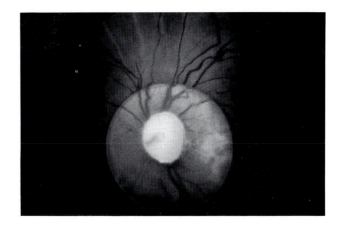

Figure 15–46. Traumatic dislocation of the lens to rest in the vitreous overlying the optic nerve. *(Courtesy of the Wills Eye Hospital slide collection.)*

capsule, leading to a small localized cataract (Fig. 15–48), to a total disruption with flocculent lens material filling the anterior chamber (Fig. 15–49).

A contusion cataract results when the lens capsule is ruptured by either a direct or contrecoup injury. In addition to lentricular opacification, affected patients also present with decreased vision, elevated intraocular pressure, and/or intraocular inflammation. The rapidity of cataract formation depends on whether the lens capsule was ruptured. In the absence of rupture, a cataract may not develop for months; with rupture the lens can become hydrated and cataractous within hours. Not every cataract is progressive; a small rent may self-seal with the development of a fibrous plaque at the site of the injury. When the visual acuity is not appreciably reduced and glaucoma or inflammation not induced, the preferred management is observation. Miotics may be helpful in reducing glare and diplopia induced by focal opacities.

Lens-induced Glaucoma

Lens-induced glaucoma can result from two mechanisms other than pupillary block (described earlier). The trabecular meshwork can be blocked by high-molecular-weight lens proteins liberated by the trauma (**lens-particle glaucoma**). Additionally, denatured lens material from a cataractous lens can leak through an intact lens capsule and be engulfed by macrophages that clog the anterior chamber angle (**phacolytic glaucoma**). Lens-particle glaucoma is suspected when a break in the lens capsule and fluffy white particles in the anterior chamber and chamber angle are seen on slit-lamp examination. Phacolytic glaucoma is suspected by the presence of iridescent particles, cells, and protein flare in the anterior chamber, on the surface of the lens capsule, and in the gonioscopically open anterior chamber angle.

Both types of lens-induced glaucoma are treated with corticosteroids, antiglaucoma medications, and

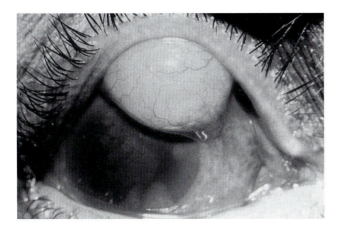

Figure 15–45. Traumatic dislocation of the lens through the sclera, under the conjunctiva. *(Courtesy of the Wills Eye Hospital slide collection.)*

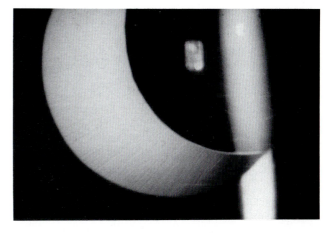

Figure 15–47. Partial dislocation (subluxation) of the ocular lens. Note the zonular fibers. *(Courtesy of the Wills Eye Hospital slide collection.)*

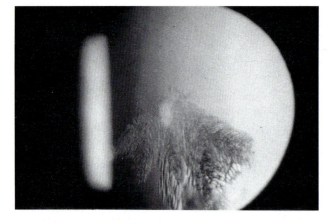

Figure 15–48. Small, localized traumatic cataract.

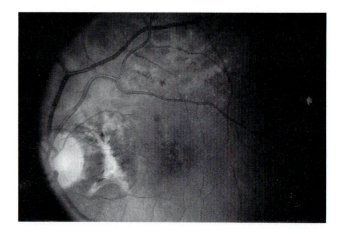

Figure 15–50. Choroidal rupture concentric with the optic disc. *(From Catalano RA: Ocular Emergencies. Philadelphia, Saunders, 1992, p 167, with permission.)*

topical cycloplegia. Cataract extraction is performed after the intraocular pressure has been brought under control (usually within 24 to 36 hours).

Injuries to the Choroid

The choroid is very susceptible to concussive injury because it lacks the strength of the sclera and the elasticity of the retina. The horizontal expansion of the posterior eye that accompanies anteroposterior compression tears the relatively inelastic Bruch's membrane of the choroid, creating a **choroidal rupture.**

Visual dysfunction occurs immediately upon injury; the visual acuity is often reduced below 20/200. Transection through the foveal area, and extensive pigmentary changes in the macular areas, portend poorly for visual acuity. A multitude of visual field abnormalities can also occur depending on the site of rupture, but often fail to correlate with the ophthalmoscopic findings. Late complications of choroidal rupture include the development of a subretinal neovascular membrane (SRNM) and atrophy of the overlying ret-

ina. No treatment for a choroidal rupture exists, but some SRNM's are amenable to laser photocoagulation.

Choroidal ruptures usually occur due to a contrecoup injury. Although hemorrhage may obscure the characteristic findings at presentation, they are eventually recognized as crescent-shaped, yellow-white, curvilinear streaks, usually concentric with the optic disc (Fig. 15–50). The macular region is often involved (Fig. 15–51). Rarely multiple or radially oriented ruptures occur.

Vitreous Hemorrhage

Vitreous hemorrhage following blunt ocular trauma suggests a retinal tear, choroidal rupture, avulsion of the optic nerve head, or an occult foreign body (Fig. 15–52). If the hemorrhage prevents adequate examination, an ultrasound examination should be performed. Retinal examination with scleral depression to examine the anterior retina for dialyses and tears should be performed as soon as it is evident that an occult scleral laceration is not present.

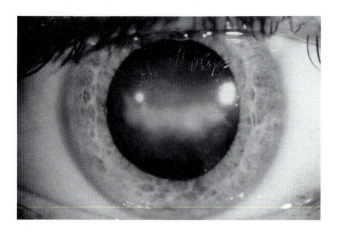

Figure 15–49. Larger, flocculent, traumatic cataract.

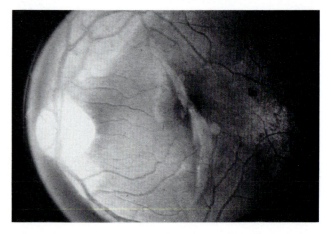

Figure 15–51. Choroidal rupture through the macula.

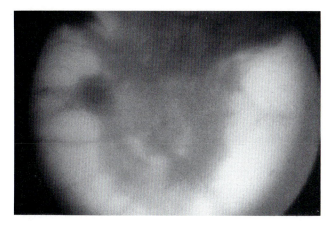

Figure 15–52. Vitreous hemorrhage obscuring visualization of the retina.

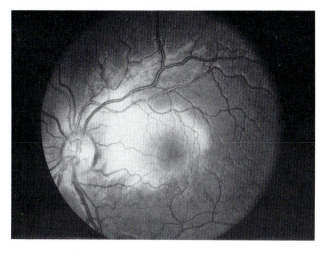

Figure 15–54. Commotio retinae involving the macular area.

Injuries to the Retina

Commotio Retinae

Commotio retinae (retinal edema, concussion edema, Berlin's edema) typically involves the retina opposite the side of an anterior segment impact (contrecoup injury). Minutes to hours after the impact, edematous swelling of the involved outer retina becomes manifest. It is recognized as a white opacification with ill-defined borders. A geographical pattern of involvement is common; the peripheral retina, macula, peripapillary area, or any combination of areas may be affected (Fig. 15–53). If the entire posterior pole is involved, a pseudo-cherry red macular spot may be present (Fig. 15–54). Normal blood flow through the inner retinal vessels easily differentiates this from a central retinal artery occlusion.

Macular involvement is manifest by an acute loss of central vision with a potential reduction in acuity of up to 20/400. Peripheral commotio retinae may be asymptomatic. The appearance of retinal opacification sub-sides over several weeks and visual function usually gradually returns to its pretrauma level. A permanent loss of vision, however, is not unusual, and can be associated with changes in the retinal pigment epithelium.

Retinitis Sclopetaria

Retinitis sclopetaria (chorioretinitis sclopetaria, chorioretinitis proliferans) is a concussive injury to the posterior eye resulting from shock waves produced by orbital penetration of a high-velocity missile (often a BB pellet). The missile does not penetrate the eye but ruptures the choroid and retina in the area adjacent to its path. Extension into the macula and concussive optic nerve injury are frequent. Initially, extensive intraocular hemorrhage is seen; retinal destruction and proliferation become apparent with resorption (Fig. 15–55). The visual acuity is almost always poor.

Traumatic Macular Holes

Traumatic macular holes can follow commotio retinae, choroidal ruptures, and subretinal hemorrhages. They

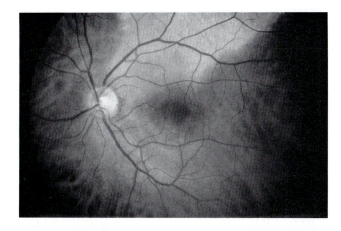

Figure 15–53. Commotio retinae involving the superior temporal quadrant of the retina. *(From Catalano RA: Ocular Emergencies. Philadelphia, Saunders, 1992, p 168, with permission.)*

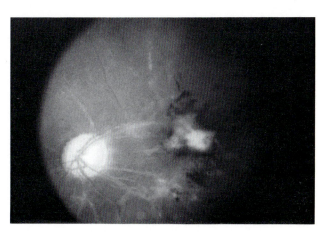

Figure 15–55. Retinitis sclopetaria with optic atrophy.

can also occur with whiplash-type injuries of the eye. The latter result from the firm adherence of the vitreous to the retina in the macular areas. Sudden deceleration creates traction, causing the vitreous and the adherent inner retina to detach from the outer retina.

Similar to idiopathic macular holes, those due to trauma have sharp, well-demarcated margins (Fig. 15–56). The hole may be partial (lamellar) or full thickness. The vision with full-thickness holes is usually reduced to 20/80 to 20/200. The majority of affected patients should be followed conservatively unless and until progressive detachment occurs. Vitrectomy, scleral buckle, and laser photocoagulation can then be performed in an attempt to preserve peripheral vision.

Traumatic Retinal Breaks and Detachments

Traumatic retinal breaks and detachments result from the same forces that cause choroidal ruptures. Anteroposterior compression of the eye expands the equatorial diameter of the globe, creating traction at the vitreous base. This traction is transmitted to the peripheral retina, which is firmly adherent to the vitreous. Consequent injuries include avulsion of the vitreous base, dialysis of the retina, peripheral retinal tears, and irregular retinal holes. Large, irregular tears can also occur from direct shearing forces. These usually occur in the temporal retina and are associated with intraretinal hemorrhages and edema.

Avulsion of the vitreous base may be asymptomatic, or the patient may note flashes (photopsia) and/or a few floaters. Vitreous base avulsion does not need to be treated, but the patient should be warned of the signs of retinal detachment (the onset of a shower of new floaters, photopsia, and/or a progressive loss of visual field similar to a curtain being drawn over the eye).

A **retinal dialysis** is a disinsertion of the peripheral retina from its anterior-most attachments at the ora

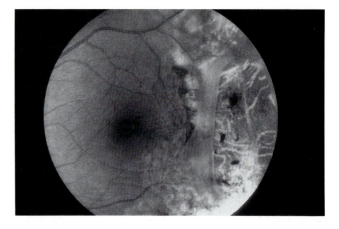

Figure 15–57. Retinal dialysis. *(Courtesy of the Wills Eye Hospital slide collection; from Catalano RA: Ocular Emergencies. Philadelphia, Saunders, 1992, p 171, with permission.)*

serrata (Fig. 15–57). A small dialysis is recognized as a slit-like separation of the retina at the ora, and is best appreciated using indirect ophthalmoscopy with scleral depression. The dialysis usually occurs on impact, but the patient may note only photopsia, floaters, or mildly disturbed vision at this time. Especially in children, these symptoms may go unheeded until the detachment progresses posterior to the equator and a visual field loss is noted.

Retinal tears due to blunt trauma include small peripheral holes without apparent vitreoretinal traction (Fig. 15–58), larger irregular-shaped holes (usually at the direct site of impact), macular holes (see "Traumatic Macular Holes," above), and tractional horseshoe tears. Retinal tears usually produce symptoms of floaters and photopsia, and may be accompanied by vitreous and retinal hemorrhage. With the exception of macular holes, tears are more likely than dialyses to progress to retinal detachment (Fig. 15–59).

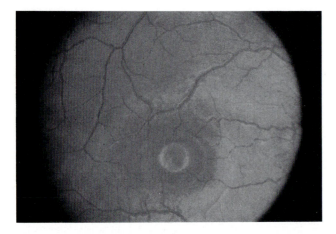

Figure 15–56. Traumatic macular hole.

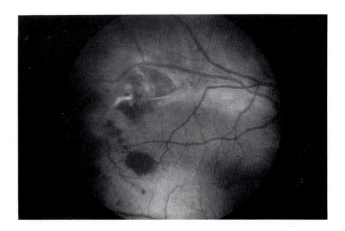

Figure 15–58. Small peripheral retinal hole without vitreoretinal traction.

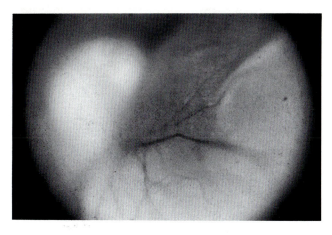

Figure 15–59. Bullous retinal detachment.

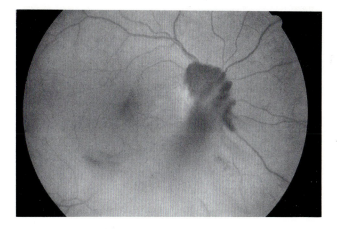

Figure 15–60. Intraocular hemorrhage emanating from the optic nerve suggesting an optic nerve laceration or avulsion. *(From Catalano RA: Ocular Emergencies. Philadelphia, Saunders, 1992, p 173, with permission.)*

The time interval between ocular contusion and **retinal detachment** is variable. Nearly half of all traumatic retinal detachments are apparent within 1 month of injury and the majority occur within 2 years of injury. A giant retinal tear is one that extends more than 90 degrees of the circumference of the globe (involves more than one quadrant). Giant tears occur especially in traumatized myopic eyes. They are usually circumferentially located at the border of the vitreous base, and may be associated with retinal necrosis at the site of impact. Signs are acute and dramatic, and include floaters, photopsia, and decreased vision.

Optic Nerve Injury

Optic Nerve Laceration or Avulsion

An optic nerve laceration or avulsion usually results from a direct penetrating orbital injury. Occasionally, blunt orbital trauma can fracture the optic canal, and the resultant bony fragments can lacerate the optic nerve. Alternatively, blunt trauma can thrombose, compress, or tear the vascular supply to the optic nerve. The most common site of impact for blunt forces causing optic nerve injury is the lateral brow.

When obtaining the history, it is essential to note whether loss of vision was immediate, suggesting an avulsion or laceration of the optic nerve, or whether it occurred after a brief period of vision. The latter suggests optic nerve contusion or central retinal vein compression. In addition to the immediate decrease in vision, intraocular hemorrhage emanating from the optic nerve suggests laceration or avulsion (Fig. 15–60). Neuroimaging can confirm this diagnosis. No treatment exists for completely avulsed nerves.

Traumatic Optic Neuropathy

Traumatic optic neuropathy is usually characterized by optic disc swelling and partial or complete central

retinal vein occlusion (Fig. 15–61). Without treatment, vision rarely improves, but dramatic improvement has been reported with optic nerve sheath decompression.

Occasionally, posterior traumatic optic neuropathy is suspected based upon an acute reduction of vision with a normal-appearing optic disc. Without treatment, vision spontaneously improves in 20 to 35 percent of affected patients (Seiff, 1991). Vision has been reported to spontaneously return, albeit with some residual defects, even in patients with no light perception at presentation (Wolin & Lavin, 1990). Many clinicians, however, advocate optic nerve decompression and/or megadose systemic corticosteroid therapy for these patients, to improve the prognosis. Megadose steroids are never recommended for the routine treatment of orbital fractures.

Intraocular Foreign Body

The possibility of an intraocular foreign body should always be considered whenever evaluating a patient with ocular trauma. A history of being struck by a pro-

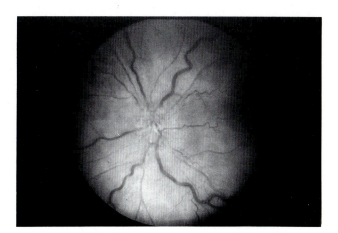

Figure 15–61. Traumatic optic neuropathy.

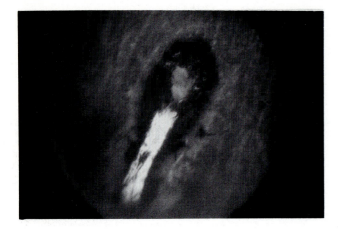

Figure 15–62. Intraocular foreign body.

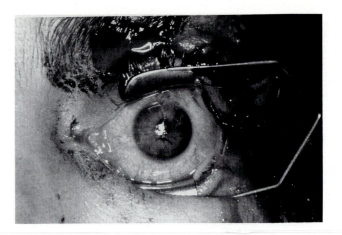

Figure 15–63. Ruptured globe demonstrating shallow anterior chamber, irregular pupil, and hyphema.

jectile, or striking metal against metal, is especially suspicious.

The history is also helpful in identifying the type of material. Many foreign bodies are relatively inert (glass, stone, high-quality plastic, stainless steel, and other quality alloys) and tolerated by the eye with minimal reaction. Organic material, iron, low-quality alloys, copper, magnesium, aluminum, and low-grade plastic, however, are potentially toxic to the eye. Iron and copper can especially cause widespread ocular destruction.

If the ocular exam reveals a local area of conjunctival injection, hyphema, localized cataract, and/or iris injury, the patient needs a thorough indirect ophthalmologic exam to search for a foreign body (Fig. 15–62). When blood in the optical media precludes an accurate assessment, orbital x-rays and/or CT scanning should be used. Although ultrasound is an effective method of determining the presence of intraocular masses, its use requires direct contact with the eyelid on the globe. As such, it is of limited use in unrepaired traumatized eyes. Orbital x-rays are helpful in demonstrating the number and shape of radiopaque foreign bodies (see Fig. 15–18). CT scanning is useful in delineating their relationship to the globe (see Fig. 15–20). MRI scanning should never be used to rule out a potentially metallic foreign body; the magnetic pull may cause movement of the foreign body, exacerbating the injury.

TABLE 15–9. SIGNS OF A POTENTIALLY RUPTURED GLOBE

Shallowing or deepening of the anterior chamber
An asymmetric reduction in intraocular pressure
A positive Seidel test
Irregularity or peaking of the pupil
Subconjunctival pigmentation due to prolapsed uveal tissue
Bullous conjunctival hemorrhage and/or chemosis
Decreased visual acuity
Hyphema

Ruptured Globe

Even in the absence of a projectile, severe trauma can result in laceration of the cornea and/or sclera (a ruptured globe). The signs of a ruptured globe are reviewed in Table 15–9; several are demonstrated in Figure 15–63. Computed tomographic signs include air within the globe (Fig. 15–64) and the loss of intraocular contents (Fig. 15–65).

Thermal and Chemical Burns

Thermal Burns

Because of reflex closure of the eyelids, the majority of thermal injuries affect only the eyelashes, eyebrows, and surrounding skin. A first-degree skin burn is very superficial, involving only the epidermis. Signs include erythema, edema, pain to touch, warmth, and singed eyebrows and eyelashes (Figs. 15–66 and 15–67). A second-degree burn involves the epidermis and part of the dermis. Pain and blisters are usually present, but

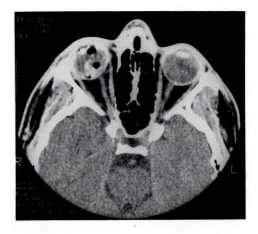

Figure 15–64. Computed tomography scan demonstrating air within a ruptured right globe.

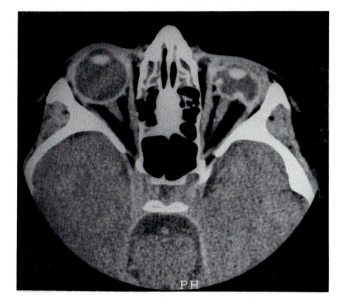

Figure 15–65. Computed tomography scan demonstrating loss of ocular contents in a ruptured left globe. *(From Catalano RA: Ocular Emergencies. Philadelphia, Saunders, 1992, p 66, with permission.)*

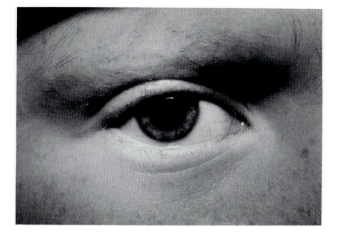

Figure 15–67. Singed eyelashes and eyebrows following first-degree thermal burn.

the skin heals with minimal scarring. A third-degree burn involves the full thickness of the dermis with charring of the skin (Fig. 15–68). Pain and blisters are absent because the nerves and vascular supply are destroyed.

The first priority in treating a thermal burn is to remove the person from the heat source and cool the tissues as rapidly as possible. This is best accomplished with cool compresses such as sterile towels soaked in an ice bath. Analgesics including parenteral narcotics may be necessary to relieve pain. The ophthalmologic examination should be performed as early as possible because the eyelids become very edematous within 24 to 48 hours of most burns.

The treatment of eyelid burns includes the topical application of silver sulfadiazine or bacitracin oint-

ment to the skin. Some studies have suggested that prophylactic ocular treatment may lead to conjunctival colonization with virulent gram-negative bacteria. Initially, therefore, ocular lubricants alone should be used. Repeated cultures of the burned area and conjunctiva should indicate whether an ocular antibiotic should be used. Elevation of the head may reduce swelling. Treatment of corneal exposure is best performed using lubricating ointments and a "Saran-wrap" moisture chamber (Fig. 15–69).

Chemical Burns

Chemical burns of the cornea and adnexal tissue are among the most urgent of ocular emergencies. They occur commonly because strong alkalies and acids are found in many common household and industrial products (Table 15–10). Alkali burns are usually more

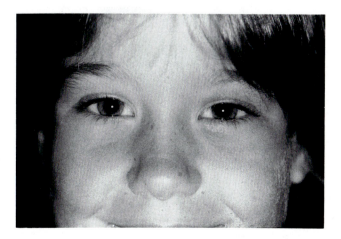

Figure 15–66. First-degree burn to the periocular area.

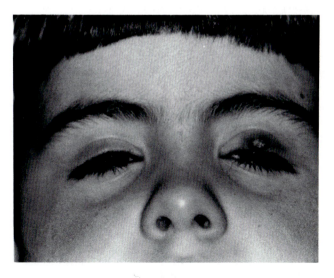

Figure 15–68. Localized third-degree burn of the left upper eyelid in a boy who inadvertently walked into a cigarette dangling from the hand of an adult.

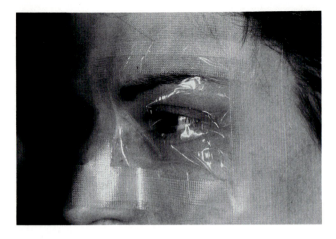

Figure 15–69. "Saran-wrap" moisture chamber to protect the cornea from desiccation following thermal injury to the eyelids. *(From Catalano RA: Ocular Emergencies. Philadelphia, Saunders, 1992, p 128, with permission.)*

destructive than acid burns. Alkalies react with fats to form soaps, which damage cell membranes, allowing further penetration of the alkali into the eye. The severity of the injury is related to the volume and concentration of the chemical, and how rapidly it diffuses through the cornea. The following alkalies are listed in order of their speed of penetration, from slowest to fastest: calcium hydroxide (mortar and plaster), potassium hydroxide (drain cleaner), sodium hydroxide (drain and oven cleaners), and ammonium hydroxide (ammonia). Calcium hydroxide does not penetrate well because the calcium soaps formed upon saponification are relatively insoluble and precipitate out, forming a barrier to further penetration.

Acids generally cause less severe, more localized tissue damage. The corneal epithelium offers moderate protection against weak acids, and little damage is seen unless the pH is 2.5 or less. Most stronger acids precipitate tissue proteins, creating a physical barrier against

their further penetration. Buffering by surrounding tissue proteins also helps localize the damage to the initial area of contact. Exceptions include hydrofluoric acid, and acids containing heavy metals, which rapidly penetrate the cornea.

Mild acid or alkali burns are characterized by conjunctival injection and swelling, and mild corneal epithelial erosions (Fig. 15–70). The corneal stroma may be mildly edematous and the anterior chamber may have mild to moderate cell and flare. With strong acids the cornea and conjunctiva rapidly become white and opaque (nitric and chromic acids, however, turn tissue yellow-brown). The corneal epithelium may slough, leaving a relatively clear stroma; this appearance may initially mask the severity of the burn. Very severe acid burns also cause complete corneal anesthesia, limbal pallor, and uveitis. Severe alkali burns are characterized by corneal opacification (Fig. 15–71) and limbal ischemia. They are classified according to the damage they cause to the limbus, as this is the single most important factor in determining the prognosis for recovery.

Substantial changes in intraocular pressure have been demonstrated following chemical burns. From experimental studies it is likely that there is an acute rise in intraocular pressure due to collagen shrinkage in alkali burns of pH 11 or higher. A second pressure elevation occurs within the first few hours, most likely due to the intraocular release of prostaglandins. A similar subsequent pressure response can also be seen with moderate and severe acid burns.

Treatment of Chemical Burns. Unlike thermal burns, chemical burns usually injure the eye as well as the adnexa. Emergency treatment consists of copious, immediate irrigation with water or saline (Table 15–11). Local debridement and removal of foreign particles should be performed while still irrigating. If the nature of the chemical injury is unknown, the use of

TABLE 15–10. COMMON ACIDS AND ALKALIES

Product	Chemical	pH
▪ *ACIDS*		
Toilet cleaner	Sulfuric acid (80%)	1.0
Battery fluid	Sulfuric acid (30%)	1.0
Pool cleaners	Sodium or calcium hypochlorite (70%)	1.0
Bleaches	Sodium hypochlorite (3%)	1.0
▪ *ALKALIES*		
Drain cleaner	Sodium or potassium hydroxide	14.0
Ammonia	Ammonium hydroxide (9%)	12.5
Dishwasher detergent	Sodium tripolyphosphate	12.0
Oven cleaners	Sodium hydroxide	14.0

Modified from Catalano RA: Ocular Emergencies. Philadelphia, Saunders, 1992, p 180, with permission.

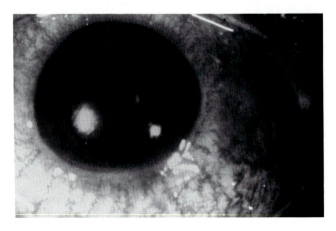

Figure 15–70. Mild acid burn to the eye.

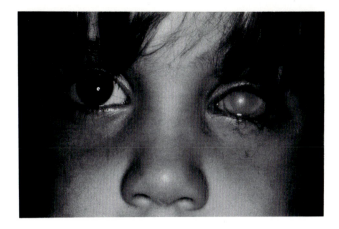

Figure 15–71. Severe alkali burn to the left eye resulting in corneal opacification.

pH paper is helpful in determining whether the agent was basic or acidic. Irrigation should continue for at least 30 minutes or 2 liters of irrigant in mild cases, and 2 to 4 hours or 10 liters of irrigant in severe cases. At the end of irrigation, the pH should be within a normal range (7.3 to 7.7). The pH should be checked again approximately 30 minutes after irrigation to ensure that it has not changed. This is particularly important in alkali burns in which particulate matter can slowly dissolve and cause a persistent elevation in the pH.

All but the mildest chemical burns are associated with intraocular inflammation. To relieve pain, adequate cycloplegia is essential. Atropine 1% or scopolamine 0.25%, two or three times daily, are the drugs of

TABLE 15–11. SUMMARY OF THE ACUTE TREATMENT OF CHEMICAL BURNS TO THE EYE

1. Copious irrigation with saline or water for at least 30 minutes, or 2L of irrigant. Analgesics, anesthetics, and a lid speculum may be necessary
2. Debridement of any retained particles.
3. Atropine 1% or scopolamine 0.25% topically 1–3 times daily for cycloplegia
4. Topical corticosteroids as needed in the first 5–7 days to control the inflammatory response.
5. Acetazolamide 5 mg/kg every 6 hours, and/or a topical beta blocker (e.g., Timoptic, Betagan, Betoptic) as needed to control elevated intraocular pressure.
6. Antibiotic ointment and semipressure patches to prevent infection and promote epithelialization. Mild cases should require only a daily application of a cycloplegic, antibiotic, and steroid with continuous patching.
7. Ascorbic acid (5–10 g) and doxycycline (100 mg twice daily) may be given orally.
8. Daily evaluation of inflammatory response, intraocular pressure, and epithelialization.
9. Severe cases are started on topical 10% sodium citrate hourly.

Modified from Catalano RA: Ocular Emergencies. Philadelphia, Saunders, 1992, p 185, with permission.

choice. The mydriatic phenylephrine is contraindicated because its vasoconstricting properties can worsen already preexisting perilimbal ischemia. Elevated pressure in the initial postburn period can be managed with carbonic anhydrase inhibitors (acetazolamide 5 mg/kg every 6 hours) and/or topical beta blockers.

Following adequate irrigation, antibiotic ointment (tetracycline may have a theoretical advantage) and a semipressure patch are applied. The goal is to promote epithelialization as rapidly as possible. The eyes are examined daily and the fluorescein staining pattern noted. In moderate to severe inflammation, corticosteroid drops are applied (for example, prednisone acetate, phosphate, or dexamethasone). In all but the mildest cases, the use of oral ascorbic acid should be considered. Exact dosages are not defined, but pharmacological doses (5 to 10 g daily) are recommended.

Sports-related Ocular Injuries

Although sports injuries occur in all age groups, far more children and adolescents participate in high-risk sports than adults. The greater number of participating children, their athletic immaturity, and the increased likelihood of their using inadequate or improper eye protection, accounts for their disproportionate share of sports-related eye injuries.

The sports with the highest risk of eye injury are those in which no eye protection can be worn. These include boxing, wrestling, and martial arts. High-risk sports include those that use a rapidly moving ball or puck, bat, stick, racket, or arrows (baseball, hockey, lacrosse, racquet sports, and archery), or involve aggressive body contact (football and basketball). Low-risk sports include swimming, track and field, and gymnastics. Related to both risk and frequency of participation, the highest percentage of eye injuries are seen in basketball and baseball.

Protective eyewear, designed for a specific activity, is available for most sports. For basketball, racquet sports, and other recreational activities that do not require a helmet or face mask, molded polycarbonate sports goggles that are secured to the head by an elastic strap, are suggested (Fig. 15–72). For hockey (goalie), football, lacrosse, and baseball (batter), specific helmets with polycarbonate faceshields and guards are available (Fig. 15–73). Children should also wear sports goggles under the helmets. For baseball, goggles and helmets should be worn for batting, catching, and base running; goggles alone are usually sufficient for other positions. For hockey the goalie, forwards, and defensemen should wear goggles and a helmet; other players should wear goggles. The appropriate helmet for hockey is shown in Figure 15–73; the molded "Jason" style hockey mask does not provide adequate ocular or orbital protection. For football, the helmet

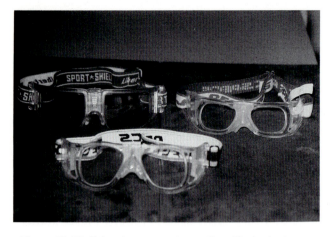

Figure 15–72. Polycarbonate sports goggles with elastic straps.

should have an attached polycarbonate face guard. Other sports for which a helmet and eye protection is advisable include horseback riding, ski racing, cycling, motorcycling, fencing, and snowmobiling. Finally, orthodontic headgear should never be worn while playing sports. The typical metallic bow, strapped to the head and anchored in the mouth, can slip with an impacting force, penetrating the eye.

Many optical and sporting good stores sell sports goggles and helmets. Table 15–12 lists the names and addresses of firms that manufacture sports eyewear.

In addition to eye protection, the ophthalmologist is often asked to suggest guidelines for sports participation by amblyopic children. Jeffers (1990) defines a functionally one-eyed athlete as one who has less than 20/50 vision in one eye and 20/20 best corrected vision in the other eye. He suggests that with appropriate eye protection these children can participate in most sports. However, participation in boxing, wrestling, and martial arts, or any other sport without eye protection, is forbidden. Jeffers adds that even for everyday

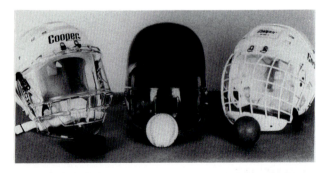

Figure 15–73. Sport-specific helmets for hockey (left), baseball (middle), and lacrosse (right). *(From Jeffers JB: An ongoing tragedy: Pediatric sports-related eye injuries. Semin Ophthalmol 5:216, 1990, with permission.)*

street wear, the one-eyed individual should be fitted with polycarbonate lenses with a minimum center thickness of 3 mm and sturdy frames. Prior informed parental consent is especially important in functionally one-eyed children. The parents, physician, athlete, coach, school administration, and legal counsel should all be involved in the decision.

Child Abuse

Child abuse should be considered whenever the history is incompatible with the child's findings, especially in infants. The most common precipitating factors are inconsolable crying, toileting incidents, whining, or refusing to eat. Ophthalmologists are often asked to examine children suspected of being abused because of the frequency of ocular involvement in child abuse. The most striking and common ocular finding is intraocular hemorrhage. Prior to the use of magnetic resonance imaging, ophthalmologic examination was especially important in diagnosing abuse because retinal, preretinal, and vitreous hemorrhage often precede computed tomography and clinical findings of subdural hematoma. The detection of hemosiderin in the optic nerve or retina, on autopsy, is also useful forensically. It should be noted, however, that medicolegally the presence of hemosiderin by itself is not sufficient to indicate repeated trauma. Hemosiderin first appears 3 days after injury and may remain in tissues for 20 years. The observation of independent hemorrhages of different ages is more important in the consideration of child abuse. Table 15–13 lists additional historical, social, and physical findings in the abused child.

The shaken baby syndrome represents an important subset of abused children. This syndrome is usually seen in infants under 12 months of age; children over 3 years of age are unlikely to be shaken. The child often has no overt signs of abuse, and is brought to the emergency room in a depressed state of consciousness, or in status epilepticus. The perpetrator is usually a parent, a babysitter, or boyfriend of a babysitter. The most telling intracranial manifestation of shaking is bilateral subdural hematomas, especially involving the interhemispheric fissure in the parieto-occipital region (Fig. 15–74). Diffuse cerebral swelling is also common. Subarachnoid hemorrhage is uncommon and intracerebral bleeding is very rare. Blindness, spastic hemiplegia or quadriplegia, mental retardation, and death can all occur from this whiplash-type injury.

Ocular findings in the shaken baby syndrome include scattered, round, almost confluent retinal and nerve fiber layer hemorrhages (some with white centers, depending on their age). Preretinal hemorrhages, often with dome-like elevations of the internal limiting membrane, are almost pathognomonic of a shaking injury. Involvement of the posterior pole, especially the

TABLE 15–12. MANUFACTURERS OF SPORTS EYEWEAR

Liberty Optical	**LST Leader Sports**	**Viking Sports**
380 Verona Avenue	P.O. Box 591	5355 Sierra Road
Newark, NJ 07014	Essex, NY 12936	San Jose, CA 95132
800–879–9992	800–847–2001	800–535–3300
Ektelon	**Herslof Optical**	**Face Guard Inc.**
8929 Aero Drive	12000 W. Carmen Avenue	P.O. Box 8425
San Diego, CA 92123	Milwaukee, WI 53225	Roanoke, VA 24014
800–854–2958	800–558–7073	800–336–9683
Cabot Safety Co.	**Titmus Optical**	
141 Broadway	P.O. Box 191	
Norwich, CT 06360	Petersburg, VA 23804	
800–982–2828	800–446–1802	

Modified from Catalano RA: Ocular Emergencies. Philadelphia, Saunders, 1992, p 98, with permission.

macula, is most typical (Fig. 15–75). Vitreous hemorrhage is usually seen several days after the episode, following breakthrough of blood from preretinal loculations.

The differential diagnosis of retinal hemorrhages in a child includes leukemia, blood dyscrasia or anemia, cardiopulmonary resuscitation, retinal vasculitis, bacterial endocarditis, severe arterial hypertension, and birth trauma. With the exception of physical abuse, however, head trauma rarely causes massive retinal hemorrhage. The latter suggests shaking and dates the incident to within several weeks. The finding of migration of blood into the vitreous, after an initial observation of only preretinal hemorrhage, further suggests

TABLE 15–13. HISTORICAL, SOCIAL, AND PHYSICAL FINDINGS IN THE ABUSED CHILD

- **HISTORICAL FINDINGS**
  - Nature of injury incompatible with history.
  - Inconsistency between mechanism of injury and child's developmental stage.
  - Male sex; age less than 1 year.
  - History of spontaneously stopping breathing, choking, minor fall, or head getting caught in crib slats.
  - Caretaker offering no explanation at all.
  - Prior episodes of loss of appetite, irritability, seizures.
  - Previously suspected failure to thrive.
  - Multiple previous hospital admissions, for this child or siblings, at different institutions.
  - Young child pleading their affection to parent.
  - Deterioration of older child's academic performance.
  - Social withdrawal or history of running away in older child.
  - Unusually high tolerance for pain in older child.

- **SOCIAL FINDINGS**
  - Perpetrator immaturity or inclination toward violent behavior.
  - Perpetrator history of being an abused child.
  - Perpetrator history of drug or alcohol abuse or mental illness.
  - Familial financial or marital difficulties.
  - Unwed mother.
  - Cessation of new injuries during hospitalization.
  - Parental failure to visit child during hospitalization.

- **SYSTEMIC FINDINGS**
  - Fractures of different ages of long bones and ribs.
  - Fractures involving metaphysis or epiphyseal plates.
  - Linear skull fractures in the frontal or parietal region.

  - Hematoma involving the cervical spinal cord.
  - Dislocated joints.
  - Disproportionate soft tissue injuries.
  - Bruises on the trunk with the imprint of an adult hand.
  - Hot water burns or burns in the pattern of a hot plate, heating grate, or cigarette.
  - Burns involving only the buttocks or genitalia.
  - A burn of a single hand or foot above the wrist or ankle.
  - Vomiting, abdominal distension, absent bowel sounds, and abdominal tenderness (ruptured liver, spleen, intestinal perforation).

- **OCULAR FINDINGS**
  - Subconjunctival hemorrhages.
  - Intraocular hemorrhages.
    Retinal and preretinal.
    Vitreous.
    Hyphema.
  - Lid lacerations/ecchymosis/proptosis.
  - Gonococcal and chlamydial conjunctivitis.
  - Corneal laceration/abrasion/ulcer/opacification.
  - Traumatic mydriasis/sphincter tear/iris disinsertion.
  - Subluxated lens/cataract.
  - Purtscher retinopathy with fat emboli from long bone fractures.
  - Retinal detachment/retinodialysis/retinal folds/retinoschisis.
  - Chorioretinal scarring.
  - Optic disc edema/optic atrophy/optic nerve avulsion.
  - Nystagmus/strabismus/cranial nerve palsy.
  - Complete loss of eye movements and pupillary function.
  - Cortical blindness.

Modified from Catalano RA: Ocular Emergencies. Philadelphia, Saunders, 1992, p 100, with permission.

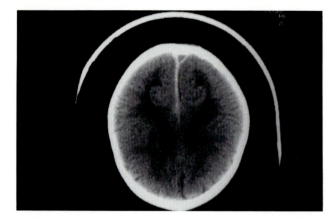

Figure 15–74. Computed tomography demonstrating acute subdural hematoma in the posterior interhemispheric fissure and over the cerebral convexity in the shaken baby syndrome. *(From Catalano RA: Ocular Emergencies. Philadelphia, Saunders, 1992, p 101, with permission.)*

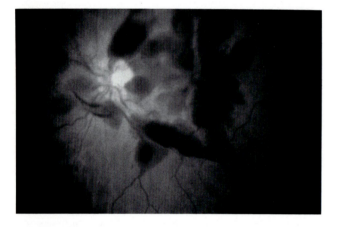

Figure 15–75. Very extensive, almost confluent, preretinal and retinal hemorrhages, principally involving the macular area, in the shaken baby syndrome. *(From Catalano RA: Ocular Emergencies. Philadelphia, Saunders, 1992, p 101, with permission.)*

that the episode occurred a few days earlier. Eventually, the fundus may appear normal, but pigment epithelial disturbances, retinal gliosis, and vascular attenuation may occur as late findings. Optic nerve injury is seen initially as disc edema and subsequently as optic atrophy. In general, preservation of the pupillary light reflex is a favorable prognostic sign.

REFERENCES

Anesthesia

Alpert CC, Salazar FG: Chloral hydrate sedation in children. Am J Ophthalmol 90:877, 1980.

Carabelle RW: Chloral hydrate. A useful pediatric sedative. Am J Ophthalmol 51:834, 1961.

Fox BES, O'Brien CO, Kangas KJ, Murphree AL, Wright KW: Use of high dose chloral hydrate for ophthalmic exams in children: A retrospective review of 302 cases. J Pediatr Ophthalmol Strabismus 27:242, 1990.

Jastak JT, Pallasch T: Death after chloral hydrate sedation: Report of a case. J Am Dent Assoc 116:345, 1988.

Judisch GF, Anderson S, Bell WE: Chloral hydrate sedation as a substitute for examination under anesthesia in pediatric ophthalmology. Am J Ophthalmol 89:560, 1980.

Nathan JE: Management of the refractory young child with chloral hydrate: Dosage selection. J Dent Child 54:93, 1987.

O'Malley PJ: Approach to the emergency pediatric patient. In Wilkins EW Jr (ed): Emergency Medicine. Baltimore, Williams & Wilkins, 1989, pp 485–486.

Whitacre MM, Ellis PP: Outpatient sedation for ocular examination. Surv Ophthalmol 28:643, 1984.

Burns—Chemical

Belin MW, Krachmer JH: Chemical burns of the cornea. In Easty DL, Smolin G (eds): External Eye Disease. London, Butterworth, 1985, pp 304–305.

Burns FR, Gray RD, Paterson CA: Inhibition of alkali-induced corneal ulceration by a thiol peptide. Invest Ophthalmol Vis Sci 31:197, 1990.

Burns FR, Stack MS, Gray RD, Paterson CA: Inhibition of purified collagenase from alkali-burned rabbit corneas. Invest Ophthalmol Vis Sci 30:1569, 1989.

Levison RA, Paterson CA, Pfister RR: Ascorbic acid prevents corneal ulceration and perforation following experimental alkali burns. Invest Ophthalmol Vis Sci 15:986, 1976.

Perry HD, Kenyon KR, Lamberts DW, et al: Systemic tetracycline hydrochloride as adjunctive therapy in the treatment of persistent epithelial defects. Ophthalmology 93:1320, 1986.

Pfister RR: Chemical injuries of the eye. Ophthalmology 90:1246, 1983.

Pfister RR, Nicolaro ML, Paterson CA: Sodium citrate reduces the incidence of ulcerations and perforations in extreme alkali burned eyes. Invest Ophthalmol Vis Sci 21:486, 1981.

Purdue GF, Hunt JL: Adult assault as a mechanism of burn injury. Arch Surg 125:268, 1990.

Ralph RA: Chemical burns of the eye. In Tasman W (ed): Duane's Clinical Ophthalmology. Philadelphia, Harper & Row, 1989, vol 4, pp 1–25.

Ralph RA, Slansky HH: Therapy of chemical burns. Int Ophthalmol Clin 4:171, 1974.

Seedor JA, Perry HD, McNamara TF, et al: Systemic tetracycline treatment of alkali-induced corneal ulceration in rabbits. Arch Ophthalmol 105:268, 1987.

Stone M: Assault by burning and its relationship to social circumstances. Burns 14:461, 1988.

Tenn PF, Fijikawa LS, Dweck MD, et al: Fibronectin in alkaliburned rabbit cornea: Enhancement of epithelial wound healing. Invest Ophthalmol Vis Sci 29(suppl):92, 1988.

Thoft RA: Keratoepithelioplasty. Am J Ophthalmol 97:1, 1984.

Thoft RA: Conjunctival transplantation. Arch Ophthalmol 95:1425, 1977.

Burns—Thermal, Electrical, and Radiation

Burns CL, Chylack LT: Thermal burns: The management of thermal burns of the lids and globes. Ann Ophthalmol 11:1358, 1979.

Gladstone GJ, Tasman W: Solar retinitis after minimal exposure. Arch Ophthalmol 96:1368, 1978.

Johnson EU, Kline LB, Skalka HW: Electrical cataracts: A case report and review of the literature. Ophthalmic Surg 18:283, 1987.

Marrone AC: Thermal eyelid burns. In Hornblass A, Hanio CT (eds): Oculoplastic, Orbital and Reconstructive Surgery, vol 1. Eyelids. Baltimore, Williams & Wilkins, 1988, pp 443–447.

Peterson HD: Eyelids. In Baswick JA Jr (ed): The Art and Science of Burn Care. Rockville, MD, Aspen, 1987, pp 339–345.

Tso MM, LaPiana RG: The human fovea after sungazing. Trans Am Acad Ophthalmol Otolaryngol 79:788, 1975.

Child Abuse

Alexander RC, Crabbe L, Sato Y, et al: Serial abuse in children who are shaken. Am J Dis Child 144:58, 1990.

Alexander RC, Schor DP, Smith WL: Magnetic resonance imaging of intracranial injuries from child abuse. J Pediatr 109:975, 1986.

Caffey J: The whiplash shaken infant syndrome: Manual shaking by the extremities with whiplash-induced intracranial and intraocular bleedings, linked with residual permanent brain damage and mental retardation. Pediatrics 54:396, 1974.

Elner SG, Elner VM, Arnall M, Albert DM: Ocular and associated systemic findings in suspected child abuse. Arch Ophthalmol 108:1094, 1990.

Friendly DS: Ocular manifestations of physical child abuse. Trans Am Acad Ophthalmol Otolaryngol 75:318, 1971.

Gaynon MW, Koh H, Marmor MF, Frankel LR: Retinal folds in the shaken baby syndrome. Am J Ophthalmol 106:423, 1988.

Giangiacomo J, Barkett KJ: Ophthalmoscopic findings in occult child abuse. J Pediatr Ophthalmol Strabismus 22:234, 1985.

Gilliland MGF, Luckenbach MW, Massicotte SJ, Folbert R: The medicolegal implications of detecting hemosiderin in the eyes of children who are suspected of being abused. Arch Ophthalmol 109:321, 1991.

Greenwald MJ: The shaken baby syndrome. Semin Ophthalmol 5:202, 1990.

Jensen AD, Smith RE, Olson MI: Ocular clues to child abuse. J Pediatr Ophthalmol Strabismus 8:270, 1971.

Levin AV: Ocular manifestations of child abuse. Ophthalmol Clin North Am 3:249, 1990.

Levin AV, Magnusson MR, Rafto SE, Zimmerman RA: Shaken baby syndrome diagnosed by magnetic resonance imaging. Pediatr Emerg Care 5:181, 1989.

Levy I, Wysenbeek YS, Nitzan M, et al: Occult ocular damage as the leading sign in the battered child syndrome. Metabol Pediatr Systemic Ophthalmol 13:20, 1990.

Ludwig S, Warman M: Shaken baby syndrome: A review of 20 cases. Ann Emerg Med 13:104, 1984.

Merten DF, Carpenter BLM: Radiologic imaging of inflicted injury in the child abuse syndrome. Pediatr Clin North Am 37:815, 1990.

Newton RW: Intracranial hemorrhage and non-accidental injury. Arch Dis Child 64:188, 1989.

Rao N, Smith RE, Choi JH, et al: Autopsy findings in the eyes of fourteen fatally abused children. Forensic Sci Int 39:293, 1988.

Reece RM, Grodin MA: Recognition of nonaccidental injury. Pediatr Clin North Am 32:41, 1985.

Riffenburgh RS, Sathyavagiswaran L: Ocular findings at autopsy of child abuse victims. Ophthalmology 98:1519, 1991.

Spaide RF, Swengel RM, Scharre DW, Mein CE: Shaken baby syndrome. Am Fam Physician 41:1145, 1990.

Tomasi LG, Rosman NP: Purtscher retinopathy in the battered child syndrome. Am J Dis Child 129:1335, 1975.

Wilkinson WS, Han DP, Rappley MD, Owings CL: Retinal hemorrhage predicts neurological injury in the shaken baby syndrome. Arch Ophthalmol 107:1472, 1989.

Williams DF, Meiler WF, Williams GA: Posterior segment manifestations of ocular trauma. Retina 10(suppl):S35, 1990.

Childhood and Sports-related Eye Injuries

Bowen DI, Magauran DM: Ocular injuries caused by airgun pellets: An analysis of 105 cases. Br Med J 1:133, 1973.

Burke MJ, Sanitato JJ, Vinger PF, et al: Soccerball-induced eye injuries. JAMA 249:2682, 1983.

Caveness LS: Ocular and facial injuries in baseball. Int Ophthalmol Clin 28:238, 1988.

Committee on Accident and Poison Prevention, American Academy of Pediatrics: Ocular hazards. In: Injury Control for Children and Youth. Elk Grove Village, IL, AAP, 1987, pp 226–234.

Committee on Sports Medicine, American Academy of Pediatrics: Eye injuries. In: Sports Medicine: Health Care for Young Athletes. Evanston, IL, AAP, 1983, pp 282–296.

DeRespinis P, Caputo A, Fiore P, Wagner R: A survey of severe eye injuries in children. AJDC 143:711, 1989.

Elman M: Racket-sports ocular injuries. Arch Ophthalmol 104:1453, 1986.

Grin TR, Nelson LB, Jeffers JB: Eye injuries in childhood. Pediatrics 80:13, 1987.

Guyer B, Gallagher SS: An approach to the epidemiology of childhood injuries. Pediatr Clin North Am 32:5, 1985.

Jeffers JB: An ongoing tragedy: Pediatric sports-related eye injuries. Semin Ophthalmol 5:216, 1990.

LaRoche GR, McIntyre L, Schertzer RM: Epidemiology of severe eye injuries in childhood. Ophthalmology 95:1603, 1988.

Liggett PE, Pince KJ, Barlow W, et al: Ocular trauma in an urban population. Review of 1132 cases. Ophthalmology 97:581, 1990.

Nelson LB, Wilson TW, Jeffers JB: Eye injuries in childhood: Demography, etiology and prevention. Pediatrics 84:438, 1989.

Pashby T: Eye injuries in Canadian amateur hockey. Can J Ophthalmol 20:2, 1985.

Rapoport I, Romen M, Kinek M, et al: Eye injuries in children in Israel: A nationwide collaborative study. Arch Ophthalmol 108:376, 1990.

Simmons S, Krohel G, Hay P: Prevention of ocular gunshot injuries using polycarbonate lenses. Ophthalmology 91:977, 1984.

Sternberg P, de Juan E Jr, Green WR, et al: Ocular BB injuries. Ophthalmology 91:1269, 1984.

Strahlman E, Elman M, Daub E, Baker S: Causes of pediatric eye injuries. A population based study. Arch Ophthalmol 108:603, 1990.

Vinger PF: The eye in sports medicine. In Duane TD (ed): Clinical Ophthalmology. Philadelphia, Harper & Row, 1986, vol 5.

Young DW, Little JM: Pellet-gun eye injuries. Can J Ophthalmol 20:9, 1985.

Choroidal and Iris Injuries

Aguilar JP, Green WR: Choroidal rupture: A histopathologic study of 47 cases. Retina 4:269, 1984.

Hilton GF: Late serosanguinous detachment of the macula after traumatic choroidal rupture. Am J Ophthalmol 79:997, 1975.

Hornblass A: Pupillary dilation in fractures of the floor of the orbit. Ophthalmic Surg 10:44, 1979.

Maberley AL, Carvounis EP: The visual field in indirect traumatic rupture of the choroid. Can J Ophthalmol 12:147, 1977.

McCannel MA: A retrievable suture idea for anterior uveal problems. Ophthalmic Surg 7:98, 1976.

Paton D, Craig J: Management of iridodialysis. Ophthalmic Surg 4:38, 1973.

Peli E: Functional difficulties resulting from traumatic anisocoria. Am J Optom Physiol Opt 61:548, 1984.

Smith RE, Kelly JS, Harbin TS: Late macular complications of choroidal ruptures. Am J Ophthalmol 77:650, 1974.

Corneal and Scleral Injuries

Binder PS, Waring GO III, Arrowsmith PN, Wang C: Histopathology of traumatic corneal rupture after radial keratotomy. Arch Ophthalmol 106:1584, 1988.

Cherry PMH: Indirect traumatic rupture of the globe. Arch Ophthalmol 96:252, 1978.

Cibis GW, Weigeist TA, Krachmer JH: Traumatic corneal endothelial rings. Arch Ophthalmol 96:485, 1978.

Deg JK, Zavala EY, Binder PS: Delayed corneal wound healing following radial keratotomy. Ophthalmology 92:734, 1985.

Farley MK, Pettit TH: Traumatic wound dehiscence after penetrating keratoplasty. Am J Ophthalmol 104:44, 1987.

Forstot SL, Damiano RE: Trauma after radial keratotomy. Ophthalmology 95:833, 1988.

Maloney WF, Colvard M, Bourne WM, Gardon R: Specular microscopy of traumatic posterior annular keratopathy. Arch Ophthalmol 97:1647, 1979.

Raber IM, Arentsen JJ, Laibson PR: Traumatic wound rupture following successful penetrating keratoplasty. Arch Ophthalmol 98:1407, 1980.

Russell SR, Olsen KR, Folk JC: Predictors of scleral rupture and the role of vitrectomy in severe blunt ocular trauma. Am J Ophthalmol 105:253, 1988.

Simmons KB, Linsalata RP: Ruptured globe following blunt trauma after radial keratotomy: A case report. J Refract Surg 4:132, 1988.

Slingsby JG, Forstot SL: Effect of blunt trauma on the corneal endothelium. Arch Ophthalmol 99:1041, 1981.

Wellington DP, Johnstone MA, Hopkins RJ: Bull's eye corneal lesion resulting from war game injury. Arch Ophthalmol 107:1727, 1989.

Eyelid Injuries

Beyer-Machule CK, Shapiro A: Skin wound repair in orbital and periorbital trauma. In Hornblass A (ed): Oculoplastic, Orbital and Reconstructive Surgery. Baltimore, Williams & Wilkins, 1988, vol 1, pp 415–421.

Bruce RA Jr, McGoldrick K, Oppenheimer P: Anesthesia for ophthalmology. Birmingham, AL, Aesculapius, 1982.

Callaham M: Controversies in antiobiotic choices for bite wounds. Ann Emerg Med 9:79, 1988.

Deutsch TA, Feller DB: Paton and Goldberg's Management of Ocular Injuries, ed 2. Philadelphia, Saunders, 1985, pp 9–36, 93–103, 145.

Dortzbach RK, Angrist RA: Silicone intubation for lacerated lacrimal canaliculi. Ophthalmic Surg 16:639, 1985.

Edlich RF, Spengler MD, Rodeheaver GT, et al: Emergency department management of mammalian bites. Emerg Med Clin North Am 4:595, 1986.

Engrav LH, Heimbach DM, Walkinshaw MD, et al: Excision of burns of the face. Plast Reconstr Surg 77:774, 1986.

Frank A, Wachtel T: The early treatment and reconstruction of eyelid burns. J Trauma 23:874, 1983.

Friedlaender MH: Contact allergy and toxicity in the eye. Int Ophthalmol Clin 28:317, 1988.

Garber PF, MacDonald D, Beyer-Machule CK: Management of trauma to the eyelids. In Smith BC (ed): Ophthalmic Plastic and Reconstructive Surgery. St. Louis, Mosby, 1987, vol 1, pp 437–469.

Gonnering RS: Orbital and periorbital dog bites. In Bosniak SL, Smith BC (eds): Advances in Ophthalmic Plastic and Reconstructive Surgery. Elmsford, NY, Pergamon, 1988, vol 7, part 2, pp 171–180.

Gonnering RS: Eyebrow reconstruction. In Hornblass A (ed): Oculoplastic, Orbital and Reconstructive Surgery. Baltimore, Williams & Wilkins, 1988, vol 1, pp 291–297.

Green BF, Kraft SP, Carter KD, et al: Intraorbital wood: Detection by magnetic resonance imaging. Ophthalmology 97:608, 1990.

Hawes MJ: Canalicular lacerations. In Linberg JV (ed): Oculoplastic and Orbital Emergencies. Norwalk, CT, Appleton & Lange, 1990, pp 15–27.

Herman DC, Bartley GB, Walker RC: The treatment of animal bite injuries of the eye and ocular adnexa. Ophthal Plast Reconstr Surg 3:237, 1987.

Holley HP Jr: Successful treatment of cat-scratch disease with ciprofloxacin. JAMA 265:1563, 1991.

Kalb R, Kaplan MH, Tenebaum MJ, et al: Cutaneous infection at dog bite wounds associated with fulminant DF-2 septicemia. Am J Med 78:687, 1985.

Kaplan AP: The pathogenesis of urticaria and angioedema: Recent advances. Am J Med 70:755, 1981.

Konovitch B: Anesthesia. In Smith BC (ed): Ophthalmic Plastic and Reconstructive Surgery. St. Louis, Mosby, 1987, vol 1, pp 405–414.

Kulwin DR, Kersten RC: Acute eyelid and periocular burns. In Linberg JV (ed): Oculoplastic and Orbital Emergencies. Norwalk, CT, Appleton & Lange, 1990, pp 77–85.

Marrone AC: Thermal eyelid burns. In Hornblass A (ed): Oculoplastic, Orbital and Reconstructive Surgery. Baltimore, Williams & Wilkins, 1988, vol 1, pp 433–447.

McNab AA, Collin JRO: Eyelid and canthal lacerations. In Linberg JV (ed): Oculoplastic and Orbital Emergencies. Norwalk, CT, Appleton & Lange, 1990, pp 1–13.

Mindlin AM, Nesi FA, Silver B, Lisman RD: Basic concepts in eyelid repair. In Smith BC (ed): Ophthalmic Plastic and Reconstructive Surgery. St. Louis, Mosby, 1987, vol 1, pp 417–436.

Montandon D, Maillard GF, Morax S, Garey LJ: Plastic and Reconstructive Surgery of the Orbital Region. New York, Churchill Livingstone, 1991.

Mustardé JC (ed): Repair and Reconstruction in the Orbital Region, ed 3. New York, Churchill Livingstone, 1991.

Ordog GJ, Balasubramanium S, Wassaberger J: Rat bites: Fifty cases. Ann Emerg Med 14:126, 1985.

Roen JL, Della Rocca RC: Basic principles of ophthalmic plastic surgery. In Smith BC (ed): Ophthalmic Plastic and Reconstructive Surgery. St. Louis, Mosby, 1987, vol 1, pp 345–356.

Spoor TCV, Nesi FA: Management of Ocular, Orbital and Adnexal Trauma. New York, Raven, 1988.

Tsur H: Eyelid burns: A general plastic surgeon's approach. In Hornblass A (ed): Oculoplastic, Orbital and Reconstructive Surgery. Baltimore, Williams & Wilkins, 1988, vol 1, pp 448–454.

Zolli CL: Microsurgical repair of lacrimal canaliculus in medial canthal trauma. In Hornblass A (ed): Oculoplastic, Orbital and Reconstructive Surgery. Baltimore, Williams & Wilkins, 1988, vol 1, pp 426–432.

Zook EG, Miller M, Van Beek AL, et al: Successful treatment protocol for canine fang injuries. J Trauma 20:243, 1980.

Hyphema

Agapitos PJ, Noel LP, Clarke WN: Traumatic hyphema in children. Ophthalmology 94:1238, 1987.

Belcher CD, Brown SVL, Simmons RJ: Anterior chamber washout for traumatic hyphema. Ophthalmic Surg 16:475, 1985.

Cassel GH, Jeffers JB, Jaeger EA: Wills Eye Hospital traumatic hyphema study. Ophthalmic Surg 16:441, 1984.

Collet BI: Traumatic hyphema: A review. Ann Ophthalmol 14:52, 1982.

Crouch ER, Frenkel M: Aminocaproic acid in the treatment of traumatic hyphema. Am J Ophthalmol 81:355, 1976.

Deutsch TA, Weinreb RN, Goldberg MF: Indications for surgical management of hyphema in patients with sickle cell trait. Arch Ophthalmol 102:566, 1984.

Dieste MC, Hersch PS, Kylstra JA, et al: Intraocular pressure increase associated with epsilon–aminocaproic acid therapy for traumatic hyphema. Am J Ophthalmol 106:383, 1988.

Edwards WC, Layden WF: Traumatic hyphema. Am J Ophthalmol 75:110, 1973.

Farber MD, Fiscella R, Goldberg MF: Aminocaproic acid versus prednisone for the treatment of traumatic hyphema. A randomized clinical trial. Ophthalmology 98:279, 1991.

Ganley JP, Geiger JM, Clement JR, et al: Aspirin and recurrent hyphema after blunt ocular trauma. Am J Ophthalmol 96:797, 1983.

Gilbert HD, Jensen AD: Atropine in the treatment of traumatic hyphema. Ann Ophthalmol 5:1297, 1973.

Goldberg MF: Sickled erythrocytes, hyphema, and secondary glaucoma. Ophthalmic Surg 10:17, 1979.

Goldberg MF: Antifibrinolytic agents in the management of traumatic hyphema. Arch Ophthalmol 101:1029, 1983.

Howard GM: Spontaneous hyphema in infancy and childhood. Arch Ophthalmol 68:615, 1962.

Kennedy RH, Brubaker RF: Traumatic hyphema in a defined population. Am J Ophthalmol 106:123, 1988.

Kraft SP, Christianson MD, Crawford JS, et al: Traumatic hyphema in children. Treatment with epsilon-aminocaproic acid. Ophthalmology 94:1232, 1987.

Kutner B, Fourman S, Brein K, et al: Aminocaproic acid reduces the risk of secondary hemorrhage in patients with traumatic hyphema. Arch Ophthalmol 105:206, 1987.

Loewy DM, Williams PB, Crouch ER Jr, Cooke WJ: Systemic aminocaproic acid reduces fibrinolysis in the aqueous humor. Arch Ophthalmol 105:272, 1987.

McGetrick JJ, Jampol LM, Goldberg MF, et al: Aminocaproic acid decreases secondary hemorrhage after traumatic hyphema. Arch Ophthalmol 101:1031, 1983.

Palmer DJ, Goldberg MF, Frenkel M, et al: A comparison of two dose regimens of epsilon aminocaproic acid in the prevention and management of secondary traumatic hyphemas. Ophthalmology 93:102, 1986.

Pilger IS: Medical treatment of traumatic hyphema. Surv Ophthalmol 20:28, 1975.

Read J, Goldberg MF: Comparison of medical treatment for traumatic hyphema. Trans Am Acad Ophthalmol Otolaryngol 78:799, 1974.

Rynne MV, Romano PE: Systemic corticosteroids in the treatment of traumatic hyphema. J Pediatr Ophthalmol Strabismus 17:141, 1980.

Spoor TC, Hammer M, Belloso H: Traumatic hyphema: failure of steroids to alter its course: A double blind prospective study. Arch Ophthalmol 98:116, 1988.

Spoor TC, Kwitko GM, O'Grady JM, Ramocki JM: Traumatic hyphema in an urban population. Am J Ophthalmol 109:23, 1990.

Thomas MA, Parrish RK, Feuer WJ: Rebleeding after traumatic hyphema. Arch Ophthalmol 104:206, 1986.

Uusitalo RJ, Ranta-Kemppainen L, Tarkkanen A: Management of traumatic hyphema in children. Arch Ophthalmol 106:1207, 1988.

Vangsted P, Nielsen PJ: Tranexamic acid and traumatic hyphema. Acta Ophthalmol 618:447, 1983.

Weiss JS, Parrish RK, Anderson DR: Surgical therapy of traumatic hyphema. Ophthalmic Surg 14:343, 1983.

Williams DF, Han DP, Abrams GW: Rebleeding in experimental traumatic hyphema treated with intraocular tissue plasminogen activator. Arch Ophthalmol 108:264, 1990.

Wilson FM: Traumatic hyphema: Pathogenesis and management. 87:910, 1980.

Wright KW, Sunal PM, Urrea P: Bed rest versus activity ad lib in the treatment of small hyphemas. Ann Ophthalmol 20:143, 1988.

Yasuna E: Management of traumatic hyphema. Arch Ophthalmol 91:190, 1974.

Lens Injuries

Chandler PA, Grant WM: Mydriatic–cycloplegic treatment in malignant glaucoma. Arch Ophthalmol 688:353, 1962.

Epstein DL, Jedziniak JA, Grant WM: Obstruction of aqueous outflow by lens particles and heavy-molecular weight soluble proteins. Invest Ophthalmol Vis Sci 17:272, 1978.

Hemo Y, Ben Ezra D: Traumatic cataracts in young children: Correction of aphakia by intraocular lens implantation. Ophthalmic Pediatr Genet 8:203, 1987.

Illiff CE, Kramer P: A working guide for the management of dislocated lenses. Ophthalmic Surg 2:251, 1971.

Jarrett WH: Dislocation of the lens: A study of 166 hospitalized cases. Arch Ophthalmol 78:289, 1967.

Kutner BN: Acute angle closure glaucoma in nonperforating blunt trauma. Arch Ophthalmol 106:19, 1988.

Nelson LB, Maumenee IH: Ectopia lentis. Surv Ophthalmol 27:143, 1982.

Nelson LB, Szmyd SM: Aphakic correction in ectopia lentis. Ann Ophthalmol 17:445, 1985.

Sellyei LF Jr, Barraquer J: Surgery of the ectopic lens. Ann Ophthalmol 5:1127, 1973.

Tchah H, Larson RS, Nichols BD, Lindstrom RL: Neodymium:Yag laser zonulysis for treatment of lens subluxation. Ophthalmology 96:230, 1989.

Optic Nerve Injuries

Anderson RL, Panje WR, Gross CE: Optic nerve blindness following blunt forehead trauma. Ophthalmology 89:445, 1982.

Giovinazzo VJ: The ocular sequelae of blunt trauma. Adv Ophthalmic Plast Reconstr Surg 6:107, 1987.

Guy J, Sherwood M, Day AL: Surgical treatment of progressive visual loss in traumatic optic neuropathy. J Neurosurg 70:799, 1989.

Joseph MP, Lessell S, Rizzo J, Momose J: Therapy for traumatic optic neuropathy: In reply. Arch Ophthalmol 109:610, 1991.

Joseph MP, Lessell S, Rizzo J, Momose J: Extracranial optic nerve decompression for traumatic optic neuropathy. Arch Ophthalmol 108:1091, 1990.

Lessell S: Indirect optic nerve trauma. Arch Ophthalmol 107:382, 1989.

Miller N: The management of traumatic optic neuropathy. Arch Ophthalmol 108:1086, 1990.

Petro J, Tooze FM, Bales CR, et al: Ocular injuries associated with periorbital fractures. J Trauma 19:730, 1979.

Seiff SR: Therapy for traumatic optic neuropathy. Arch Ophthalmol 109:610, 1991.

Seiff SR: High dose corticosteroids for treatment of vision loss due to indirect injury to the optic nerve. Ophthalmic Surg 21:389, 1990.

Wolin MJ, Lavin PJM: Spontaneous visual recovery from traumatic optic neuropathy after blunt head injury. Am J Ophthalmol 109:430, 1990.

Orbital Injuries

Beyer CK, Fabian RL, Smith B: Naso-orbital fractures: Complications and treatment. Ophthalmology 89:456, 1982.

Chole RA, Yee J: Antibiotic prophylaxis for facial fractures: A randomized clinical trial. Arch Otolaryngol Head Neck Surg 113:1055, 1987.

Cruse CW, Blevins PH, Luce ES: Naso-ethmoid-orbital fractures. J Trauma 20:551, 1980.

Dutton J, Slamovits T: Management of blowout fractures of the orbital floor. Surv Ophthalmol 35:279, 1991.

Fujino T, Makino K: Entrapment mechanism and ocular injury in orbital blowout fracture. Plast Reconstr Surg 65:571, 1980.

Goldfarb MS, Hoffman DS, Rosenberg S: Orbital cellulitis and orbital fractures. Ann Ophthalmol 19:97, 1987.

Green RP Jr, Peters DR, Shore JW, et al: Force necessary to fracture the orbital floor. Ophthalmic Plast Reconstr Surg 6:211, 1990.

Greenwald HS, Keen AH, Shannon GM: A review of 128 patients with orbital fractures. Am J Ophthalmol 78:655, 1974.

Grove AS Jr: Computed tomography in the management of orbital trauma. Ophthalmology 89:433, 1982.

Grove AS Jr, McCord C: Acute orbital trauma, diagnosis and management. In McCord C, Tanenbaum M (eds): Oculoplastic Surgery. New York, Raven, 1987.

Hawes MJ, Dortzbach RK: Surgery on orbital floor fractures: Influence of time of repair and fracture size. Ophthalmology 90:1066, 1983.

Healy JF: Computed tomography of orbital trauma. CT 6:1, 1984.

Jones SEP, Evans JNG: Blowout fractures of the orbit: Investigation into their anatomical basis. J Laryngol 81:109, 1967.

Jordan DR et al: Orbital emphysema: A potentially blinding complication following orbital fractures. Ann Emerg Med 17:853, 1988.

Kersten RC, Rice CD: Subperiosteal orbital hematoma: Visual recovery following delayed drainage. Ophthalmic Surg 18:423, 1987.

Krohel GB, Wright JE: Orbital hemorrhage. Am J Ophthalmol 88:254, 1979.

Linberg JV: Orbital compartment syndromes following trauma. Adv Ophthalmic Plast Reconstr Surg 6:51, 1987.

McLachan DL, Flanagan JC, Shannon GM: Complications of orbital roof fractures. Ophthalmology 89:1274, 1982.

Millman AL et al: Steroids and orbital blowout fractures: A new systematic concept in medical management and surgical decision-making. Adv Ophthalmic Plast Reconstr Surg 6:291, 1987.

Nelson LB, Catalano RA: Atlas of Ocular Motility. Philadelphia, Saunders, 1989, pp 2–23.

Pfeiffer RL: Traumatic enophthalmos. Adv Ophthalmic Plast Reconstr Surg 6:301, 1987.

Putterman AM, Stevens T, Urist M: Non-surgical management of blowout fractures of the orbital floor. Am J Ophthalmol 77:233, 1974.

Silkiss RZ, Baylis HI: Management of traumatic ptosis. Adv Ophthalmic Plast Reconstr Surg 7:149, 1987.

Smith BC (ed): Ophthalmic Plastic and Reconstructive Surgery. St. Louis, Mosby, 1987, vol. 1.

Waring GO III, Flanagan JC: Pneumocephalus: A sign of intracranial involvement in orbital fracture. Arch Ophthalmol 98:847, 1975.

Wilkins RB, Havins WE: Current treatment of blowout fractures. Ophthalmology 89:464, 1982.

Zismor J, Noyek A: Radiologic diagnosis of orbital fractures. In Aston SJ, Meltzer MA, Rees TD (eds): Third International Symposium of Plastic and Reconstructive Surgery of the Eye and Adnexa. Baltimore, Williams & Wilkins, 1982.

Retinal and Vitreous Injuries

Aaberg TM, Blair CJ, Gass JDM: Macular holes. Am J Ophthalmol 69:555, 1970.

Appiah AP, Hirose T: Secondary causes of premacular fibrosis. Ophthalmology 96:389, 1989.

Assaf A: Traumatic retinal detachment. J Trauma 25:1085, 1985.

Blight R, Hart JCD: Structural changes in the outer retinal layers following blunt mechanical nonperforating trauma to the globe: An experimental study. Br J Ophthalmol 6:573, 1977.

Chang S, Reppucci V, Zimmerman NJ, et al: Perfluorocarbon liquids in the management of traumatic retinal detachments. Ophthalmology 96:785, 1989.

Cox MS, Freeman HM: Traumatic retinal detachment. In Freeman HM (ed): Ocular Trauma. New York, Appleton-Century-Crofts, 1979, pp 285–293.

Cox MS, Schepens CL, Freeman HM: Retinal detachment due to ocular contusion. Arch Ophthalmol 76:678, 1966.

De Juan E Jr, Hickingbotham D, Machemer R: Retinal tacks. Am J Ophthalmol 99:272, 1985.

Delori F, Pomerantzeff O, Cox MS: Deformation of the globe under high-speed impact: Its relation to contusion injuries. Invest Ophthalmol 8:290, 1969.

Dumass JJ: Retinal detachment following contusion of the eye. Int Ophthalmol Clin 7:19, 1967.

Federman JL, Shakin JL, Lanning RC: The microsurgical management of giant retinal tears with trans-scleral retinal sutures. Ophthalmology 89:832, 1982.

Fuller B, Gitter KA: Traumatic choroidal rupture with late serous detachment of macula: Report of successful argon laser treatment. Arch Ophthalmol 89:354, 1973.

Glaser BM: Treatment of giant retinal tears combined with proliferative vitreoretinopathy. Ophthalmology 93:1193, 1986.

Glaser BM, Cardin A, Biscoe B: Proliferative vitreoretinopathy: The mechanism of development of vitreoretinal traction. Ophthalmology 94:327, 1987.

Goffstein R, Burton TC: Differentiating traumatic from nontraumatic retinal detachment. Ophthalmology 89:361, 1982.

Han DP, Mieler WF, Schwartz DM, Abrams GW: Management of traumatic hemorrhagic retinal detachment with pars plana vitrectomy. Arch Ophthalmol 108:1281, 1990.

Hart JCD, Frank HJ: Retinal opacification after blunt nonperforating concussional injuries to the globe. Trans Ophthalmol Soc UK 95:94, 1975.

Hutton WL, Fuller DG: Factors influencing final visual results in severely injured eyes. Am J Ophthalmol 97:715, 1984.

Kelly JS, Hoover RE, George T: Whiplash maculopathy. Arch Ophthalmol 96:834, 1978.

McCuen BW II, Hida T, Sheta SM: Transvitreal cyanoacrylate retinopexy in the management of complicated retinal detachment. Am J Ophthalmol 104:127, 1987.

Michels RG, Rice TA, Blakenship G: Surgical techniques for selected giant retinal tears. Retina 3:139, 1983.

Richards RD, West CE, Meisels AA: Chorioretinitis sclopetaria. Am J Ophthalmol 66:852, 1968.

Ross WH: Traumatic retinal dialysis. Arch Ophthalmol 99:1371, 1981.

Sipperley JO, Quigley HA, Gass JDM: Traumatic retinopathy in primates: The explanation of commotio retinae. Arch Ophthalmol 96:2267, 1978.

Zion VM, Burton TC: Retinal dialysis. Arch Ophthalmol 98:1971, 1980.

APPENDIX

RESOURCES FOR IMPAIRED CHILDREN AND THEIR FAMILIES

Disorder	Agency Resource(s)
Cancer	American Cancer Society 261 Madison Avenue New York, NY 10016 (212)–599–3600

	The Candlelighters Childhood Cancer
	    Foundation
	1901 Pennsylvania Ave. NW,
	    Suite 1001
	Washington, DC 20006
	(202)–659–5136

Cerebral Palsy	United Cerebral Palsy Association, Inc. 66 East 34th Street New York, NY 10016 (212)–947–5770
Down Syndrome	Down's Syndrome Society 666 Broadway New York, NY 10012 (800)–221–4602
	Easter Seal Society 70 East Lake Street Chicago, IL 60601 (800)–221–6827
Genetic Diseases	National Clearinghouse for Human Genetic Diseases 805 15th Street NW, Suite 500 Washington, DC 20005 (202)–842–7617
	Health Information Clearing House P.O. Box 1133 Washington, DC 20013 (800)–336–4797

Disorder	Agency Resource(s)
Glaucoma	Glaucoma Support Network 490 Post Street San Francisco, CA 94102 (800)–245–3005
Learning Disability	ACLD Inc. 4156 Library Road Pittsburgh, PA 15234 (412)–344–0224
	Council for Learning Disabilities P.O. Box 40303 Overland Park, KS 66204 (913)–492–8755
	Foundation for Children with Learning Disabilities 99 Park Avenue New York, NY 10016 (212)–687–7211
	Orton Dyslexia Society 724 York Road Baltimore, MD 21204 (301)–296–0232
Neurofibromatosis	The National Neurofibromatosis Foundation, Inc. 141 Fifth Avenue, Suite 7S New York, NY 10010 (800)–323–7938
Retinitis Pigmentosa	Retinitis Pigmentosa Association International P.O. Box 900 Woodland Hills, CA 91365 (800)–344–4877

Disorder	Agency Resource(s)
Retinoblastoma	Retinoblastoma Support News c/o The Institute for Families of Blind Children Childrens Hospital of Los Angeles P.O. Box 54700 Los Angeles, CA 90054 (213)–669–4649
Sturge–Weber Syndrome	The Sturge–Weber Foundation P.O. Box 460931 Aurora, CO 80015 (303)–693–2986

Visual Impairment	American Council of Parents of Blind
	  Children
	Route A, Box 78
	Franklin, LA 70538
	
	American Foundation for the Blind
	15 W. 16th Street
	New York, NY 10011
	(800)–232–5463
	
	The Blind Childrens Center
	4120 Marathon Street
	P.O. Box 29159
	Los Angeles, CA 90029
	(213)–664–2153
	
	Library of Congress Division for the
	  Blind and Visually Handicapped
	1291 Taylor Street NW
	Washington, DC 20213
	(202)–376–6289

Disorder	Agency Resource(s)

Visual Impairment
(continued)
	The Lighthouse
	Low Vision Products
	36-02 Northern Boulevard
	Long Island City, NY 11101
	(292)–393–3666
	
	National Association for Parents of the
	  Visually Handicapped
	2011 Hardy Circle
	Austin, TX 78757
	(800)–562–6265
	
	National Association for the Visually
	  Handicapped, Inc
	22 W. 21st Street
	New York, NY 10010
	(212)–889–3141
	
	National Federation of the Blind
	1800 Johnson Street
	Baltimore, MD 21230
	(301)–659–9314
	
	TeleSensory Systems, Inc.
	455 N. Bernardo
	P.O. Box 7455
	Mount View, CA 94043
	(800)–227–8418
	
	Vision Foundation, Inc.
	818 Mt. Auburn Street
	Watertown, MA 02172
	(617)–926–4232

INDEX

Pages numbers followed by *t* and *f* indicate tables and figures, respectively.